OFFICE-BASED COSMETIC PROCEDURES AND TECHNIQUES

IN THE LAST TWENTY YEARS, there has been an explosion of new cosmetic surgery procedures developed for a large base of office-based dermatologists, cosmetic surgeons, plastic and reconstructive surgeons, and otolaryngologists. Tricks and techniques are swapped across the globe, with practitioners in Europe, Asia, and North and South America. This is a practical, simple manual of those tricks and techniques, with input from specialists around the world. This book is aimed at practitioners who want to add new procedures to their scope of practice and learn new methods of application. A wide range of procedures, from fillers and neurotoxins to suture suspension and chemical peels, are covered here in a comparative format and are accompanied by more than two hundred color illustrations. In addition to detailing the procedures, chapters also cover anesthetic techniques and brands. This book is designed to be an easy and useful reference for the beginning practitioner or more senior physician. More than fifty internationally renowned dermatologists, plastic surgeons, facial plastic surgeons, and cosmetic surgeons have contributed to this text.

Sorin Eremia, MD, is Associate Clinical Professor of Medicine and Director of the Cosmetic Surgery Unit in the Division of Dermatology at the University of California, Los Angeles.

OFFICE-BASED COSMETIC

PROCEDURES AND TECHNIQUES

Edited by

Sorin Eremia

University of California, Los Angeles

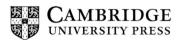

CAMBRIDGE UNIVERSITY PRESS

CAMBRIDGE UNIVERSITY PRESS
Cambridge, New York, Melbourne, Madrid, Cape Town, Singapore,
São Paulo, Delhi, Dubai, Tokyo

Cambridge University Press
32 Avenue of the Americas, New York, NY 10013-2473, USA

www.cambridge.org
Information on this title: www.cambridge.org/9780521706520

First published 2010

Printed in China by Everbest

A catalog record for this publication is available from the British Library.

Library of Congress Cataloging in Publication data

Office-based cosmetic procedures and techniques / edited by Sorin Eremia.
p. ; cm.
Includes bibliographical references and index.
ISBN 978-0-521-70652-0 (hardback)
1. Surgery, Plastic.   2. Dermatology.   3. Ambulatory medical care.   I. Eremia, Sorin, 1951–   II. Title.
[DNLM: 1. Cosmetic Techniques.   2. Skin – surgery.   3. Ambulatory Surgical Procedures – methods.
WR 650 O32 2009]
RD118.O34   2009
617.9′5 – dc22   2009019259

ISBN 978-0-521-70652-0 Hardback

Contents

Preface

TOGETHER WITH the help of many of my friends and colleagues, I have attempted to provide the reader of this textbook with practical, up-to-date information on the broad range of cosmetic procedures that are generally performed in an office setting.

This textbook is focused on the common cosmetic applications of fillers; neurotoxins; laser, light, radiofrequency, and ultrasound devices; chemical peels; and microdermabrasion. Supporting chapters on anatomy, anesthesia, minimally invasive suture suspension lifts, and mesotherapy round out the text.

This is an international, multispecialty, multiauthored textbook. The fifty senior contributing authors include experts in various topics from the fields of dermatology, facial and general plastic surgery, and cosmetic surgery and medicine and hail from the United States, Canada, Europe, South America, and Asia. Because the United States lags far behind the rest of the world with respect to the variety of options available for fillers and neurotoxins, American readers can benefit greatly from such author diversity.

The sections on lasers and other energy devices for resurfacing, skin tightening, and treatment of fat and cellulite attempt to cover some of the most recent devices available, with some short sections devoted to specific individual brands. Brand names are frequently mentioned in this text, not to promote the products but to make it easy for readers to identify the products discussed.

The book is divided into five parts. Part One, "Anatomy and the Aging Process," is limited to discussions of the anatomy of the aging face and neck and is written by Dr. Pierre Nicolau, a well-known, Paris-based general plastic surgeon trained in both France and England, with a strong interest and background in fillers. For a more detailed study of anatomy, readers are referred to any of a number of detailed textbooks on the subject. In general, face lift and blepharoplasty textbooks offer some of the best and most detailed clinically practical information on face and neck anatomy. Needless to say, a strong understanding of anatomy is essential to performing any cosmetic procedure. Because nothing beats hands-on study of anatomy, an excellent weeklong course is offered annually at the University of California, San Diego, called the Greenway Superficial Anatomy Course.

Part Two, "Anesthesia and Sedation for Office Cosmetic Procedures," provides detailed and practical information on local, topical, nerve block, and mild to moderate anesthesia methods that are applicable to the procedures covered in this textbook. I particularly recommend that less surgically oriented practitioners learn the art of nerve blocks. That chapter is written by Dr. Joseph Niamtu III, a highly experienced cosmetic surgeon with an oral and maxillofacial surgery background.

Part Three is called "Fillers and Neurotoxins." The filler chapters attempt to cover, in as much practical detail as possible, the various classes of fillers currently in use, including hyaluronic acid; collagen; hydroxyapatite; polylactic acid; various permanent fillers, including silicone; and finally, fat. Understanding why and how fillers work is essential, so I strongly recommend the chapters on how structure affects function: Chapter 7, by Dr. Johannes Reinmüller, a German plastic surgeon with a strong interest in fillers, on hyaluronic acid fillers and Chapter 19, by Dr. Pierre Nicolau, on long-lasting and permanent fillers. The introductory chapter, by Drs. Eric Williams, David J. Kouba, and Ronald L. Moy, provides excellent background information and a list of various fillers available in the United States or in the Food and Drug Administration (FDA) pipeline.

Multiple sections by various authors, including Derek Jones, Hayes B. Gladstone, Michael H. Gold, C. William Hanke, Rhoda S. Narins, B. Kent Remington, and Neil S. Sadick, from the field of dermatology, cover individual products such as the Restylane, Juvéderm, and Puragen families of nonanimal stabilized hyaluronic acid fillers; collagens; Sculptra; Radiesse; Artecoll; and silicone. American and international facial plastic and general plastic surgeons' perspectives are provided by Drs. Andrew B. Denton, Taro Kono, Devinder S. Mangat, Arturo Prado, and Constantin Stan.

Fat grafting is extensively covered by Drs. Mark Berman, Kimberly J. Butterwick, and William P. Coleman III, and the European perspective on commercial fillers versus fat is covered by Dr. Stan.

BOTOX and Dysport, the latter of which is now finally available in the United States, are the main focus of the neurotoxins section of Part Three. The Dysport chapter is written by one of the deans of French cosmetic dermatology, Dr. Bernard Rossi. Drs. Prado and Kono also provide excellent discussions of these and other neurotoxins (and fillers) available around the world in their respective chapters. A novel device for minimally invasive corrugator muscle denervation is discussed by Stanford facial plastic surgeon Dr. James Newman.

Part Four is devoted to laser, broadband light, radiofrequency, and ultrasound devices. The senior author for the chapter on treatment of vessels and vascular lesions, and for the chapter on aminolevulinic acid, is one of the foremost authorities in that field, Dr. Mitchel P. Goldman. Other well-known senior authors include Dr. Christopher B. Zachary, writing on fractional CO_2 lasers; Dr. Thomas Rohrer, writing on hair removal; and Dr. E. Victor Ross, writing on the treatment of acne and acne scars with energy devices. Individual devices or treatment techniques are discussed by multiple authors, including laser experts Drs. Tina S. Alster, Michael H. Gold, Gregory S. Keller, Vic A. Narurkar, Javier Ruiz-Esparza, and Neil S. Sadick.

Together with my old friend and University of California, Los Angeles (UCLA) colleague Dr. Bernard I. Raskin, and with the assistance of Drs. Edgar F. Fincher and Joseph F. Greco, we share our extensive experience in chapters on classic ablative laser resurfacing and nonablative infrared lasers. The new fractional laser systems and the latest in radiofrequency systems are also thoroughly covered.

Dr. Mat Avram, from Harvard, covers recent advances in fat and cellulite treatment devices. The two eagerly awaited ultrasonic fat reduction devices now available in Europe and Latin America, UltraShape and LipoSonix, are covered by Dr. Karyn Grossman, with assistance from Mexico City plastic surgeon Dr. Ernesto Gadsden, principal investigator for LipoSonix.

Part Five is devoted to three topics:

1. Minimally invasive suture suspension techniques are briefly discussed. Although ContourThreads, the U.S. patented version of barbed sutures, has been pulled off the market, if new versions become available, the same principles of use would apply. APTOS sutures remain widely available in the rest of the world. I summarize my five years of experience with the larger cogged, slowly absorbable multianchor sutures (AnchorSuture), and Dr. Nicanor Isse discusses the FDA-approved intermediate-type cogged suture, Silhouette Sutures, the only cogged suture actively marketed in the United States as of June 2009.

2. A section on chemical peels and microdermabrasion is headed by a chapter authored by Dr. Suzan Obagi, who needs no introduction.

3. A section on mesotherapy comprises a chapter written by Dr. Adam M. Rotunda, the foremost American scientific authority on the subject.

I hope this brief road map for the textbook will help direct the reader to his or her area of greatest interest.

A special mention goes to my UCLA colleagues Dr. Gary Lask, Dr. Jenny Kim, Dr. Fred Beddinfield, Dr. Bernard Raskin, and Dr. Teresa Soriano, who not only helped contribute to this book but also provided great moral support for this project. Special thanks go to Dr. Ron Moy, Dr. Mitch Goldman, and Dr. Neil Sadick for their always-friendly encouragement over the years and for their support for this book as well. Special thanks also go to Ms. Sharon Sausedo for her assistance with the images for the text.

Eternal gratitude goes to my late wife, Dr. Susie Van-Holten, and our son Dylan, for their understanding of the time my academic pursuits have taken away from our family life.

Sorin Eremia
Associate Clinical Professor of Medicine
Director, Cosmetic Surgery Unit
Division of Dermatology
University of California
Los Angeles

Contributors

Maria Teresa Aguilar, MD
Plastic Surgery Division
Hospital Central Militar
Hospital Torre Medica
Mexico City, Mexico

Tina S. Alster, MD
Director, Washington Institute of Dermatologic Laser
    Surgery
Clinical Professor of Dermatology
Georgetown University Medical Center
Washington, DC

Patricio Andrades, MD
Division of Plastic Surgery
School of Medicine
Clinical Hospital JJ Aguirre
University of Chile
Santiago, Chile

Mat Avram, MD, JD
Director, Dermatology Laser and Cosmetic
    Center
Massachusetts General Hospital
Harvard Medical School
Boston, Massachusetts

Frederick C. Beddingfield III, MD, PhD
Vice President and Therapeutic Area Head
Dermatology Clinical Research and Development
Allergan, Inc.
Assistant Clinical Professor
Division of Dermatology
David Geffen School of Medicine
University of California, Los Angeles
Los Angeles, California

Mark Berman, MD, FACS
Department of Otolaryngology (Facial Plastic
    Surgery)
University of Southern California School
    of Medicine
Los Angeles, California

David P. Beynet, MD, MS
Clinical Instructor
Division of Dermatology
David Geffen School of Medicine
University of California, Los Angeles
Los Angeles, California

Kimberly J. Butterwick, MD
Dermatology and Cosmetic Surgery (private practice)
La Jolla, California

Lina M. Cardona, MD
Research Associates Skin Care Research, Inc.
The Dermatology and Aesthetic Center
Boca Raton, Florida

Paul J. Carniol, MD
Facial Plastic and Reconstructive Surgery (private
    practice)
Summit, New Jersey

Henry H. L. Chan, MD
Dermatology (private practice)
Hong Kong, China

F. Landon Clark, MD, MPH
Department of Dermatology
Stanford University Medical Center
Stanford, California

Kyle M. Coleman, MD
Department of Dermatology
Tulane University Health Sciences Center
New Orleans, Louisiana

William P. Coleman III, MD
Editor in Chief, Dermatologic Surgery
Clinical Professor of Dermatology
Adjunct Professor of Surgery
   (Plastic Surgery)
Tulane University Health Sciences Center
New Orleans, Louisiana

Giuseppe Curinga, MD
Department of Plastic and Reconstructive
   Surgery
University of Rome "La Sapienza"
Rome, Italy

Michel Delune, MD
Dermatology (private practice)
Brussels, Belgium

Andrew B. Denton, MD, FRCSC
Assistant Professor
Division of Otolaryngology
Department of Surgery
University of British Columbia
Vancouver, British Columbia, Canada

David Duffy, MD
Clinical Professor of Medicine
Division of Dermatology
University of Southern California
Assistant Clinical Professor
Division of Dermatology
David Geffen School of Medicine
University of California, Los Angeles
Los Angeles, California

Sorin Eremia, MD
Associate Clinical Professor of Medicine
Director, Cosmetic Surgery Unit
Division of Dermatology
David Geffen School of Medicine
University of California, Los Angeles
Los Angeles, California

Doug Fife, MD
Department of Dermatology
University of California, Irvine
Irvine, California

Edgar F. Fincher, MD, PhD
Dermatology (private practice)
Los Angeles, California

Ernesto Gadsden, MD
Chief of Plastic Surgery Division
Hospital Central Militar
Principal Investigator for LipoSonix
   in Mexico
Mexico City, Mexico

Paul H. Garlich, MD
Otolaryngology and Facial Plastic Surgery (private
   practice)
Gainesville, Georgia

Hayes B. Gladstone, MD
Director, Division of Dermatologic Surgery
Associate Professor
Stanford University
Stanford, California

Michael H. Gold, MD
Medical Director, Gold Skin Care Center
Tennessee Clinical Research Center
Clinical Assistant Professor
Department of Medicine and Department of
   Dermatology
Vanderbilt University School of Medicine
Vanderbilt University School of Nursing
Nashville, Tennessee

Mitchel P. Goldman, MD
Medical Director, La Jolla Spa
Volunteer Clinical Professor of Dermatology and
   Medicine
University of California, San Diego
San Diego, California

Joseph F. Greco, MD
Assistant Clinical Professor
Division of Dermatology
David Geffen School of Medicine
University of California, Los Angeles
Los Angeles, California

Karyn Grossman, MD
Chief, Division of Dermatology
St. John's Medical Center
Santa Monica, California
Attending, Division of Dermatology
University of Southern California
Los Angeles, California

C. William Hanke, MD, FACP, MPH
Professor of Dermatology
University of Iowa Carver College of Medicine
Iowa City, Iowa
Clinical Professor of Otolaryngology–Head and Neck
    Surgery
Indiana University School of Medicine
Indianapolis, Indiana

Nicanor Isse, MD
Assistant Clinical Professor
    (Plastic Surgery)
University of California Irvine
Irvine, California

Derek Jones, MD
Assistant Clinical Professor
Division of Dermatology
David Geffen School of Medicine
University of California, Los Angeles
Los Angeles, California

Rebecca A. Kazin, MD
Medical Director
Johns Hopkins Cosmetic Center
Assistant Professor of Dermatology
Johns Hopkins University
Baltimore, Maryland

Gregory S. Keller, MD, FACS
Associate Clinical Professor of Surgery
    (Head and Neck)
David Geffen School of Medicine
University of California, Los Angeles
Los Angeles, California

Jane G. Khoury, MD
Dermatology (private practice)
Ladera Ranch, California

David Kiken, MD
Division of Dermatology (private
    practice)
University of California, San Diego
La Jolla, California

Jenny Kim, MD, PhD
Assistant Professor of Medicine
Division of Dermatology
David Geffen School of Medicine
University of California, Los Angeles
Los Angeles, California

Taro Kono, MD
Assistant Professor and Chief of Laser Unit
Department of Plastic and Reconstructive Surgery
Tokyo Women's Medical University
Tokyo, Japan

David J. Kouba, MD, PhD
Chief of Cosmetic Dermasurgery
Assistant Professor of Dermatology
Henry Ford Health System
Detroit, Michigan

Patricio Leniz, MD
Division of Plastic Surgery
School of Medicine
Clinical Hospital JJ Aguirre
University of Chile
Santiago, Chile

Cathy A. Macknet, MD
Dermatology and Dermatologic Surgery (private practice)
Loma Linda, California

Devinder S. Mangat, MD, FACS
Associate Professor, Facial Plastic and Reconstructive
    Surgery
University of Cincinnati Medical Center
Cincinnati, Ohio

Grigoriy Mashkevich, MD
Instructor, Surgery (Head and Neck)
David Geffen School of Medicine
University of California, Los Angeles
Los Angeles, California
Facial Plastic and Reconstructive Surgery
New York Eye and Ear Infirmary
New York City, New York

Abby Meltzer
Wellesley College
Wellesley, Massachusetts

Greg S. Morganroth, MD
Assistant Clinical Professor of Dermatology
University of California–San Francisco
San Francisco, California
Adjunct Clinical Assistant Professor of
    Otolaryngology/Head and Neck Surgery
Stanford University
Stanford, California

Ronald L. Moy, MD
Clinical Professor of Medicine
Division of Dermatology
David Geffen School of Medicine
University of California, Los Angeles
Los Angeles, California

Rhoda S. Narins, MD
Director, Dermatology Surgery and Laser Center
Clinical Professor of Dermatology
New York University Medical School
New York City, New York

Vic A. Narurkar, MD
Assistant Clinical Professor of Dermatology
University of California, Davis School of Medicine
Sacramento, California

Andrew A. Nelson, MD
Department of Dermatology
Harvard Medical School
Boston, Massachusetts

James Newman, MD, FACS
Assistant Clinical Professor
Division of Facial Plastic and Reconstructive Surgery
Stanford University
Stanford, California

Joseph Niamtu III, DMD
Department of Oral and Maxillofacial Surgery
Virginia Commonwealth University
Richmond, Virginia

Pierre Nicolau, MD
Plastic Surgery (private practice)
Paris, France

Suzan Obagi, MD
Assistant Professor of Dermatology
Director, The Cosmetic Surgery and Skin Health Center
Department of Dermatology
University of Pittsburgh School of Medicine
Pittsburgh, Pennsylvania

Mariana Pinzon-Plazas, MD
Research Associates Skin Care Research, Inc.
The Dermatology and Aesthetic Center
Boca Raton, Florida

Arturo Prado, MD
Division of Plastic Surgery
School of Medicine
Clinical Hospital JJ Aguirre
University of Chile
Santiago, Chile

Bernard I. Raskin, MD
Assistant Clinical Professor of Medicine
Division of Dermatology
David Geffen School of Medicine
University of California, Los Angeles
Los Angeles, California

Kelley Pagliai Redbord, MD
Dermatology (private practice)
Vienna, Virginia

Johannes Reinmüller, MD
Plastic Surgery (private practice)
Klinik am Sonnenberg
Wiesbaden, Germany

B. Kent Remington, MD
Dermatology (private practice)
Calgary, Alberta, Canada

Marta I. Rendon, MD
Clinical Associate Professor
Department of Dermatology
Miller School of Medicine, University of Miami
Miami, Florida
Department of Dermatology
Florida Atlantic University
Boca Raton, Florida

Thomas Rohrer, MD
Clinical Associate Professor of Dermatology
Boston University School of Medicine
Boston, Massachusetts

E. Victor Ross, MD
Director, Laser and Cosmetic Dermatology Center
Scripps Clinic
La Jolla, CA
Assistant Clinical Professor
Dermatology Division
School of Medicine
University of California, San Diego
San Diego, California

Bernard Rossi, MD
Department of Dermatology
Hôpital Charles Nicolle
University of Rouen
Rouen, France
Lecturer
Department of Dermatology
University of Paris V
Paris, France

Adam M. Rotunda, MD
Dermatology (private practice)
Newport Beach, California

Deborshi Roy, MD
Department of Facial Plastic and Reconstructive
   Surgery
Lenox Hill Hospital
New York City, New York

Javier Ruiz-Esparza, MD
Associate Clinical Professor
University of California, San Diego
San Diego, California

Neil S. Sadick, MD
Associate Professor of Dermatology
Cornell University Medical College
New York City, New York

Sogol Saghari, MD
Dermatology (private practice)
Beverly Hills, California

Antonio Rusciani Scorza, MD
Department of Plastic Surgery
    (private practice)
Catholic University of Sacred Heart
Rome, Italy

Joseph Sedrak, MD
Department of Dermatology
Loma Linda University School of Medicine
Loma Linda, California

Nael Shoman, MD
Division of Otolaryngology
Department of Surgery
University of British Columbia
Vancouver, British Columbia, Canada

Michelle Zaniewski Singh, MD, FACP
Cosmetic Medicine and Endocrinology
    (private practice)
Houston, Texas

Teresa Soriano, MD
Assistant Professor of Medicine
Department of Dermatology
David Geffen School of Medicine
University of California, Los Angeles
Los Angeles, California

Constantin Stan, MD
Plastic Surgery (private practice)
Bacau, Romania

Zeina Tannous, MD
Department of Dermatology
Harvard Medical School
Boston, Massachusetts

Ahmet Tezel, PhD
Research and Development

Allergan Inc.
Santa Barbara, California

Abel Torres, MD, JD
Professor and Chairman
Division of Dermatology
Loma Linda University School of
    Medicine
Loma Linda, California

Joshua A. Tournas, MD
Department of Dermatology
University of California, Irvine
Irvine, California

Jean Francois Tremblay, MD
Department of Dermatology
University of Montreal
Montreal, Quebec, Canada

Molly Wanner, MD
Clinical Instructor of Dermatology
Department of Dermatology
Harvard Medical School
Massachusetts General Hospital
Boston, Massachusetts

Eric Williams, MD
Division of Dermatology
David Geffen School of Medicine
University of California, Los Angeles
VA West LA Medical Center
Los Angeles, California

Mark Willoughby, MD
Dermatology (private practice)
San Diego, California

Katrina Wodhal, MD
Dermatology (private practice)
La Jolla, California

Paul S. Yamauchi, MD
Division of Dermatology
David Geffen School of Medicine
University of California, Los Angeles
Los Angeles, California

Christopher B. Zachary, MD
Professor and Chair
Department of Dermatology
University of California, Irvine
Irvine, California

PART ONE

ANATOMY
AND
THE AGING
PROCESS

CHAPTER 1

Anatomy and the Aging Changes of the Face and Neck

Pierre Nicolau

With aging, all facial elements undergo specific modifications. This results in an appearance typical for a specific age group, well recognizable by others. These signs of aging, most of which are demonstrated by Figure 1.1, which shows, split-face, the same man at ages twenty-three and fifty-one, include the following:

- loss of forehead skin elasticity and subcutaneous fat, which, along with increased depressor muscles tonus, results in apparent skin redundancy and pronounced frown lines
- brow ptosis
- wider and deeper orbital appearance
- distortion of the superolateral upper orbital rim with excess upper eyelid skin and fat (hooding)
- distortion of the inferomedial orbital rim: protrusion and sagging of fat, muscles, and skin
- prominent nasolabial folds
- deeper and more vertically sloped nasolabial crease
- loss of jawline contour with formation of jowls due to skin laxity and fat ptosis
- loss of submental cervical angle: midline platysma separation and band formation, skin ptosis

These changes result in loss of the arches of the face that define the youthful appearance noted in Figure 1.2.

Such massive structural and morphological changes involve all the tissues, but each in a different way. Laxity of the skin and subcutaneous tissues accounts only for a part. Loss of volume, due to fat atrophy and bone remodeling, also contributes significantly to the aging process. Let us examine the roles of bone, fat, and muscle changes during the aging process and their consequences on appearance.

ROLE OF BONE

Human bone goes through remodeling throughout the lifetime. Maximum bone mass is reached between fifteen and twenty-five years of age, at which age, women have about 20% less bone mass than men. By the age of sixty, 25% of bone mass will be lost. There is an acceleration of bone disappearance in women at menopause, then a slowing down of the process, while men show a steady decrease in bone mass. Men catch up gradually to women, and both end with the same loss.

Several studies have shown that craniofacial bones do not undergo disappearance, but rather, they show continuous growth throughout life, with enlargement of facial height and width. However, bone of dermal origin, like facial bone, differs in its evolution from bone of endoskeletal origin (postcranial skeleton). They present with permanent zones of bone deposition or resorbtion that modify their shape, as can be seen with the global transverse enlargement at the malar and zygomatic arch levels.

Studies of the evolution of facial dimensions and structures with age give contradictory results. In transversal studies (Pessa 2000; Shaw and Kahn 2007), individuals of different age groups are studied at a given time. The authors' conclusions are that there is a marked decrease of the midfacial vertical maxillary dimension and posterior sliding, associated with a deepening of the inner part of the inferior orbital rim. This allows Pessa (2000) to describe a clockwise rotation of the face.

These conclusions are totally contradicted by a longitudinal study based on Behrents's atlas, from the original work of Bolton, who followed almost six thousand subjects yearly from 1928 to the 1970s. Levine et al. (2003) states that bone resorption at the orbital rim and maxilla ridge is responsible, through disappearance of the maxillary concavity, for an increase in the vertical length of the maxilla with anterior maxillary wall displacement, under the forces generated by the descent of the soft tissues of the midface.

Clinical and therapeutic conclusions are therefore completely different. In the first case, bone posterior displacement would be responsible for the sliding downward and forward of the malar fat pad, increasing the thickness and

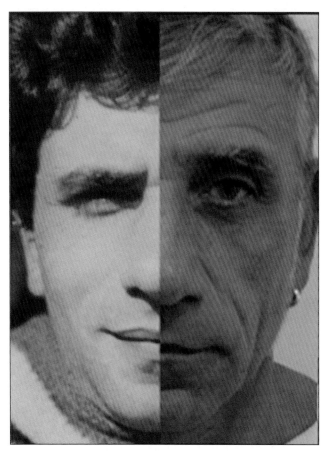

FIGURE 1.1: The signs of aging: same man, age twenty-three and age fifty-one.

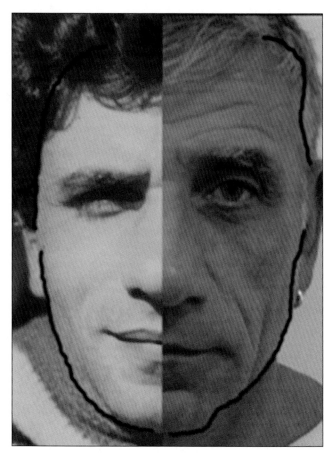

FIGURE 1.2: Loss of convexities of the once youthful curvatures of the face.

volume of the nasolabial fold, thus inducing a reactional muscular retraction. Youthful appearance would then be best achieved by restoring the bone dimensions of youth, with bone apposition or osteotomies and deep, subperiosteal face lifts.

In contrast, according to Levine et al. (2003), it is the loss of soft tissue volume and position, unmasking underlying skeletal contours, that is responsible for the aging appearance. Muscle tone is increased by the pull of soft tissues and the lengthening of underlying bones. Rejuvenation will be best achieved by restoring soft tissue volume and repositioning, hence the role of facial fillers and superficial face lifts.

We know that bone remodeling is induced by forces applied on the periosteum, and the rotation effect described might be an illusion, as it could be based, not on the backward movement of the lower maxilla, but on its vertical descent. This could explain why we do not see the functional consequences such a clockwise rotation should have on the nasopharyngeal area, which should be diminished and impaired.

The true consequences of bone remodeling on facial aging are still to be demonstrated and quantified. Longi-

tudinal studies are currently under way to try to shed light on this very important issue.

ROLE OF FAT

There are two layers of subcutaneous fat. The first is a superficial one, between the dermis and fascia superficialis (upper layer of the SMAS), corresponding to the hypodermis and being fairly evenly distributed. Its role is protective, mechanically and chemically. A deeper layer, deep in the SMAS, is found around or under the muscles. It improves the gliding of tissue planes during muscle movement (Dumont et al. 2007). These layers are further divided into several fat compartments well limited by septa, which can fuse in a membrane corresponding to the facial retaining ligaments and within which can be found the feeding vessels to the skin (Rohrich and Pessa 2007).

Aging seems to occur differently between these layers. The deep, perimuscular fat layer is not very much affected by variations in weight of individuals, whereas the volume of the superficial, subcutaneous layer relates more to overall body fat content and weight variations. The variations in fat volume present in the superficial compartments are responsible for the thin (skinny) or heavy (fatty) appearance of an aging face.

Muscles also play a part in fat distribution, as with aging, fat is displaced from being deep to superficial around the muscles in the deep layer, and this accentuates fat and skin sliding in the superficial layer, and all of this in a different way for each compartment.

Fat distribution, including fat distribution around the muscles, is very important to understand. The true goal is to re-create the appearance of youth, not just to blindly add volume to an aging face. When injecting a dermal or subdermal filler, including autologous fat, to produce the desired effect, the depth of this injection is of primary importance to re-creating the appearance of youth, and not just its volume.

ROLE OF MUSCLES

Although it seems common sense that there is lengthening of facial muscles with age, numerous studies show that the actual muscle tone increases, with shortening of the amplitude of movement, muscle tone at rest staying closer to maximum contracture tone. According to some authors, this is due to a reactional adaptation to bone resorbtion, and according to others, it is due to the lengthening of the bone bases. There is also a marked decrease in muscle mass, well proven in the lower eyelid. It is possible that this might increase the tone of the remaining muscle mass. Whatever the cause, Le Louarn (2007) has well demonstrated this tightening of the muscles of the face, the permanent contracture of which results in shifting of the underlying fat, accentuation of skin creases, and permanent skin wrinkling.

This is well observed in facial nerve palsy, in which the absence of movement results in the disappearance of wrinkles and the nasolabial fold. The best way to treat this contracture could be through the use of botulinum toxin, but it cannot be used easily or without unpleasant side effects everywhere in the face.

CONSEQUENCES FOR EACH FACIAL AREA

Forehead

There is bone loss with a verticalization of the forehead and a flattening of the supraorbital ridge. This results in an apparent lengthening of the forehead skin, further increased by recession of the hairline. The thinning of the subcutaneous fat in all compartments contributes to the thinning of the skin and the marked hollowing of the temple area. Increased muscular tone results in permanent wrinkling, horizontal lines by the frontalis, and glabellar frown lines by the corrugators and superior orbicularis oculi.

Botulinum toxin is efficient for treating the wrinkles, with care being taken to leave the inferior third of the frontalis muscle untreated. If skin laxity is important, with marked descent of the eyebrows, a forehead lift is indicated, as releasing the muscle contracture will further accentuate drooping eyebrows. Superficial fillers will give good results for suprazygomatic and temple hollowing.

Upper and Lateral Orbit

Bone changes are major here, with flattening of the supraorbital ridge, bone loss at the nasion, and oblique lengthening of the orbital diameter, with bone resorption on the superolateral rim contributing to brow ptosis. A combination of all factors – bone resorbtion, skin relaxation, muscle contracture and volume loss, and fat displacement – results in ptosis of the brow and upper eyelid, with hollowing of the upper part of the eyelid and protrusion of the inner orbital fat, medial to the levator muscle. Contracture of the lateral orbicularis oculi muscle results not only in crow's feet, but also, at its lower external portion, in marked displacement of the suborbicularis oculi fat pad (SOOF).

Lower Eyelid and Nasolabial Fold

There is marked bone resorbtion on the inferomedial orbital rim and major changes of the anterior maxilla, with resorbtion and verticalization. Contracture of the palpebral part of the orbicularis oculi is responsible for wrinkling of the palpebral skin, while the orbital, peripheral part of the muscle pushes away the deep fat pads, some parts of the muscle showing marked volume loss. The orbital septum slackens, together with the orbicularis retaining ligament, resulting in orbital fat herniation and lower-eyelid lengthening. The subcutaneous fat superficial to the orbital part of the orbicularis muscle slides downward and inward, deepening the tear trough. It pushes on the nasolabial fat compartment, thus creating or thickening the nasolabial fold and deepening the crease. Laterally, sliding of the SOOF, together with skin and muscle, is stopped by the superficial malar fat compartment, resulting in so-called malar bags.

Orbital rim changes can be treated with deep permanent or long-lasting fillers to replace orbital rim losses, lifting up the brows and filling the tear-trough deformity. Muscle contracture is released with botulinum toxin, but skin excess and displacement need tightening, repositioning, or resection, and fat protrusion is best treated with surgical procedures. For the eyelids proper, in the opinion of the author, there is no indication for superficial fillers since a variety of complications can result from superficial placement of the fillers, whether subcutaneous or injected within the orbicularis muscle.

Displaced malar and lower orbital subcutaneous fat should be repositioned surgically. Fillers can only be used to replace volume loss. If fillers are injected superficially without prior repositioning of the sagging deeper tissues, the result is an abnormal-looking cheek and malar volume when smiling. The problem can be avoided by injecting the filler deep, under the muscular layer, around the periosteum of the maxilla, so that the filler is not subject to muscle movements. The result is a natural, youthful appearance.

Lips and Perioral Region

Apart from major changes induced by tooth loss, normal aging is characterized by thinning of the lips due to loss of muscle volume; permanent superficial orbicularis oris contracture, resulting in vertical perioral wrinkles; and deepening of the chin crease through the combined effect of muscle and fat volume loss and bone resorbtion. These changes can be treated with fillers, skin resurfacing, and, if done very carefully, with neurotoxin.

Jowls and Marionette Lines

Marionette lines are due, in their superior part, to the permanent contracture of the depressor anguli oris, with a pull downward of the corner of the mouth, unbalanced by the weakened lip levator muscles. This can be released with botulinum toxin. In their lower part, like the nasolabial fold, they correspond to a ligamentous border separating the ptotic cheek skin and its fairly thick subcutaneous fat from the lip, where there is very little subcutaneous fat. This jowl fat seems to be within a distinct anatomical compartment. Therefore jowl treatment could probably be better achieved by surgery than by filling the lip or by liposuction of the fold.

Lower Face and Neck

Skin and muscle laxity are responsible for a sliding of the teguments of the cheek, with an anterior and downward rotation. As we have seen, the obstacle represented by the labiomental crease will stop this sliding, creating the anterior fold of the jowl. The contracture of the platysma increases this effect and is responsible for the submental vertical folds, or platysmal bands. Platysmaplasty with submental horizontal platysma muscle release and midline suture allows for the creation of a platysmal sling, which defines the cervicomental angle and repositions the medial submental fat pad. Platysmaplasty is even more critical for patients with visible platysmal bands due to a separation of the medial platysma borders. Deep placement of appropriate fillers or implants (subcutaneous or along the periosteum) is an excellent nonsurgical alternative for restoring the jawline and blunt jowls. Placement should be along the mandibular border, at the lower end of the labiomental

crease, corresponding to the ligament of Furnas. Botulinum toxin has been used to release the platysma bands, but results are short-lived, it is very costly, and it can have undesirable side effects; thus it has limited usefulness in this area. Numerous surgical techniques have been described to try to correct the platysmal muscle bands and tighten the skin in the anterior neck region, which means that none can be entirely satisfactory or helpful for all cases. Jowls and lateral neck laxity, however, respond far more predictably to lifting procedures.

The availability of new and improved fillers, neurotoxins, and various tissue tightening and skin resurfacing methods and devices, discussed in this textbook, can provide alternatives or supplementation to classic surgical techniques. In conclusion, a good understanding of anatomy and how it changes with the aging process, and careful analysis of each patient's morphology, is mandatory to define for each individual what will be the best combination of treatments.

SUGGESTED READING

Levine RA, Garza JR, Wang PTH, et al. Adult facial growth: applications to aesthetic surgery. *Aesthetic Plast. Surg.* 2003;27:265–8.

Pessa J. An algorithm of facial aging verification of Lambros' theory by three dimensional stereolithography with reference to the pathogenesis of midfacial aging, scleral show and the lateral suborbital trough deformity. *Plast. Reconstr. Surg.* 2000;106:479–88.

Pessa JE, Yuan C. Curve analysis of the aging orbital aperture. *Plast. Reconstr. Surg.* 2002;109:751–5.

Shaw RB, Kahn DM. Aging of the midface bony elements: a three-dimensional computed tomographic study. *Plast. Reconstr. Surg.* 2007;119:675–81.

Suggested Reading about Fat

Coleman SR, Grover R. The anatomy of the aging face: volume loss and changes in 3-dimensional topography. *Aesthetic Surg. J.* 2006;26(Suppl):S4–S9.

Dumont T, Simon E, Stricker M, et al. Analysis of the implications of the adipose tissue in facial morphology, from a revue of the literature and dissections of 10 half faces. *Ann. Chir. Plast. Esthet.* 2007;52:196–205.

Rohrich RD, Pessa JE. The fat compartments of the face: anatomy and clinical implications for cosmetic surgery. *Plast. Reconstr. Surg.* 2007;119:2219–27.

Suggested Reading about Muscles

Le Louarn C. Botulinum toxin and the Face Recurve® concept: decreasing resting tone and muscular regeneration. *Ann. Chir. Plast. Esthet.* 2007;52:165–76.

PART TWO

ANESTHESIA AND SEDATION FOR OFFICE COSMETIC PROCEDURES

CHAPTER 2

Local Anesthetics

Cathy A. Macknet
Greg S. Morganroth

BASICS OF LOCAL ANESTHESIA

Mechanism of Action

Local anesthetics block Na^+ influx during depolarization of the nerve cell membrane. The result is the blockade of the action potential and subsequent anesthesia.

Order of Blockade

The blockade proceeds from pain through temperature, touch, pressure, vibration, propioception, and motor function:

- First affected are the small, unmyelinated C-type nerve fibers (which transmit pain and temperature).
- Last affected are the largest, myelinated A-type fibers (which transmit pressure sensations and motor fibers).

Patients may have anesthesia but still feel pressure and may have the ability to move because the A-type fibers are unblocked.

Composition

Anesthetics are weak organic bases that exist in two forms:

- The ionized form is an active form that blocks nerve conduction. The ionized form is water-soluable, therefore allowing injection. At physiologic pH, 80% is in the ionized form.
- The nonionized form is the lipid-soluable form that facilitates diffusion into tissues and nerve cell membranes.

Chemical Structure

The chemical structure has three components:

- The aromatic portion is usually composed of a benzene ring (lipophilic).
- The intermediate chain is either an ester or an amide linkage (determines class).
- The amine is hydrophilic (water solubility).

Lipid solubility is important because it enables diffusion through the lipophilic nerve membrane. Lipophilicity is directly related to potency.

Duration of Anesthesia

Duration is directly related to the degree of protein binding of the anesthetic receptors along the nerve cell membrane (determined by amine structure).

Potency

Potency is determined by lipid solubility.

Speed of Onset

Speed of onset relies on the pKa (the fraction of anesthetic that is active at physiologic pH). This is determined by the aromatic structure. An anesthetic with a low pKa will have a rapid onset of action. Alkalinization of the anesthetic solution with sodium bicarbonate will speed the onset of action.

TECHNIQUES FOR PAINLESS ANESTHESIA

- Verbal reassurance and distraction
- If anxious, could consider premedication
  - Ambien 5–10 mg, sl 30 minutes prior (short-acting, 4-hour effect)
  - Valium 5–10 mg, sl 30 minutes prior
  - Demerol, Vistaril
- Mechanical distraction
- Use small-gauge needle (30 gauge) and syringes (larger syringes result in more pressure and increase pain)

- Cryoanesthesia: fluorethyl, frigiderm, ethyl chloride, ice cube, smart cool (–5°C)
- Warm anesthetic to body temperature
- Inject slowly, first subcutaneously and then dermally
- Inject through previously anesthetized tissue
- Increase pH with bicarbonate 1:10
- Plain lidocaine, if possible
- Preoperative EMLA

ADDITIVES TO LOCAL ANESTHETICS

When choosing an additive, one should consider the desired effect and weigh the risk versus the benefits. Additives may potentiate hemostasis and/or prolong or shorten the duration or onset of anesthesia. Because additives alter the pH of the anesthetic, this may result in more or less patient discomfort. Tissue irritation is related to the acidity of the infiltrated solution. Epinephrine and bicarbonate affect acidity and alter the associated discomfort.

- prolongs anesthesia by 100% to 150%
- hemostatic up to 1:500,000 or 1:1,000,000
- available at premixed concentrations of 1:100,000 and 1:200,000 with lidocaine
- Risks
  - systemic effects
  - possible tissue necrosis, increased if used for ring blocks
  - interacts with tricyclic antidepressants (HTN, tachycardia, ventricular tachycardia) and nonselective beta blockers (propranolol; hypertension and bradycardia)
  - increased risk for rapid absorption in vascular areas (e.g., glans penis)
  - concentrations greater than 1:200,000 are usually not necessary for dermatologic surgery and concentrations greater than 1:100,000 are at increased risk for side effects
  - should not exceed 1 mg (100 mL of 1:100,000)

	pH	Comments
1% lidocaine	5.5–7.0	- close to physiologic pH, resulting in less pain
1% lidocaine + epinephrine	3.5–5.0	- A more acidic pH is necessary to preserve the epinephrine; this results in increased pain
"Buffered" Anesthetic 1% lidocaine + epinephrine (10 parts) with 8.4% sodium bicarbonate (1 part) 10:1 ratio	7.3–7.5 (very close to physiologic pH)	- bicarbonate helps neutralizes pH, thereby decreasing pain - bicarbonate decreases hemostatic effect of epinephrine - good for only 1 week because bicarbonate degrades epinephrine, which results in loss of vasoconstriction after 1 week - stable at room temperature for approximately 24 hours (must be refrigerated) - faster onset but decreased duration of anesthesia
"Fresh" Anesthetic: 50 mL 1% lidocaine 0.025 mL of 1:1,000 epinephrine → 1% lidocaine with 1:200,000 epinephrine	50 mL of 1% lidocaine 0.5 mL of 1:1,000 epinephrine → 1% lidocaine with 1:100,000 epinephrine	Close to physiologic pH	- does not have acidic preparations that manufacturers use to preserve epinephrine

Author's Tips: You may initially use buffered lidocaine + epinephrine to avoid the burning sensation, then follow this with nonbuffered lidocaine + epinephrine to improve hemostasis. So-called fresh anesthetic is preferred.

Additives to Local Anesthetics

Epinephrine

- Benefits
  - has vasoconstrictive effect
  - less anesthetic is required to obtain anesthesia, therefore there is less toxicity from the anesthetic

- pregnancy category C

Hyaluronidase (Widase)

- Mechanism
  - hydrolyzes hyaluronic acid in the connective tissue and facilitates diffusion of the anesthetic

- Benefits
  - increases the spread of anesthesia, decreases the duration of action of the anesthetics because it increases absorption
  - USE: to decrease distortion of the surgical site, the addition of hyaluronidase is useful for nerve blocks and procedures around the orbit
- usual dilution is 150 U in 30 mL of anesthetic
- Risks:
  - potential for allergy – contraindicated in patients with a known allergy to bee stings
  - contains the preservative thimerosal
  - recommended intradermal test dose
  - increases the potential for toxicity of the anesthetic

CLASSIFICATION OF ANESTHETICS

Anesthetics are classified into two groups, depending on the linkage in the intermediate chain: the ester group and the amide group. This structural difference affects metabolism and allergic potential.

Amides

- Two "i"s in their name
- Hydrolyzed in the liver by hepatic microsomal enzymes p450 3A4 (p450 3A4 inhibitors will increase half-life of anesthetic)
- Metabolites are excreted by the kidneys
- Patients with severe liver disease may be at increased risk of amide anesthetic toxicity

Generic name (trade name)	Relative Potency	Onset (min)	Duration (hours)	Max Dose "Plain" (mg, for 70-kg male)	Max Dose "with Epi" (mg, for 70-kg male)	Other
Bupivicaine hydrochloride (Marcaine)	8	2.0–10.0 slow	2–4 long	175	225	• cannot be buffered due to precipitation with bicarbonate • more intense injection burn • greater cardiac toxicity than lidocaine: ventricular arrhythmias and cardiovascular collapse • ideal for long procedure (bupivicaine 0.25% ± 1:200,000 epinephrine)
Etidocaine (Duranest)	6	3–5 med	3.0–5.0 long	300	400	
Leubopivicaine hydrochloride (Chirocaine)		2–10	2.0–4.0	150	not available	
Lidocaine (Xylocaine) 0.5%, 1%, 2%	2	Rapid	0.5–2.0 med	350	500 (3,500 dilute)	• maximum dose without epi = 4.5 mg/kg • maximum dose with epi = 7.0 mg/kg • tumescent = 55 mg/kg • buffered: 1 mL 8.4% $NaHCO_3$ + 10 mL anesthetic (increases pH to 7.3) • 2% lidocaine may produce a larger concentration gradient, promoting diffusion into the nerve
Mepivacaine (Carbocaine)		3–20	0.5–2.0	300	500	
Prilocaine hydrochloride (Citanest)	2	5–6	0.5–2.0	400	600	• metabolized to orthotoluidine metabolite, causing methemoglobinemia
Prilocaine/lidocaine (EMLA)			short			• topical
Ropivacaine (Naropin)		1–15	2.0–6.0	200	not available	
Dibucaine (Nupercaine)			short			• topical

Esters

- metabolized/hydrolyzed by pseudocholinesterases in plasma
- metabolized to PABA and therefore may cross-react with sulfonamides, sulfonureas, PABA, paraphenylene diamine (PPD), PAS, thiazides
- excreted renally (therefore contraindicated with severe renal failure)
- allergic reactions are infrequent but more common than seen with amides

Generic Name (trade name)	Relative Potency	Onset (min)	Duration (hours)	Max Dose "plain" (mg, for 70-kg male)	Max Dose "with Epi" (mg, for 70-kg male)	Other
Benzocaine (Anbesol)			short			• topical • may induce methemoglobinemia
Chloroprocaine hydrochloride (Nesacaine)	1	5–6	0.5–2.0	800	1,000	
Procaine (Novocaine)	1	5	1.0–1.5	500	600	• risk of methemoglobinemia
Tetracaine (Pontocaine)	8	7	2.0–3.0	100	not available	

Author's Tips:

- Blepharoplasty: 1% lidocaine with epinephrine injected locally
- Lip augmentation with fillers: gingival mucosal block using 1% lidocaine ± epinephrine
- TCA chemical peel: supraorbital, infraorbital, and mental nerve blocks 2–3 mL (amide-type anesthetics; may use 2% lidocaine to enhance diffusion; may use vasoconstrictor [epinephrine 1:200,000] to slow absorption of anesthetic and prolong duration of anesthesia)

Risk of methemoglobinemia: (prilocaine ≫ lidocaine, procaine [Novocaine], benzocaine)

- Iron molecule in Hg oxidizes from ferrous $2+$ to ferric $3+$ state, which decreases ability to bind, transport, and deliver oxygen
- Increased risk in premature infants given >500 mg
- Treatment: stop drug, give oxygen, methylene blue 1–2 mg/kg over five minutes (mix 7 mg/kg ± IV glucose)
- Increased risk in patients taking Tylenol, sulfa, dapsone, benzocaine, chloroquine, phenobarbital, phenytoin
- Note that lidocaine and procaine may also cause it, but less commonly: 0.5% = 0.5 g/100 mL → 5 mg/cc 1% = 1g/100 mL → 10 mg/cc 2% = 2 g/100 mL → 20 mg/cc

Tumescent Anesthesia and Tumescent Liposuction Solutions

Tumescent anesthesia	
Uses	• liposuction, face lifts, reconstruction, ambulatory phlebectomy, ablative laser resurfacing, hair transplantation, endovenous radiofrequency ablation
Benefits	• increases maximum safe dose of lidocaine to 55 mg/kg • dilute epinephrine results in vasoconstriction of subepidermal vessels, resulting in hemostasis and decreased absorption
Formula	
Lidocaine 1%	50–100 mL
Epinephrine 1:1,000	1 mL
Sodium bicarbonate 8.4%	10 mL
Normal saline 0.9%	900–950 mL
Hyaluronidase 150 U/mL	6 mL (optional)
Triamcinolone acetonide 40 mg/mL	0.25 mL (optional)

- A final concentration of 0.05% to 0.1% lidocaine with 1:1,000,000 is prepared
- Peak plasma levels of lidocaine at 12 hours postinfusion (CNS toxicity at blood levels of 5–6 µg/mL)

Tumescent liposuction solutions

	0.05%	0.075%	0.1%
Lidocaine 1%	50 mL (= 500 mg)	75 mL (= 750 mg)	100 mL (= 1,000 mg)
Sodium chloride 0.9%	1,000 mL	1,000 mL	1,000 mL
Epinephrine 1:1,000	1 mL	1 mL	1 mL
Sodium bicarbonate 8.4%	10 mL	10 mL	10 mL

Author's Tips: Tumescent anesthesia in cosmetic procedures

Full-face laser resurfacing	0.3% tumescent solution with 1:1,000,000 epinephrine infiltration following supraorbital, infraorbital, and mental nerve blocks with 1% lidocaine with 1:100,000 epinephrine
Neck liposuction	0.075% to 0.1% tumescent solution with 1:1,000,000 epinephrine
Body liposuction	0.05% to 0.075% tumescent solution with 1:1,000,000 epinephrine
Face lift/neck lift	0.3% tumescent solution with 1:500,000 epinephrine

SIDE EFFECTS AND PRECAUTIONS

Patient selection is important when considering which anesthetic is appropriate for use. There are contraindications for the use of both local anesthetics and epinephrine. It is also important to be aware of the total amount of anesthetic used as both lidocaine and epinephrine have associated systemic toxicities.

Contraindications
Contraindications to local anesthetics

- Severe blood pressure instability
- History of true anesthetic allergy
- Psychological instability
- For amides: severe liver compromise (amides metabolized by liver but excreted by kidney)
- For esters: severe renal compromise

Contraindications to epinephrine

- Absolute
  - uncontrolled hyperthyroidism
  - pheochromocytoma
  - severe peripheral vascular occlusive disease
- Relative (dilute to 1:500,000 and use sparingly)
  - hypertension
  - heart disease
  - pregnancy (concern regarding premature labor)
  - phenothiazines, MAO inhibitors, tricyclics, amphetamines, digitalis

- beta blockers (especially with nonselective beta 1 & 2) result in HTN and bradycardia
- narrow-angle glaucoma
- acral areas: digits, penis
- peripheral vascular disease

Maximal Safe Doses of Lidocaine

	Max Dose	Max Volume
1% lidocaine	4.5 mg/kg	30 cc
1% lidocaine in a child	*1.5–2.5 mg/kg*	
1% lidocaine with 1:100,000 epi	7.0 mg/kg	50 cc
1% lidocaine with 1:100,000 epi in a child	*3.0–4.0 mg/kg*	
0.1% lidocaine with 1:1,000,000 epi (tumescent)	35.0 mg/kg (or 55.0 mg/kg)	2,500 cc

Side Effects of Local Anesthetics
Local reactions

- Pain and burning (immediate and temporary)
- Ecchymosis
- Hematoma (rare)
- Infection (rare)
- Direct trauma to nerve resulting in paresthesias or transient motor nerve paralysis (twenty to thirty minutes after injection)
- Intravascular injection

	Symptoms	Treatment
Systemic reactions		
Vasovagal episode	excess parasympathetic tone; diaphoresis, hyperventilation, nausea, hypotension, bradycardia	Trendelenburg, cold compress reassurance
Epinephrine reaction	excess α- and β-adrenergic receptor stimulation; palpitations, hypertension, tachycardia, diaphoresis, angina, tremors, and nervousness; serious effects include arrhythmias, ventricular tachycardia, ventricular fibrillation, cardiac arrest, and cerebral hemorrhage	reassurance (usually resolves within minutes), phentolamine, propranolol
Anaphylactic reaction	peripheral vasodilation with reactive tachycardia; stridor, bronchospasm, urticaria, angioedema	epinephrine 1:1,000 0.3 mL SC, antihistamines, fluids, oxygen, airway maintenance
Lidocaine toxicity: first central nervous system, then respiratory, then cardiac		
• Treatment: most important to give O$_2$ to decrease seizure threshold		
1–6 µg/mL	circumoral and digital paresthesias, restlessness, drowsiness, euphoria, lightheadedness	observe patient
6–9 µ/mL	nausea, vomiting, muscle twitching, tremors, blurred vision, tinnitus, confusion, excitement, psychosis	maintain airway, consider diazepam
9–12 µ/mL	seizures, cardiopulmonary depression	respiratory support
>12 µ/mL	coma, cardiopulmonary arrest	CPR/ACLS; may need prolonged CPR to allow lidocaine to pass through system

Anesthetic allergies exist and are extremely rare, especially with amide local anesthetics. Allergic reactions can be either type 1 (i.e., anaphylactic) or type 4 (i.e., delayed-type hypersensitivity).

Anesthetic Allergy

Ester allergy

• Type 1 reactions are usually caused by ester-type anesthetics; ester anesthetics have a much greater allergenic potential than the amide group

• Pseudocholinesterases break down esters to produce the highly allergenic metabolic product PABA

• Reactions to preservatives, specifically methylparaben and sodium metabisulfate (found in multiple-dose vials), may cause adverse reactions in a patient who is allergic to an ester-type anesthetic

• Cross-reactivity exists among ester anesthetics; avoid all anesthetics in this structural group

• Not likely a cross-reaction between esters and amides; substitute amide anesthetic

Amide allergy

• Extremely rare, usually related to preservatives (bisulphites or parabens)

• Preservative-free single-dose vials of lidocaine are available for use if an amide anesthetic is to be used in a patient with a true hypersensitivity reaction to ester-type anesthetics

Alternatives to ester and amide anesthetics

• Benadryl 12.5 mg/mL may be substituted for a biopsy (this concentration is different from the packaged concentration and therefore must be diluted to avoid skin necrosis [packaged as 50 mg/mL])

• Promethazine, normal saline

• Bacteriostatic saline: benzyl alcohol is anesthetic (must get peau d'ange appearance for anesthesia to take effect)

• Skin testing of various local anesthetics and preservatives recommended

SUGGESTED READING

Huether MJ, Brodland DG. Local anesthetics. In: Wolverton SE, ed., *Comprehensive Dermatologic Drug Therapy*. Philadelphia: W. B. Saunders; 2007:825–49.

Nouri K, Leal-Khouri S, Khouri R. Local and topical anesthesia. In: Nouri K, Leal-Khouri S, eds., *Techniques in Dermatologic Surgery*. New York: Mosby; 2003:47–50.

Soriano TT, Lask GP, Dinehart SM. Anesthesia and analgesia. In: Robinson JK, Hanke CW, Sengelmann RD, Siegel DM, eds., *Surgery in the Skin*. Philadelphia: Elsevier; 2005:39–58.

CHAPTER 3

The Concept of Tumescent

Mark Willoughby

Sorin Eremia

Tumescent anesthesia is used today for various surgical procedures on the skin. Although most commonly used for liposuction and for harvesting fat for use as an autologous filler, the technique has been applied to various other procedures, including laser resurfacing, laser tattoo removal, endovenous ablation of varicose veins, and various medical and cosmetic surgical procedures. Tumescent anesthesia is achieved by injecting relatively large volumes of dilute neutralized lidocaine solution with epinephrine into the subcutaneous tissue. Tumescent anesthesia allows procedures that previously required conscious sedation or general anesthesia to be performed more safely, while patients are awake or mildly sedated. Commonly, it decreases or eliminates the need for narcotic analgesics or IV sedation for many cosmetic procedures. Tumescent lidocaine solutions have also been attributed antibacterial effects, possibly accounting for the very low rate of infection seen with tumescent liposuction. The use of dilute epinephrine in the tumescent solution further increases the safety of procedures, including liposuction, by decreasing blood loss. When used for resurfacing procedures, distending the skin can better expose the base of wrinkles to the resurfacing procedure.

Tumescent anesthesia, which revolutionized liposuction, was developed in the mid-1980s by dermatologic surgeon Dr. Jeffery Klein, who was able to demonstrate that lidocaine serum levels remained within safe limits following the injection of what were then considered high doses of lidocaine in terms of milligrams per kilogram, while at the same time achieving excellent anesthetic effect, if the lidocaine was delivered as large volumes of very dilute (0.05%) solution into fatty tissue. Prior to that time, lidocaine had not been commonly used in concentrations less than 0.25%. Typical volumes of 0.25% lidocaine used for face lifts were in the 150–250 cc range, designed not to exceed the Food and Drug Administration (FDA)-specified maximum safe dose of lidocaine of 7 mg/kg. There were no scientific studies supporting the FDA-recommended 7 mg/kg

lidocaine limit, especially with respect to li... into subcutaneous tissue. On the other hand, serum levels of lidocaine at which toxicity begin... well established. The key factor with tumescent ... is the slow absorption of the lidocaine from poorl... larized subcutaneous tissue to serum, which allows t... of the larger milligram per kilogram doses. Several s... ies have shown that peak serum levels are reached betwe... four and fourteen hours after injection of tumescent solu... tion into adipose tissues and that doses of 35 mg/kg are quite safe. In practical terms, this means that for a 70-kg individual, it is safe to use five 50-cc bottles of 1% lidocaine to make 5 L of 0.05% lidocaine tumescent solution. A single study has shown levels of 55 mg/kg to be free of toxicity in sixty patients. Lidocaine concentrations currently used in tumescent anesthesia commonly range from 0.05% to 0.15%. Slightly higher concentrations can be used for procedures in more fibrous and/or sensitive areas. Just remember that the higher the lidocaine concentration of the tumescent solution and the more vascular the area injected, the lower the total milligrams per kilogram dose of lidocaine should be. For example, we would not recommend using more than 500 cc of a 0.2% solution (about 15 mg/kg) for face and neck tumescent anesthesia in an average-weight patient.

To prepare the tumescent solution, 1% or 2% lidocaine is usually injected into bags of 0.9% normal saline. For example, 50 cc of 1% lidocaine (a total of 500 mg of lidocaine since 1% solution means 1 g = 1,000 mg per 100 cc) added to 950 cc of saline will make 1,000 cc of 0.05% tumescent solution. The solution is neutralized by adding sodium bicarbonate (10 mEq/L), making it less painful to infiltrate than the otherwise acidic solution. Epinephrine (1:1,000,000) is added, which prolongs the anesthetic effect and slows the absorption of lidocaine by vasoconstriction of the local vasculature. Fresh epinephrine, which usually comes in 1-cc vials of 1:1,000, has a more predictable effect and is preferred for preparing large volumes of tumescent

the use of 1% lidocaine with epinephrine
the base solution for dilution is quite adequate.
mescent solution was used chilled, but many
ow prefer body-temperature solution. Neutral
solutions (by addition of Na bicarbonate) are
o less painful injection. For most of the proce-
ered in this textbook, relatively low volumes, well
,000 cc, and often under 500 cc, of tumescent solu-
e used. Infiltration can be performed with a 30- to
syringe using an infiltration canula or spinal needle.
se of a peristaltic infusion pump allows for easier and
ker infiltration of large volumes of anesthetic solutions,
n as for liposuction, for which 3,000–5,000 cc is often
e norm.

Tumescent anesthesia has been developed and advanced
ver the past twenty years, providing a very safe and
effective method for anesthesia for dermatologic procedures. Potential applications of the technique are broad,
and the technique will likely be used in a wide range of
procedures.

SUGGESTED READING

Klein JA. Anesthesia for liposuction in dermatologic surgery. *J. Dermatol. Surg. Oncol.* 1988;14:1124–32.

Klein JA. Tumescent technique for regional anesthesia permits lidocaine doses of 35 mg/kg for liposuction. *J. Dermatol. Surg. Oncol.* 1990;16:248–63.

Klein JA. *Tumescent Technique: Tumescent Anesthesia and Microcannular Liposuction.* St. Louis: Mosby; 2000.

Lillis PJ. Liposuction surgery under local anesthesia: minimal blood loss with minimal lidocaine absorption. *J. Dermatol. Surg. Oncol.* 1988;14:1145–8.

Ostad A, Kageyama N, Moy RL. Tumescent anesthesia with a lidocaine dose of 55 mg/cc is safe for liposuction. *Dermatol. Surg.* 1996;22:921–7.

Stewart JH, Cole GW, Klein JA. Neutralized lidocaine with epinephrine for local anesthesia. *J. Dermatol. Surg. Oncol.* 1989;15:1081–3.

Yang, CH, Hsu HC, Shen SC, Juan WH, Hong HS, Chen CH. Warm and neutral tumescent anesthetic solutions are essential factors for a less painful injection. *Dermatol. Surg.* 2006;32:1119–22.

CHAPTER 4

Nerve Blocks

Joseph Niamtu III

Minimally invasive cosmetic surgery has become extremely attractive for patients and cosmetic practitioners. These procedures allow noninvasive correction of a variety of aging problems. They appeal to patients due to the quick result and minimal downtime. The era of lunchtime procedures has truly arrived.

One significant problem that still exists, despite the new technology, is procedural pain. BOTOX, fillers (especially lip), broad band light treatments (BBL), hair removal, radiofrequency skin tightening, vascular lasers, light chemical peels, and lasers are all examples of popular procedures that are painful to patients. Some practitioners adapt the so-called frown and bear it technique, but these clinicians will risk losing patients to a more compassionate doctor. It is very common in my practice for a new patient to present for fillers or other procedures that he or she has been doing traditionally at another office. When these patients realize that they have been enduring unnecessary pain, they usually praise our compassion, stay with our practice, and send their friends. All it takes is one woman at the tennis club telling her friends about her new positive experience, and others will usually follow. This compassion involves many factors, including a calming environment, physical touch, and verbal relaxation by the doctor and staff – and, of course, pain control. Finding the correct mixture of the preceding factors is an unbelievable marketing influence for a practice. We can use dentistry as a model. All of us have heard of patients seeking a certain dental practice because of the painless procedures. On the converse, many of us have personally left a dentist, or have friends who have done so, because the dentist was rough or used painful procedures.

While the focus of this chapter is nerve blocks for head and neck procedures, new topical anesthetic mixtures are also available that cause excellent topical cutaneous anesthesia and profound mucosal anesthesia. They are often used in combination with injection nerve blocks. My topical anesthetic of choice is so-called BLT, which is a mixture of 20% benzocaine, 6% lidocaine, and 4% tetracaine that can be formulated from most local pharmacies (e.g., Bayview Pharmacy, Baltimore, Maryland, [410] 633-6262). When applied to the skin, this mixture provides adequate anesthesia for most small procedures such as BOTOX injection, injectable fillers (excluding the lips), spider veins, IPL, hair removal, and so on. I use it mostly for cutaneous filler injection such as nasolabial folds. This mixture can also be used judiciously on the lips and perioral mucosa. When a patient arrives for lip fillers, his or her lips and the mucosa to the oral sulcus are coated with a layer of the BLT mixture. After five to ten minutes, the patient rinses out his or her mouth and is ready for phase 2, which is local anesthetic injection. Before discussing local anesthesia, it should be noted that toxic levels of anesthetics can be absorbed through the skin and/or mucous membranes, and every practitioner should be aware of toxic levels and modes of administration.

LOCAL ANESTHETIC BLOCKS FOR FACIAL PROCEDURES

Local anesthetic blocks are extremely effective for minimally invasive cosmetic procedures. Positive features include the ability to anesthetize large areas with a single injection and the fact that a remote local anesthetic block does not distort the target treatment area. Negative features of local anesthetic blocks are that they usually need to be performed bilaterally and often simultaneously in the upper and lower face. This can leave the patient with a totally numb face and the inability to normally animate, and can last for hours. Many patients do not appreciate these extended effects. Before discussing local anesthetic blocks, I will discuss mini-blocks, which, in reality, are regional infiltrative techniques.

MINI-BLOCK TECHNIQUE FOR LIP ANESTHESIA

This technique is designed to provide adequate local anesthesia of the lips and perioral regions and is most commonly

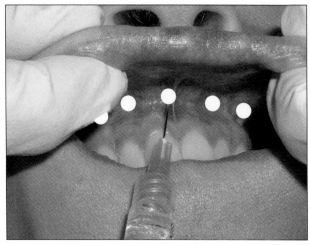 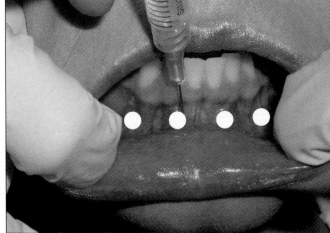

FIGURE 4.1: Mini-block technique for lip anesthesia.

used for lip and perioral filler injection, but it can be adapted for other procedures such as biopsy. The first step is to coat the lips and intraoral mucosa (including the sulcus) with the BLT topical anesthetic mixture. After approximately five to ten minutes, small infiltrations of local anesthesia (0.25–0.5 cc of 2% lidocaine with 1:100,000 epinephrine) are injected with a ½ inch, 32-gauge needle across the lip mucosa (just below the sulcus in the upper lip and just above the sulcus in the lower lip; Figure 4.1). Placing four to five injections from the canine tooth on one side to the canine tooth on the other side will usually provide sufficient anesthesia for lip filler injection and frequently will extend to most of the nasolabial fold. If the filler is to be injected all the way to the oral commisures, an additional injection may be required at the premolar area.

UPPER FACIAL NERVE BLOCKS: SCALP AND FOREHEAD

The frontal nerve exits through a notch (in some cases, a foramen) on the superior orbital rim approximately 27 mm lateral to the glabellar midline (Figure 4.2). This supraorbital notch is readily palpable in most patients. After exiting the notch or foramen, the nerve traverses the corrugator supercilli muscles and branches into a medial and lateral portion. The lateral branches supply the lateral forehead and the medial branches supply the scalp. The supratrochlear nerve exits a foramen approximately 17 mm from the glabellar midline (Figure 4.2) and supplies sensation to the middle portion of the forehead. The infratrochlear nerve exits a foramen below the trochlea and provides sensation to the medial upper eyelid, canthus, medial nasal skin, conjunctiva, and lacrimal apparatus (Figure 4.2).

When injecting this area, it is prudent to always use a free hand to palpate the orbital rim to prevent inadvertent

injection into the globe. To anesthetize this area, the supratrochlear nerve is measured 17 mm from the glabellar midline and 1–2 cc of 2% lidocaine 1:100,000 epinephrine is injected (Figure 4.3, left). The supraorbital nerve is blocked

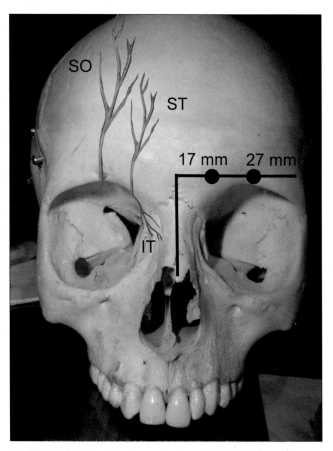

FIGURE 4.2: The supraorbital nerve (SO) exits about 27 mm from the glabellar midline, and the supratrochlear nerve (ST) is located approximately 17 mm from the glabellar midline. The infratrochlear nerve (IT) exits below the trochlea.

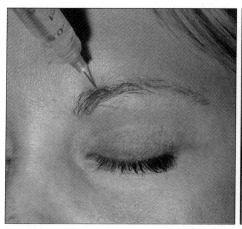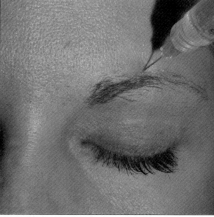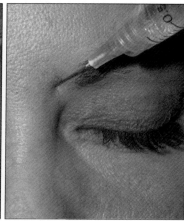

FIGURE 4.3: *The forehead and scalp are blocked by a series of injections from the central to the medial brow.*

by palpating the notch (and/or measuring 27 mm from the glabellar midline) and injecting 2 cc of local anesthetic solution (Figure 4.3, center). The infratrochlear nerve is blocked by injecting 1–2 cc of local anesthetic solution at the junction of the orbit and the nasal bones (Figure 4.3, right). In reality, one can block all three of these nerves simply by injecting 2–4 cc of local anesthetic solution from the central brow proceeding to the medial brow. Figure 4.4 shows the regions anesthetized from the preceding blocks.

The most versatile block in the upper face is the infraorbital nerve block. The infraorbital nerve is a branch of the second division of the trigeminal nerve and supplies the unilateral lower eyelid, lateral nose, hemi upper lip, and medial cheek (Figure 4.5A). The block is achieved by depositing the local anesthetic solution at or about the infraorbital foramen. The block can be performed transcutaneously with a ½ inch, 32-gauge needle (my preferred technique; Figure 4.5B) or intraorally with a 1½ inch, 27-gauge needle (Figure 4.5C). The infraorbital foramen is located 5–8 mm below the infraorbital rim in the pupillary midline. By injecting 1–2 cc of 2% lidocaine with 1:100,000 epinephrine at or near the foramen, the entire hemi midface is anesthetized, obviating a bilateral block for the full lip.

MIDFACE LOCAL ANESTHETIC BLOCKS

Two often overlooked nerves in facial local anesthetic blocks are the zygomaticotemporal and zygomaticofacial nerves. These nerves represent terminal branches of the zygomatic nerve. The zygomaticotemporal nerve emerges through a foramen located on the anterior wall of the temporal fossa. This foramen is actually behind the lateral orbital rim posterior to the zygoma at the approximate level of the lateral canthus (Figure 4.6). The injection technique

involves sliding a 1½ inch needle behind the concave portion of the lateral orbital rim. It is suggested that one closely examine this area on a model skull prior to attempting this injection as it will make the technique simpler. To orient for this injection, the doctor needs to palpate the lateral

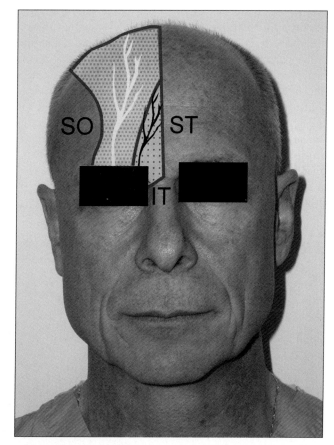

FIGURE 4.4: *The shaded areas indicate the anesthetized areas from SO, ST, and IT blocks.*

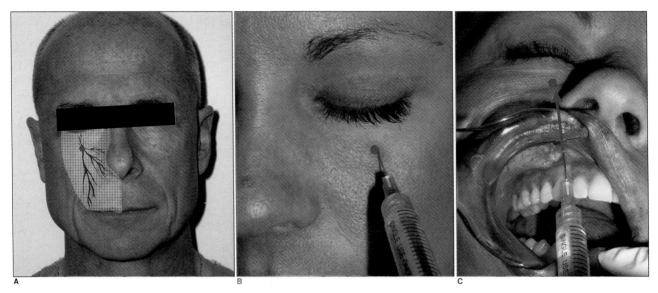

FIGURE 4.5: **A,** *The infraorbital nerve. The foramen is located 5–8 mm below the inferior orbital rim in the pupillary midline.* **B,** *Transcutaneous block with a* $^1/_2$ *inch, 32-gauge needle.* **C,** *Intraoral block with a* $1^1/_2$ *inch, 27-gauge needle.*

orbital rim at the level of the frontozygomatic suture (which is frequently palpable). With the index finger in the depression of the posterior lateral aspect of the lateral orbital rim (inferior and posterior to the frontozygomatic suture), the operator places the needle just behind the palpating finger (which is about 1 cm posterior to the frontozygomatic suture; Figure 4.6). The needle is then walked down the concave posterior wall of the lateral orbital rim to the approximate level of the lateral canthus. After aspirating, 1–2 cc of 2% lidocaine 1:100,000 epinephrine is injected in this area with a slight pumping action to ensure deposition of the local anesthetic solution at or about the foramen. Again, it is important to hug the back concave wall of the lateral orbital rim with the needle when injecting. Blocking the zygomaticotemporal nerve causes anesthesia in the area

superior to the nerve, including the lateral orbital rim and the skin of the temple, from above the zygomatic arch to the temporal fusion line (Figure 4.7).

The zygomaticofacial nerve exits through a foramen (or foramina in some patients) in the inferior lateral portion of the orbital rim at the zygoma. If the surgeon palpates the junction of the inferior lateral (the most southwest portion of the right orbit, if you will) portion of the lateral orbital rim, the nerve emerges several millimeters lateral to this point. By palpating this area and injecting just lateral to the finger, this nerve is successfully blocked with 1–2 cc of local anesthesia (Figure 4.8). Blocking this nerve will result in anesthesia of a triangular area from the lateral canthus and the malar region along the zygomatic arch and some skin inferior to this area (Figure 4.7).

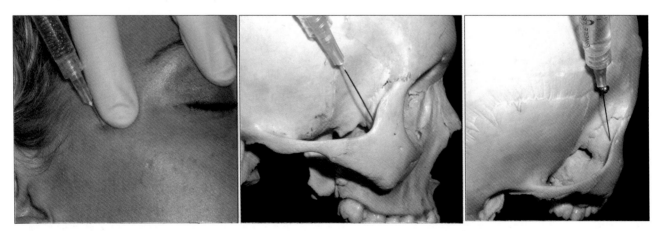

FIGURE 4.6: *The zygomaticotemporal nerve is blocked by placing the needle on the concave surface of the posterior lateral orbital rim.*

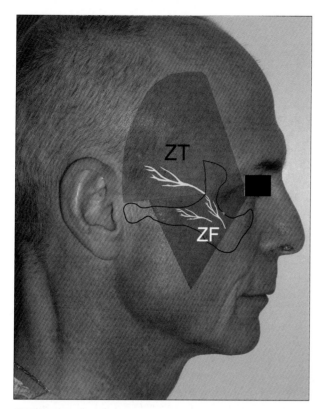

FIGURE 4.7: Zygomaticotemporal (ZT) and zygomaticofacial (ZF) nerve blocks.

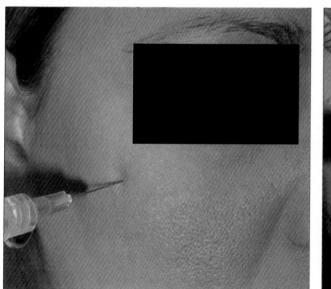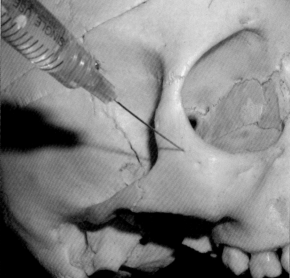

FIGURE 4.8: The ZF nerve(s) are blocked by injecting the inferior lateral portion of the orbital rim.

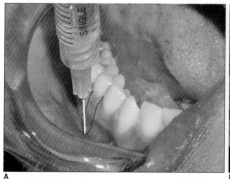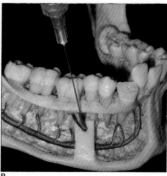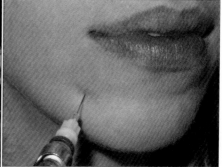

A   B   C

FIGURE 4.9: A, Mental nerve block through the intraoral route. B, The foramen located at the base of the second premolar. C, Transcutaneous route of injection.

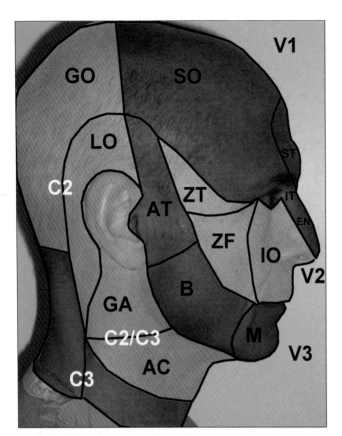

FIGURE 4.10: The major sensory dermatomes of the head and neck. AC = anterior cervical cutaneous colli; AT = auriculotemporal; B = buccal; EN = external (dorsal) nasal; GA = greater auricular; GO = greater occipital; IO = infraorbital; IT = infratrochlear; LO = lesser occipital; M = mental; SO = supraorbital; ST = supratrochlear; ZF = zygomaticofacial; ZT = zygomaticotemporal.

LOWER FACIAL BLOCKS

The central portion of the lower face is most easily blocked by performing bilateral mental nerve blocks. The mental nerve is a branch of the inferior alveolar nerve, which is a branch of the third division of the trigeminal nerve. Blocking this nerve will provide anesthesia of the hemi lower lip and a portion of the chin. This is an easily performed block to anesthetize the lower lip. This block can also be performed transcutaneously (Figure 4.9C) or intraorally (my preferred technique; Figure 4.9A). After mucosal topical anesthesia, a 1½ inch, 32-gauge needle is inserted through the sulcus to the base of the mandibular second premolar (Figure 4.9B); then, 1–2 cc of 2% lidocaine 1:100,000 epinephrine is injected at or about the mental foramen, which lies just below the lower second premolar. When choosing the local anesthetic block technique, bilateral infraorbital and mental blocks are performed (assuming both lips are to be treated). The surgeon has the option to use a lower percentage of local anesthetic or local without epinephrine to decrease the duration of the anesthesia.

In conclusion, the entire sensory apparatus of the face is supplied by the trigeminal nerve and several cervical branches. There exist many patterns of nerve distribution anomaly, cross-innervation, and individual patient variation; however, by following the basic techniques outlined in this chapter, the cosmetic surgeon should be able to achieve pain control of the major dermatomes of the head and neck. A basic dermatomal distribution is illustrated in Figure 4.10 and can serve as road map to local anesthesia of the head and neck.

CHAPTER 5

Topical Anesthesia

Mark Willoughby

The development of topical anesthetics began with the description of topical cocaine in the nineteenth century. However, it took many decades to develop safe, effective topical anesthetics. An ideal agent would provide rapid, complete anesthesia for a short period of time, while being free of local or systemic side effects. With the increasing number of laser and surgical skin procedures being developed and performed, the need for and use of topical anesthetics have grown steadily. More recent advances, including eutectic mixtures and liposomal membranes, have led to the availability of multiple effective local anesthetics.

PHARMACOLOGY, METABOLISM, AND ABSORPTION

Topical anesthetics comprise three main components: an aromatic ring, an intermediate ester or amide linkage, and a tertiary amine. The amide anesthetics have an amide linkage, whereas the ester anesthetics have an ester linkage between the intermediate chain and aromatic ring. The amide anesthetics are metabolized by microsomal enzymes in the liver, whereas ester anesthetics are primarily metabolized by plasma cholinesterase.

The sensation of pain relies on neural transmission. Electrical stimuli are transmitted along nerve fibers via an ionic gradient based on differential electrolyte concentrations between intracellular (low Na^+, high K^+) and extracellular (high Na^+, low K^+) fluid. Without stimuli, the outer membrane is positively charged relative to the intracellular environment due to the action of the Na^+/K^+ adenosine triphosphatase pump as well as the outer membrane's poor permeability to Na^+ ions. When the nerve is stimulated, Na^+ permeability of the outer membrane increases, allowing Na^+ ions to travel into the cell, causing depolarization. Depolarization causes a shift in electrical potential across the neural membrane, which is propagated down the nerve fiber as an action potential. Topical anesthetics inhibit depolarization of the nerve by inhibiting the influx of Na^+ ions. By inhibiting Na^+ influx, the threshold for nerve excitation increases, preventing the development of an action potential. This, in turn, prevents transmission of nerve impulses, providing cutaneous analgesia.

The stratum corneum is the rate-limiting step in delivery of topical anesthetic to underlying free dermal nerve endings, known as nociceptors. The stratum corneum contains both water and lipids. The lipids represent the main permeability barrier to the diffusion of all substances through the skin surface. These polar and nonpolar lipids are composed of ceramides, fatty acids, and cholesterol. The lipids are deposited in the interstitial spaces within the stratum corneum. The stratum also contains water. Due to this composition, the horny layer preferentially absorbs lipid-soluble molecules in an aqueous base.

Cutaneous absorption represents penetration of a drug or other substance into the skin. Percutaneous absorption refers to absorption through the skin into the blood. Ideally, a topical anesthetic would be absorbed into the dermis to act on nociceptors without diffusing into the blood.

TYPES OF TOPICAL ANESTHETICS

Topical anesthetics may be divided into two main categories: physical and chemical (Table 5.1). Two physical methods have been developed to enhance the absorption of topical anesthetics. Iontophoresis uses electric current, whereas phonophoresis uses sound waves to increase penetration and absorption of local anesthetics. These physical methods are not commonly employed in clinical practice. Various chemical methods have been developed to enhance absorption of anesthetic molecules. Pure anesthetic molecules usually exist as solids. The solids must be converted to a liquid form. Topically applied salts proved to be ineffective, whereas topical anesthetics dissolved in organic solvents (e.g., DMSO) had an unacceptable side effect profile. Other chemical methods, including eutectic mixtures and liposomal technology, have proven more successful. Eutectic compounds represent liquids that have a lower melting point than any of their individual

TABLE 5.1: Types of Chemical Topical Anesthetics

Physical
Iontophoresis (electric current)
Phonophoresis (sound waves)
Chemical
Eutectic mixtures
Liposomal membrane
Dissolve anesthetic in water
Dissolve anesthetic in alcoholic solvent

components, allowing higher concentration of anesthetic. Liposomes mimic lipid bilayers of cell membranes, allowing enhanced penetration of the stratum corneum. These methods will be discussed in more detail with the products that utilize the techniques.

PRODUCTS

Eutectic mixture of local anesthetics (EMLA) is the most widely used topical anesthetic. EMLA (AstraZeneca) is a eutectic of 2.5% lidocaine and 2.5% prilocaine. The active anesthetic ingredients are combined with an emulsifier, thickener, and distilled water. Euctectic mixtures are liquids that melt at temperatures lower than any of the individual components. They contain higher concentrations of the active ingredient than standard oil in water emulsions. The product was approved by the Food and Drug Administration (FDA) in 1993. EMLA has been shown to be effective for intact and diseased skin for a variety of clinical procedures, including superficial surgery, split-thickness skin grafts, removal of molluscum contagiosum and venereal lesions, painful ulcers, alleviation of pain when inserting a needle, pain induced by pulsed-dye and argon lasers, and removal of hair (lasers, wax, electrolysis).

On intact skin, the cream should be applied in a thick layer under occlusion for sixty to ninety minutes prior to clinical procedure. Dermal analgesia has been shown to increase with up to two hours of application and may increase further for fifteen to sixty minutes after removal of cream.

The most common side effects are redness and blanching at application sites due to vasoconstriction. As both lidocaine and prilocaine are amide anesthetics, topical contact hypersensitivity is rare but has been reported. Plasma concentrations may become elevated when EMLA is applied to diseased skin or mucous membranes. The reported levels were not high enough to cause systemic toxicity, but shorter application periods (five to thirty minutes) should be used in these areas. The most significant concern with use of EMLA is the development of methemoglobinemia, which is a known complication of prilocaine. Methemoglobinemia involves the oxidation of the hemoglobin molecule from the ferrous (Fe^{2+}) to ferric (Fe^{3+}) state, making it

unable to transport oxygen. Cyanosis appears at a level of 10%, while breathlessness occurs at 35%. Levels greater than 80% may result in death. A single case has been reported in a three-month-old after application of EMLA for five hours. As long as the package insert is followed, EMLA is safe to use in infants older than three months.

LMX (Ferndale Laboratories Inc.), previously named Elamax, contains 4% or 5% lidocaine in a liposomal delivery system. Both products are FDA approved. The 5% formulation is indicated for the temporary relief of anorectal pain, itching, and burning. LMX has been shown to be an effective anesthesia for lasers and medium-depth chemical peels. A liposomal delivery system utilizes lipid bilayers to facilitate penetration of skin and enhance delivery of anesthetic to the dermis. The liposomes also protect the lidocaine molecule from being degraded, prolonging the duration of action. The recommended application time is fifteen to sixty minutes, with no occlusion required. Local application site erythema, edema, and pruritus may occur; more serious adverse advents have not been reported.

Tetracaine 4% gel (Ametop, Smith-Nephew), previously known as amethacaine in the United Kingdom, has been reported to have a more rapid onset and longer duration compared to EMLA. The gel should be applied to intact, unbroken skin under occlusion for thirty to forty-five minutes. The contents expellable from a single tube (approximately 1 g) are sufficient to cover and anesthetize an area of up to 30 cm^2. The gel should not be used on mucous membranes. Analgesia is maintained for four to six hours, and longer application periods are unnecessary. The product has been shown to provide effective anesthesia for pulsed-dye laser treatment of port-wine stains and prior to venipuncture.

Allergic reactions to tetracaine and other ester anesthetics are relatively common. Ester hydrolysis results in the metabolite para-aminobenzoic acid (PABA), which may cause allergic reactions. Use of topical ester anesthetics is contraindicated in patients with allergies to hair dyes, PABA, and sulfonamides. The medication is contraindicated in patients with a known hypersensitivity to ester-type anesthetics as well as in premature infants and full-term infants less than one month old, in whom the tetracaine metabolic pathway may not be fully developed. Application site edema, erythema, and pruritus have been reported; more serious adverse events have not. The compound has not been FDA approved and can only be obtained from the manufacturer.

Betacaine-LA, formerly eutectic-LA, ointment contains lidocaine, prilocaine, and the vasoconstricting compound phenylephrine. Recommended application time is thirty to forty-five minutes, with no occlusion required. The concentrations of the ingredients have not been revealed by the manufacturer. EMLA and LMX were both found to be more effective than Betacaine-LA thirty minutes after removing the compound following a sixty-minute

TABLE 5.2: Topical Anesthetics

	Ingredients	Vehicle	Application Time (min)	FDA	Complications	Max Adult Dose
Betacaine-LA	lidocaine, prilocaine, dibucaine	petroleum jelly	30–45	no	see FDA warning letter discussion	300 cm^2
LMX	4% lidocaine	liposomal	60	yes	local	600 cm^2
LMX 5%	5% lidocaine	liposomal	30	yes	local	600 cm^2
EMLA	2.5% lidocaine, 2.5% prilocaine	eutectic mixture	60–90[a]	yes	methemoglobinemia	20 g per 200 cm^2
Tetracaine gel	4% tetracaine	gel	30–45[a]	no	ester anesthetic	not established
Topicaine gel	4% lidocaine	microemulsion	30–60	yes	local	600 cm^2
Pliaglis	7% tetracaine	7% lidocaine, eutectic mixture	30–60	yes	ester anesthetic	not available

[a] Under occlusion.

application. In December 2006, the FDA recommended that Betacaine-LA and several other unapproved compounded topical anesthetics no longer be manufactured (see the section on unapproved compounded anesthetics).

Topicaine (Esba Laboratories Inc.) is 4% lidocaine in a gel microemulsion drug delivery system. Recommended application time is thirty to sixty minutes under occlusion. Topicaine is FDA approved for the temporary relief of pain and itching in normal, intact skin and is available without a prescription. Adverse events have been limited to localized application site erythema, blanching, and edema.

Pliaglis (Zars Inc.), previously named S-Caine Peel, is a eutectic mixture of 7% lidocaine and 7% tetracaine. The product is a cream that is applied for thirty to sixty minutes and forms a pliable peel on the skin when exposed to air. It is removed as a flexible membrane after it dries. Pliaglis has been shown to provide adequate anesthesia for pulsed-dye, long-pulsed Nd:YAG, Q-switched Nd:YAG, and diode lasers. The unique eutectic mixture avoids the need for occlusion and reduces application times. Table 5.2 contains a summary of this and the preceding products.

UNAPPROVED PHARMACY COMPOUNDED TOPICAL ANESTHETICS

In December 2006, the FDA sent letters to five firms asking them to stop compounding and distributing various topical anesthetic compounds. Products cited included Lasergel (10% lidocaine, 10% tetracaine), Lasergel Plus 10/10 (10% lidocaine, 10% tetracaine, 0.5% phenylephrine), Photocaine gel (lidocaine, tetracaine), Betacaine-LA ointment (lidocaine, prilocaine, and phenylephrine),

Betacaine Plus ointment, Anesthetic Skin Lotion (10% lidocaine and 2% prilocaine), Tetracaine 6% in DMSO gel, Triple Kwick Anesthetic Gel (benzocaine, lidocaine, and tetracaine), NEW topical anesthetic (30% lidocaine, 2% prilocaine, 4% tetracaine), Kwick Anesthetic Gel (benzocaine, lidocaine, tetracaine, and DMSO), Lidocaine and Tetracaine Demi Gel, Anesthetic Skin Gel 3+ (lidocaine, prilocaine, and tetracaine), and Extra Strength Triple Anesthetic Cream (20% benzocaine, 6% lidocaine, 4% tetracaine).

The agency is concerned with the public health risks associated with the compounding and sale of products that contain high doses of lidocaine and/or tetracaine. There have been at least two nonfatal reactions and two deaths attributed to the use of compounded topical local anesthetic creams containing high doses of local anesthetics. Local anesthetics may be toxic at high doses, and this toxicity can be additive. Furthermore, there is a narrow difference between the optimal therapeutic dose of these products and the doses at which they become toxic (low therapeutic index).

Adverse events consistent with high systemic exposures to these products include seizures and cardiac arrhythmias. Specifically, risks of systemic adverse events from tetracaine products include (1) a systemic allergic response to PABA, which, at worst, could lead to cardiac arrest, and (2) excessive systemic absorption following repetitive or extensive application, especially for 4% and 6% tetracaine products, which could ultimately lead to convulsions. Tetracaine is associated with a higher incidence of allergic reactions than other anesthetics such as lidocaine. The risk of systemic toxicity is greatest in small children and in patients with preexisting heart disease. Factors that may increase systemic exposure are time and surface area of exposure, particularly when the area of application is covered by an occlusive dressing. Benzocaine and prilocaine have an additional toxicity not seen with lidocaine. This toxicity, which is called *methemoglobinemia*, is an acquired disease in the oxygen-carrying capacity of the red blood cells. Furthermore, patients with severe hepatic disease are at greater risk of developing toxic plasma concentrations of local anesthetics because of their inability to metabolize them.

CONCLUSION

This chapter reviewed the several topical anesthetics available for dermatologic use. The anesthetic compounds and delivery methods vary, leading to a wide range of potential side effects and toxicities. Knowledge of the pharmacologic properties of these agents, methods of application, and potential adverse events is important to the practicing cosmetic surgeon to maximize results and safety. The use of liposomes and eutectic mixtures has led to the development of several effective agents and a promising future for topical anesthesia.

SUGGESTED READING

Bryan HA, Alster TS. The S-Caine Peel: a novel topical anesthetic for cutaneous laser surgery. *Dermatol. Surg.* 2002;28:999–1003.

Bucalo BD, Mirikitani EJ, Moy RL. Comparison of skin anesthetic effect of liposomal lidocaine, nonliposomal lidocaine and EMLA using 30-minute application time. *Dermatol. Surg.* 1998;24:537–41.

Chen BK, Eichenfield LF. Pediatric anesthesia in dermatologic surgery: when hand-holding is not enough. *Dermatol. Surg.* 2001;27:1010–18.

Chen JZ, Alexiades-Armenakas MR, Bernstein LJ, Jacobsen LG, Friedman PM, Geronemus RG. Two randomized, double-blind, placebo-controlled studies evaluating the S-Caine peel for induction of local anesthesia before long pulsed Nd:YAG laser therapy for leg veins. *Dermatol. Surg.* 2003;29:1012–18.

Friedman PM, Fogelman JP, Nouri K, Levine VJ, Ashinoff R. Comparative study of the efficacy of four topical anesthetics. *Dermatol. Surg.* 1999;25:950–4.

Friedman PM, Mafong EA, Friedman ES, Geronemus RG. Topical anesthetic update: EMLA and beyond. *Dermatol. Surg.* 2001;27:1019–26.

Huang W, Vidimos A. Topical anesthetics in dermatology. *J. Am. Acad. Dermatol.* 2000;43:286–98.

Jih MH, Friedman PM, Sadick N, Marquez DK, Kimyai-Asadi A, Goldberg LH. 60-minute application of S-Caine Peel prior to 1,064 nm long-pulsed Nd:YAG laser treatment of leg veins. *Lasers Surg. Med.* 2004;34:446–50.

Juhlin L, Evers H. EMLA: a new topical anesthetic. *Adv. Dermatol.* 1990;5:75–92.

Koay J, Orengo I. Application of local anesthetics in dermatologic surgery. *Dermatol. Surg.* 2002;28:143–8.

Lener EV, Bucalo BD, Kist DA, Moy RL. Topical anesthetic agents in dermatologic surgery. *Dermatol. Surg.* 1997;23:673–83.

Lycka BA. EMLA: a new and effective topical anesthetic. *Dermatol. Surg.* 1992;18:859–62.

PART THREE

FILLERS
AND
NEUROTOXINS

INTRODUCTION

CHAPTER 6

Fillers: Past, Present, and Future

Eric Williams

David J. Kouba

Ronald L. Moy

Aside from the advances made in laser and light-based technologies, no other subset of dermatology has expanded or advanced in the past two decades as much or as quickly as the field of tissue fillers. As we will discuss in this chapter, early products used were rudimentary, often allergenic, and cosmetically inferior when compared to the products that are available in the U.S. and European markets now as well as those in late-stage development at the time this chapter was written. In fact, advances in hypoallergenicity; stability though cross-linking; and newer, more biocompatible filling agents are coming through the pipeline so quickly that the reader may see only a brief lag after reading this chapter to a time when agents covered in our "Future Directions" section become available in certain global aesthetic markets.

In the following discussion, we will first provide a historical backdrop for the development of early filling agents, their uses, benefits, and drawbacks. We feel it is important for current practitioners who may not have used earlier products to know how the field has evolved. This becomes quite important when we see, like many fashions, that trends in tissue filling agents come and go, and some become reborn again in the future because of advances in science that eliminate certain side effects or drawbacks to a particular product. We will then discuss the wide range of products currently available both in the U.S. and in global markets – which frequently are more expansive than in the U.S. system, controlled by the Food and Drug Administration (FDA). We have divided this main discussion between those fillers that are permanent and those that degrade in vivo, resulting in a transient cosmetic result.

Finally, we will discuss some of the very exciting science behind future developments that are early in the pipeline and that may someday become a reality. These products are being designed to harness the body's own ability to create the tissue substances lost with natural aging as well as in pathologic processes that result in atrophy or dermal or subcutaneous structures.

HISTORICAL OVERVIEW

Physicians have been working to perfect the science of injectable fillers since the late nineteenth century, when Neuber first used transplanted fat from the arm to fill depressed facial scars. Shortly thereafter, in 1899, Gersuny injected paraffin into the scrotum of a patient as a prosthesis for a testicle that had been lost as a complication of tuberculosis. In the years subsequent to this, physicians started noticing undesirable granulomatous inflammatory reactions (paraffinomas) resulting from the injection of paraffin. By the end of the 1920s, the injection of paraffin decreased significantly.

The development of new fillers then slowed until the mid-1930s, when Dr. J. F. Hyde of Dow Corning Corporation began his research into silicone and silicone rubber. The first use of liquid silicone as a cosmetic filler was reported by Uchida in 1961, when he documented his experience using silicone for the cosmetic treatment of pectus excavatum, muscle atrophy, and also breast and cheek augmentation. Unfortunately, silicone was also noted to produce foreign body granulomas and occasionally to migrate away from the site of injection, especially when larger amounts were injected. These drawbacks, combined with its near impossibility of removal and the absolute permanence of silicone have made injection of this material less popular until recently. Now, the use of the microdroplet technique, by which small microdroplets are injected over many visits, and the FDA approval of silicone for ophthalmologic uses has increased the acceptance of this filler material.

While some continue to use silicone precisely because it is permanent, others shy away from silicone and instead opt for the less permanent materials that have since emerged. These materials have an easier learning curve, and minor mistakes in injection volume and placement are only temporary. The first temporary injectable filler was collagen, which first became popular in 1977 with the introduction of a bovine collagen preparation (Zyderm I). While bovine collagen had a natural feel and lacked the problems associated with the permanence of silicone, allergenicity and reports of skin necrosis when injected into the glabella, and rapid dissolution within tissue, were clearly drawbacks to its continued presence in the market. The array of injectable collagens has continued to widen with the introduction of cadaveric and allogenic collagens (Cosmoderm, Cosmoplast), which do not require allergy testing prior to injection. More recently developed fillers include the hyaluronic acids, first available in the mid-1990s, and newer, more biocompatible semipermanent and permanent fillers, including calcium hydroxyapatite, polymethylmethacrylate, and poly-L-lactic acid.

CURRENT FILLERS

The vast array of available fillers can appear daunting. Fillers currently FDA approved for use inside the United States are listed in Table 6.1, and the much broader array of products available on the world market are categorized in Table 6.2. In this portion of the chapter, we will discuss the so-called ideal filler, investigate some of the current filling materials available, and draw some useful distinctions between broad categories of products. The discussion will separate the available filling materials based on permanence: temporary fillers, lasting a few months; semipermanent fillers, lasting a year or longer; and those products with a permanent effect. The sheer volume of available filling products makes discussion of all individual products infeasible, and thus the discussion will focus on these three broad categories and the subdivisions of products within them. The individual fillers and techniques necessary to correctly use them will receive greater coverage in the subsequent chapters of this book.

TABLE 6.1: FDA-Approved Fillers and Fillers Not Requiring FDA Approval for Use within the United States

Type	Composition	Available Forms
Collagen	bovine	Zyderm I
		Zyderm II
		Zyplast
	human	Cosmoderm I
		Cosmoplast
		Dermologen
		Isologen
Acellular dermal matrix	human	Cymetra
		Autologen
Hyaluronic acid	rooster comb	Hylaform
	bacterial	Captique
		Restylane
		Restylane Fine Lines
		Perlane
		Juvéderm Ultra
		Juvéderm Ultra Plus
Semipermanent	calcium hydroxyapatite	Radiesse
	autologous fat	
	poly-L-lactic acid	Sculptra
Permanent	bovine collagen with lidocaine and polymethyl-methacrylate beads	ArteFill
	silicone	Adatosil 5000
		Silikon 1000

The ideal filler for all applications does not yet, and, in fact, may never, exist. The ideal filler would require only a single treatment and be permanent but easily reversible or removable, if desired. It would be inexpensive, highly elastic, easily stored for long periods of time, and easy to inject. The ideal filler would be suitable for all patients because it would be nonallergenic and noninflammatory. While many available fillers are painful to inject, and may cause bruising, the ideal filler would not have these qualities. The ideal filler would not migrate away from the site of injection, would not form beads or cysts, and would not cause necrosis of tissues. Moreover, the ideal filler would be different for different locations, applications, and patients. The practitioner would most likely desire a low-viscosity filler that is easy to inject through a very fine needle for the fine lines of the glabella, periorbital area, and perioral areas. For lip augmentation, the deeper lines of the melolabial fold and marionette lines, a more viscous material that would provide some volume correction as well as wrinkle reduction, but would not migrate away from the injection

TABLE 6.2: Fillers Available Worldwide

Collagens	Hyaluronic Acids	Semipermanent	Permanent
Atelocollagen	Ac-Hyal	Bioinblue DeepBlue	Adatosil 5000
Autologen	Belotero Soft, Basic	Bioinblue Lips	Amazing Gel
Cosmoderm 1, 2	Captique	Fibroquel	Argiform
Cosmoplast	Esthelis		Aquamid
CosmetaLife	Hyacell	Laresse	ArteFill
Cymetra	Hyal 2000 Injection	Matridur	Artecoll
Dermicol	Hyal-System	Matridex	Arteplast
Dermalogen	Hyaluderm	Profill	Bio-Alcamid
Endoplast	Hydrafill Grade 1, 2, 3	Radiesse	Biocell Ultravital
Evolence	Hydrafill Softline	Reviderm	Bioformacryl
Fibrel	Hydrafill Softline Max	Sculptra	Bioplastique
Isolagen	Hylaform Fine Lines		Coaptitie
Koken	Hylaform		DermaCellagen
Permacol Injection	Hylaform Plus		DermaLive
Resoplast	Isogel 1, 2, 3		DermaDeep
Rofilan	Juvéderm 18, 24, 30		Evolution
Zyderm I, II	Juvelift Corneal		Formacryl
Zyplast	Mac Dermol		Kopolymer
	Macrolane		Med
	Matridur		MetaCril
	Matridex		Metrex
	Puragen		Novasoft
	Restylane		Outline
	Restylane Perlane		PMS 350
	Restylane SubQ		Profill
	Restylane Touch		Rhegecoll
	Reviderm Intra		Silicone 1000
	Rofilan		Surgisis
	Surgiderm 18, 30		Surgisis ES
	Surgiderm 24, 30XP		
	Surgilips		
	Surgilift Plus		
	Teosyal 27 g, 30 g		
	Teosyal Meso, Kiss		
	Varioderm		
	Viscontour		
	Visagel		
	Zetavisc L		
	Voluma Corneal		

site, would be ideal. For the filling of large defects from the loss of facial soft tissue related to age, muscle atrophy from neurological disease, and advanced HIV, a very viscous material that allows a greater deal of volume correction and sculpting, and thus not suitable for use in other areas, would likely be most advantageous. Scientists and physicians are diligently researching new technologies as well as variations on existing technologies in the hope of finding this ideal filler, and the area will likely continue to progress exponentially in coming years.

Collagen products are the original temporary filler. While it may seem undesirable for a filler to be temporary, it is not necessarily so. Consider what would be the ramifications of a patient who decides that he or she feels or looks "overfilled" after treatment with a permanent filler.

As an analogy, consider the trend of patients receiving lip liner tattoos in the early 1990s – now that this fashion is passé, many of these patients are very unhappy. Current fashion for the degree of soft tissue correction or augmentation may also change, and surgical removal of implanted permanent fillers can be extraordinarily difficult. The collagen injectables currently available include bovine-derived (Zyderm/Zyplast), porcine-derived (Evolence), and human collagen (Cosmoderm/Cosmoplast) products that also may be either cadaveric (Dermologen/Cymetra/Fascian) or autologously (Isologen) derived. The bovine products require skin testing to help reduce the incidence of allergic reactions to the filler material, but porcine-derived materials are thought to be nonallergenic because of the close homology between porcine and human collagen. The human-derived products are suitable for those allergic to bovine collagen or those who desire to have treatment performed without delay, but have no additional benefit. The main downside for collagen products is that they provide little or no volume restoration and are best used for the treatment of finer lines, and their effect may last as little as two to three months. One product whose duration of effect is not clear is Isologen, which is composed of the patient's own extracellular matrix, cultured from a punch biopsy of the patient's skin. Unfortunately, the multistep process involved in harvesting the skin from the patient, growing and purifying the extracellular matrix, and then injection makes this product somewhat cumbersome to use.

Hyaluronic acid is a naturally occurring, protein-free, glycosaminoglycan composed of thousands of repeating glucuronic acid/N-acetylglucosamine dimers. It is a major binder of water in normal human dermis, able to bind up to a thousand times its weight in water, and is identical in all species, unlike collagens. Current hyaluronic acid products are derived from the rooster comb or recombinant streptococcal sources. There are rare reports of hypersensitivity reactions and angioedema to specific hyaluronic acid products, but manufacturers still do not recommend allergy testing. Hyaluronic acid is colorless and thus will usually not cause discoloration of tissues, even with superficial injection. Unmodified hyaluronic acid is rapidly cleared from the body by the action of the ubiquitous hyaluronidases. To slow the action of hyaluronidases, manufacturers have developed multiple different ways of joining, or cross-linking, hyaluronic acids. This slows the action of the hyaluronidases and leads to prolongation of clinical effect. The other consequence of cross-linking hyaluronic acid products is an increase in the viscosity of the material. As was discussed earlier, a more viscous material is desirable when volumetric correction is desired but makes superficial injection, and thus the correction of fine rhytids, more difficult. Variation in the size of particles also influences the usefulness and ease of use of hyaluronic acids, with smaller particle sizes (and higher concentrations) being more useful for the treatment of fine lines through fine needles. For the treatment of deeper rhytids, and for volumetric correction, a larger particle is more desirable as it is more likely to stay where injected when used in higher volumes, and fine control over injected volume is unnecessary. Such sites include the nasojugular groove, and filling this area involves the placement of small droplets at the bone level to gain volume of this tear-trough deformity.

Newer fillers with a longer duration of effect than collagen and hyaluronic acid have recently become available. Many of these permanent and semipermanent fillers rely on a nondegradable or slowly degradable compound suspended in a carrier vehicle that can either be water, gel, or collagen based. Some of these preparations also include lidocaine in the formulation to ameliorate the pain associated with injection. Treatment with these materials requires an experienced hand as incorrect placement or overcorrection will last for much longer and be difficult to reverse.

Poly-L-lactic acid (New-Fill or Sculptra) is a semipermanent filler currently approved by the FDA only for the treatment of HIV-associated facial lipoatrophy but is approved in Europe for the treatment of rhytids. This type of material is not new to dermasurgeons as commonly used absorbable sutures, such as Vicryl (Ethicon Inc.) and Dexon (Syneture Corp.) are made of the same material. Because the material works by inciting a delayed inflammatory reaction, and because it is difficult to inject, requiring a larger-caliber needle, poly-L-lactic acid is unsuitable for intradermal injection. In fact, the most common side effect, nodule formation, frequently occurs when the material is injected too superficially in the dermis or is unevenly distributed. Instead, the material is injected at the deepest dermis, or better, in the subcutaneous layer to stimulate skin thickening, thereby affecting both volume and correction of rhytids. We prefer to perform cheek augmentation not with the traditional multiple puncture transcutaneous approach, but rather, with a single entry per cheek at the oral commissure, using a long, 22-gauge needle, repeatedly fanning out within the subcutaneous plane to fill all areas of the midface, a technique that closely mimics fat injection.

Radiesse is a semipermanent filler composed of calcium hydroxyapatite particles suspended in a gel mixture of cellulose, glycerin, and water. The filler was approved by the FDA in January 2006 for the treatment of moderate to severe rhytids but previously had been used extensively off-label in the United States as well as outside the United States. The particles are thought to remain in place after injection and act as a scaffold for the ingrowth of recipient fibroblasts and the production of native collagen. The implant remains soft and flexible, even though it is composed of the same material found in bone. Furthermore, the expected longevity of this product is greater than twelve months, making it a good alternative to hyaluronic acid for patients who want longer-lasting effects. A potential downside of this compound is that it is radioopaque and thus makes X-ray imaging of underlying structures difficult or impossible to interpret. Furthermore, if the injections are too superficial, the implant will be visible and result in a palpable nodularity. It is inappropriate for use in lip augmentation.

Aquamid is a permanent filler composed of cross-linked polyacrylamide polymer in a water vehicle. While it is not approved by the FDA as of the time this chapter was written, it is approved for use in many countries outside the United States for the treatment of deep rhytids. It is easy to inject, and like the semipermanent fillers previously discussed, it is designed to be used in the subcutis. One potential downside of Aquamid and other polyacrylamide fillers is that there is an increased risk of infection surrounding the implant, even years after injection. Of a recent survey of 251 patients treated with Aquamid, there were no long-term adverse events, and the product showed stability of effect even at twelve-month evaluation.

Highly purified medical grade silicone is a permanent filler used extensively for cosmetic purposes outside the United States and off-label by many U.S. practitioners. The early formulations of silicone were more prone to creating unattractive foreign body reactions due to contaminants like olive oil and through the use of large volumes of injection. Today, these complications are avoided through using small volumes of highly purified silicone, which is injected over multiple treatment sessions.

ArteFill (the successor to Artecoll) is a permanent filler composed of polymethylmethacrylate beads suspended in a bovine collagen and lidocaine carrier. It is used worldwide for the treatment of nasolabial folds but requires pretreatment allergy testing to decrease the risk of reaction to the bovine collagen carrier vehicle. In the United States, a multicenter study comparing ArteFill to bovine collagen found superior efficacy to collagen at six months, with sustained efficacy at twelve months. In analyzing adverse event data at five years after injection, 2.2% of patients had adverse lumpiness, rated as mild, and one patient had severe nodularity (0.7%). Because the parent company has recently filed for bankruptcy, the future of ArteFill is uncertain.

Bio-Alcamid is a permanent filler that contains polymeric polyalkylimide gel in water. It is classified as an endoprosthesis because it becomes encapsulated in host collagen shortly after injection. The implant can be surgically removed at any time. The encapsulation is thought to decrease migration of the material but could also make removal of this material more difficult with time. It is approved for use in Europe but is not yet FDA approved. A recent case series of eighteen adverse events demonstrated a delayed infection in ten patients that was triggered by unrelated medical procedures that were performed in the vicinity of the implant. These reports underscore the importance of strict aseptic technique when injecting this product and of warning patients about the risk of delayed infection.

Fat is a very convenient agent for semipermanent to permanent filling because of its ubiquity. Every patient who desires some volume correction will have adequate stores of autologous fat, which can be easily harvested and minimally processed in preparation for injection. Fat will tend to last longer in areas with limited movement, like the buccal area, as opposed to areas like the lips, which are involved in frequent motion. Studies in the literature, largely uncontrolled reports, all show extreme variability in the longevity of autologously transplanted fat. Many clinicians find the percentage of patients who get a long-term, viable correction to be low; in our experience, the figure is somewhere in the range of 50% after three treatments. Other cosmetic surgeons report a higher percentage of patients with excellent results.

FUTURE DIRECTIONS

New discoveries are rapidly occurring within the science of fillers, and much of them are coming from the orthopedic and plastic surgical fields. Because these products are potentially huge sources of income for the companies that successfully bring them to market, it is understandable that most of the developments in this field will not see publication until late in their testing, many years after they have been developed. With that in mind, several emerging technologies appear quite promising.

As is evident from Tables 6.1 and 6.2, the number of companies creating filling substances and the sheer number of worldwide injectable fillers are daunting. New technologies are always on the horizon. At the benchtop, some interesting discoveries in filling substances are pushing the envelope of routine fillers. A group from the Middle East (Uysal et al. 2006) has used fibrin glue to fashion harvested porcine hair into soft tissue implants. This kind of innovative thinking may provide some of tomorrow's more creative aesthetic augmentation products.

Practitioners in the area of aesthetic correction have globally recognized the importance of treating age-related lipoatrophy. Therefore improvements in techniques to augment subcutaneous tissue are of paramount importance. If fat transfer had any reliability in terms of longevity, it likely would expand into a much more widely embraced corrective modality. Recent research from University of Wisconsin scientists (Piasecki et al. 2007) has attempted to optimize cell viability after harvesting fat grafts. The researchers have found that applying a regimen of collagenase digestion followed by centrifugation and washing of harvested adipocytes optimized cell viability upward of 90%. While this research is exciting from the standpoint of improving initial adipocyte loss, it does not address the issue of improving the long-term integration of living adipocytes to the donor site.

There has been significant controversy in the literature regarding the longevity of autologously transplanted fat if used fresh from harvest or after being frozen. This question was recently approached by a group from California (Butterwick et al. 2006) studying aesthetic improvement in a side-by-side comparison of fresh versus prefrozen autologously transplanted fat to the dorsal hand. This group found significant superiority in the prefrozen fat side. Could it be that this simple modification may improve the longevity of fat grafts? Another, more sophisticated approach to improving subcutaneous tissue would be to induce the body to create new fat cells.

Some very exciting research from biologists in Sweden (Huss et al. 2007) was performed by using gelatinous, porous microspheres injected into soft tissues. Interestingly, the microspheres had been preseeded by cultured pre-adipocytes or fibroblasts. The greatest volume correction occurred with the microspheres seeded with preadipocytes or fibroblasts and was associated with neoangiogenesis. This concept of regrowing new adipocytes or matrix-producing fibroblasts is an exciting one in biofiller science. While this research was successful, it was performed in mice, and translation to humans may be difficult. The main obstacle to overcome likely will be having to use a system similar to that used in the creation of Isologen, in which preadipocytes and fibroblasts would have to be harvested from each patient and then reinjected back into the patient to prevent disease transmission from random tissue donors.

SUGGESTED READING

Andre P, Lowe NJ, Parc A, Clerici TH, Zimmermann U. Adverse reactions to dermal fillers: a review of European experiences. *J. Cosmet. Laser Ther.* 2005;7:171–6.

Broder KW, Cohen SR. An overview of permanent and semipermanent fillers. *Plast. Reconstr. Surg.* 2006;118(3 Suppl):7S–14S.

Butterwick KJ, Bevin AA, Iyer S. Fat transplantation using fresh versus frozen fat: a side-by-side two-hand comparison pilot study. *Dermatol. Surg.* 2006;32:640–4.

Eppley BL, Dadvand B. Injectable soft-tissue fillers: clinical overview. *Plast. Reconstr. Surg.* 2006;118:98e–106e.

Humble G, Mest D. Soft tissue augmentation using silicone: an historical review. *Facial Plast. Surg.* 2004;20:181–4.

Huss FR, Junker JP, Johnson H, Kratz G. Macroporous gelatine spheres as culture substrate, transplantation vehicle, and biodegradable scaffold for guided regeneration of soft tissues. In vivo study in nude mice. *J. Plast. Reconstr. Aesthetic Surg.* 2007;60:543–55.

Piasecki JH, Gutowski KA, Lahvis GP, Moreno KI. An experimental model for improving fat graft viability and purity. *Plast. Reconstr. Surg.* 2007;119:1571–83.

Uysal A, Ulusoy MG, Sungur N, et al. Combined use of hair and fibrin glue for soft tissue augmentation: experimental study. *Aesthetic Plast. Surg.* 2006;30:469–73.

CHAPTER 7

Hyaluronic Acid Fillers: How Structure Affects Function

Johannes Reinmüller

HISTORY OF DERMAL FILLERS

Soft tissue augmentation is an important tool in present-day cosmetic treatment. First attempts at soft tissue augmentation were made early in the last century with more or less inappropriate material, such as wax, but became more effective and frequent due to the invention of silicone oil by Eugene G. Rochow in 1940. In the 1950s and 1960s, silicone oil was used for various indications, including breast augmentation, body shaping, and wrinkle treatment of the face. This synthetic material showed some intriguing features, such as ease of application and longevity of results, but in the long term, it turned out to be hazardous because of migration, fat tissue damage, granuloma formation, and ulcerations. In the 1970s, purified bovine collagen was available for wrinkle treatment of the face; this marked a change in paradigm from the use of technical products to biological preparations. Collagen was effective and easy to administer, but its duration in the skin was limited to several months, and there was a risk of allergic reaction. Therefore pretesting was mandatory prior to treatment. Nevertheless, collagen remained the most commonly used filler for the treatment of wrinkles of the face for more than twenty years. Finally, early in the 1990s, collagen was replaced as a dermal filler by derivatives of hyaluronic acid (HA). Since then, there has been parallel development of new so-called permanent and semipermanent filler materials, but the use of permanent filler materials still raises the same problems and issues known from past use (and, in some cases, present use) of silicone.

HISTORY OF HA-BASED BIOMATERIALS

HA was first isolated and purified by Karl Meyer and John Palmer in 1934 from the bovine vitreous body. In 1964, T.C. Laurent described the first cross-linking of HA by Bis-epoxid as a cross-linking agent. Andre Balazs was successful in isolating a highly purified, high-molecular-weight HA from the rooster's comb for medical use, which was primarily introduced in ophthalmic surgery as a

substitute for the vitreous body and, later, as a lubricant in cataract surgery to facilitate the insertion of artificial lenses. The use of HA in medicine has increased steeply since 1980. To protect the water-soluble native HA from biodegradation, Balazs stabilized native HA by a cross-linking procedure, using divinylsulfone (DVS) as a cross-linking agent, and originated a water-insoluble gel, or hydrogel. Because of increased elasticity from the cross-linking process, this hydrogel had to be crushed into small pieces to be injected through a needle into arthritic joints for pain relief and lubrication. The preparation is known as Hylan G-F 20, and the corresponding remedy was introduced to medicine in Europe around 1990. At that time, and parallel to a clinical study carried out in Germany, the first attempts were made to substitute Hylan B for collagen in the treatment of wrinkles, and first results were reported in 1992. Meanwhile, a variety of different preparations of cross-linked HA were available for cosmetic treatment, which differed by source of the HA (avian or bacterial), applied cross-linking agent, cross-linking procedure, and hydrogel properties (particulated or nonparticulated). A chronicle of developments is given in Table 7.1.

BIOCHEMISTRY

HA is, like collagen, a biomolecule. It is a main component of the connective tissue of all vertebrates and is found in some bacterial strains. Unlike collagen, HA has a chemically identical structure throughout the entire biology, which is why its structure is independent from its source of isolation. The total contents of HA in a human body of an average weight of 70 kg is about 15 g. More than 30% of it is in the dermis. HA is an unbranched chain molecule of high thermal stability composed of multiple disaccharide units consisting of N-acetyl-glucosamine and glucoronic acid linked with a beta-glycosidic junction and molecular weight (MW) reaching 10 million Da. Short chains with low MW and long chains with high MW have different functions in the bioorganism. Unique features of HA are

TABLE 7.1: Historical Perspective of Hyaluronic Acid Products

Generation	Trademark	Source	Cross Linker	Technique	State	Start
GO	Healon	rooster's comb	no		solution	1966
GO	Synvisc	rooster's comb	divinylsulfon	single	particles	1988
GI	Hylaform	rooster's comb	divinylsulfon	single	particles	1990
G2	Restylane	streptococcus	BDDE	single	particles	1994
G3	Puragen	streptococcus	DEO	double	particles	2001
G4	Belotero	streptococcus	BDDE	CPM	polydense matrix	2004

the extremely high water-binding capacity and the biosynthesis at the cell surface without linkage to a protein, which contributes to purity when HA is isolated from various biological sources. For HA-based fillers, the material is isolated either from avian or from streptococcal sources. With respect to biocompatibility, it should be noted that growth of streptococci needs animal substrata. Therefore the production of HA from streptococci is, in fact, not a nonanimal procedure, except for transgenic bacterial species.

BIODEGRADATION OF HA

Native HA injected in the human organism is rapidly degraded, depending on the injection site. Half-life in the dermis is about twenty-four hours. The degradation needs specific enzymes, hyaluronidases, which are membrane-bound at the cell surface or in the lysosomes inside the cell. Knowledge of the cleaving of the HA chain is mostly derived from in vitro observation. Therefore we do not know with certainty the in vivo pathway of degradation, but the main route of biodegradation is presumably through binding to cell surfaces, engulfment by the cell membrane, internalization, and processing inside the cell (liver endothelial cells, macrophages) into various low-molecular end products. The same route of biodegradation can be hypothesized for the in vivo degradation of HA derivatives, especially the cross-linked species (XLHA). Whether looking at biphasic (particulated) or monophasic gels, degradation likely takes place at the interface of the implant with the macrophages. Since particles larger than 20 μm cannot be surrounded and engulfed by a single macrophage, histological sections of the HA particle degradation process also contain multinucleated giant cells.

BIOLOGICAL FUNCTIONS OF HA

In living organisms, HA has various functions. It contributes to the extracellular matrix (ECM), and in this function, it may act as a wrap for the fiber network, with excellent hydrating properties serving to preserve the native structure of collagen. Moreover, as there are specific HA binding receptors at the cell surface, HA is a signaling molecule, triggering or modulating cell functions. Furthermore, there are specific HA binding proteins that are able to bind to HA and, together with specific cell surface receptors, form a network in the different tissues by a kind of natural cross-linking. The simple cross-linking of HA by chemicals as it is used to generate hydrogels for cosmetic HA-based products is therefore already anticipated by nature but cannot really be compared with that complex natural process. The injection of a cosmetic HA-based dermal filler is neither a substitution of natural HA nor a replacement therapy. It is implantation of a HA-derived biomaterial. There is evidence that under certain circumstances, the injection of HA-based filler material can trigger new collagen formation and stimulate skin remodeling.

TYPES OF HA-BASED FILLERS

It is of great importance to discriminate preparations of non-cross-linked HA for medical use from preparations of filler material for aesthetic treatment. The latter are categorized as dermal implants, and that is, in fact, what they are.

HA-based fillers may consist of the following:

- precipitated unsoluble HA (no chemical cross-linking)
- chemically cross-linked and particulated HA (biphasic)
- chemically cross-linked, nonparticulated HA (monophasic)

Non-cross-linked material usually has a low viscosity and can easily pass through narrow needles. The first generations of cross-linked material and the double-cross-linked material were stiff hydrogels with a high viscosity. Such gels are not able to pass through a 30- or even 27-gauge, needle. Therefore they are crushed to smaller pieces and supplemented with native HA, which serves as a lubricant. Such a composition is called *biphasic* because two physical states of HA are combined: a solid state (the gel) and a liquid state (the solubilized HA and/or free water). The particle sizes of different preparations vary over a broad range, and

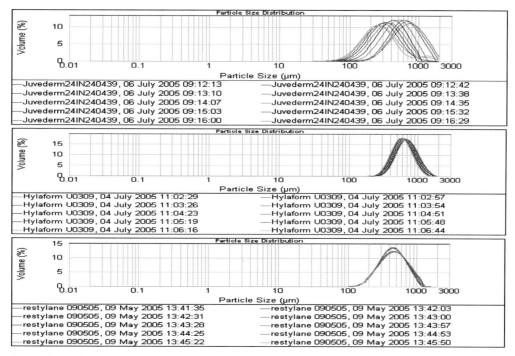

FIGURE 7.1: Gel particle diameter.

even in a single product, there is usually a broad distribution of particle sizes around the indicated mean diameter (Figure 7.1 and Table 7.2). As small particles are rapidly phagocytized or tend to migrate, partial loss of correction may occur. This may explain the need for so-called touch-up injections two weeks after initial treatment. Since adding neurotoxin injections to intradermal applications of biphasic filler material increases the duration of correction, it is reasonable to assume that muscle movement–induced migration of the particulated material also plays a significant role in how well the implanted material remains in place.

In contrast, in the *monophasic* products, the cross-linking process is carried out in a more stepwise procedure to achieve gels with low elasticity, so that such gels can pass through smaller-diameter needles without the need to be crushed to pieces. It is not easy to be certain to what degree such gels fragment into pieces as they pass through the needle during the implantation procedure; however, with the exception of the newer, cohesive polydensified matrix (CPM) gels, some degree of fragmentation of HA gels during injection is very likely to occur and is supported by histological observations in thin sections of treated skin.

By a new cross-linking technology (CPM technology), the gels can be made less elastic and are capable of passing through narrow needles without the need for fragmentation. The resulting gel product is characterized by a CPM. In contrast to the biphasic predecessor products, the monophasic CPM gels have a different distribution in the dermis, which can be demonstrated by thin sections of biopsies. Whereas the biphasic material fills the dermis by forming clusters (Figure 7.2), the monophasic material

TABLE 7.2: Variations in Particle Size

Hylaform	Restylane	Puragen
692 μm	525 μm	240 μm

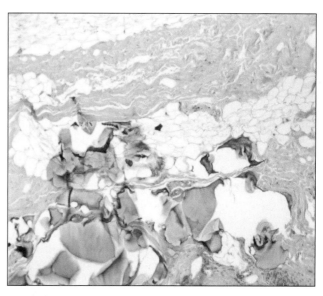

FIGURE 7.2: Biphasic material fills the dermis by forming clusters.

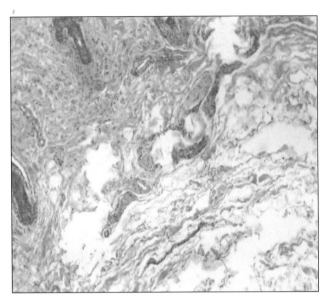

FIGURE 7.3: *Monophasic material spreads and forms layers.*

spreads and forms layers (Figure 7.3), which has consequences for the injection technique: the dermis should be filled in a more punctual way, comparable to a hydrodissection.

How does one discriminate between these two types of gel? Take a gel specimen, put it in a Petri dish, and add several milliliters of water. The particulated (biphasic) gels will decompose to visible particles. The precipitated and monophasic gels will stay coherent. This test is called the *Petri dish test* and is easily performed in the office.

VISCOELASTIC PROPERTIES OF CROSS-LINKED HA GELS

Non-cross-linked HA and the cross-linked (XL) species have viscoelastic properties, which means that physically, they behave like both fluids and solids, depending on the testing conditions. When exposed to shear forces, they behave like fluids, decreasing in viscosity with increasing shear force. When exposed to deformation forces, they act like solids. This behavior is significant with respect to injection and distribution in the ECM. Injection through a small-gauge needle generates high shear force and renders the XLHA more fluid. Deposed in the tissue gaps, the XLHA is exposed to more or less concentric remodeling force by the elastic fibers, thus changing its properties to a solid mass acting against compression and, in fact, contributing to volume as a filler.

To characterize the viscoelastic properties of XLHA, several physical parameters can be measured:

- $\tan(\delta)$ is an indicator for the degree of cross-linking and structuring in the gel; a low value indicates a rigid structure, whereas a high value is found in flexible preparations

TABLE 7.3: Comparison of Viscoelastic Properties of XLHA Products

	tan (δ)	G' (0.628)	η (0.628)	% elasticity
Belotero Basic	0.70	38.7	61.6	58.8
Juvéderm 30HV	0.27	51.5	81.9	78.7
Puragen	0.24	591.7	941.8	80.4
Restylane	0.28	334.5	532.4	78.2
Perlane	0.30	305.6	486.4	77.2
Restylane Lip	0.18	753.5	1,199.0	84.9

Note: Data adapted from Falcone SM, Doerfler AM, Berg RA. Poster presented at: Facial Aesthetic Conference and Exhibition; 29th June-1st July 2007; London.

- G' (0.628) indicates the elastic modulus and is a measure of the overall stiffness of the material
- ν (0.628) indicates the magnitude of the complex viscosity
- percentage elasticity describes the relation between the elastic modulus (overall stiffness) and viscous modulus and may be an indicator of the clinical performance of a product

A comparison between different filler materials is presented in Table 7.3. It is obvious from these data that the CPM product Belotero is characterized by the least inner structure and highest flexibility, the lowest overall stiffness, and the lowest viscosity, resulting in a low percentage elasticity value and accounting for the ability to produce a so-called blanching effect. In contrast, Restylane Lip shows the most rigid inner structure, the highest overall stiffness, and the highest viscosity, resulting in an extremely high percentage elasticity value, indicating a limited distribution in the tissue and a high lifting capacity.

CONSEQUENCES OF INJECTION TECHNIQUES

What goes on in the dermis when a hydrogel is injected? First, there is tissue injury. The needle hits the microvessels in the dermis and dermal papillae, which initiates an inflammatory reaction, the first step of wound healing. Placing pressure on the plunger of the syringe generates a degree of hydrostatic pressure, which extends uniformly to the inside walls of the syringe and the needle. At the tip of the needle, the open end of the system, the pressure acts against the remodeling forces of the ECM and its interconnecting fibrils. When the pressure exceeds the remodeling force, the filler material is pushed between the tissue layers. The connecting fibrils break, and the filler penetrates into the developing gaps between collagen bundles, thus forming cavities filled with the implant material. This procedure of forcing open an artificial space inside the dermis is the main cause of the sensations of pain experienced by the patient. In the case of high remodeling forces of the dermis or in the

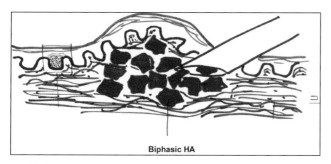

FIGURE 7.4: *Injecting biphasic material.*

case of high viscosity of the gel or gel particles, the spreading of the material can be facilitated by cutting the tissue with a sharp needle, an application even more traumatic to the tissue known as the tunnel technique, fan technique, or layering technique.

The result of the filling process is strongly influenced by the properties of the filling material, especially its viscoelastic properties. With monophasic gels, the viscosity is usually low and the elasticity is low, which allows for easy placement in the tissue. Low viscosity is a condition for easy spreading of the implant material in the dermis and a blanching effect visible at the surface of the skin, much like the effect previously noted with injection of collagen fillers. The tissue augmentation occurs more or less in three dimensions (Figure 7.4). For the biphasic gels with much higher viscoelastic properties, the distribution in the dermis is limited by high viscosity, high elasticity, and, finally, by the size of the particles. Large particles are more bulky and cannot easily penetrate the dermal layers. Therefore they have a very limited radius of distribution but a high ability to lift the skin surface (Figure 7.5). They have a more pronounced *lifting capacity* and thus are prone to forming visible bumps on the skin surface, which are, in most cases, transient.

There is a broad variety of different types of filler on the market. Many possible combinations are available. This is of particular importance because success of the treatment is not only dependent on the properties of the filler, but also, and to an equal extent, on the status of the patient's

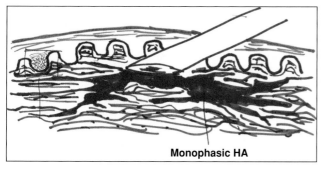

Monophasic HA

FIGURE 7.5: *Injecting monophasic material.*

dermis. Remodeling forces inside connective tissue, especially in the dermis, are widely variable and are measured as having greater or lesser resistance to the injection of filler. Therefore it is important to choose the right material for a particular skin type. Given these considerations, manufacturers usually offer the same basic filler with different grades of cross-linking of the gel, different HA contents, and different particle sizes, all marketed with a common branded or trademarked name. The reader is again reminded that most biphasic fillers have a broad range of particle sizes (Figure 7.1), which means that they are mixtures of smaller and larger particles in one preparation, with the smaller particles compensating for the limited distribution of the larger particles, facilitating injection and placement in the tissue, and contributing to an acceptable result. The CPM filler material, in contrast, combines dense and less dense zones in a monophasic gel and therefore tends to spread in a self-regulating way.

EFFICACY AND LONGEVITY

Efficacy of treatment with HA-based dermal fillers has been demonstrated in many clinical studies and is comparable to the efficacy of collagen fillers. The duration of the filling effect exceeds that of collagen preparations. The loss of HA-based fillers in biological tissues is due to biodegradation and, presumably, to migration. Migration has never been investigated meticulously. It is a passive movement of the implant material driven by gravitational and muscular forces, which generate unidirectional pressure on the artificial material. It is a common phenomenon of all fillers and may also be referred to as dislocation of the filler. In vivo biodegradation of HA and XLHA seems to be primarily cell-dependent because the degrading enzymes (several different hyaluronidases) are linked to cells. The degradation of HA and XLHA by oxygen radicals is also cell-dependent because the cells generate the radicals. In the dermis, macrophages seem to be primarily responsible for the breakdown of fillers. Macrophages can be seen in histological sections engulfing the gel portions. Therefore it is assumed that the degradation process of XLHA takes place at the interface between the gel product and macrophages and that it is a function of the overall surface available. As a rule of physics, the surface-to-volume ratio of a relatively spherical particle increases exponentially as the particle size decreases, which means that smaller particle sizes translate to faster loss of material. As a result of these considerations, it is easy to understand that a large particle size with a relatively low surface-to-volume ratio has enhanced stability in the biological environment. But it is more difficult to properly distribute these larger particles in the dermis because of the limited spreading properties of large particles. For these reasons, small particles, such as those utilized in filler products designed specifically for treatment of very superficial, fine line–type wrinkles, are more rapidly degraded. In fact, particles below 20 μm diameter can be completely phagocytized by single macrophages and digested inside the cell into different end products of the HA catabolism.

The so-called isovolumetric degradation, claimed for nonanimal stabilized hyaluronic acid (NASHA) products, is sheer imagination and more or less a marketing ploy. There is no theoretical or experimental proof of that kind of biodegradation.

Enhancement of resistance to enzymatic degradation without loss of performance is achieved by double-cross-linking with a new type of cross-linking agent, diepoxy-octane. Thus it is possible to make a gel with improved longevity and reduced particle size. The corresponding third-generation double-cross-linked product is characterized by a mean particle size of about 250 μm, less than half the size of standard second-generation gel particles. Longevity and efficacy have been proved in a clinical study to be at least similar to single-cross-linked products with a mean particle size of about 700 μm.

Except for the European-based CPM technology products, we have no data available for the sustainability of monophasic products. It is difficult to assess the surface area of these products available to attack by macrophages in vivo because of the uncertainty of fragmentation during injection. In a recent clinical study, the longevity of the CPM product turned out to be at least comparable to the biphasic products. A blinded study using a 1–5 wrinkle severity grading scale yielded an improvement of at least one grade in 82% of the subjects after six months (Table 7.3).

No data are available for the unsoluble precipitated HA fillers. Assessments of their longevity in vivo by clinical observations suggest significant underperformance compared to the chemically cross-linked material.

SAFETY

As a biomaterial, HA is nontoxic and biodegradable. HA-based fillers presently available are highly purified products, whether bacterial or avian derived. Endotoxin contents are reduced to the limits of measurement. In rare cases, there may be allergic reaction (dependent on the product source) to chicken egg white or streptococcal proteins. The rate of allergic reaction for HA fillers is assumed to be 0.02% which is low compared to animal-derived collagen fillers, which have a rate of allergic reaction of 0.05 to 0.02%. Therefore pretesting for HA fillers is usually not required. Minor reactions to the injection procedure are common for all dermal fillers and are reported to some degree in up to 90% of patients during the first two weeks, then drop drastically. In some patients, granulomas develop after injection and vanish within three months. NASHA has a pronounced tendency to granuloma formation, which may persist for

several years. Such granulomas are underreported and, in some cases, have been erroneously interpreted as neocollagenesis, but in fact, they constitute an adverse event that can impair the cosmetic outcome. Except for these types of generally minor and self-limited reactions, the overall safety profile of HA-based fillers is considered excellent. This assessment of safety of XLHA products is strictly linked to proper placement of the material in the dermis. It is a matter of fact that administration in the subcutaneous space may generate special hazards, for example, injecting vessels may cause necrosis in downstream tissue. Such problems are more likely in the periorbital and nasolabial zones.

CONCLUSIONS

HA-based dermal fillers are safe and efficacious in the treatment of aging skin. Composition and structure affect filler function with respect to placement and diffusion in the dermis and longevity. Proper patient selection, matching the correct filler(s) to the type of wrinkles present, and the overall condition and characteristics of the patient's skin are important for the final cosmetic result. With increasing numbers of available fillers, a good understanding of filler properties, along with physician skill and experience, will be required to select the optimal filler for any given individual.

SUGGESTED READING

Carruthers A, Carey W, De Lorenzi C. Randomized, double-blind comparison of the efficacy of two hyaluronic acid derivatives, Restylane, Perlane and Hylaform, in the treatment of nasolabial folds. *Dermatol. Surg.* 2005;31(11 Pt 2): 1591–8.

Carruthers J, Carruthers A. A prospective, randomized, parallel group study analyzing the effect of BTX-A (Botox) and nonanimal sourced hyaluronic acid (NASHA, Restylane) in combination compared with NASHA (Restylane) alone in severe glabellar rhytides in adult female subjects: treatment of severe glabellar rhytides with a hyaluronic acid derivative compared with the derivative and BTX-A. *Dermatol. Surg.* 2003;29: 802–9.

Coleman S. Crosslinked hyaluronic acid fillers. *Plast. Reconstr. Surg.* 2006;117:661–5.

Daugherty SH. Microbiology of infection in prosthetic devices. In: Wadström T, Eliasson I, Holder I, Ljungh A, eds., *Pathogenesis of Wound and Biomaterial-Associated Infections*. London: Springer; 1990:375–90.

Day DJ, Littler CM, Swift RW, Gottlieb S. The Wrinkle Severity Rating Scale. *Am J. Clin. Dermatol.* 2004;5:49–52.

DeLustro F, Smith TS, Sundsmo J, Salem G, Kincaid S, Ellingsworth L. Reaction to injectable collagen: results in animal model and clinical use. *Plast. Reconstr. Surg.* 1987;79: 581–92.

Duranti F, Salti G, Bovani B, Calandra M, Rosati ML. Injectable hyaluronic acid gel for soft tissue augmentation: a clinical and histological study. *Dermatol. Surg.* 1998;24:1317–25.

Entwistle J, Hall CL, Turley EA. HA receptors: regulators of signaling to the cytoskeleton. *J. Cell. Biochem.* 1996;61: 569–77.

Falcone SJ, Berg RA. Crosslinked hyaluronic acid dermal fillers: a comparison of rheological properties. *J. Biomed. Mater. Res.* 2008;87(1):264–71.

Falcone SJ, Palmeri DM, Berg RA. Rheological and cohesive properties of hyaluronic acid. *J. Biomed. Mater. Res. A.* 2006;76:721–8.

Ferry JD. *Viscoelastic Properties of Polymers.* 3rd ed. New York: John Wiley; 1980.

Friedmann PM, Mafong EA, Kauvar ANB, Geronemus RG. Safety data of injectable nonanimal stabilized hyaluronic acid gel for soft tissue augmentation. *Dermatol. Surg.* 2003;28: 491–4.

Ha RY, Kimihiro N, Adams WP, Brown SA. Analysis of facial skin thickness: defining the Relative Thickness Index. *Plast. Reconstr. Surg.* 2005;115:1769–73.

Hashimoto M, Saegusa H, Chiba S, inventors. Sodium hyaluronate manufacture with *Streptococcus equi.* US patent 4 946 780, filing date 05/04/1989, publication date 08/07/1990.

Hruby K. Hyaluronsäure als Glaskörperersatz bei Netzhautablösung. *Klin. Monatsblatter Augenheilkd. Augenarztl. Fortbild.* 1961;138:484–96.

Kinney BM. Injecting Puragen Plus into the nasolabial folds: preliminary observations of FDA trial. *Aesthetic Surg. J.* 2006;26:741–8.

Knapp TR, Kaplan EN, Daniels JR. Injectable collagen for soft tissue augmentation. *Plast. Reconstr. Surg.* 1977;60(3):398–405.

Kohda D, Morton CJ, Parkar AA, et al. Solution structure of the link molecule: a hyaluronan-binding domain involved in extracellular matrix stability and cell migration. *Cell.* 1996;86:767–775.

Laurent TC. *The Chemistry, Biology and Medical Applications of Hyaluronan and First Derivatives.* Miami, FL: Potland Press; 1998.

Laurent TC, Hellsing K, Gelotte B. Cross-linked gels of hyaluronic acid. *Acta Chem. Scand.* 1964;18:274–5.

Lee JY, Spicer AP. Hyaluronan, a multifunctional, megadalton, stealth molecule. *Curr. Opin. Cell Biol.* 2000;12:581–6.

Lesley J, Hascall VC, Tammi M, Hyman R. Hyaluronan binding by cell surface CD44. *J. Biol. Chem.* 2000;275:26967–75.

Liesegang TJ. Viscoelastic substances in ophthalmology. *Surv. Ophthalmol.* 1990;34:268–93.

Lindqvist C, Tveten S, Eriksen Bondevik B, Fagrell D. A randomized, evaluator-blind, multicenter comparison of the efficacy and tolerability of Perlane versus Zyplast in the correction of nasolabial folds. *Plast. Reconstr. Surg.* 2005;115:282–9.

Lowe NJ. Arterial embolization caused by injection of hyaluronic acid (Restylane). *Br. J. Dermatol.* 2003;148:379–595.

Lowry KM, Beavers EM. Thermal stability of sodium hyaluronate in aqueous solution. *J. Biomed. Mater. Res.* 1994;28:1239–44.

Lupton JR, Alster TS. Cutaneous hypersensitivity reaction to injectable hyaluronic acid gel. *Dermatol. Surg.* 2000;2:1–2.

Morhenn VB, Lemperle G, Gallo RL. Phagocytosis of different particulated dermal filler substances by human macrophages and skin cells. *Dermatol. Surg.* 2002;28 (6):484–90.

Narins RS, Brandt F, Leyden J, Lorenc ZP, Rubin M, Smith S. A randomized, double-blind, multicenter comparison of the efficacy and tolerability of Restylane versus Zyplast for the correction of nasolabial folds. *Dermatol. Surg.* 2003;29:588–95.

Nicolau PJ. Long-lasting and permanent fillers: biomaterial influence over host tissue response. *Plast. Reconstr. Surg.* 2007;119:2271–86.

Noble PW, McKee CM, Horton MR. Induction of inflammatory gene expression by low-molecular-weight hyaluronan fragments in macrophages. In: Laurent TC, ed., *The Chemistry, Biology and Medical Applications of Hyaluronan and Its Derivatives.* London: Portland Press; 1998:219–25.

Olenius M. The first clinical study using a new biodegradable implant for the treatment of lips, wrinkles and folds. *Aesthetic Plast. Surg.* 1998;22:97–101.

Piacquadio DJ, Jarcho M, Goltz R. Evaluation of hylan B gel as a soft tissue augmentation material. *J. Am. Acad. Dermatol.* 1997;36:544–9.

Ponta H, Sherman L, Herrlich P. CD44: from adhesion molecules to signaling regulators. *Nat. Rev. Mol. Cell Biol.* 2003;4:33–45.

Rames RA, Aaroson IA. Migration of polytef paste to the lung and brain following intravesical injection for the correction of reflux. *Pediatr. Surg. Int.* 1991;6:239–40.

Rees TD, Ashley FI, Delgado JP. Silicone fluid injection for facial atrophy. *Plast. Reconstr. Surg.* 1973;52:118–27.

Reinmüller J. Die Anwendung der Hyaluronsäure als Biomaterial in der plastischen und ästhetischen Chirurgie. Paper presented at: Fifth Annual Meeting of the Deutsche Gesellschaft für Ästhetische Medizin; September 11–13, 1992; Lindau, Germany.

Reinmüller J, inventor. Medizinische Implantate aus Formkörpern. European Patent EP 0 756 475 B1, filing date 04/12/1995, publication date 12/30/1998.

Reinmüller J. Hyaluronic acid. *Aesthetic Surg. J.* 2003;23:309–11.

Reinmüller J, Lockett C. Assessing the performance and safety of CX001 (Puragen) when applied as an intradermal implant for the correction of facial wrinkles and folds, publication in preparation.

Reinmüller J, Wolters M, Steinkraus V, et al. Efficacy and tolerability of the hyaluronic acid filler Belotero Basic after single bilateral injection for correction of the nasolabial folds. Poster 4321 presented at: 21st World Congress of Dermatology; 2007, 2–5 October; Buenos Aires.

Richter AW, Ryde EM, Zetterstrom EO. Non-immunogenicity of a purified sodium hyaluronate preparation in man. *Int. Arch. Allergy Immunol.* 1988;59:45–8.

Schanz S, Schippert W, Ulmer A. Arterial embolization caused by injection of hyaluronic acid (Restylane). *Br. J. Dermatol.* 2002;146:928–9.

Schwach-Abdellaoui K, Sorensen MV, Andersen KB, Weibye M, Beck TC. Recombinant hyaluronic acid: physicochemical and thermal characterization. In: Balazs EA, Hascall VC, eds., *Hyaluronan: Structure, Metabolism, Biological Activities, Therapeutic Applications.* New Jersey: Matrix Biology Institute; 2005:89–92.

Stern R. Devising a pathway for hyaluronan catabolism: how the goo gets cut. In: Balazs EA, Hascall VC, eds., *Hyaluronan: Structure, Metabolism, Biological Activities, Therapeutic Applications*. New Jersey: Matrix Biology Institute; 2005:257–66.

Swann DA, Kuo J. Hyaluronic acid. In: Byrom D, ed., *Biomaterials*. New York: Stockton Press; 1991:285–305.

Tammi RH, Pasonen-Seppänen S, Kultti A, et al. Hyaluronan degradation in epidermis. In: Balazs EA, Hascall VC, eds., *Hyaluronan: Structure, Metabolism, Biological Activities, Therapeutic Applications*. New Jersey: Matrix Biology Institute; 2005:241–5.

Wang F, Garza LA, Kang S, et al. In vivo stimulation of de novo collagen production caused by cross-linked hyaluronic acid dermal filler injection in photodamaged human skin. *Arch. Dermatol.* 2007;143:155–63.

Yanaki T, Yamaguchi T. Temporary network formation of hyaluronate under physiological conditions: 1. Molecular-weight dependence. *Biopolymers* 1990;30:415–25.

Zao XB, Fraser JE, Alexander C, Lockett C, White BJ. Synthesis and characterization of a novel double crosslinked hyaluronan hydrogel. *J. Mater. Sci.* 2002;13:11–16.

RESTYLANE, JUVÉDERM, AND PURAGEN FAMILIES OF NONANIMAL STABILIZED HYALURONIC ACID FILLERS

CHAPTER 8

Restylane: General Concepts

Sorin Eremia

Restylane (Q-Med) was introduced in 1994 as the first nonanimal stabilized hyaluronic acid (NASHA) filler and quickly became widely used around the world. In spite of intense competition from other, newer hyaluronic acid (HA) products, Restylane remains the best-selling product today. It was the first HA product to receive Food and Drug Administration (FDA) approval, in December 2003, and is distributed in the United States by Medicis Aesthetics Inc.

Restylane is a partially (single) cross-linked HA manufactured from *Streptococcus* bacterial fermentation. It is a moderately viscous clear particulated gel (biphasic gel) that can be injected through a 30-gauge needle. Restylane, like other HA products, binds water very well. In fact, as, over time, it loses cross-linkage as it undergoes enzymatic degradation, its volume can actually increase as more water becomes bound to the exposed HA.

For this type of product, the manufacturing process can determine the gel particle size, which, at equal concentrations of HA, determines viscosity of the gel. Outside the United States, a variety of Restylane products are available, which are of variable particle size and thus of variable numbers of particles per milliliter. The number of particles per milliliter is inversely proportional to the particle size. The larger the particle size, the greater the viscosity.

Four Restylane products are available in Canada and Europe (Table 8.1). They are, in order of particle size, Restylane Fine Lines, Restylane, Perlane, and Restylane SubQ. In the United States, only Restylane and Perlane are FDA approved. The products with larger particle sizes/fewer particles per milliliter are designed for deeper use and require larger-gauge needles. If a gel containing larger particles is forced through a smaller-gauge needle than recommended, the particles break up and essentially become more like the smaller-particle product.

Restylane and Perlane are the two most popular products. When injected for lip augmentation and nasolabial folds, the correction lasts about an equivalent length of time. Perlane seems to generate a little more volume but

TABLE 8.1: Restylane Family of Products

Product	Gel Particles per Milliliter	Type of Use
Restylane Fine Lines	200,000	fine, superficial wrinkles
Restylane	100,000	lips, medium wrinkles
Perlane	8,000	deeper wrinkles
Restylane SubQ	1,000	volume augmentation

needs to be injected a little deeper into the dermis. For lips and average-depth nasolabial folds, and for tear-trough deformities, the author prefers Restylane, which is injected with a 30-gauge needle (vs. 27-gauge for Perlane). For deeper nasolabial folds, for deep lateral oral commissural folds, and for valleylike depressed scars, Perlane does a little better, but not enough to justify using a separate syringe, if more superficial areas are also treated and a single 1-cc syringe of Restylane will suffice. For cheek, chin, and prejowl area volume augmentation, Perlane is much better. Where available, Restylane Fine Lines has seen limited use since crow's feet, its primary intended market, are treated much better with neurotoxin. Resurfacing is also a much more practical long-term option for most very superficial fine lines. Captique (Allergan), another FDA-approved NASHA containing a lower concentration of HA per milliliter, and which has not gained much popularity in the United States, would be its close clinical equivalent.

Restylane SubQ was designed as a longer-lasting, deeper-placed, subcutaneous volume replacement product. Its area of use would be the cheeks, chin, and prejowl area, but many experienced and devoted Restylane family of products users still prefer Perlane for those areas over SubQ.

The Restylane family of products are not packaged with lidocaine, and intradermal injection can be quite painful. Most patients require some type of topical, local, or nerve block anesthesia. The author strongly recommends nerve block anesthesia and uses 2% plain lidocaine (without epinephrine) to decrease the injection volume, decrease the duration of the block, and avoid the tachycardia and anxiety epinephrine can produce.

More specific discussion of injection techniques for Restylane and Perlane can be found in Chapters 9 and 14.

CHAPTER 9

The Restylane Family of Fillers: Canadian Experience

B. Kent Remington

The aging face has never been so well understood, nor the treatment options so varied. Achieving optimal results – softer, smoother skin; a younger, more youthful appearance that is both harmonious and symmetrical – requires a change in the way aesthetic clinicians view the aging face and its treatment. Focusing on single lines and folds limits the range of possibilities in facial enhancement. The successful aesthetic clinician is one who examines the length, width, and depth of the folds and, most importantly, the amount of volume loss associated with each fold and crease to determine how much product is needed for adequate correction. Moreover, the concept of facial zones – and treating multiple zones with product layering in a single visit – leads to optimal results and a high rate of patient satisfaction.

FILLERS FOR FACIAL ENHANCEMENT

The face can be likened to a beach ball or partitioned rubber raft: over time, it deflates and descends unevenly. Thus each side of the aging face is a sister, rather than a twin, of the other side. Many patients are themselves unaware of volume loss in the face, particularly in the cheeks. To create great results, clinicians must have double vision: first, the ability to see the areas of volume loss (and demonstrate this loss to the patient); second, the ability to see the end result before beginning treatment.

Filling Agent

The clinician has a number of choices when considering filler material. In our clinic, we prefer products from the Restylane family (Restylane Sub-Q, Perlane, Restylane Plain, and Restylane Fine Lines). We use Restylane Fine Lines for small wrinkles and lines, Perlane for restoring volume, and Restylane Plain for folds and creases. Layering Restylane on top of Perlane leads to optimal appearance and patient satisfaction and increased longevity. Moreover,

using adequate product during the first treatment session means fewer and less frequent touch-ups or maintenance treatments.

Treatment Zones

Rather than focusing simply on individual wrinkles and lines, recognize the complex and synergistic relationships of neighboring muscles by considering treatment zones. Treating several zones over the course of one session leads to an improved aesthetic appearance and increased patient satisfaction; multiple treatments create better facial harmony and balance. Typical zones for shaping, contouring, and volume enhancement include the tear trough and lateral orbital hollowing, the cheeks, the so-called aesthetic nose, and lip augmentation, among others (Figure 9.1).

The Remington Fold-Crease Grading System

In our clinic, we base injections on the Remington Fold-Crease Grading System, in which each facial aesthetic zone is assigned a value of 0 to 5, measured by clinical judgment of the length, width, and depth of the fold, in addition to the volume loss associated with each crease and fold. The grading system allows physicians to inject the appropriate amount of dermal filler for each specific procedure performed. For example, static lines without animation can be treated by fillers alone; static lines accentuated by animation require botulinum toxin type A (BTX-A) plus fillers; and static lines, folds, and creases with animation associated with elastotic wrinkles can be diminished by a combination of BTX-A and ablative resurfacing, followed by fillers a few months after the ablation of wrinkles. It also follows that higher scores require greater attention than lower scores; thus patients with level 5 wrinkles require restoration before fillers. Injecting an adequate amount of filler to restore volume loss adds longevity to the correction, with a smaller amount of touch-up material required in the future.

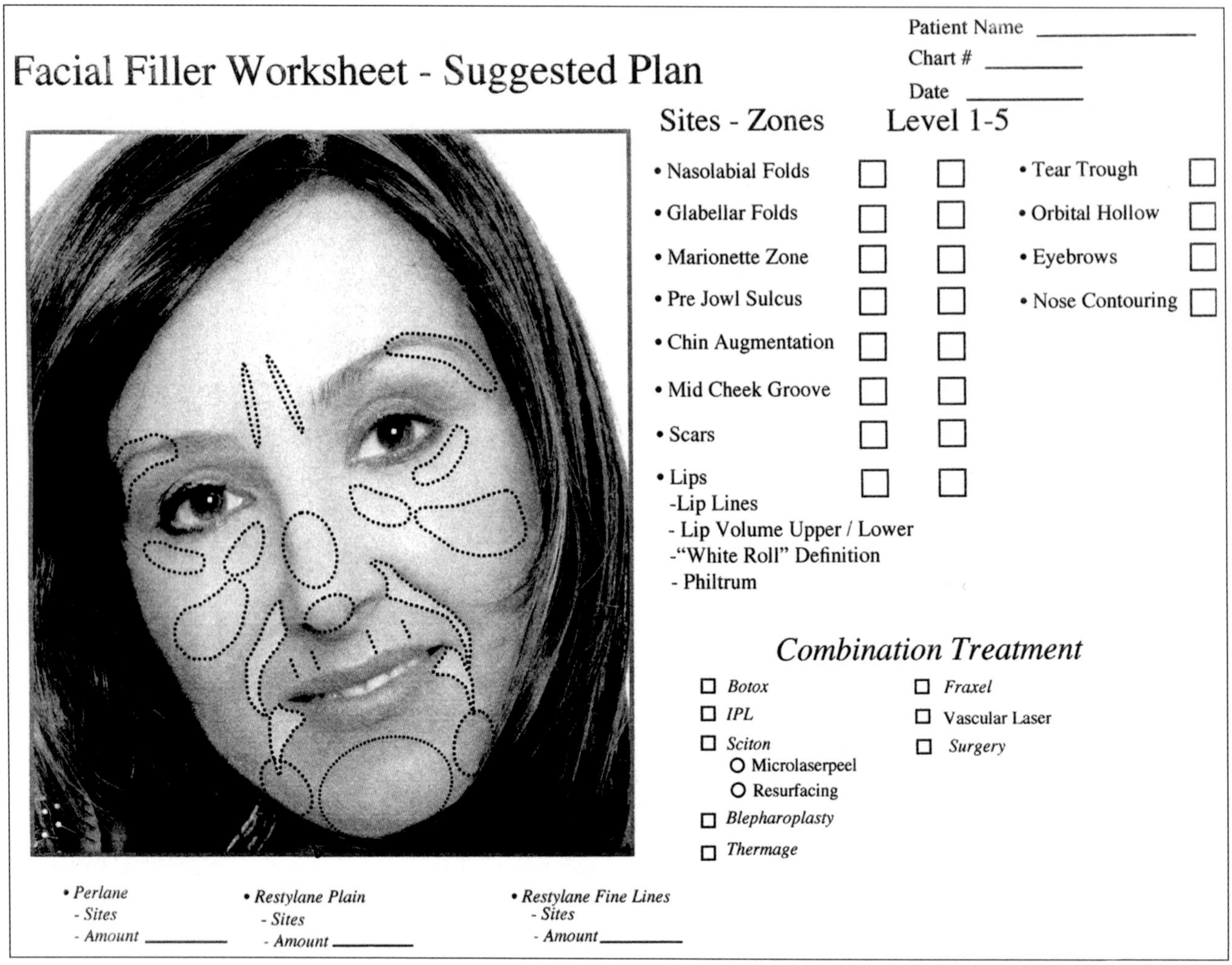

Facial Filler Worksheet - Suggested Plan

Patient Name _____

Chart # _____

Date _____

Sites - Zones   Level 1-5

- Nasolabial Folds ☐ ☐
- Glabellar Folds ☐ ☐
- Marionette Zone ☐ ☐
- Pre Jowl Sulcus ☐ ☐
- Chin Augmentation ☐ ☐
- Mid Cheek Groove ☐ ☐
- Scars ☐ ☐
- Lips ☐ ☐
  -Lip Lines
  - Lip Volume Upper / Lower
  -"White Roll" Definition
  - Philtrum

- Tear Trough ☐
- Orbital Hollow ☐
- Eyebrows ☐
- Nose Contouring ☐

Combination Treatment

☐ Botox   ☐ Fraxel
☐ IPL   ☐ Vascular Laser
☐ Sciton   ☐ Surgery
  ○ Microlaserpeel
  ○ Resurfacing
☐ Blepharoplasty
☐ Thermage

- Perlane   - Restylane Plain   - Restylane Fine Lines
  - Sites   - Sites   - Sites
  - Amount _____   - Amount _____   - Amount _____

FIGURE 9.1: Facial filler planning worksheet: potential filler injection sites.

Using the grading system, and acknowledging that higher scores require greater attention than lower scores, leads to more predictable results, harmony, and accord among facial wrinkles.

INJECTION TIPS AND TECHNIQUES

When treating specific zones, it is sometimes necessary to inject both antegrade and retrograde in the same area, whereas other areas require only one injection technique. Using a layering technique, inject Perlane deep on top of the periosteum (bone) in a grid pattern at 30- to 90-degree angles to the main lines or folds. After grid "lifting," layer Restylane Plain and Fine Lines to create the finishing touches. Volumizing requires molding and blending to ensure even results. Using cool ultrasound gel immediately after filler injection leads to enhanced proprioception and makes the postinjection massage more comfortable for the patient. In the perioral zone, place an index finger under the treated area with a gloved thumb on the outside.

Molding and blending for lip enhancement improves balance and harmony by detecting uneven areas that require more filling agent. For the tear troughs, midcheeks, eyebrows, and prejowl sulcus, mold and blend assertively over the periosteum. Nose contouring requires a firm but smooth approach.

Perlane and Restylane injectables for volume loss and improving folds and creases often complement other treatment modalities such as BTX-A, light-based therapies (intense pulsed light), ablative and nonablative resurfacing, and radiofrequency (Thermage). Combination therapy works synergistically to produce an improved aesthetic outcome of greater duration. Indeed, combination treatments often produce dramatic results (Figure 9.2).

Tear Trough and Lateral Orbital Hollowing

Most patients are unaware that tear troughs are one of the causes of dark circles under the eyes. Treating the tear trough is a simple procedure that makes a significant

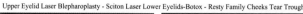

Upper Eyelid Laser Blepharoplasty - Sciton Laser Lower Eyelids-Botox - Resty Family Cheeks Tear Trough

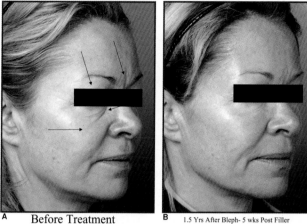

A **Before Treatment** B 1.5 Yrs After Bleph- 5 wks Post Filler
3.0 Ml Perlane Restylane
Note : Return of an Awake Bright Alert Look

FIGURE 9.2: Combination treatment – upper blepharoplasty, Er:YAG laser resurfacing, BOTOX, Restylane fillers for the tear trough and cheeks: A, pretreatment; B, posttreatment.

difference in appearance (Figure 9.2). The tear trough lies at the top end of the nasojugal groove, which runs to the top of the midcheek and is usually treated concomitantly. Baseline and follow-up photographs taken full-face, three-quarter face, and profile (both relaxed and animated) are essential. The vasoconstrictive blanching effect of topical anesthetic applied ten minutes prior to treatment decreases the chances of bruising and lessens any associated injection discomfort. Inject Restylane on top of the periosteum near the orbital rim floor, injecting antegrade to push the filler ahead (retrograde injections increase the likelihood of the Tyndall effect – discoloration of the skin – caused by dermal filler placed too superficially). Conservative injections lead to optimal results, as overcorrection or incorrect location creates a negative impression among patients. This zone requires a light touch; consider orbital contouring, rather than adding volume. For that reason, heavier or permanent fillers should be avoided. Blend immediately after injection with ultrasound gel. Animated and static lower eyelid wrinkles can be pretreated with BTX-A and ablative lasers.

The Aesthetic Nose

Most patients with contour changes of the nose are often surprised to discover that nonsurgical correction is available. In fact, only a small amount of filler is required to produce beautiful, natural-looking results. Conservative doses (1.0 mL Restylane Fine Lines), using 5-diopter (2.5 power) magnifying glasses to inject vertically through hair follicle pores, can make an immense difference in appearance. Finish with posttreatment blending, molding, and feathering with cool ultrasound gel.

Cheeks

Cheek volume is perhaps the greatest – and most subtle – sign of youth and vitality. However, most patients are unaware of volume loss (or its effects) in the face. Contouring and volumizing the cheeks with dermal fillers can be a gratifying procedure for both clinician and client. Prior to treatment, show patients their volume loss and the sites of injection using a mirror The greater the volume loss, the higher the amount of product needed; in our clinic, we use 0.5, 1.0, 2.0, and 2.5–3.0 mL Perlane for mild, moderate, moderate to severe, and severe volume loss, respectively, per cheek (Figure 9.3).

Patients receive injections in a seated position or slightly reclined (approximately 10 degrees). Inject vertically through a hair follicle pore, and inject slowly right on top of the periosteum, as if pumping up a flat tire. Do not inject too close to the lateral nasal ridge, and take care to avoid the infraorbital nerve. Proper cheek enhancement also smoothes the nasolabial fold and restores facial volume, lending previously sunken or drooping cheeks a natural vitality (Figure 9.4). Cheek enhancement will need periodic touch-ups to maintain results.

Marionette and Prejowl Sulcus Zones

The marionette and prejowl sulcus zones are often treated in conjunction with the nasolabial fold and the mid- and lateral cheek in one session. The amount of filler used increases with greater fold severity, as rated by the Remington Fold-Crease Grading System. In our clinic, we use 0.5 mL Perlane/Restylane per side for patients with level 1 severity, and up to 2.5 mL for those with level 5 severity (Figure 9.3).

Lip Enhancement

Age, genetics, sun damage, and smoking all cause the lips – the expressive focal point of the face – to change over time,

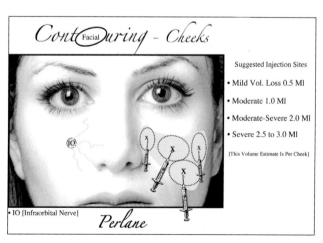

FIGURE 9.3: Volumizing the midface.

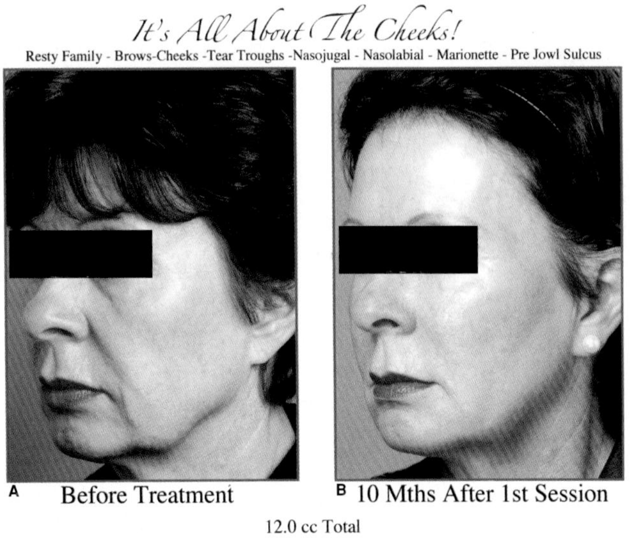

It's All About The Cheeks!

Resty Family - Brows-Cheeks -Tear Troughs -Nasojugal - Nasolabial - Marionette - Pre Jowl Sulcus

A Before Treatment   **B** 10 Mths After 1st Session

12.0 cc Total

FIGURE 9.4: *Cheek volumizing:* **A**, *pretreatment;* **B**, *after 1.5 cc Perlane per cheek.*

losing volume, shape, and definition. The height of the vermilion shrinks, the top lip flattens, and the philtrum base widens. The perioral lip zone becomes wrinkled, lipstick "bleeds" into the lip lines, and the lip corners lose their support and begin to droop. The goal of lip enhancement (versus augmentation) is to reestablish lip volume and add support, creating harmony between the upper and lower lips. Classically, the bottom lip is often fuller than the upper lip, but it is important to match lip volume and shape with each patient's age, goals, and lifestyle before beginning treatment. Regardless of shape, the lips must be symmetrical; while the upper and lower lips can be considered sisters, the right and left halves are twins and must achieve symmetrical balance.

Prior to treatment with fillers, treat any level 4 or 5 wrinkles with ablative resurfacing. Sketch fine lines before using regional nerve blocks (mepivacaine without epinephrine). Redefine the lip borders (white roll) and reestablish the philtrum ridges, which provide a more youthful and feminine appearance. A minimum amount of filler is required at the philtral columellar junction. For older patients, in whom the philtrum and base widen and splay, inject medial to each philtral column. Avoid so-called sausage lips by filling the midzone with more product, using less filler for lateral injections into the body of the lips. Finally, reestablish support of the lip corners by injecting the lateral commissures. Finish by molding and blending with cool ultrasound gel. Avoid using permanent fillers in the lips, and be conservative in the first session, allowing patients to adapt to their new lips as the tissue settles.

CONCLUSION

Successful enhancement of the face with filling agents relies not only on the clinical judgment of the length, width, and depth of each fold and crease, but also (and perhaps most importantly) on taking into account the associated volume loss when determining the optimal amount of filler needed. Moreover, the face and its imperfections can be divided into treatment zones, rather than single lines and wrinkles; treatment of multiple zones during one session creates a high level of satisfaction among both injectors and patients and results in the appealing, symmetrical face of youth.

CHAPTER 10

The Juvéderm Family of Fillers

Frederick C. Beddingfield III

Ahmet Tezel

Sorin Eremia

Dermal fillers have steadily grown in use over the years, despite the limitations of available products. Longevity without permanence and the absence of animal proteins have been desired attributes in fillers. Hyaluronic acids (HA), and in particular, the Juvéderm family of dermal fillers (Allergan), have the desired characteristics previously lacking in other available fillers.

As we age, our faces begin to show the effects of gravity, sun exposure, and years of facial muscle movement such as smiling, chewing, and squinting. The underlying tissues that keep our skin looking youthful begin to break down, often leaving laugh lines, smile lines, crow's feet, and facial creases, in addition to a general loss of volume around the face. Soft tissue fillers can help fill in these lines and creases, temporarily replenish volume loss, and restore a more youthful looking appearance. Some characteristics of an ideal filler are being nonpermanent (but long lasting), having minimal side effects, not requiring allergy testing, being easy to use/inject, being painless on injection, being reversible, and being cost effective for both the physician and the patient.

HA fillers, primarily due to their ability to bind to large amounts of water and their favorable adverse event profiles, offer an attractive solution to addressing the aging face and lifting the skin. Despite these general features, HA dermal fillers are not all the same. They differ in characteristics such as the type of cross-linker used, degree of cross-linking, gel hardness, viscosity, extrusion force, gel consistency and cohesivity, lift capacity, total HA concentration, and clinical duration in the skin. Key to the performance of an HA dermal filler is how these characteristics act in concert to deliver a product that combines ease of injection with long life and efficacy as a filler.

Juvéderm implants have been approved and used widely in Europe and Canada since 2000. Three formulations of Juvéderm HA dermal fillers (Juvéderm Ultra, Juvéderm Ultra Plus, and Juvéderm 30) were approved in the United States in 2006 for treatment of facial wrinkles and folds. These next-generation HA fillers are derived from *Streptococcus equi* bacteria and thus contain no animal proteins. In addition, they employ a high concentration of cross-linked HA to provide long-lasting, but not permanent, correction. Recent extended data from the trials used for Food and Drug Administration (FDA) approval showed that the clinical benefit of Juvéderm Ultra lasts up to nine months or longer, while the benefit of Juvéderm Ultra Plus lasts up to twelve months or longer. Indeed, Juvéderm is the only HA filler granted a label from the FDA that states that its benefits may last up to one year.

Juvéderm dermal fillers have a smooth consistency attributable to a proprietary process known as Hylacross technology. The smooth consistency of the Juvéderm dermal fillers contrasts with the granular consistency of other HA fillers such as Restylane and Perlane (Medicis), a difference that can readily be seen under magnification. The Juvéderm gels flow easily during injection and are malleable and appear smooth postinjection.

Juvéderm Ultra is available in a 0.8-mL syringe and a 30-gauge needle and is appropriate for placement in the mid-dermis to correct moderate folds and wrinkles. Juvéderm Ultra Plus injectable gel has an even higher degree of cross-linking than Juvéderm Ultra, which makes it particularly well suited for correcting deeper folds and wrinkles and adding volume. Juvéderm Ultra Plus is available in a 0.8-mL syringe and comes with a 27-gauge needle, though some clinicians report a preference for using a 30-gauge needle when using the filler for less deep injections or in areas where smaller aliquots may be more desirable (e.g., periorbitally). Patients with deep facial wrinkles and folds are generally at a disadvantage when it comes to cosmetic correction as they require a large volume of dermal filler and their correction may not be sustained, so a filler that is specifically designed to treat severe wrinkles is an important advancement. Juvéderm Ultra can also

TABLE 10.1: Summary of Relative Elastic Modulus, Cohesivity, Overall Lift, and the Correlation with Placement and Depth of Injection for Restylane and Juvéderm Families of Products

Product	G'	Cohesivity	Lift Capacity	Area on the Face	Depth of Injection
Restylane Touch	***1/2	*	**	fine lines	superficial
Restylane	****	**	***	glabellar/NL folds marionette/perioral periorbital/lips	mid to deep dermis
Perlane	*****	**	***1/2	deeper NLF cheeks/chin jaw/malar	mid to deep dermis
Hylaform/Captique	**	***	**1/2	fine lines	superficial
Juvéderm 18	*	***	**	glabellar/NL folds marionette/perioral periorbital/lips vermilion border tear trough	mid to deep dermis
Juvéderm Ultra	**	****	***	deeper NLF/lips (body) cheeks/chin/jaw/malar	mid to deep dermis
Juvéderm Ultra Plus	***	****	***1/2	volume/contouring	mid to deep dermis
Juvéderm 30	***	*****	****	volume/contouring	mid to deep dermis
Voluma	****1/2	***1/2	****	volume/contouring	subcutaneous

Note: Lift capacity is a function of both elastic modulus and cohesivity.

be layered on top of Juvéderm Ultra Plus when treating areas such as the nasolabial folds, where deeper folds may also have superficial rhytids. Results from the randomized, controlled study of three Juvéderm formulations compared with bovine collagen have been published and can be accessed at the American Society of Plastic Surgeons Web site listed below.

To better evaluate HA dermal fillers, it is helpful to have an understanding of two physical attributes, gel hardness and cohesivity, which play a key role in determining the ideal placement of a certain formulation in terms of area of treatment and depth of injection. When designing therapies for the increasing number of patients seeking facial enhancement, restoration, and rejuvenation, a deeper understanding of the science and the factors that impact the final product characteristics should be sought.

When a HA dermal filler is implanted into the skin, the natural elasticity or tension of the skin will tend to deform and flatten out the implant, reducing the initial desired correction. In principle, the lifting capacity of a dermal filler (opposing its deformation) is defined by the fluidity of the product. In return, the fluidity is primarily determined by two material properties, namely, gel hardness (elastic modulus, G') and the cohesivity of the gel. Thus lift is a function of both gel hardness and cohesivity, and both parameters play a role of equal importance

Within this context, the Restylane family of dermal filler products relies on high values of G' (resulting in harder

products) to provide the necessary lift to achieve optimal correction. However, high G' values also require the incorporation of high amounts of soluble (free) HA, which acts as a lubricant to aid the extrusion of the gel through a thin needle. As a counteraction, the addition of soluble HA[1] results in decreased cohesivity of the product.

In contrast, the Juvéderm family of dermal filler products relies on high cohesivity to provide the necessary lift to achieve optimal correction. Since Juvéderm fillers are softer (lower G' values), they only require minimal amounts of soluble HA (acting as a lubricant) to aid the extrusion of the gel through a thin needle. This results in very high gel cohesivity and therefore in gels that retain their gel structure on injection.

As explained earlier, these two different approaches are both suitable to achieve optimal lift. One approach is to have harder gels but add soluble HA, yielding a lower cohesivity to the product (Restylane family of products). The other approach is to formulate softer gels (lower G' values) that enable the use of minimal soluble HA, which, in return, results in high cohesivity (Juvéderm family of products).

Table 10.1 summarizes the authors' evaluation of lift capacity and the potential correlation with optimal treatment area and injection depth for both the Restylane and

---

[1] Soluble (free, non-cross-linked) HA lubricates the surface of HA particles, which results in decreasing the affinity of the gel particles with each other, in return resulting in lower cohesivity of the product.

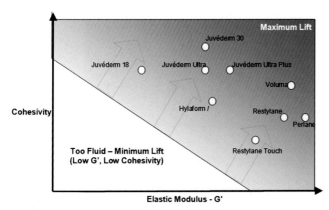

FIGURE 10.1: *The relative lift capacities of Juvéderm and Restylane families of products.*

Juvéderm families of products. Figure 10.1 shows the layout of the Juvéderm and Restylane families of products in terms of their lift capacity in reference to one of the earlier HA dermal filler formulations, that is, Hylaform. Note that Restylane and Juvéderm are comparable in terms of their lift capacities, even though the two products take two different approaches to create lift. The authors believe that some HA formulations primarily available in the European Union that are marketed as soft HA fillers do not possess lift capacities as they have low cohesivities in addition to very low elastic moduli.

Physicians often use the lift capacity in addition to the relative softness of the product as a tool to determine the appropriate choice of filler for the target area of treatment and required depth of injection. As a general rule of thumb, products that have a higher lift capacity are used

for correction of deeper wrinkles and folds, in addition to volumizing and contouring applications due to their robust nature. On the other hand, products that have higher fluidity (Restylane, Juvéderm Ultra) are more appropriate for mid- to deep dermis injections for correction of moderate to severe wrinkles and folds. Given otherwise identical products, a softer product (lower G') will be preferred for more superficial injections, in areas where the skin is very thin (such as the periorbital areas) or to avoid lumpiness where softness is particularly important (e.g., some clinicians prefer softer fillers for treating the lips).

CLINICAL APPLICATIONS OF JUVÉDERM PRODUCTS[2]

For the tear-trough deformity, Juvéderm Ultra is an excellent choice, and 0.2–0.4 cc is best injected with a 30-gauge needle into the subperiosteal or suborbicularis. Results last nine to twelve months (Figure 10.2). For malar augmentation, Juvéderm Ultra Plus is preferable and should be injected through a 27-gauge needle. For the lips, Juvéderm Ultra is easier to use, especially along the vermilion. For the nasolabial folds, lateral oral commissural folds, and chin area, either product can be used, depending on the depth of the fold and skin thickness. In some patients with deep folds, layering the products leads to the best results. Given the packaging of two 0.8-cc syringes, it is easy to split packages of Juvéderm Ultra and Ultra Plus and use one of each. For most patients, with proper intradermal

[2] This "Clinical Applications" section was contributed by Sorin Eremia.

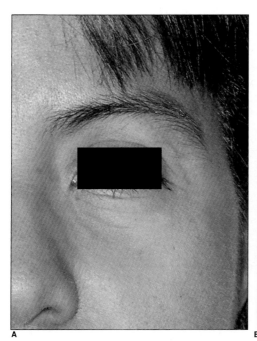
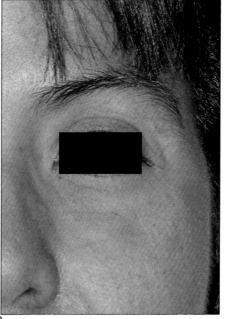

FIGURE 10.2: *Tear-trough deformity treatment:* **A**, *pretreatment;* **B**, *posttreatment with 0.3 cc Juvéderm Ultra placed on the periosteum with 30-gauge needle.*

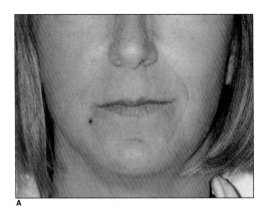 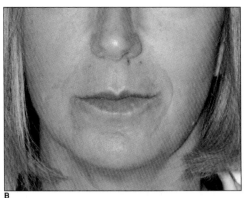

A   B

*FIGURE 10.3: Lip augmentation: **A**, pretreatment; **B**, posttreatment with 0.8 cc Juvéderm Ultra.*

placement, two 0.8-cc syringes of product is amply sufficient to treat the perioral area and the nasolabial folds. When placed intradermally, Juvéderm correction seems to last about eight to nine months (Figure 10.3), a little shorter than with subperiosteal placement. Since Juvéderm flows out of the syringe into the tissues much more readily than Restylane, care must be taken to apply less pressure on the plunger to avoid inadvertent overcorrection.

In practice, clinicians must weigh a variety of factors, such as patient characteristics, location to be treated, familiarity with the products available, and trust in both product efficacy and safety, in addition to the physicochemical properties of the dermal fillers, when deciding which dermal filler to utilize. HA fillers are good choices for dermal filling because they are natural constituents of the dermis and are well tolerated, have a long safety record, are at least partially reversible with hyaluronidase, and achieve natural-appearing and satisfying results. Although the ideal filler may not exist, HA fillers may be the best approximation of such an ideal to date.

SUGGESTED READING

American Society of Plastic Surgeons. Injectable fillers: improving skin texture. Arlington Heights, IL: American Society of Plastic Surgeons; 2006. Available at: http://www.plasticsurgery.org/public_education/procedures/InjectableFillers.cfm. Accessed June 22, 2006.

Born T. Hyaluronic acids. *Clin. Plast. Surg.* 2006;33:525–38.

Dover JS. The filler revolution has just begun. *Plast. Reconstr. Surg.* 2006;117(3 Suppl):38–40S.

Smith KC. Practical use of Juvéderm: early experience. *Plast. Reconstr. Surg.* 2007;120(6 Suppl):67–73S.

CHAPTER 11

Puragen: A New Dermal Filler

Michael H. Gold

The dermal filler market continues to see increasing growth due to longer-lasting effects of the newer fillers as compared to the original collagen, bovine-derived materials. Much of the research has focused on the hyaluronic acid (HA) class of compounds, and these compounds, taken in total, rank fifth among the most common noninvasive cosmetic procedures, according to 2006 statistics from the American Society of Plastic Surgeons.

Dermal fillers utilizing HA have become popular due to their natural properties as HA is a material found commonly in the human body. HA for dermal fillers has been derived via two sources: they are either animal based or derived via bacterial fermentation. Animal-derived HA products have not produced the consistent, long-lasting results clinicians were hoping for; therefore technology and research have focused on bacterial fermentation of these products. At the time of this writing, there are four HA products currently available in the U.S. market: Restylane, Perlane, Juvéderm Ultra, and Juvéderm Ultra Plus. There are differences among these products, including the concentration of HA included and the amount of cross-linking of HA for each of the products. In summary, Restylane and Juvéderm Ultra do not have as much cross-linking as Perlane and Juvéderm Ultra Plus, which gives these two latter products greater longevity when injected into the skin by skilled physicians and injectors. It is beyond the scope of this chapter to review each of the currently available dermal fillers.

In Europe, there are reports of over two hundred HA fillers available for clinicians to choose from for dermal filler injections. Fortunately or unfortunately, most of these products will never receive clearance from the Food and Drug Administration (FDA) for use in the United States, and only those special fillers, with decisive clinical research behind them, will see the U.S. market and be available to U.S. patients. Several new (to the United States) dermal fillers and novel compounds are currently undergoing investigation in the United States, but because of confidentiality agreements and other restrictions, comment on these molecules and products cannot be given in this chapter. Suffice to say, the dermal filler market will undergo more positive change over the next several years, as our armamentarium of filling agents available for our patients increases, ensuring new and various treatment options.

One of the products from Europe that deserves comment is Puragen (Mentor Corp.), a novel HA product that has CE clearance in Europe and, in another form, is in clinical trials in the United States and may be available for clinicians in the United States in the next year or so. Puragen utilizes what is known as DXL technology, and is the first of the HA products to utilize double-cross-linked HA technology, a process that stabilizes extremely pure HA chains using a two-stage process with two separate types of bonds. DXL uses 1,2,7,8-diepoxyoxyoctane to create both ether and ester bonds. This creates a hydrophobic environment, which increases the HA gel network physical bonding, translating into an HA that is highly stable against heat. Additionally, with the additional ester bonds found in this product, the molecular configuration may slow the degradation rate of the cross-linked HA by reducing the diffusion rate of hyaluronidase into the matrix of the filler. This is demonstrated in Figure 11.1. Puragen also uses small HA particles, around 200 μm, and a narrow distribution of the HA particles, which translates clinically into a smooth flow through the syringe into the skin. It also has a low incidence of free HA, or non-cross-linked HA, in the order of 6%. Non-cross-linked HA reabsorbs into the body fairly quickly, and because there is such a small amount of non-cross-linked HA in Puragen, many clinicians find that once injected, Puragen touch-ups are rarely required. Clinical trial work in the United States has focused on a newer form of Puragen, to be known as Puragen Plus. Puragen Plus will utilize the same DXL technology of double-cross-linked HA, but will also contain lidocaine in the syringe to make the injections themselves more comfortable for patients. As stated, clinical research with this HA product has been conducted in the United States, and data collection and FDA submission are pending at this time.

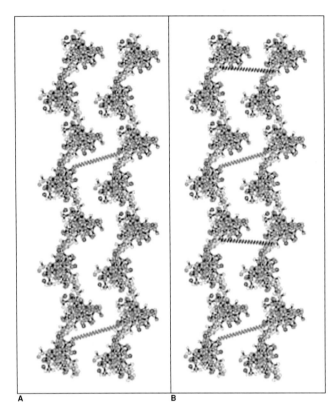

FIGURE 11.1: **A,** *Single-cross-linked fillers are held together with single hydrophilic ether-type bonds.* **B,** *The double cross-linkage between both hydrophilic ether and hydrophobic ester bonds results in more stable molecules with greater resistance to biodegradation.*

As with all the HA products currently available, Puragen Plus, once approved by the FDA, will be cleared for the treatment of dermal defects involving the nasolabial folds. Clinical trial work with all the HA products focuses on the nasolabial folds, and safety and efficacy trials are performed to determine the usefulness of HA products. As with other HA products, skin testing with Puragen and Puragen Plus is not and will not be required, as the incidence of allergic reactions associated with HA products is virtually nonexistent.

PATIENT SELECTION

Patients who have depressions of the nasolabial folds are candidates for Puragen injections. In Europe, Puragen is also available for injection into the lips for lip augmentation. Patient preparation is relatively simple. The treatment areas should be cleansed with an appropriate cleanser after an informed consent is signed by the patient and photographs of the treatment areas are taken. Skin testing with Puragen is not required for patients to receive this treatment. This is consistent with other HA products currently available.

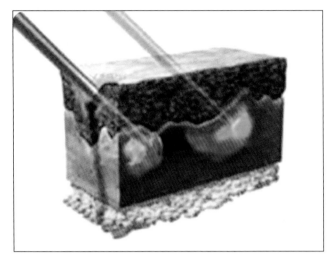

FIGURE 11.2: *Serial puncture technique.*

HOW TO PERFORM THE PROCEDURE

There are various treatment techniques available for the injection of HA. These include the serial puncture technique and the linear thread technique. Both are acceptable for Puragen injections and are shown schematically in Figures 11.2 and 11.3, respectively. This author commonly utilizes the linear threading technique when injecting HA products. The needle is placed into the mid-dermis and HA material is injected into the skin as the needle is removed. Clinical examples of Puragen injections are shown in Figures 11.4 and 11.5.

COMPLICATIONS

HA products are very safe. Allergic reactions are extremely rare. The major adverse effects from these products as a

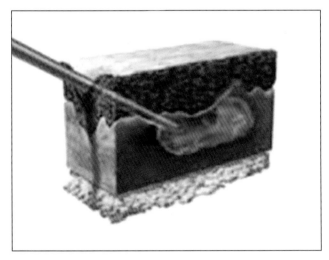

FIGURE 11.3: *Linear thread technique.*

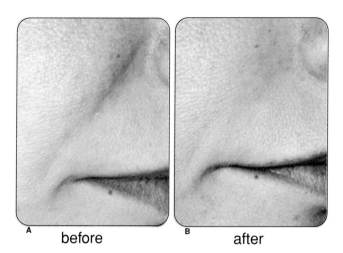
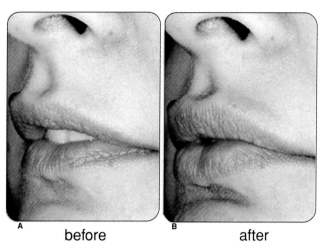

A before   **B** after

FIGURE 11.4: Clinical examples of Puragen injections: naso-labial folds, **A,** *before treatment,* **B,** *after treatment.*

A before   **B** after

FIGURE 11.5: Clinical examples of Puragen injections: **A,** *before treatment;* **B,** *after lip augmentation.*

whole, and Puragen is no exception, involve injection site reactions, which are rare and involve swelling and erythema at the treatment sites that may last from several hours to several days. Most clinicians feel that injection site reactions with the HA family of products partially involve the speed of injection into the skin, and with the newer HA products, we are all aware that slower injection techniques are required to safely deliver these more robust dermal fillers. Following an injection with HA fillers, on occasion, these fillers do not produce a smooth result. This is almost always related to injection technique, and it is prudent for all injectors to be skilled in the injection techniques described pre-

viously before beginning treatment of patients with HA fillers.

Puragen has been found to be safe in clinical trials performed in Europe, and thus far, the Puragen Plus clinical trials in the United States appear to have an excellent safety profile as well.

SUGGESTED READING

Zhao XB, Fraser JE, Alexander C, et al. Synthesis and characterization of a novel double cross linked hyaluronan hydrogel. *J. Mater. Sci. Mater. Med.* 2002;13:11–16.

CHAPTER 12

Puragen: Asian Experience

Taro Kono

Hyaluronic acid (HA) was first discovered by Meyer and Palmer in 1934. HA is a long, linear polysaccharide composed of repeating disaccharide units of N-acetylglucosamine and D-glucuronic acid. HA has potential use in skin rejuvenation, is rapidly metabolized by hyaluronidase and free radicals, and is highly soluble. By using cross-linking agents, the in vivo residence of HA can be increased. Currently various HAs are being used to rejuvenate facial skin. Animal-source single-cross-linked HA was developed in 1990; its concentration is 5.5 mg/mL, and its duration is relatively short. Non-animal-source single-cross-linked HA was developed in 1994, with a concentration of 20–24 mg/mL and a duration that is relatively longer than the animal-source HA. More recently, a non-animal-source double-cross-linked HA, Puragen, which was recently renamed Prevelle (Mentor Corp.), was developed.

WHAT IS PURAGEN?

Restylane and Puragen have the same concentration of HA (20 mg/mL); however, Puragen has different constituent properties from Restylane. First, the HA chains of Puragen are chemically cross-linked, giving in vivo stability to the product. Hylaform, Restylane, and Juvéderm are single cross-linked with ether bonds. Puragen is double cross-linked with ether bonds and ester bonds. Ester bond linkages confer increased stability and protect ether bonds during sterilization, and are hydrophobic. The novel process can be tailored to yield water-insoluble gels and films with a broad range of physical and chemical characteristics, and greater resistance to degradation by hyaluronidase and free radicals. Second, Restylane has a larger particle size (about 250–300 μm) than Puragen (about 200 μm). Third, gel hardness or rheologic properties are measured by energy stored as the gel is deformed through a syringe and are determined by particle size and cross-linking. In a gel with a low degree of cross-linking, where the HA polymer chains are loosely linked to one another, the force required for displacement is low, so gel hardness is low. As the degree of cross-linking is increased at the same overall HA concentration, the network formed by the HA polymers becomes more tightly connected, and a greater force is required to displace the gel. Both Restylane and Puragen have a greater rheologic score, but because of double cross-linking, the gel hardness of Puragen reaches nearly 1,000 Pa. Fourth, regarding the ratio of gel to soluble HA per milliliter, Puragen's ratio is relatively higher than Restylane's. Because the HA concentration of Restylane and Puragen is the same (20 mg/mL), the cross-linked HA concentration of Puragen is higher than that of Restylane. In terms of particle size, Restylane has a potential factor for longevity regarding size, but in terms of the other characteristics, Puragen has several factors contributing to increased longevity (Table 12.1). In my experience, it appears to last longer than Restylane (Figure 12.1).

PATIENT SELECTION

Patients who would like to diminish nasolabial folds, forehead lines, glabellar lines, and upper lip rhytids can attain

TABLE 12.1: Comparison of Restylane and Puragen

	Restylane	Puragen
HA source	Streptococcus equin	Streptococcus equin
HA concentration, mg/mL	20	20
Cross-linking	single	double
Particle size, μm	300	200
No. of gel particle/mL	100,000	150,000
Gel:fluid ratio	unknown	88:12
Gel hardness, Pa	unknown	1,000
Syringe volume, mL	1.0	1.0
Needle size (Gauge)	30	30

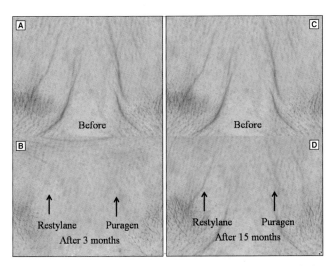

FIGURE 12.1: *Eighty-year-old female. The right side of the glabella was treated with Restylane and the left side was treated with Puragen:* **A**, *before;* **B**, *after three months;* **C**, *before;* **D**, *after fifteen months. Puragen lasts longer than Restylane.*

significant improvement with Puragen, like with other HAs. Lip augmentation has increased in popularity and Puragen is also very effective for this site.

INJECTION TECHNIQUE

Injection techniques are similar to those of other HAs. The advantages of Puragen are its longevity and low degree of swelling. Puragen should only correct to 100% of desired volume. On the other hand, a disadvantage of Puragen is its hardness.

SUGGESTED READING

Zhao XB, Fraser JE, Alexander C, Lockett C, White BJ. Synthesis and characterization of a novel double crosslinked hyaluronan hydrogel. *J. Mater. Sci. Mater. Med.* 2002;13:11–16.

Section 3

COLLAGEN FILLERS

CHAPTER 13

Review of Collagen Fillers

Andrew B. Denton

Nael Shoman

Soft tissue augmentation dates back more than 100 years, and over the past few decades, many agents and techniques have been introduced to cosmetically enhance soft tissue defects. With more patients now seeking aesthetic improvements without major surgery, the emphasis on soft tissue augmentation has received widespread acceptance among patients and physicians. With aging, reduced subcutaneous fat and dermal collagen results in soft tissue volume depletion, which may be superficial, as with facial rhytids, or involve deeper planes.

Collagen is the major insoluble fibrous protein in connective tissue and is the most abundant protein in the body. It provides the major structural component of the dermis, comprising 70% of dry skin mass. There are at least sixteen types of collagen, each denoted by a Roman numeral. Eighty to 90% of the collagen in the body consists of types I, II, and III. Type I collagen was the first to be isolated and characterized. Its fundamental structural unit is a long (300 nm), thin (1.5 nm diameter) protein that consists of three coiled subunits: two α1 chains and one α2 chain. Each chain contains 1,050 amino acids wound around one another in a characteristic right-handed triple helix. The collagen triple-helical structure contains an abundance of three amino acids, glycine, proline, and hydroxyproline, making up the characteristic repeating motif Gly-Pro-X, where X can be any amino acid. Collagen is synthesized by fibroblasts as α procollagen, and the posttranslational hydroxylation of proline residues is performed by propyl hydroxylase in the presence of ascorbic acid (vitamin C). About 96% of the chain length is helical, with nonhelical telopeptides at the amino- and carboxylter-

mini. These telopeptides contain important antigenic loci. Hydrogen bonds linking the peptide bond NH of a glycine residue with a peptide carbonyl (C=O) group in an adjacent polypeptide help hold the three chains together. Many three-stranded type I collagen molecules pack together side by side, forming fibrils with a diameter of 50–200 nm. These fibrils, roughly 50 nm in diameter and several micrometers long, are packed side by side in parallel bundles, called *collagen fibers*. All collagens were eventually shown to contain three-stranded helical segments of similar structure; the combination of 3α chains determines the type of the resulting collagen molecule.

During the embryonic period, collagen type III predominates in human skin. After birth, the ratio of collagen type I increases. Dermal collagen in adult skin is composed of type I (80 to 85%) and type III (10 to 15%), in addition to glycosaminoglycans and elastin fibers. Type I collagen remains the predominant type during childhood and early adulthood, but the proportion of type III will increase with aging. Overall, collagen production by fibroblasts decreases with age, accounting for an overall 20% reduction in dermal thickness in aged skin. Ultraviolet radiation will increase the level of matrix metalloproteinases (e.g., collagenase), which will accelerate collagen degradation and skin aging.

The first attempt at soft tissue augmentation was in 1893, when Neuber transplanted fat from the arm into facial defects. In 1899, Gersuny became the first to use an injectable material for a cosmetic deformity, when he injected paraffin into a patient's scrotum to create a testicular prosthesis. Although paraffin initially gained popularity as a filler material, the associated risk of foreign body granulomas resulted in abandonment of its use in the 1920s. Liquid silicone was later developed in the 1960s as a filler agent and was utilized widely for superficial and deep soft tissue deformities, despite lack of Food and Drug Administration (FDA) approval. Its use, however, was burdened with risks of permanent beading, migration, and granuloma formation. Silicone was largely abandoned in the early 1980s. Because of the obvious defect in collagen in aged skin, the use of collagen as a filler became popular with the introduction and FDA approval of Zyderm, a bovine collagen, in 1981. An abundance of agents were introduced over the past two decades in a continuing quest for the ideal dermal filler (Table 13.1).

XENOGENIC MATERIALS

Bovine collagen was first extracted from fresh calf skin in 1958 by Gross and Kirk at the Harvard Medical School. They later demonstrated that under physiologic conditions, collagen has the property of precipitating into a rigid gel composed of fibrils with the characteristic axial periodicity of native collagen. Studies in the 1960s demonstrated that the major immunogenic sites in native tropocollagen are the telopeptides, and as such, selective removal of the nonhelical amino- and carboxylterminal segments of the collagen molecule significantly reduced its antigenicity. Investigators at Stanford University began work in the early 1970s on developing a clinically useful collagen implant material. In 1977, they injected purified human, rabbit, and rat collagen into rats and studied the evolution of the implants over time using light and scanning electron microscopy. In that same year, they published the results of their initial clinical trials using allogenic and xenogenic (bovine) collagen injection in twenty-eight patients, involving more than six hundred individual injections. Of twenty-eight patients, there was moderate to profound improvement in twenty-four, with follow-up periods exceeding one year.

Injectable bovine collagen was first introduced to the market as Zyderm (Collagen Corp.) in 1976 and was approved by the FDA in 1981 for the treatment of facial lines and wrinkles. It is a purified, enzyme-digested bovine collagen with the telopeptide regions of the molecule removed to reduce product antigenicity. The collagen is extracted from the hides of a closed American herd to protect against the possibility of bovine spongiform encephalopathy virus or prion contamination. Zyderm I, the initial product released, comprised 96% type I collagen, with the remainder being type III collagen, suspended in phosphate-buffered physiologic saline with 0.3% lidocaine. It is 3.5% bovine dermal collagen by weight. Due to quick resorption of the collagen, Zyderm II was thereafter introduced with an increased collagen concentration of 6.5% bovine dermal collagen by weight. Zyderm II gained FDA approval in 1983.

In an effort to produce a material with a longer-lasting effect, the collagen in Zyderm was cross-linked through glutaraldehyde processing by forming covalent bridges between 10% of available lysine residues, effectively inhibiting degradation by collagenase. The resulting product, Zyplast, was FDA approved in 1985. It is 3.5% bovine dermal collagen by weight and is more viscous, more resilient to biodegradation, and less immunogenic than Zyderm.

Zyderm and Zyplast are prepackaged in 1- or 2-mL syringes, and Zyderm II is packaged in 0.5-mL syringes; all are administered through a small-gauge needle. The products are stored at low temperature (4 degrees Celsius) and consolidate into a solid gel once implanted at body temperature. Zyderm I is injected into the superficial papillary layer, Zyderm II into the middermis layer, and Zyplast into the deep dermis. Zyderm I and II are used for correction of soft distensible lesions in the face with relatively smooth margins. These would include glabellar, forehead, and periorbital rhytids as well as fine perioral rhytids, acne scars, traumatic and surgical scars, and steroid-induced atrophy. Zyderm II has more collagen and is therefore more effective in moderate to deep wrinkles. Zyplast is more valuable in treating deeper lines often unresponsive to Zyderm such as nasolabial folds, deep acne scars, and the vermilion border of the lips. With Zyderm I, overcorrection by 100% is required as it is diluted with phosphate-buffered physiologic saline, which is reabsorbed typically over two to three months. With Zyderm II, 50% overcorrection is recommended. No overcorrection is required with Zyplast. As the saline is absorbed, host connective tissue cells grow into the collagen, giving the appearance of normal tissue. Eventually, the injected collagen is detected as a foreign substance, with an ensuing inflammatory response. Overall, results, albeit variable and dependent on the facial anatomic region, injection depth, and agent used, typically last two to three months for Zyderm, with Zyplast lasting about three to four months.

Prior to the administration of these products, intradermal skin testing is required. Approximately 3 to 5% of people will display a delayed hypersensitivity response to the skin challenge, generally by forty-eight to seventy-two hours. 1 to 2% of people may be sensitized following the skin challenge, and as such, many practitioners as well as the American Academy of Dermatology recommend a second skin test a few weeks following the first. Repeated injections may result in the development of hypersensitivity to bovine collagen. In general, skin testing is necessary for any patients new to bovine collagen as well as for patients who have not received treatment with bovine collagen for over one year.

Bovine collagen injections are contraindicated in patients undergoing treatment with steroids, in those with a history of allergy to other bovine products or meat or to lidocaine, or in those with a history of an autoimmune

TABLE 13.1: Summary of Collagen Fillers

Name	FDA	Ingredient	Duration of Effect (months)	Allergy Tests Needed	Storage: Shelf Life	Sizes Available	Rhytid Size: Indicated	Degree of Overcorrection
Zyderm I	yes	bovine collagen	3–4	two skin tests 2–4 weeks apart; may treat 4 weeks after second skin test	35 mg/mL; refrigerated 3 years	0.5, 1.0, and 1.5 cc syringes	fine lines	1.5–2.0 times
Zyderm II	yes	bovine collagen	3–4	two skin tests 2–4 weeks apart; may treat 4 weeks after second skin test	65 mg/mL; refrigerated 3 years	0.5 and 1.0 cc syringes	fine lines	1.5–2.0 times
Zyplast	yes	cross-linked bovine collagen	3–5	two skin tests 2–4 weeks apart; may treat 4 weeks after second skin test	35 mg/mL; refrigerated 3 years	0.5, 1.0, 2.0, and 2.5 cc syringes	large folds	no overcorrection
Cosmoderm I	yes	human collagen	3–4	no skin test	35 mg/mL; room temperature shelf life unknown	1.0 cc syringes	fine lines	100% overcorrection
Cosmoderm II	yes	human collagen	3–4	no skin test	65 mg/mL	0.5 cc only	fine lines	no overcorrection
Cosmoplast	yes	cross-linked human collagen	3–4	no skin test	35 mg/mL; refrigerated 3 years	1.0 and 1.5 cc syringes	large folds	no overcorrection
Autologen	yes	autologous collagen fibrils, elastin, fibronectin, and glycosaminoglycans	4–9	no skin test	50–120 mg/mL; frozen (kept with manufacturer) 5 years	3 mL syringes	moderate to deep defects	20% to 30% overcorrection
Isolagen	no	autologous cultured fibroblasts	unclear	test dose done 2 weeks prior to treatment	frozen (kept with manufacturer)	1–1.5 mL syringes	superficial to moderate defects	
Dermalogen	no	cadaveric suspension of types I and III collagen				1.0 mL syringes		20% to 30% overcorrection
Alloderm	yes	allogenic matrix of collagen, elastin, and glycosaminoglycans	12–24		sheets of different sizes (1 × 2 cm; 4 × 12 cm); room temperature 2 years	sheets	deep defects and scars	up to 200% overcorrection
Cymetra	yes	injectable form of Alloderm	3–6		330-mg powder in 5-cc syringe; room temperature 2 years	5 cc syringes	deep defects and scars	30% overcorrection
Fascian	yes	allogenic preserved particulate fascia	3–6	contraindicated with gentamicin allergy	80 mg/2 mL; room temperature 2 years	0.25, 0.5, 1.0, and 2.0 ug particles; 80 mg in each 3 cc syringe	deep defects and scars	
Evolence	no	cross-linked porcine collagen	12	no skin test	35 mg/ml; room temperature 3 years	1.0 cc syringe	moderate to deep lines and folds, lips	no overcorrection

disorder, particularly a collagen vascular disease. Zyplast is contraindicated for the treatment of glabellar rhytids due to the possibility of central retinal artery occlusion. Bruising, scarring, and infection may appear postinjection. Localized necrosis occurs with an incidence of 0.09%, with the glabellar area at higher risk due to its dependence on the supratrochlear vessels for perfusion. Reactivation of herpes is possible with lip injections, and as such, patients with a positive history need antiviral prophylaxis. Approximately 0.5% of patients may experience systemic symptoms with flulike symptoms, paresthesias, or difficulty breathing.

BIOENGINEERED HUMAN COLLAGENS

The human-derived collagens Cosmoderm and Cosmoplast were FDA approved in March 2003 for cosmetic indications and contain types I and III human bioengineered collagen. They do not require skin tests prior to treatment.

Dermal fibroblasts are harvested from bioengineered human skin cells qualified by extensive testing for viruses, retroviruses, cell morphology, karyology, isoenzymes, and tumorigenicity. The cells are seeded onto a three-dimensional mesh that is then cultured in a bioreactor under conditions simulating those found in the human body. The fibroblast cells attach to the mesh within the reactor, replicate, and secrete collagen and extracellular proteins. The developing dermal tissue on the mesh is identical to the human dermis but lacks immunological cells and melanocytes. The extracellular type I and type III collagen is isolated from the resulting dermal tissue and is capable of binding with hyaluronic acid and other molecules to provide structure to the skin. As with Zyplast, Cosmoplast has gluteraldehyde cross-linking the lysine residues to make it more resilient to degradation by collagenase.

Cosmoderm I contains 35 mg/mL of collagen dispersed in a phosphate buffered saline solution and 0.3% lidocaine. Cosmoderm II is similar but contains about twice the collagen concentration. Cosmoplast is similar to Cosmoderm I but is cross-linked with gluteraldehyde. These products are prepackaged in 1-mL syringes and should be refrigerated (4 degrees Celsius) but not frozen. They are typically injected using a 30-gauge needle. The manufacturer recommends administration with an accurate depth gauge assist device on the needle, adjusted so that a 2-mm length of the needle tip is exposed.

Cosmoderm is injected into the superficial papillary dermis, and Cosmoplast is injected into the mid- to deep dermis. Cosmoderm is best suited for correcting fine lines and acne scars, and Cosmoplast is best suited for the correction of deeper rhytids, for smoothing scars, and for lip enhancement. Overcorrection by 150 to 200% is necessary with Cosmoderm because it is diluted with saline, which is reabsorbed. A lesser degree of overcorrection is needed for Cosmoderm II than for Cosmoderm I, and no overcorrection is needed with Cosmoplast. Results seen with these products are immediate, and the duration of effect is typically three to six months.

The use of these products is contraindicated in patients with a lidocaine allergy, and they should be used cautiously in patients with autoimmune diseases such as rheumatoid arthritis.

AUTOLOGOUS HUMAN COLLAGENS

In the late 1980s, a research and development biomedical lab (Autogenesis Technologies) investigated the feasibility of extracting intact human collagen fibers for injection from skin obtained electively during aesthetic plastic surgical procedures. Results reported with injectable autologous collagen varied, and further development of this product resulted in Autologen (Collagenesis Inc.).

Autologen is a dermal matrix dispersion derived from the patient's own skin, predominantly composed of intact collagen fibrils of types I, III, and IV. Processing of the specimen allows for isolation of collagen fibrils, elastin, fibronectin, and glycosaminoglycans. Syringes are returned to the physician after three to four weeks. Unlike bovine collagen, which is treated to remove the telopeptide allogenic units, Autologen contains only human proteins, and no such treatment is required. The collagen concentration ranges from 50 to 120 mg/mL. Only a limited amount of collagen tissue persists with each injection, and usually, three or more injections are given over a period of several weeks to fully correct most dermal defects. Overcorrection of approximately 30% is recommended during each treatment. The tight collagen fibrils and lack of xenoproteins are thought to result in minimal inflammatory response, with tissue augmentation relying mostly on the injected collagen. On average, 1.0 mL of 5% Autologen requires 2 square inches of skin (excluding skin obtained from blepharoplasty). Harvested skin can be stored at Collagenesis BioBank if immediate use is not needed or uncertain. Autologen is available in 1.0-mL syringes and is stored under refrigeration for up to six months.

Skin testing is not needed with the use of Autologen. Its autologous nature further eliminates the potential for donor-to-recipient disease transmission. While the concept of Autologen may be very attractive for patients undergoing skin excision procedures, those who are not must subject themselves to a skin harvesting procedure. The injectable material is not prepared with lidocaine and so the injections are more painful, and may necessitate nerve blocks or topical anesthesia. Autologen augmentation can last three to six months; however, a recent study showed no statistically significant difference between Autologen and Zyplast in implant persistence over a twelve-week period.

ALLOGENIC HUMAN COLLAGENS

The advantages of Autologen compared to other intradermal injectable biomaterials were offset by the need for an elective surgical procedure during which skin was removed. As such, the search continued for an allogenic injectable human collagen available prepackaged from tissue donors. Central to this search is the concept that intraspecies collagen is identical, and as such, an economically available and safe allogenic collagen product could be harvested that is essentially identical to autologous collagen.

Dermalogen (Collagenesis Inc.) is a dermal filler derived from human cadavers at tissue banks accredited by the American Association of Tissue Banks. The skin is deep-ithelialized and aseptically processed to provide an acellular suspension of collagen fibers and human collagen tissue matrix. The product is structurally identical to Autologen, but without the need for the preliminary harvesting and prolonged processing. The donors' past medical and social histories are thoroughly reviewed; blood samples are taken for viral testing; and skin specimens are tested for bacterial, fungal, or viral contamination. A sterilization protocol is followed despite negative screening for known pathogens. The final product is supplied in boxes of six 1.0-mL syringes that can be refrigerated for six months.

Skin testing prior to treatment with Dermalogen is not required but is recommended to ensure that no hypersensitivity to the delivery vehicle or by-products of processing exists. Intradermal injections of Dermalogen supplied in separate containers for this purpose are typically administered to the volar forearm, and absence of a reaction at seventy-two hours excludes a hypersensitivity response. A single test is sufficient. Dermalogen is injected into the middermis, with 20 to 30% overcorrection recommended. The results with Dermalogen have been generally satisfactory, with a duration lasting approximately three to six months.

Alloderm (LifeCell Corp.) is an acellular processed human dermal allograft matrix derived from cadaveric skin at tissue banks and has been in use since 1992. A freeze-drying process eliminates all cells and leaves a matrix of collagen and dermal elements, including laminin, elastin, and proteoglycans. No class I or II histocompatibility antigens were shown using immunohistochemical staining. Alloderm has the capacity to incorporate into the surrounding tissue, acting as a framework to allow ingrowth of native tissue and allowing for revascularization. It is manufactured as sheets and, following rehydration, is inserted through an incision or dissected dermal tunnels. It may be used for treating full-thickness burns, surgical defects, and acne scars as well as for soft tissue augmentation. Alloderm sheet volume persistence is significantly greater than Zyplast during the first three months after placement. Overcorrection is needed and will depend on the size of the defect, but up to 200% may be necessary.

Cymetra (LifeCell Corp.), available since 2000, is a micronized form of Alloderm for injectable use. Strips of homogenized Alloderm sheets are cut out, dried, and packed as 330 mg of product in 5-cc syringes that may be refrigerated for up to six months. The freeze-dried particles are mixed with 1 mL of lidocaine or saline up to two hours prior to injection. Once injected, host fibroblast and collagen ingrowth as well as neovascularization ensue. Overcorrection by 30% is recommended, and multiple treatments may be warranted. The duration of response is generally noted to be longer than bovine collagen, lasting approximately four to six months. As with Alloderm, skin testing is not required.

Fascia has been extensively utilized in the past for numerous applications, including suture material, dura repair, tendon and ligament repair, and tympanic membrane replacement. Clinical response persists for years following implantation, with minimal complications. Native collagen ultimately replaces implanted fascial grafts, as consistently demonstrated by histological studies. Dermatologic applications were first adopted by Burres in 1994, who utilized the material for volume replacement. His work on acne scars and, later, on lip augmentation led the development of preserved particulate fascia (Fascian, Fascia Biosystems), first distributed as an injectable filler material in 1998. The fascia in Fascian comes primarily from human cadaveric donor gastrocnemius fascia. Following processing through sterilized baths, the material is freeze-dried to a water content of less than 6%, and is then sterilized with gamma radiation and ethylene oxide. The graft is then particulated and loaded into vacuum-packed syringes. Syringes of five different particle sizes (0.1, 0.25, 0.5, 1, and 2 mm) are available, each containing 80 mg. Because the material is freeze-dried, it may be stored at room temperature for up to five years. Fascian particulate and 1.5–2.0 mL of 0.5% lidocaine are mixed in the syringes for one minute. The finer particles may be injected with a 20- to 25-gauge needle, but the larger particles may require a 14- to 18-gauge needle. No skin testing or refrigeration is required; however, trace amounts of polymyxin B, bacitracin, and/or gentamicin may be present in Fascian and may trigger a hypersensitivity response in allergic recipients. Injections should only be made in healed defects without active inflammation. Fascian may be injected intradermally, subdermally, or in the subcutaneous tissue. After injection, the graft matrix is digested over the ensuing several months. New collagen is then laid down by invading fibroblasts, a process termed *recollagenation* by Burres, and as such, preserved fascia grafts may result in longer-lasting tissue augmentation. Although the exact duration remains largely unknown, one study found Fascian still persistent three to four months following injection.

EVOLENCE AND EVOLENCE BREEZE

Evolence and Evolence Breeze (ColBar LifeScience Ltd.) are the latest products available in the evolution of collagen-derived fillers. Both Evolence and Evolence Breeze are produced from the same porcine collagen and are formulated at a collagen concentration of 35 mg/mL. The products differ in their rheologic properties, which are reflected in their viscosity and injectability properties. The viscosity of Evolence Breeze is approximately 60% of the viscosity of Evolence and is injectable through a 30-gauge needle. Evolence has been available in Europe and Canada for a couple years, and it appears to be a far superior product in terms of duration of results than the Zyplast/Cosmoplast products, and at least comparable to Restylane/Perlane, Juvéderm, and Radiesse. Evolence became available in the United States in late 2008, and Evolence Breeze is expected in early 2009. Both are discussed in more detail in Chapter 15. Table 13.1 summarizes collagen-based products.

SUGGESTED READING

Baumann L, Kaufman J, Saghari S. Collagen fillers. *Dermatol. Ther.* 2006;19:134–40.

Eppley BL, Dadvand B. Injectable soft-tissue fillers: clinical overview. *Plast. Reconstr. Surg.* 2006;118:98e–106e.

Fagien S. Facial soft tissue augmentation with autologous and homologous injectable collagen. In: Klein AW, ed., *Tissue Augmentation in Clinical Practice: Procedures and Techniques.* New York: Marcel Dekker; 1998:88–124.

Klein AW. Skin filling: collagen and other injectables of the skin. *Dermatol. Clin.* 2001;19:491–508.

Knapp TR, Luck E, Daniels JR. Injectable collagen for soft tissue augmentation. *Plast. Reconstr. Surg.* 1977;60:398–405.

Lowe NJ, Maxwell CA, Patnaik R. Adverse reactions to dermal fillers: review. *Dermatol. Surg.* 2005;31(11 Pt 2):1616–25.

Matton G, Anseeuw A, De Keyser F. The history of injectable biomaterials and the biology of collagen. *Aesthetic Plast. Surg.* 1985;9:133–40.

Skouge J, Diwan R. Soft tissue augmentation with injectable collagen. In: Papel I, Nachlas N, eds., *Facial Plastic and Reconstructive Surgery.* St Louis: Mosby Year Book; 1992;203–12.

CHAPTER 14

Human and Bovine Collagen-Based Fillers

Sogol Saghari

Derek Jones

Dermal matrix in adult skin is composed of type I (80 to 85%) and type III collagen (10 to 15%), in addition to glycosaminoglycans and elastin. Decreased collagen synthesis and increased levels of matrix metalloproteinases, including collagenase, result in reduction and alteration in dermal collagen. The art of soft tissue augmentation was directed toward collagen implants in the 1970s at Stanford University, where researchers first studied bovine- and human-derived collagen as injectable implants. In recent years, significant growth has been observed both in the development of newer dermal implants and in patients' interest in treatment with these products.

This chapter will discuss the available animal- and human-derived collagen products, in addition to their clinical applications, advantages, and disadvantages.

BOVINE-DERIVED COLLAGEN IMPLANTS

Bovine-derived collagen implants were introduced in the 1970s for correction of facial lines and were the most popular dermal implants for about two decades in the United States. These products include Zyderm I, Zyderm II, and Zyplast. Zyderm I and Zyderm II contain 35 mg/cc and 65 mg/cc of bovine collagen, respectively, dispersed in a phosphate-based solution and lidocaine. Zyplast is composed of 35 mg/cc of bovine collagen and is cross-linked by 0.0075% gluteraldehyde in addition to lidocaine. Zyderm I and II are intended for correction of superficial, etched-in rhytids and are expected to provide a duration of correction of two to three months. The cross-linked collagen in Zyplast provides more resistance to degradation and extends the duration of correction to four to five months. Zyplast is indicated for the correction of nasolabial folds, melolabial folds, and the vermilion border of the lip. It is contraindicated in the glabella due to an increased risk of glabellar necrosis. Zyderm I, Zyderm II, and Zyplast were approved by the Food and Drug Administration (FDA) in 1981, 1983, and 1985, respectively. These products are required to be stored at refrigerator temperature.

Skin testing is required prior to injections of bovine collagen. It is recommended that patients receive double skin tests. The skin test is performed by intradermal injection of 0.1 mL of the collagen implant test syringe in the volar aspect of the forearm. If the first test is negative, there is still a 1.3 to 6.2% chance of developing an allergic reaction to the product. Therefore a second test is recommended at four weeks. A positive reaction is manifested by delayed development of erythema and induration, commonly associated with pruritus. Although two negative skin tests decrease the chance of allergic hypersensitivity developing, a very small risk still remains in 0.5% of patients. Allergic reactions to bovine collagen resolve spontaneously within a few months and may be treated with topical or oral corticosteroids. There is one report of a patient with hypersensitivity who improved within eighteen days when treated with oral cyclosporine. Bovine collagen implants, due to hypersensitivity reactions and relatively short duration of correction, have recently lost their popularity, since human-based collagen and hyaluronic acid fillers have been introduced to the market.

Artecoll is composed of 80% bovine collagen and 20% polymethylacrylate (PMMA) microspheres, in addition to lidocaine. After injection, the bovine collagen is degraded and gradually replaced by native collagen, which forms secondary to fibroplasia around the durable PMMA microspheres. The nonbiodegradable nature of PMMA particles provides a sustained correction of the folds. Since this product is bovine derived, pretesting of the skin is required prior to injection.

HUMAN-BIOENGINEERED COLLAGEN

Possible hypersensitivity reactions to animal-derived collagen implants led to the development of human-derived collagen fillers. Human-bioengineered collagen implants include Cosmoplast, Cosmoderm I, and Cosmoderm II (Inamed Corp.). Dermal fibroblasts derived from human skin cells are cultured in a fibroblast growth media,

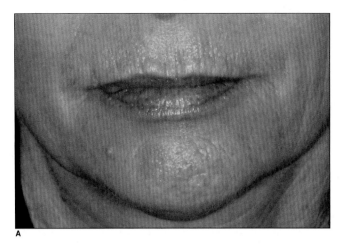 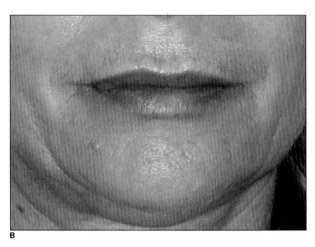

FIGURE 14.1: *Cosmoplast and Zyplast are intended for correction of deeper folds such as nasolabial folds, melolabial folds, and vermilion border of the lips:* **A**, *before;* **B**, *after.*

simulating growth factors in human skin, which generates types I and III collagen. Cosmoderm I and Cosmoderm II contain 35 mg/cc and 65 mg/cc human-based collagen, respectively, along with 0.3% lidocaine. They are most appropriate for the correction of superficial, etched-in lines of the face, such as perioral and glabellar lines, and are expected to provide correction for two to three months. Cosmoplast also contains 35 mg/cc human-based collagen but is cross-linked by gluteraldehyde in a phosphate-based solution and 0.3% lidocaine. The cross-linked collagen provides more resistance to degradation. Cosmoplast is most suitable for medium to deep facial wrinkles, such as nasolabial and melolabial folds, and the vermilion border of the lips and is expected to provide correction for three to four months. Like Zyplast, it is contraindicated in the glabella as it may be associated with an increased chance of glabellar necrosis. Human-derived collagen fillers do not require skin testing prior to injection. Cosmoplast, Cosmoderm I, and Cosmoderm II were FDA approved in the United States in March 2003. As with Zyplast and Zyderm, these products require refrigeration.

INJECTION TECHNIQUE

Patient education and obtaining informed consent are key aspects of treatment. It is recommended that the patient be placed in an upright position. Due to gravity, facial lines and folds are more defined in an upright position when compared to a reclined position. Patients' comfort and pain management play an important role in an easier process of injection. Topical anesthesia may be applied to the area of injection fifteen to thirty minutes prior to the procedure. Collagen implants containing lidocaine provide some pain control with injection. In addition, when used in combination and prior to hyaluronic acid injections, the lidocaine grants a painless hyaluronic acid injection process. Regional blocks may be used on sensitive patients. Injections should be performed using a 30-gauge needle at a 45 degree angle with the skin, medial to the fold or wrinkle. Cosmoderm and Zyderm are used in the correction of superficial facial lines such as perioral, glabellar, and periocular lines. They are injected superficially in the papillary dermis using the serial puncture technique. The blanching effect of the skin after injection confirms the correct level of injection. Cosmoplast and Zyplast are intended for correction of deeper folds such as nasolabial folds, melolabial folds, and the vermilion border of the lips (Figure 14.1). They are injected slightly deeper in the middermis using the linear threading technique. If injected too superficially, the material may become visible and cause beading of overlying skin. Overcorrection of the folds is recommended with most collagen fillers. The swelling and edema caused by injection will resolve in a few hours.

Artecoll/ArteFill should be injected with 27- and 26-gauge needles, respectively, and placed in the junction between the dermis and subcutaneous fat using a tunneling technique. Overcorrection is not recommended with these products.

ADVERSE EVENTS

Ecchymoses, edema, reactivation of herpes virus, beading, cyst and abscess formation, allergic reactions, and local necrosis are among the side effects of collagen implants. Bruising may be minimized by avoidance of aspirin, NSAIDs (nonsteroidal anti-inflamatory drugs), vitamin E, anticoagulants, and other medications and natural supplements that make patients prone to bleeding.

Patients with a history of herpes labialis may warrant prophylaxis with antiviral medications. Local necrosis has been reported in the glabellar area and is believed to be secondary to vascular occlusive injury due to intravascular injection or extravascular compression. It is recommended that the physician inject only Zyderm and Cosmoderm in the glabellar lines and that he or she avoids injecting Zyplast and Cosmoplast in the glabella. There are reports of granulomas following Artecoll injection. Therefore selecting appropriate areas for injection and the correct level of material placement is important when injecting Artecoll.

The possibility of an increased risk of developing autoimmune disorders (in particular, dermatomyositis) after collagen implants has been a subject of debate. Hanke et al. (1996) demonstrated that the incidence rate of dermatomyositis in subjects who received bovine collagen was not higher than in a controlled match population. Development of cross-reacting antibodies, especially with animal-derived collagen, is theoretically possible, but studies have shown such risks to be unlikely.

SUMMARY

Collagen implants replenish the collagen lost due to aging. Human-derived collagen fillers are considered safe and effective and carry a low side effect profile when used appropriately. Although the popularity of bovine and human collagen products has declined since the introduction of hyaluronic acid implants, Cosmoderm and Zyderm are still the most effective fillers for treating superficial, etched in lines that may be too superficial to be injected with hyaluronic acids without creating beading.

SUGGESTED READING

Alcalay J, Alkalay R, Gat A, Yorav S. Late-onset granulomatous reaction to Artecoll. *Dermatol. Surg.* 2003;29:859–62.

Baumann L. Soft tissue augmentation. In: Baumann L, ed., *Cosmetic Dermatology Principles and Practice*. New York: McGraw-Hill; 2002:155–72.

Baumann LS, Kerdel F. The treatment of bovine collagen allergy with cyclosporin. *Dermatol. Surg.* 1999;25:247–51.

Castrow FF, Krull EA. Injectable collagen implant – update. *J. Am. Acad. Dermatol.* 1983;9:889–99.

Hanke CW, Higley HR, Jolivette DM, Swanson NA, Stegman SJ. Abscess formation and local necrosis after treatment with Zyderm or Zyplast collagen implant. *J. Am. Acad. Dermatol.* 1991;25:319–26.

Hanke CW, Thomas JA, Lee WT, Jolivette DM, Rosenberg MJ. Risk assessment of polymyositis/dermatomyositis after treatment with injectable bovine collagen implants. *J. Am. Acad. Dermatol.* 1996;34:450–4.

Kim KJ, Lee HW, Lee MW, Choi JH, Moon KC, Koh JK. Artecoll granuloma: a rare adverse reaction induced by micro-implant in the treatment of neck wrinkles. *Dermatol. Surg.* 2004;30(4 Pt 1):545–7.

Klein AW, Elson ML. The history of substances for soft tissue augmentation. *Dermatol. Surg.* 2000;26:1096–105.

Rosenberg MJ, Reichlin M. Is there an association between injectable collagen and polymyositis/dermatomyositis? *Arthritis Rheum.* 1994;37:747–53.

Siegle RJ, McCoy JP, Schade W, et al. Intradermal implantation of bovine collagen: humoral immune responses associated with clinical reactions. *Arch. Dermatol.* 1984;120:183–9.

CHAPTER 15

Porcine Collagen: Evolence

Andrew B. Denton

Nael Shoman

Evolence and Evolence Breeze (ColBar LifeScience Ltd.) are the latest products available in the evolution of collagen-derived fillers. Both Evolence and Evolence Breeze are produced from the same porcine collagen and are formulated at collagen concentrations of 35 mg/mL. The products differ in their rheologic properties, which are reflected in their viscosity and injectability properties. The viscosity of Evolence Breeze is approximately 60% of the viscosity of Evolence and is injectable through a 30-gauge needle. The force that is needed to inject Evolence Breeze from the syringe (extrusion force) through a 30-gauge needle at a flow rate of 1 mL/min is 10 N. Evolence exhibits a similar extrusion force as Evolence Breeze of about 10 N when tested on a 27-gauge needle.

During production, collagen from porcine tendons is broken down into collagen molecules. Next, the antigenic telopeptides are removed from the molecules, which are then purified. Following purification, the monomeric collagen is polymerized to create collagen fibers, which are then cross-linked using d-ribose in a proprietary technique known as Glymatrix Technology. ColBar LifeScience contends that by using a natural and nontoxic cross-linking agent (d-ribose), a higher degree of cross-linking can be achieved than is possible with the use of other agents (e.g., formalin and glutaraldehyde), which are limited by toxicity.

Evolence is indicated for the treatment of moderate to deep facial lines and wrinkles as well as for lip augmentation. Evolence Breeze is well suited to the treatment of fine lines and wrinkles and effacement of the nasojugal fold area (Figures 15.1 and 15.2). Current experience suggests aesthetic improvement for a period of up to twelve months following treatment, which, if validated by comparative clinical studies, is significantly longer than any previously available collagen-derived injectable filler. Furthermore, because porcine collagen is highly compatible with the human immune system, no allergy skin test is required prior to treatment.

TECHNIQUE

For those accustomed to using the hyaluronic acid family of fillers, some modifications in technique are necessary to

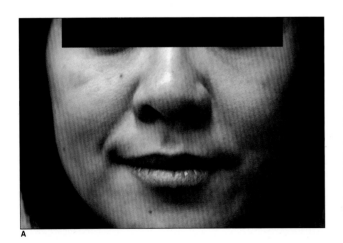
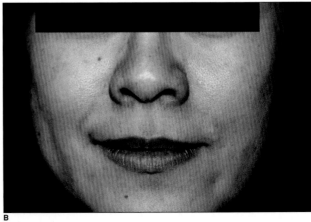

FIGURE 15.1: *Evolence for nasojugal folds:* **A,** *before;* **B,** *after treatment.*

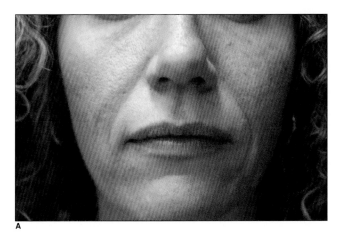 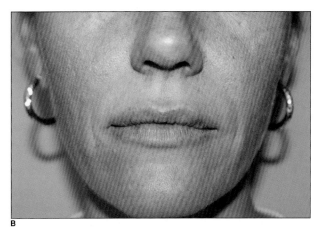

FIGURE 15.2: *Evolence for nasojugal folds:* **A**, *before;* **B**, *after treatment.*

achieve optimal results with Evolence and Evolence Breeze. Both fillers are supplied in 1-mL ergonomic syringes with a rotating finger support to allow viewing of the syringe calibration at all times. Prior to connecting the needle to the syringe, the product present in the terminal lumen should be expressed and discarded to reduce the risk of needle plugging. Evolence is injected using a 27-gauge needle, and Evolence Breeze is injected through either a 27-gauge or 30-gauge needle. Evolence is placed in the mid- to deep dermis and Evolence Breeze in the mid-dermis. The flow characteristics are less consistent than when using hyaluronic acid, and variations in the amount of force applied to the plunger are necessary. Needle plugging may occur, albeit much less commonly than when the product was initially introduced. If this occurs, do not attempt to force the issue and simply change the needle. We recommend regional blocks of the infraorbital and mentalis nerves using 1% lidocaine without epinephrine prior to treatment. A 27-gauge, 1¼ inch needle on a 3-cc syringe is ideal for this purpose. Icing the area prior to treatment

will also reduce the risk of bruising. It is very important to massage the product immediately after placement to mold and smooth the contour. This is critical to achieve optimal results, and we recommend using either a gloved finger or a clean cotton-tipped applicator. No overcorrection is required. Posttreatment edema is minimal.

Thus far, results have been favorable and patient satisfaction high. Some patients have commented on the palpability of the product, particularly in the oral commissural area; however, with appropriate pretreatment education, this has not been a problem. We have yet to use either product in a patient with a documented allergy to bovine collagen and would recommend proceeding very carefully in such a case.

SUGGESTED READING

Baumann L, Kaufman J, Saghari S. Collagen fillers. *Dermatol. Ther.* 2006;19:134–40.

Eppley BL, Dadvand B. Injectable soft-tissue fillers: clinical overview. *Plast. Reconstr. Surg.* 2006;118:98e–106e.

Section 4

CALCIUM HYDROXYLAPATITE (RADIESSE)

CHAPTER 16

Calcium Hydroxylapatite (Radiesse): A Facial Plastic Surgeon's Approach

Paul H. Garlich

Devinder S. Mangat

With their safety, effectiveness, and longevity increasing, public interest in soft tissue fillers is proportionally increasing. Patients not yet ready for traditional cosmetic surgery are looking for simpler means to correct the gravitational and deleterious effects of aging. Be it the atrophy of facial fat, the thinning of lips, the furrowing of the middle and lower face, or the deepening of the melolabial (nasolabial) folds, soft tissue fillers offer an immediate and relatively uncomplicated corrective measure. Calcium hydroxylapatite (Radiesse, Bioform Inc.) is a recent entry into the cosmetic surgery practitioner's armamentarium.

CaHA is a biocompatible material that has the important qualities of being latex-free, nontoxic, nonmutagenic, nonantigenic, and nonirritating. It is a semisolid, cohesive implant material consisting of CaHA microspheres that range from 25 to 45 μm in diameter, suspended in a gel consisting of water, glycerin, and carboxymethylcellulose. CaHA is an inorganic component normally found in teeth and bone, thus its attractive safety profile. CaHA, which should be injected in a subdermal plane, has been shown to elicit no foreign body reaction or toxicity.

Although it has been used safely, and with Food and Drug Administration (FDA) approval, in laryngeal augmentation; soft tissue marking; and oral, maxillofacial, and dental defects for many years, it was not until January 2007, after extensive off-label use and study, that it was FDA approved for cosmetic facial soft tissue augmentation.

As with all procedures, the patient should be counseled regarding the risks of CaHA injection, specifically bleeding, ecchymoses, and edema. The patient's history should be taken to assess for bleeding tendencies. Patients with skin infections, a history of keloid scars, or collagen disorders should not be treated with CaHA or other soft tissue fillers. Photographs of the patient should be taken prior to injections. Since gravitational forces often create the facial features to be corrected, the patient should always be marked in an upright or seated position.

Depending on the patient's pain threshold, local anesthesia should be considered. Due to its subdermal plane of injection, topical anesthetics (i.e., EMLA) are of little use. Instead, for those patients who request anesthesia, either a regional or nerve block should be performed (1% lidocaine with 1:100,000 epinephrine). Adequate time for vasoconstriction and anesthesia should be allowed. The practitioner should be aware that the injected local anesthetic volume could alter the soft tissue volume at the treatment site.

The senior author has found that a 1½ inch, 27-gauge needle is ideal for most injection sites. In addition, smaller

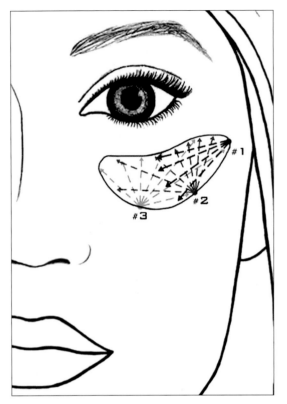

FIGURE 16.1: *Diagram representing fanning and cross-hatching vectors for Radiesse injection into the cheek.*

areas of treatment do well with a 1/2 inch, 27-gauge needle. The pattern of injection should be tailored to the location being augmented. Threading of the CaHA is useful for long, narrow areas of need such as the melolabial folds, whereas fanning or cross-hatching of the CaHA is useful for wider, larger areas of correction. Bimanual massaging of the treated area creates a softer, more evenly distributed result.

The melolabial folds are the most readily treated areas with CaHA. The folds should be augmented in a parallel, threading fashion. Depending on the depth and width of the fold, two to four passes should be used. This can amount to 0.5–1.3 cc per fold. These passes span the length of the fold; however, additional, smaller, shorter passes may be needed at the deeper portion of the fold adjacent to the alar crease. The goal of this treatment is to soften the transition of the cheek to the upper lip.

Additionally, the infracommissural folds, or marionette lines, should be addressed in a similar fashion. Typically, these folds are not as long or as deep as the aforementioned melolabial folds, and therefore a volume of 0.3–0.5 cc is sufficient for standard treatment.

The lips, which develop radial rhytid formations at the vermilion border, loss of overall volume, and loss of mucosal show with aging, are ideal for CaHA injection. However, it is important to note that CaHA injection into

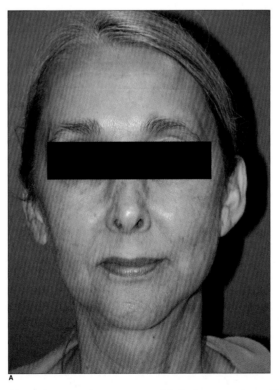

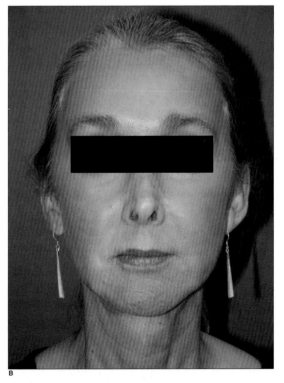

FIGURE 16.2: **A,** *Pretreatment with Radiesse: patient with prominent melolabial (nasolabial) and infracommissural (marionette line) folds.* **B,** *Posttreatment with Radiesse 1.3-cc syringe injected into the melolabial and infracommissural folds.*

the lips is only recommended for the experienced practitioner of facial aesthetic surgery. The ideal height ratio of 2:1 for the lower and upper lips should be kept in mind when injecting the lips. Each half of the lip, both upper and lower, should be addressed with injection from the corner of the mouth, which allows for equal and even CaHA deposition in the lip. The cupid's bow and the philtrum columns should be injected separately. One single thread of material should be placed in the deep, muscular plane, followed by a second parallel thread, if necessary, for desired lip volume. Massaging of CaHA is paramount in the lips to avoid coalescence of the CaHA and resultant submucosal nodules. Often no more than 0.7–1 cc is necessary for each lip.

With fat atrophy and soft tissue descent, a volume loss occurs in the midface and infraorbital region. Increasing numbers of HIV-positive patients being well controlled on antiretroviral therapy has led to an increasing number of patients with associated midface lipoatrophy. Also, anomalous and congenital facial soft tissue and bony defects are appropriate for augmentation. CaHA can serve as a prelude or substitute for malar or midface alloplastic augmentation. Fanning and cross-hatching (Figure 16.1) are best suited for these larger areas such as the cheek and malar region. Volume loss will dictate the amount of CaHA needed, though, on occasion, up to 4–5 cc has been used in each larger area.

If the practitioner is well versed in nasal anatomy and ideal nasal aesthetics, CaHA can be used for nasal augmentation. This is especially the case in postoperative rhinoplasty patients, who need small and subtle, yet lasting soft tissue augmentation. However, due to relative lack of muscular activity in the nose, CaHA deposition has a much longer lasting effect. This should be done with a 1/2 inch 27-gauge needle in small increments, so as not to overcorrect.

Patients should be advised to apply cool compresses after injection to reduce edema and ecchymoses. Due to its longevity – twelve to twenty-four months of correction – care should be taken not to overcorrect areas of the face. Instead, judicious correction should be followed by reevaluation in four to six weeks. At that time, more CaHA may be used for correction, if necessary.

CaHA is a predictable, safe soft tissue filler that can provide a long-lasting, but temporary, augmentation. Once knowledgeable regarding its use, the cosmetic surgery practitioner will find it a valuable tool in his or her facial cosmetic practice (Figure 16.2).

SUGGESTED READING

Havlik RJ. Hydroxylapatite. *Plast. Reconstr. Surg.* 2002;15:1176–9.

Jacovella, PF. Calcium hydroxylapatite facial filler (Radiesse™): Indications, technique and results. *Clin. Plast. Surg.* 2006;33: 511–23.

Tzikas TL. Evaluation of the Radiance soft tissue filler for facial soft tissue augmentation. *Arch. Facial Plast. Surg.* 2004;6: 234–9.

CHAPTER 17

Calcium Hydroxylapatite (Radiesse): A Dermasurgeon's Approach

F. Landon Clark

Hayes B. Gladstone

With a soaring increase in the U.S. aging population, there has been a parallel increase in interest in cosmetic procedures. Many people interested in rejuvenation are not prepared to undergo aggressive surgical interventions and elect for less invasive, yet aesthetically appreciable rejuvenation techniques. Soft tissue fillers have become increasingly popular given their ease of administration, immediate aesthetic enhancement capabilities, safety profiles, and relative affordability. Calcium hydroxylapatite (CaHA), manufactured as Radiesse, is one of the more versatile injectables.

THE PRODUCT

Radiesse is composed of 30% CaHA microspheres (25–45 μm diameter) suspended in a gel carrier composed of carboxymethylcellulose, glycerin, and water. CaHA is an inorganic compound with a chemical structure identical to components found in bone and teeth. Hence CaHA injectables are considered nonimmunogenic, minimizing any risk of allergic reaction to the product.

While approved for laryngeal augmentation and correction of urinary incontinence, CaHA was used safely as a soft tissue filler until December 2006, when it gained Food and Drug Administration (FDA) approval for this purpose. It is manufactured in 1.3-cc and 0.3-cc correction-sized syringes.

PATIENT INDICATIONS

CaHA is FDA approved for nasolabial folds and for lipoatrophy secondary to HIV. However, because of its viscosity and length of duration, it has many off-label indications. It is particularly effective for deeper nasolabial folds. In most patients, one syringe is sufficient, and the results will last for nearly twelve months. It can also be used for the marionette lines and, with care, the glabellar crease. As we have gained more experience using CaHA over the past several years, its indications have expanded. For experienced injectors,

CaHA can be very effective in filling the tear-trough deformity and the prejowl sulcus as well as building up the nasal bridge and the chin. For general volume enhancement, it can be injected into the cheeks, and also into the submalar region to elevate the malar eminence. While the authors do not recommend CaHA for lip enhancement, it can be used as an adjunct to hyaluronic acid or collagen by using it in the commissure region, where other less viscous fillers will become lost.

TECHNIQUE

When injecting, it is important for the patient to be sitting so that gravity's full effect can be easily discerned. After marking the entry site, the authors prefer direct injection with 1% lidocaine with 1/100,000 epinephrine, rather than a nerve block. For instance, 1 cc of anesthetic is injected along each nasolabial fold. The epinephrine will result in local vasoconstriction, thus reducing the risk of ecchymosis. Pain on injection is generally less with this technique.

The authors prefer using a 27-gauge, $\frac{1}{2}$ inch needle. The product flows through this gauge with firm pressure on the plunger. The short needle allows for accurate placement via the multiple puncture technique, though threading can be performed even with a $\frac{1}{2}$ inch needle. Often the authors will use a combination of these two techniques while injecting in a retrograde fashion. The product should be placed at the dermal-subcutaneous border. Placing it too superficially will result in prolonged lumpiness. While injecting into the subcutis will unlikely result in any adverse effects, it will also give a suboptimal correction. Following injection, molding can be performed initially by the physician, and then by the patient over the next forty-eight hours. The patient should be instructed to gently pat the skin along the injection line two to three times per day.

When injecting into the tear trough, it is important to place the CaHA submuscular to avoid nodules. In this area, the product should be injected very judiciously. For both the cheeks and marionette lines, a fanning or cross-hatching

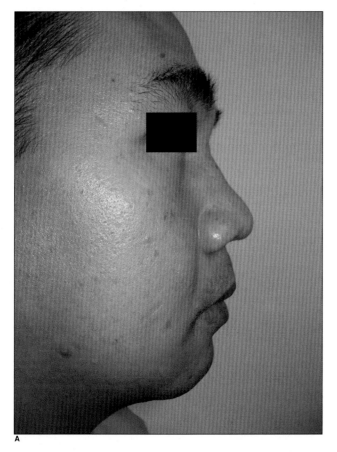 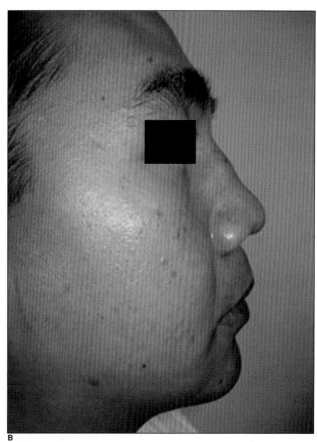

FIGURE 17.1: **A,** *Pre-Radiesse injection of chin and nose, profile view.* **B,** *Post-Radiesse injection of 1.3 cc into the mentum and 0.3 cc into the nasal dorsum. Note significantly improved chin projection and nasal contour.*

technique should be used. For the cheeks, it will provide a more even distribution; for the marionette lines, it will provide a buttress. For the prejowl sulcus, injecting deep and in a fanning motion will result in a more even distribution. Chin augmentation with CaHA can be very satisfying, but the product must be placed in small amounts and in two to three sessions (Figure 17.1). When building up the nasal dorsum, a threading technique, in which thin lines of material are laid down, will provide the most even results (Figure 17.1).

COMPLICATIONS

Postprocedure complications are limited, and the most common adverse effect is posttreatment edema (Table 17.1). This may be controlled, in part, by placing ice packs at the injection site immediately after the procedure. Other common, and expected, postprocedure complications include erythema and ecchymoses. As with any procedure, abstaining from any antiplatelet agents for two weeks before the procedure can help with this complication. Visible tissue nodules may be seen as a complication when, as described earlier, the filler is placed too superficially.

While FDA approval for soft tissue augmentation is more recent, Radiesse has been widely used off-label for these purposes, and serious complications seen with other fillers, like hypersensitivity and granuloma formation, have not, to date, been reported. Theoretical risks, expected for any filler, including intravascular injection, still remain.

TABLE 17.1: Adverse Effects

- Injection site erythema: 1–2 days
- Bruising: 1–4 days
- Hematoma: 0
- Seroma: 0
- Infection: 0
- Lumpiness: mild
- Granulomas: 0
- Migration: 0
- Extrusion: 0

Note: Data adapted from a study, n = 35, by H. B. Gladstone and G. S. Morganroth, presented at the annual American Society for Dermatologic Surgery Meeting, 2004.

WHERE CALCIUM HYDROXYLAPATITE FITS IN OUR PRACTICE

CaHA is a very versatile filler. We most commonly use it for prominent nasolabial folds. Because of its substance and 1.3-cc syringes, this product can fill most nasolabial folds without any touch-up. As an additional benefit, the malar fat pads are raised secondary to the volume displacement. Since it lasts nearly a year or more, it is also the most cost-effective. We also like this product for filling the cheeks and raising the malar eminences. For similar reasons, it is better than other fillers for the prejowl grooves. While many practitioners prefer a hyaluronic acid for the tear-trough deformity, we prefer CaHA because of its substance and ability to mold it in this area. Again, placing it at the correct depth is imperative. The only disadvantage of CaHA is that it is not suitable for lip augmentation – we prefer hyaluronic acid. While CaHA clearly plays a role in cheek augmentation, for those patients with HIV lipoatrophy, we still prefer l-polylactic acid. More recently, Radiesse has also been used for the dorsum of the hand. This is discussed separately in Chapter 18.

SUGGESTED READING

Ahn MS. Calcium hydroxylapatite: Radiesse. *Facial Plast. Surg. Clin. North Am.* 2007;15:85–90.

Alam M, Yoo SS. Technique for calcium hydroxylapatite injection for correction of nasolabial fold depressions. *J. Am. Acad. Deramtol.* 2007;56:285–9.

Calcium Hydroxylapatite for Hand Volume Restoration

Marta I. Rendon

Mariana Pinzon-Plazas

Lina M. Cardona

Facial enhancement has long interested dermatologists and plastic surgeons. Other anatomical areas, such as the dorsum of the hands, have more recently become popular sites for enhancement because these areas can show signs of aging, such as lack of fullness, skeletinization, wrinkles, and tortuous veins, thereby reflecting true age.

The exponential growth of cosmetic procedures has resulted from the introduction of new products that last longer and produce superior results. These have been developed in response to increased demand for minimally invasive and cost-effective aesthetic treatments, an aging U.S. population, and a growing emphasis on self-image driven by the media.

A survey conducted by the American Society of Plastic Surgeons using digital photographs of hands identified factors that determine the age of the hands' appearance. The researchers concluded that specific factors characterize aging hands, including wrinkles, lack of fullness, veins, prominent joints, thin skin, deformities, and age spots. As a result, a patient's age can be estimated by viewing the hands alone.

According to the American Society for Aesthetic Plastic Surgery, the so-called hand lift will soon be one of the top most requested procedures. Multiple dermatological procedures are available for hand rejuvenation, including chemical peels, microdermabrasion, laser therapy (ablative and nonablative), sclerotherapy, dermal fillers, and fat augmentation. Dermal fillers are widely used for volume restoration and can be expected to produce a natural, smooth appearance.

Patients who present with volume loss over the dorsum of their hands are candidates for hand volume restoration with calcium hydroxylapatite (CaHA), manufactured by BioForm Medical USA and marketed under the name Radiesse – a semipermanent filler. It is biodegradable and dissipates over time. Patients may require more than one treatment for full correction. Optimal results occur two to four weeks after injection and last for twelve to eighteen months.

CaHA is supplied in sterile 1.3-mL and 0.3-mL syringes. The product is ready to use after opening. There is no need for skin testing because the product is biocompatible. An unopened package has a shelf life of two years.

GENERAL CONSIDERATIONS

The ability to properly and optimally inject fillers is an evolutionary process that improves with experience. Four important aspects must be taken into consideration when injecting any filler: injection technique (tunneling, depot, threading, serial puncture, fanning, tenting), injection depth (superficial, middle, or deep into the dermal layer), specific syringe (gauge and length), and the volume of the product to be injected.

INJECTION TECHNIQUE

Before injection with CaHA, the dorsum of the hand is anesthetized with topical anesthetic cream (20% to 30% lidocaine, prilocaine, or tetracaine) for a period of twenty to thirty minutes. The area is then cleaned using a surgical preparation base of chloroxylenol USP 3% (Care-Tech Laboratories Inc.).

In a 3-mL syringe, 0.15–0.20 mL of lidocaine 10% (10 mg/mL) without epinephrine is mixed with the CaHA using a sterile rapid-fill connector (luer lock fitting). CaHA is injected into the deep dermal plane using a 27-gauge needle (1/2 to $1\frac{1}{2}$ inch), pulling the skin up between the second and fifth intermetacarpal spaces. The syringe should be inserted with an angle between 20 and 30 degrees to the skin. The product is delivered slowly deep into the dermis to form a large reservoir or bolus with an approximately 0.65–1.3 mL vial per hand, depending on the defect being corrected. The technique used is single puncture and syringe withdrawal, producing a globular deposit that must be massaged with moisturizer cream to achieve a uniform distribution and to mold the material in the desired area. A Q-tip dampened with aluminum chloride-hexahydrate

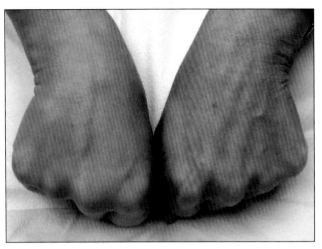

FIGURE 18.1: *Right hand treated with Radiesse; left hand untreated.*

20% (Drysol, Person and Covey Inc.) can be used to arrest the minimal blood flow resulting from the site of puncture.

AFTERCARE

After the injection, ice packs should be applied for five to ten minutes, and the area should be washed with soap and water. Topical antibiotic ointment should be applied on the injection site daily until it has healed.

It is also highly recommended that the skin be kept well hydrated and protected from the sun with a moisturizer containing SPF 15 or greater.

COMPLICATIONS

No studies on the safety of injecting CaHA in the dorsum of the hand have been published. Studies of CaHA in other anatomical locations have revealed few complications. In rare cases, hematoma, ecchymosis (5% incidence), minimal edema, and bruising have occurred. The possibility of pruritus, persistent bruising, infections, intravascular product placement, ulcerations, and filler migration must be considered. Palpable subcutaneous nodules occurring from injection in the lips can be easily treated with surgical resection.

CONCLUSION

Restoring youthful fullness to the hands can be accomplished with different treatments that do not require downtime. CaHA offers a full correction of the aged hand with immediate results (Figure 18.1), long duration, and minimal side effects. In our personal experience, CaHA appears to be as equally safe and effective in the dorsum of the hands as with facial restoration; however, more data are needed to confirm the longevity and lack of side effects of CaHA treatment in the dorsum of the hands.

SUGGESTED READING

Broder KW, Cohen SR. An overview of permanent and semipermanent fillers. *Plast. Reconstr. Surg.* 2006;118(3 Suppl):7S–14S.

Butterwick KJ. Rejuvenation of the aging hand. *Dermatol. Clin.* 2005;23:515–27.

Deborshi R, Sadick N, Mangat D. Clinical trial of a novel filler material for soft tissue augmentation of the face containing synthetic calcium hydroxylapatite microspheres. *Dermatol. Surg.* 2006;32:1134–9.

Jacovella P, Peiretti C, Cunille D, et al. Long-lasting results with hydroxylapatite (Radiesse) facial filler. *Plast. Reconstr. Surg.* 2006;118(3 Suppl):15S–21S.

Jakubietz RG, Jakubietz MG, Kloss D, Gruenert JG. Defining the basic aesthetics of the hand. *Aesthetic Plast. Surg.* 2005;29:546–51.

Jansen DJ, Gravier MH. Evaluation of a calcium hydroxylapatite-based implant (Radiesse) for facial soft tissue augmentation. *Plast. Reconstr. Surg.* 2006;118(3 Suppl):22S–30S, discussion 31S–33S.

Silvers SL, Eviatar JA, Echavez MI, Pappas AL. Prospective open label 18-month trial of calcium hydroxylapatite (Radiesse) for facial soft tissue augmentation in patients with HIV-associated lipoatrophy: one year durability. *Plast. Reconstr. Surg.* 2006;118(3 Suppl):34S–45S.

LONG-LASTING FILLERS

CHAPTER 19

Long-Lasting Fillers: How Structure Affects Function

Pierre Nicolau

Whatever substance is injected within human tissues, it will start a series of reactions that must be known. These reactions are part of the normal healing process, with the aim of removing or isolating the foreign body from the host tissue. They follow three phases: recognition of the foreign body, removal or isolation, and a final healing phase. But these reactions can be either reduced or enhanced by the structure of the injected filler. Therefore it seems important to well understand these mechanisms to choose, if not the best, then the least harmful product available.

FOREIGN BODY REACTION: THE INFLAMMATORY PROCESS

Phase 1: The Foreign Body Must Be Identified

Identification is the role of the monocytes from the bloodstream, activated into macrophages by factors released through the wound, even a minimal puncture, by platelets coming into contact with the extracellular matrix (ECM).

Adhesion

Macrophages must adhere to the foreign body. This adhesion is the most important aspect of the cellular interaction. It is mediated by *adsorption*, the deposition of glycoproteins from the ECM and/or plasma on the surface of the foreign body. The more the proteins cover the surface, the more cell adhesion, spreading, and proliferation will be efficient.

Recognition

These deposited proteins start a specific recognition by monocyte/macrophage surface cell receptors. There is also a nonspecific interaction between cell surface molecules (oligosaccharides), the adsorbed proteins, and the implant surface.

Phase 2: The Foreign Body Must Be Removed

Removal is accomplished through phagocytosis from:

monocytes/macrophages

neutrophils/polymorphonuclears

keratinocytes, if the implant is superficial (papillary dermis).

These cells have the capacity to absorb the foreign body, transport it, and destroy it, but phagocytosis does not always occur.

If the implant is not recognized as a foreign element, phagocytic cells will go into apoptosis:

It is the self-destruction of inefficient phagocytic cells.

It is a specialized form of cellular death, with shrinkage of the cell, condensation of its chromatin, and fragmentation into apoptotic bodies that will be removed by phagocytosis.

The result is a cleaning up without inflammation or damage to local tissues.

The implant will be surrounded by a thin fibrillar membrane with very few cells.

If the implant is recognized as a foreign body but is too large to be phagocytosed, macrophages fuse into foreign body giant cells (FBGCs). These are specific to foreign body granulomas. They show well over twenty nuclei, scattered within the cytoplasm. Nonphagocytosed elements are surrounded by macrophages and FBGCs, but no lymphocytes.

They are found at the host-implant interface and will remain for the duration of the implant. If it is a permanent implant, then these cells will be found throughout the lifetime. They can be compared to a peace corps of sorts, surrounding the implant for an armed truce. The rate of cell turnover is not well known, but could be as often as every forty-eight hours.

From the cells are created podosomal structures, which join the host to the implant. Many microfibrils and microvesicules can be seen at the interface of host and implant, thus enhancing the capacity of destruction and phagocytosis to become more efficient than isolated macrophages. Their role is to concentrate, at the host-implant interface, the necessary degradation enzymes, the oxidizing oxygen ions, and chemotactic proteins to enroll more competent cells.

Phase 3: The Foreign Body Must Be Isolated

Phase 3 occurs when the foreign body cannot be removed. Macrophages also secrete growth factors to regulate the change from the inflammatory phase, for cleaning, into the proliferative phase, for reconstruction. Initially, the fibroblasts secrete type I collagen, immature fluid gel, into the ECM, then type III, mature collagen. This maturation phase starts with collagen reticulation, which then leads to collagen contraction, which tightens the net and brings back strength to the tissues. The implant is therefore isolated with a strong fibrous collagenous capsule, with fibroblasts changing into mature fibrocytes. Each foreign particle should be encapsulated independently from the others. This prevents it from being displaced, that is, mechanically moved from the original implantation site. This is not to be confused with migration, which is an active transportation process through phagocytic cells.

It is therefore possible to define two types of filler, according to the reactions they induce. Either the agent is recognized as a foreign body, and its role will be to induce good capsule formation to fill up the tissue defect, or it is accepted without reactions, and it is the injected volume that will produce the result sought (Table 19.1). The first type can be considered a *biological stimulator*, whereas the second is a *volumizer* (Table 19.2).

TABLE 19.1: Effect of Cellular Adhesion on Injected Filler

If Cellular Adhesion, Recognition	If Little or No Adhesion, No Recognition
Phagocytosis, by	no phagocytosis
Monocytes/macrophages	
Polynuclears	
Keratinocytes if implant is superficial (papillary dermis)	
or fusion into FBGC: Concentration at the implant-host interface of degradation enzymes oxidizing O_2 ion chemotactic proteins	**apoptosis: elimination of "inefficient" cells**
Thick, strong isolating fibrous capsule	**thin fibrillar membrane with few cells**

HOW STRUCTURE OF THE IMPLANT INFLUENCES THESE REACTIONS

Size and Volume of Implant

Particles over 40 μm are not phagocytosed. The smaller the size of the particles, the faster they will be phagocytosed; the smaller the size of the particles, the more

TABLE 19.2: Types of Permanent Fillers

Biological Stimulators	Volumizers
Aim: induce a reaction from the body; to stimulate creation of sustaining tissues; mainly collagen matrix; for a filling, immediate but temporary, then secondary and persisting	Aim: bring an immediate volume; with no reaction of the body; for immediate filling
The biological reaction is sought for and should be favorable	**The biological reaction is not wanted and unfavorable**
It is necessary to obtain	
For the biological stimulators,	for the volumizers,
a good cell adhesion	no cell adhesion
no phagocytosis	no phagocytosis
good encapsulation for fixation and isolation, which will stop the inflammatory reaction	no fragmentation of the agent, ending up with a thin encapsulation

inflammation they will induce, which can lead to local necrosis; and the smaller the size of the particles, the more migration, that is, active transportation by phagocytic cells, sometimes causing dramatic complications at a distance. Therefore a particulate implant should be over 40 μm in size.

For fluid implants, liquid or gel, there is a light reaction around the bulk, but a strong reactivation of the inflammatory process can be seen around each detached microdroplet. This explains why inflammation may occur sometimes months or years after injection of low-grade-viscosity silicon oil or polyacrylamid gel, and why inflammatory processes can be activated when injecting another substance close to the same location. For fluid implants, as there will be only a thin encapsulation, mechanical displacement can occur more easily, especially if the substance is injected in a mobile area, as within muscle, or in large volume. Furthermore, the implant can diffuse into the surrounding tissues, forming digitations, which will make the implant impossible to remove surgically in case of an adverse reaction. This is why I do not recommend the use of large amounts of material, even if the material has been advocated as a possible material for injectable prostheses (e.g., polyacrylamid gels, BioAlcamid).

Morphology of Implant

Spherical shapes induce less enzymatic activity, with less inflammatory reaction (Artecoll, ArteFill, Radiesse, New-Fill). Smooth surfaces induce more collagen secretion, which is the aim for particulate implants, but porous or irregular surfaces induce a more severe foreign body reaction. The fibrous capsule is often irregular, thicker on flat surfaces, and thinner over the edges.

Surface Area

There is a critical value for a particle surface area, above which the inflammatory response increases spectacularly. It has been shown that for a given mass, the largest particles induce more inflammation, and a spherical particle induces less inflammation than an irregularly shaped one, as it has the smallest surface for the largest mass. But for a given mass, 100-μm beads induce 56% collagen formation, and 40-μm beads induce 78% collagen formation. This is understandable since the total surface area for the same mass composed of the smaller microspheres is larger.

This concept of threshold surface area could also explain why particles of irregular or porous surfaces induce more inflammatory reactions, as porosity increases their total surface area. It is well known that the gradual degradation of polylactic acid implants, such as microscrews and plates, induces strong inflammatory reactions after thirty to sixty months. This gradual degradation increases their surface area, causing them to reach the threshold value. Inflammation will resume gradually with the disappearance of the product. It is possible to imagine that the same could be seen with Radiesse or New-Fill.

Chemical Composition

Hydrophobic implants induce more fibronectin adsorption and more macrophage adhesion, therefore starting a stronger foreign body reaction. Carboxylic groups activate C3, inducing specific macrophage recognition. Dermalive and Dermadeep are made of irregularly shaped microparticles combining these two chemicals, whose properties make them very recognizable by specific macrophages. They therefore have a potential for a strong inflammatory reaction. This is confirmed by up to 11% of patients presenting with complications, including as much as 5.5% secondary granulomas.

Electric Charge

Positively charged beads attract and/or activate macrophages. Positive surface charges induce greater FBGC formation. Positive surface charges induce faster reorientation of collagen bundles. Positive surface charges result in thicker connective tissue. Negative surface charges could repel negatively charged bacteria. The only available positively charged implants are Beautisphere and Reviderm, composed of dextran microspheres with hyaluronic acid. But despite this potential for strong collagen activation, its effects do not seem to last longer than a year.

Implantation Site

The complication rate is less in chin and malar areas, but it is greater in nose and ears. This seems to be related to thickness and tension of the overlying skin. Furthermore, it has been shown that the fibrous capsule is thicker on the surface toward the skin and thinner on the surface facing depth. Implantation within muscles (lip) can break the implant into small masses, leading to displacement and nodule formation.

THE QUEST FOR THE IDEAL LONG-LASTING, PERMANENT FILLER

Considering the preceding elements, it is possible to define which characteristics will promote the best effect.

Particulate Implants: Biostimulators

Efficacy is due to the injected volume and the promotion of collagen it will induce. Particles, ideally, should be (1) spherical (2) with a perfectly smooth surface and (3) a positive surface charge, (4) over 40 μm in diameter, and (5) show no migration or displacement and therefore able to

TABLE 19.3: Looking for the Ideal Particulate Implant

Name	>40 μ	Spherical	Smooth Surface	+ Surface Charge	No Degradation of Particules	No Migration or Displacement	Total
Artecoll/ArteFill	+	+	+	(−)	+	+	+ : 5 − : 1
Radiesse	+	+	(−)	(−)	(−)	+	+ : 3 − : 3
Reviderm/Beauti sphere	+	+	(−)	+	(−)	(−)	+ : 3 − : 3
New-Fill/Sculptra	+	+	(−)	(−)	(−)	(−)	+ : 2 − : 4
Dermalive/Dermadeep	+	(−)	(−)	(−)	+	(−)	+ : 2 − : 4

TABLE 19.4: Looking for the Ideal Fluid/Gel Implant

Name	Porosity	No Monomer Release	No Fragmentation	No Degradation or Dehydration	No Migration or Displacement	Total
Outline	+	+	+	(−)	(−)	+ : 3 − : 2
Bio Alcamid	+/−	+	(−)	(−)	(−)	+ : 2 − : 4
Silicone gel	+	(−)	(−)	+	(−)	+ : 2 − : 3
Aquamid PAAG	+/−	(−)	(−)	(−)	(−)	+ : 1 − : 5

be placed in a carrying medium viscous enough to last for about two to three months, allowing for good local collagen encapsulation (see Table 19.3).

Fluid Implant: Volumizer

The filling effect is due only to the implanted volume. Its porosity (molecular network) should prevent penetration of its bulk by cells. It should show the following: (1) no release of free monomers, as acrylic monomers are carcinogenic; (2) no enzymatic or chemical degradation over time, unless gradual disappearance is sought; (3) no fragmentation into droplets or particles; and (4) no migration or displacement (see Table 19.4).

CONCLUSION

Long-lasting or permanent injectable implants could be effective and safe, provided that we understand their characteristics and respect three treatment technique guidelines emerging from these well-documented characteristics: (1) for either type, particulate or fluid, always practice deep injection (below the papillary dermis) to avoid phagocytosis by keratinocytes and infection through skin adnexae, and avoid injections in muscles or mobile areas, unless the area

can be immobilized for at least nine to twelve days, to prevent mechanical displacement (e.g., low-dose botulinum toxin to the lips); (2) for fluid implants, avoid bulk injections to prevent displacement, facilitated by the lack of a strong enough capsule; and (3) for particulate implants, always inject as deep as possible, well below the dermis, to try to minimize the clinical consequences of an eventual inflammatory reaction.

SUGGESTED READING

Comprehensive Review of the Different Fillers and Comprehensive Bibliography

Nicolau PJ. Long lasting and permanent fillers: biomaterial influence over host tissue response. *Plast. Reconstr. Surg.* 2007:119;2271–86.

Size and Volume of Implant

Morhenn VB, Lemperle G, Gallo RL. Phagocytosis of different particulate dermal filler substances by human macrophages and skin cells. *Dermatol. Surg.* 2002;28:484–90.

Morphology of Implant

Misiek DJ, Kent JN, Carr RF. Soft tissue response to hydroxylapatite particles of different shapes. *J. Oral Maxillofacial Surg.* 1984;42:150–60.

Surface Area

Gelb H, Schumacher HR, Cukler J, et al. In vivo inflammatory response to polymethylmethacrylate particulate debris: effect of size, morphology and surface area. *J. Orthop. Res.* 1994;12:83–92.

Rubin JP, Yaremchuck MJ. Complications and toxicities of implantable biomaterials used in facial reconstructive and aesthetic surgery: a comprehensive review of the literature. *Plast. Reconstr. Surg.* 1997;100:1336–53.

Chemical Composition

Saylan Z. Facial fillers and their complications. *Aesthetic Surg. J.* 2003;23:221–4.

Smetana KJ. Cell biology of hydrogels. *Biomaterials* 1993;14:1046–50.

Electric Charge

Eppley BL, Summerlin D-J, Prevel CD, et al. Effects of positively charged biomaterial for dermal and subcutaneous augmentation. *Aesthtic Plast. Surg.* 1994;18:413–16.

Implantation Site

Li D-J, Ohsaki K, Ii P-C, et al. Thickness of fibrous capsule after implantation of hydroxyapatite in subcutaneous tissue in rats. *J. Biomed. Mater. Res.* 1999;45:322–6.

CHAPTER 20

Acrylic Particle–Based Fillers: ArteFill

Rhoda S. Narins

Rebecca A. Kazin

ARTEFILL HISTORY AND PATHOPHYSIOLOGY

Polymethymethacrylate (PMMA) was first synthesized by Roehm in 1902 and patented as Plexiglas in 1928. It has been used in dentures, prosthetic devices, and intraocular lenses and as a carrier for antibiotics. In 1985, PMMA was studied by G. Lemperle for soft tissue augmentation.

ArteFill is classified as a permanent soft tissue implant composed of 20% homogenous PMMA microspheres evenly suspended in an 80% mixture of 3.5% purified bovine collagen, 0.3% sodium chloride, and 0.3% lidocaine. The PMMA microspheres stimulate fibroblasts to produce autologous collagen, which then encapsulates each PMMA microsphere. The bovine collagen component of the filler serves as a carrier for deep dermal implantation that prevents clumping on injection and stimulates tissue ingrowth. Following injection, the collagen carrier is degraded by collagenases within one to four months and is replaced by the body's own collagen, ensuring a steady rate of augmentation consisting of 80% autologous connective tissue and 20% PMMA.

PMMA fillers have evolved substantially from Arteplast to Artecoll, now ArteFill. Predecessors of ArteFill had PMMA microspheres of less than 20 μm in size, while those in ArteFill are virtually all 30–42 μm. This optimum size is large enough to avoid phagocytosis, thus facilitating connective tissue encapsulation, but small enough to allow injection into the deep dermis through a 26-gauge needle. Additionally, the PMMA is washed and coated with high-viscosity bovine collagen (versus the Tween 80 or gelatin medium in Arteplast), which reduces the rate of foreign body granuloma formation from 2.5% with Arteplast to 0.01% reported with Artecoll.

In 2003, the Food and Drug Administration (FDA) advisory panel recommended that Artecoll receive U.S. marketing approval after the 2001 completion of the U.S. clinical trial of 251 patients, which reported that Artecoll was superior to collagen (Zyderm II or Zyplast) at three, six, and twelve months in wrinkles of the nasolabial area, glabella,

radial lip lines, and oral commissures. Adverse events and immunoglobulin G levels were similar in both groups. Five-year studies have confirmed the permanence of this product.

ArteFill, produced by Artes Medical Inc., is a recent PMMA filler approved by the FDA for cosmetic facial volume restoration. The bovine collagen in ArteFill is from a closed U.S. herd of cows that is processed in a dedicated plant in San Diego, which has translated into a lower reported allergy rate (0.1% in the trials versus the 3.4% reported from the previous collagen produced in France). The allergenic peptide ends of the collagen are removed with pepsin, and it is processed with 1 N sodium hydroxide to protect against bovine spongiform encephalopathy and many other viruses.

PATIENT SELECTION AND REALISTIC EXPECTATIONS

ArteFill is the first and only permanent injectable skin filler FDA approved for cosmetic purposes. Patients inquiring about the procedure will typically report injection, or so-called credit card, fatigue; however, physicians are ultimately responsible for accurately selecting appropriate patients for this procedure.

Patients need to have realistic expectations of benefits and limitations of the product and be able to give informed consent. Exclusion criteria from the Artecoll/Zyplast study are listed in Table 20.1, but absolute contraindications include collagen or lidocaine allergy and history of keloid formation.

ArteFill is indicated primarily for facial volume restoration. Nasolabial folds and marionette lines are treated most commonly, but other indications are being examined, including acne scars, defects after rhinoplasty, and nipple reconstruction. The Artecoll study included patients seeking correction in the glabella, nasolabial folds, radial lip lines, or oral commissures. Physicians with injection

TABLE 20.1: Exclusion Criteria from the U.S. Artecoll/Zyplast Study

Pregnancy
Wrinkle treatment within six months
Ultraviolet light therapy
Chemotherapy or steroids within three months
Anticoagulation medication
Autoimmune disorders
Atrophic skin disease
Thin and flaccid facial skin
Keloid formation
Lidocaine hypersensitivity
Collagen or beef allergy
Positive collagen skin test

experience caution against injection of the body of the lip secondary to bunching of the product and nodule formation. Glabellar injection should also be cautioned as the viscous product could increase the risk of necrosis at this site.

Temporary fillers may be used as a trial to a permanent filler to give patients an idea of what can be accomplished and the amount of product that may be needed.

ArteFill is injected into the dermal-subdermal junction just above the subcutaneous fat to splint or support the overlying wrinkle. It is used for deep lines and cannot be injected into the papillary dermis for finer lines.

Patients need to be aware that they may need other nonpermanent fillers, either layered on top of ArteFill for complete wrinkle correction or in other areas of the face with finer wrinkles that require more superficial fillers.

HOW TO DO IT

Currently patients need to be skin tested for allergy to bovine collagen one month before utilizing this filler. After a negative skin test is confirmed and the patient is deemed appropriate for injection by the treating physician, topical anesthetic or nerve blocks can be placed to improve patient comfort during the procedure.

ArteFill must be refrigerated prior to use. Each kit contains three syringes of 0.8 cc and two syringes of 0.4 cc of ArteFill. A 26-gauge, 3/4 needle is used to implant the filler into the deep dermal-subdermal plane with a tunneling technique. This technique involves moving the needle in a linear fashion back and forth just beneath the wrinkle. Be aware that the high-viscosity product requires higher constant pressure on the syringe than injection of hyaluronic or collagen fillers. Before injection, proper flow can be tested by squeezing a drop of ArteFill out of the needle tip – be sure that the needle is locked tightly to the syringe.

Nasolabial fold augmentation has been very successful with ArteFill in both female (Figure 20.1) and male (Figure 20.2) patients. When treating this area, it is important to stay approximately 1 mm medial to the crease when injecting the product to avoid lateral dislocation by facial movement. Nasolabial creases are best supported by inserting the needle at a 20 degree angle parallel to the length of the fold and placing two or three linear strands of product. A second injection is often necessary at one to three months. Deep nasolabial folds may take up to 2 cc of product in three or more sessions two to three months apart. Touch-up treatments should be done in the space between the crease and the first implant. Subdermal fanning is indicated only in the upper triangle adjacent to the nose.

Oral commissures and marionette lines may be more difficult to treat but, when done appropriately, can yield excellent results. First augment the lower lip white roll horizontally approximately 1 cm in length from the oral commissure. Use a crisscross technique of five to ten threads of product to augment the oral commissures and marionette lines. This supports the region and can slightly lift the corners of the mouth. Superficial injection in these sites can cause overlying telangectasia. Ideally, ArteFill should

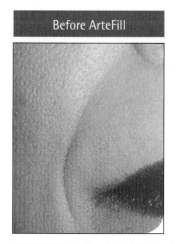
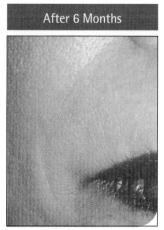
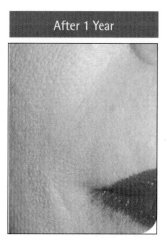

Before ArteFill | After 6 Months | After 1 Year

FIGURE 20.1: *Nasolabial fold before and at six and twelve months after treatment with ArteFill: female.*

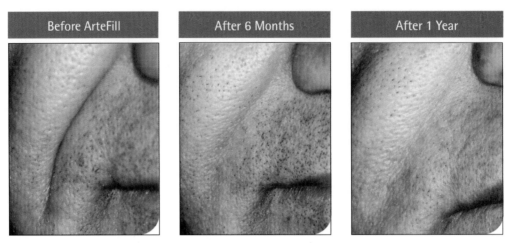

FIGURE 20.2: *Nasolabial fold before and at six and twelve months after treatment with ArteFill: male.*

be implanted in many different tunnels in two or more treatments. Care should be taken in the triangle below the oral commissure as there is almost no fat between the dermis and orbicularis oris. Implanting into muscle will almost always result in submucosal nodules inside the lip because the muscle will compress the injected strand into a lump.

Radial lip lines are often a concern for patients. In younger patients with adequate maintenance of the upper lip white roll, each radial lip line can be injected individually. In patients with four or more radial lip lines and in whom the white roll projection is diminished, ArteFill can be injected along the natural pocket in the deep dermis between the white roll and the orbicularis oris. Then each radial line can be injected separately. It is best to inject the lip lines in a cephalad direction to avoid excessive deposition of product at the vermilion. Perioral injections may be painful, and dental blocks are often warranted. Care should be taken not to inject ArteFill into the orbicularis oris as formation of nodules has been reported.

If ArteFill is injected too superficially into the papillary dermis, causing a blanching effect, the injection should be stopped, the area massaged, and the needle repositioned to a deeper plane in the skin. In patients with thin skin, superficial injections may cause overlying erythema for several months, and the implant may be visible as small white granules.

At the end of treatment, the implant should be evenly massaged to ensure even distribution of the product.

AFTERCARE

Patients are advised that there will be some swelling for the first twelve to twenty-four hours, and erythema along injection sites may be present for two to five days. They are also advised to minimize facial movement and refrain from smoking (especially if injected around the mouth) for one

to two days as ArteFill could be dislocated during the first several days posttreatment. Placing clear tape over treatment areas may reinforce this restriction.

INDICATIONS VERSUS OTHER MODALITIES

As more fillers are available for cosmetic usage, careful consideration must be taken by the treating physician to select the optimal filling agent for the site being treated as well as to consider other factors such as a patient's expectations and understanding of the risks and benefits of the procedure. Semipermanent and permanent products are often more economical for patients over the long term, but if done improperly by less experienced injectors, complications can arise.

Often the best overall cosmetic result will result from multiple fillers used on the same patient, each with its own benefit in specific areas for specific concerns. Deeper fillers like ArteFill can be used to form a scaffold under the wrinkle that lasts from months to years, while other more temporary fillers may be layered on top for finer lines or used in areas like the lip, where ArteFill is not advised. Patients need to understand that there is not one filler that works best for every indication.

COMPLICATIONS AND PREVENTION AND MANAGEMENT OF COMPLICATIONS

As stated earlier, PMMA implants have been utilized in other sites for decades. There have been no reports of harmful side effects like carcinoma arising from years of usage in fields like orthopedics. Since the PMMA microspheres are not phagocytosed and are encapsulated by autologous collagen (unlike liquid silicone, which evokes little encapsulation), late dislocation to lymph nodes and distant sites has not been detected.

Side effects from ArteFill are usually secondary to technical mistakes such as superficial injection, uneven distribution, or overfilling. These errors can result in lumps or nodules that often can be alleviated by massage.

Nodules that appear in the areas of injection may be due to inappropriate amounts of product, inappropriate accumulations of product due to muscular activity, or true foreign body granulomas. The incidence of foreign body granulomas has been examined in depth with ArteFill and its predecessors. Original PMMA cosmetic implant Arteplast had an unacceptable rate of close to 2.5% foreign body granuloma formation, but improvements in manufacturing techniques, such as ultrasonic baths and wet sieving through a metallic grid, resulted in smooth, uniform microspheres used to create Artecoll, with reports of less than a 0.01% rate of true foreign body granuloma formation. Granulomas that do form often respond to intralesional triamcinolone injections (10–40 mg/mL).

ArteFill has significant risk of lumpiness and nodularity when injected into the lips, and therefore it is recommended that alternatives be considered for lip enhancement. PMMA implants are designed for deep dermal injection and are not suitable for injection into muscle such as the orbicularis oris. A review of fifty-three patients who received Artecoll injection into the body of the lip as well as the vermilion demonstrated that twenty-seven of fifty-three patients (51%) had some palpable granularity or nodules in the lips. Some of these nodules were treated successfully with intralesional triamcinolone to shrink the nodule, while others required excision.

SUGGESTED READING

Broder KW, Cohen SR. ArteFill: a permanent skin filler. *Expert Rev. Med. Devices* 2006;3:281–9.

Broder KW, Cohen SR, Holmes RE. ArteFill: a long-lasting injectable wrinkle filler material – summary of the U.S. Food and Drug Administration trials and a progress report on 4- to 5-year outcomes. *Plast. Reconstr. Surg.* 2006;118:64S–76S.

Cohen SR, Holmes RE. Artecoll: a long-lasting injectable wrinkle filler material: report of a controlled, randomized, multicenter clinical trial of 251 subjects. *Plast. Reconstr. Surg.* 2004;114:964–76.

Lemperle G, Holmes RE, Cohen SR et al. A classification of facial wrinkles. *Plast. Reconstr. Surg.* 2001;108:1735–50.

CHAPTER 21

Poly-L-Lactic Acid Fillers

Kelley Pagliai Redbord

C. William Hanke

INTRODUCTION

Poly-L-lactic acid (PLLA) is a biodegradable, biocompatible synthetic polymer from the alpha-hydroxy-acid family. Injectable poly-L-lactic acid, marketed as Sculptra (Dermik Laboratories) is used for the treatment of subcutaneous volume restoration. Injection of PLLA into the subcutis results in expansion of the area through a foreign body reaction that elicits increased collagen production from fibroblasts.

The Food and Drug Administration approved PLLA for the treatment of HIV lipoatrophy in August 2004. PLLA is used off-label for the correction of facial lipoatrophy secondary to the normal aging process. PLLA has been available in Europe since 1999 under the trade name New-Fill.

The use of injectable PLLA is growing. Treatment is safe and effective. Precise injection technique is essential for good results and to avoid complications.

PATIENT SELECTION

The best candidates for treatment with PLLA are those seeking volumetric correction secondary to aging or medical conditions such as HIV. On initial evaluation of the patient, facial volume, concavities, and tissue quality should be assessed. Treatment with PLLA involves a series of injections every four to six weeks.

MATERIAL RECONSTITUTION

Each PLLA vial is reconstituted with 3 mL of sterile water on the evening before the procedure. On the day of the procedure, an additional 2 mL of plain lidocaine is added for a total dilution of 5 mL. Some physicians utilize an even greater dilution. The material is stored at room temperature before and after reconstitution. The vials are thoroughly shaken with a laboratory vortex before suspension is drawn up into syringes. The material is drawn into a 3-mL syringe with an 18-gauge needle and is transferred to a 25-gauge 1-inch needle for injection.

PREPROCEDURE

Photographs should be obtained before beginning treatment, at each subsequent visit, and at full correction. Informed consent should be obtained. Skin testing is not required prior to use.

Prior to injection, the patient's cheeks are prepped with isopropyl alcohol and the areas of concavity are outlined with a wax marking pencil. Additional dots are marked within the outlined area to indicate injection sites for anesthesia and PLLA.

The areas to be treated are anesthetized with 1 mL of 1% lidocaine with 1:100,000 epinephrine to each marked dot. A total of 4–8 mL of anesthetic is injected per cheek to four to eight areas on each cheek. One half of the amount is injected into the dermis and one half into the subcutaneous tissue.

Following injection of the local anesthesia, facial landmarks can be distorted; however, the areas to be treated have been previously outlined for accurate injection of PLLA.

TECHNIQUE

Immediately prior to and during injection, the material is vigorously shaken to obtain a uniform suspension and to prevent settling. The PLLA suspension is injected with a 25-gauge, 1-inch needle into the subcutaneous tissue using precise fanlike sweeps with the needle into the outlined areas. The material is injected evenly during needle withdrawal, avoiding superficial injection into the dermis.

Treatment volumes vary depending on the patient's severity. On average, one half to one vial of PLLA to each cheek is required. Treatment intervals are four to six weeks.

POSTPROCEDURE

After the injection, vigorous massage and manual sculpting are performed for five to ten minutes to both cheeks to evenly distribute the material. Application of ice packs to

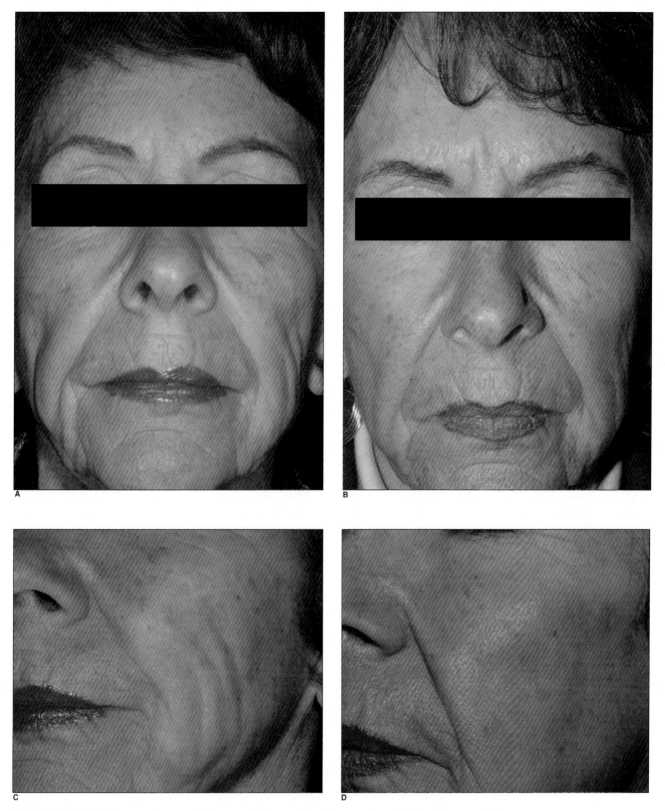

FIGURE 21.1: **A, C,** *Seventy-six-year-old woman with age-related lipoatrophy of both malar areas.* **B, D,** *The malar areas demonstrate improvement following four treatment sessions with PLLA.*

the injected areas is recommended for fifteen minutes of every hour while awake over the next twelve to twenty-four hours to minimize bruising and swelling.

Immediate postprocedure appearance of apparent full correction is not lasting. Tissue edema and mechanical volume effect from the anesthesia and PLLA suspension create the apparent correction. This is a preview of full correction with continued treatment and will dissipate in a few days and return to baseline.

RESULTS

Patients treated with PLLA for subcutaneous volume loss secondary to aging achieve full correction with two to three treatments using a total of three to four vials of PLLA. Patients fully correct on an average of seventeen weeks. Figure 21.1 demonstrates before and after photographs of successful results.

Results are long lasting. Gradual resorption occurs over a two- to three-year period. Studies are under way to determine the durability of PLLA over a five-year period. Patients are very satisfied with their treatment and report improved quality of life.

COMPLICATIONS

The most common treatment-related complications include bruising, erythema, swelling, and hematoma formation at the site of injection. No systemic complications from PLLA have been reported in the literature. Subcutaneous papule formation is the most common adverse event associated with PLLA therapy. Subcutaneous papules can be prevented by following precise techniques: thorough mixing, using a 5-mL or greater dilution, injection into the subcutis, avoiding injection of the thin skin of the orbital rim, and manual massage after injection.

PLLA COMPARED TO FAT TRANSFER

Clinical results following tissue augmentation with PLLA are equivalent to fat transfer, but PLLA provides more predictable and long-lasting results. Fifty percent of injected fat disappears after six months, while PLLA lasts two years or longer. PLLA treatment is simpler because surgical harvesting and storage of fat is unnecessary.

SUMMARY

PLLA is an injectable filler that corrects soft tissue volume loss secondary to lipoatrophy of aging and HIV lipoatrophy. Proper technique is critical for successful results.

SUGGESTED READING

Leonard AL, Hanke CW. A protocol for facial volume restoration with poly-L-lactic acid. *J. Drugs Dermatol.* 2006;5:872–7.

Leonard AL, Hanke CW. Surgical pearl: the use of a laboratory vortex for poly-L-lactic acid injection. *J. Am. Acad. Dermatol.* 2006;55:511–12.

Woerle B, Hanke CW, Sattler G. Poly-L-lactic acid: a temporary filler for soft tissue augmentation. *J. Drugs Dermatol.* 2004;3:385–9.

CHAPTER 22

Poly-L-Lactic Acid (Sculptra) for Hand Volume Restoration

Marta I. Rendon

Mariana Pinzon-Plazas

Lina M. Cardona

INTRODUCTION

Hand rejuvenation with minimally invasive, nonsurgical procedures has become increasingly popular to minimize the discrepancy between a rejuvenated facial appearance and the aged appearance of the hands. The dorsum of the hand is the most important target for rejuvenation due to its visibility and how it reflects the process of aging, from volume loss due to skeletinization to muscular atrophy, tortuous veins, and solar damage.

Multiple dermatological procedures are available for hand rejuvenation, including chemical peels, microdermabrasion, laser therapy (ablative and nonablative), sclerotherapy, dermal fillers, and fat augmentation. Dermal fillers are widely used for volume restoration because they can be expected to produce a natural, smooth appearance.

POLY-L-LACTIC ACID

Poly-L-lactic acid (PLLA) is semipermanent filler that is biocompatible and biodegradable. It is a synthetic polymer with microparticles of poly-L-lactic acid supplied in a clear glass vial as a sterile, freeze-dried preparation for injection. A carton of PLLA contains two vials, each containing 367.5 mg of powder. PLLA can be stored at room temperature up to 30 degrees Celsius during and after hydration. The manufacturer recommends that any remaining material be discarded seventy-two hours after reconstitution; however, we have found that the product can be safely stored for up to three weeks when it is mixed with bacteriostatic water.

PLLA is reconstituted by hydrating the powder with 4 mL of bacteriostatic water plus 1–2 mL of local anesthetic (lidocaine 1%). For injection in the hands, we prefer a greater dilution, with 8 mL of bacteriostatic water and 1–2 mL local anesthetic (lidocaine 1%). This is in line with recently published studies indicating a preference for dilution with 6–12 mL of sterile water. Following the addition of bacteriostatic or sterile water, the vial should be allowed to stand for at least two hours to ensure complete hydration of the microparticles, before the vial is agitated with an electrical shaker or simply shaken manually to obtain a uniform translucent suspension. It is important to keep the product well shaken to avoid foaming in the vial.

PATIENT SELECTION

Patient selection is based on patient product preference, anatomical place, price, longevity of results, and physician experience. PLLA is manufactured in Italy and distributed as Sculptra by Dermik Laboratories, a division of Sanofi-Aventis USA. It offers good results that last twenty-four to thirty-six months; however, it is more expensive than calcium hydroxylapatite. PLLA is appropriate for patients presenting with volume loss in the dorsum of their hands, revealing wrinkles, veins, prominent joints, extensor tendons, and thin skin. Patients who desire cosmetic enhancement and a balanced appearance in the age of their face and hands are good candidates for this product. Three to six treatments given two to four weeks apart are usually needed for full correction, depending on the degree of volume loss and degree of patient satisfaction.

GENERAL CONSIDERATIONS

The ability to properly and optimally inject fillers is an evolutionary process that improves with experience. Four important aspects must be taken into consideration when injecting any filler: injection technique (tunneling, depot, threading, serial puncture, fanning, tenting), injection depth (superficial, middle, or deep into the dermal layer), specific syringe (gauge and length), and the volume of the product to be injected.

INJECTION TECHNIQUE

Before injection with PLLA, the dorsum of the hand is anesthetized with topical anesthetic cream (20 to 30%

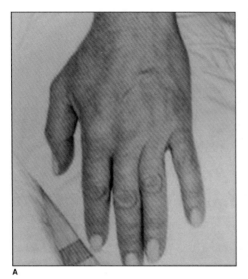 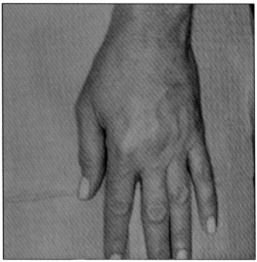

A   **B**

FIGURE 22.1: **A,** *Pretreatment.* **B,** *Results three months following PLLA injection.*

lidocaine, prilocaine, or tetracaine) for a period of twenty to thirty minutes. The area is then cleaned using a surgical preparation based on chloroxylenol USP 3% (Care-Tech Laboratories Inc.). The product is injected using a 26.5-gauge, 1-inch needle inserted at an angle of 30–40 degrees into the deep dermis or subcutaneous plane. A reflux maneuver should be performed before injecting the material to ensure that a blood vessel has not been involved. A volume of 0.1–0.2 mL per site is injected using the threading technique: injecting the material as the skin is pulled out and stretched to control the depth of the injection. Typically, we use one half to three fourths of the vial per hand per session. PLLA must be injected at the dermal, subcutaneous level and in small amounts in each intermetacarpal space. A Q-tip dampened with aluminum chloride-hexahydrate 20% (Drysol, Person and Covey Inc.) can be used to arrest the minimal blood flow resulting from each puncture. Moisturizer cream should be applied to the entire area and massaged periodically to obtain an even distribution of the microparticles. The intermittent use of ice pads can help slow the inflammation process. An average of three treatments are required for cosmetic enhancement, depending on desired effect.

AFTERCARE

The patient should be instructed to massage the area three times a day for five days to promote a natural-looking correction and optimal results. Massaging is crucial to prevent papule formation. Topical antibiotic ointment should be applied at each injection site until complete healing has occurred. The skin should be kept well hydrated and protected from the sun with a moisturizer containing SPF 15 or greater.

COMPLICATIONS

In clinical trials and in our practice, PLLA has demonstrated safety, with no evidence of systemic adverse effects or immunologic responses and a minimal (5%) incidence of hematoma and ecchymosis, which can last up to two weeks after treatment. In the hands of an inexperienced physician, the risk of temporary severe bruising, asymmetric correction, textural change, visible nodules, and granulomas is increased. In a retrospective study of twenty-seven patients with an average age of 65.9 years, conducted to assess the safety of PLLA for cosmetic hand rejuvenation, no significant side effects were seen; however, one case of fine, unnoticeable nodulation was noted, and seven patients were unsatisfied with the results.

CONCLUSION

Hand rejuvenation is gaining popularity in the aesthetic field as standard techniques, such as dermal fillers, have improved. PLLA has shown successful results in patients with lipoatrophy and HIV and was approved by the Food and Drug Administration in 2004. It has demonstrated efficacy by increasing dermal thickness up to three times the baseline value, which correlates with a clinically visible volume deficit correction. Cosmetic contouring of hands and face with PLLA has produced very good results, and more studies should be forthcoming to reveal the safety, efficacy, and tolerability of PLLA over time. Figure 22.1 demonstrates typical results.

SUGGESTED READING

Bains RD, Thorpe H, Southern S. Hand aging: patients' opinions. *Plast. Reconstr. Surg.* 2006;117:2212–18.

Broder K, Cohen S. An overview of permanent and semipermanent fillers. *J. Am. Soc. Plast. Surg.* 2006;118(Suppl 3):7S–14S.

Buford GA, Burgess CM, Lacombe VG, et al. The role of stimulatory fillers in aesthetic facial rejuvenation. *J. Cosmet. Dermatol.* 2007;20(Suppl 5):4–18.

Butterwick KJ. Rejuvenation of the aging hand. *Dermatol. Clin.* 2005;23:515–27.

Medical Insight Inc. Executive summary: global market for dermal fillers 2005–2011. Available at: http://www.miinews.com/exec_summaries/Global%20Market%20for%20Dermal%20Fillers%20Executive%20Summary%20022106.pdf. Accessed November 30, 2007.

Parker P. Hand lift plastic surgery. Available at: www.parkercenter.net/plastic_surgery_procedures_hand_lift.html. Accessed November 30, 2007.

Redaelli A. Cosmetic use of polylactic acid for hand rejuvenation: report on 27 patients. *J. Cosmet. Dermatol.* 2006;5:223–38.

Vleggaar D. Soft-tissue augmentation and the role of poly-L-lactic acid. *Plast. Reconstr. Surg.* 2006;118(Suppl 3):46S–54S.

CHAPTER 23

Bioalkamide

Andrew B. Denton

Bio-Alcamid (Polymekon) is a nonresorbable polymeric material composed of 4% alkylimide-amide group and 96% apyrogenic water. Alkylimide belongs to the family of acryl derivatives, and its polymeric structure does not contain free monomers. Histologic studies have shown that following implantation, the material is quickly surrounded by a thin collagen capsule, which stabilizes the material and protects it from the host tissues. Bio-Alcamid is indicated for the treatment of congenital and acquired areas of soft tissue depletion. It has been used successfully in the treatment of postliposuction skin irregularities, HIV facial lipoatrophy, Poland's syndrome, pectus excavatum, and posttraumatic soft tissue deficits. Increasingly, Bio-Alcamid is playing an important role in the armamentarium of the aesthetic physician as an alternative to surgical malar and chin augmentation as well as the correction of deep nasolabial folds. Unlike other injectable fillers currently available, Bio-Alcamid can be used to permanently correct large-volume deficits in a single treatment session. Contraindications include cutaneous collagen disease, uncompensated diabetes, and active infectious processes in the area of the implant. Patients are begun on antibiotic therapy aimed at gram-positive organisms one day prior to treatment and for seven days posttreatment. It is recommended that patients avoid direct sun exposure in the area of the implant for six weeks following the procedure to reduce the risk of bruising and edema. It is recommended that patients stop any blood thinning agents two weeks prior to and for one week following treatment.

TECHNIQUE

After photographs are taken, the areas to be treated are sterilized with an alcohol swab and outlined in the upright sitting position with a skin marker. Using a 3-cc syringe and a 30-gauge needle, the treatment areas are infiltrated with 1% lidocaine with 1:100,000 epinephrine. If avail-able, 0.3 cc of hyaluronidase added to each 3-cc syringe of lidocaine will dramatically decrease anesthetic-related soft tissue distortion. Following the onset of vasoconstriction, as evidenced by blanching of the skin (approximately ten minutes), the treatment may begin. It is recommended that the patient remain in the upright position during the injections. The product is delivered in sterile 5-cc luer lock syringes and is transferred to the 1-cc treatment syringes via a luer lock stopcock. The material is then injected into the subcutaneous tissue using a 1½ inch, 20-gauge needle. The material should never be injected into the dermis or directly into muscle. Treatment superior to the infraorbital rim and medial to the infraorbital foramen should also be avoided. Critically, the material is not threaded, as are many other soft tissue filling products, but is rather placed in contiguous aliquots of 0.3–0.5 cc until the desired correction is achieved. Smaller aliquot volumes have been shown not to become surrounded by an endogenous collagen capsule and are eventually degraded by the host tissue. The implant is then firmly massaged to smooth the contour – this is of particular importance in thinner-skinned individuals and in thin-skinned areas such as the temple. Despite the relatively large needle used, bleeding during the procedure and posttreatment bruising are both rare because of the vasoconstriction. The patient is told to expect mild swelling and redness of the treated areas, which typically settle over the first one to three days. As is the case following any facial procedure, keeping the head of the bed elevated and the use of cold compresses are helpful.

During the first posttreatment visit at one week, the areas are examined for visible or palpable irregularities, which are treated with firm massage. At this time, although the collagen capsule has already begun to form, it can be disrupted, allowing contour manipulation. Any small touch-up injections that may be required are carried out approximately six weeks later. Prophylactic antibiotic coverage is not used for touch-up treatments. Unlike any other

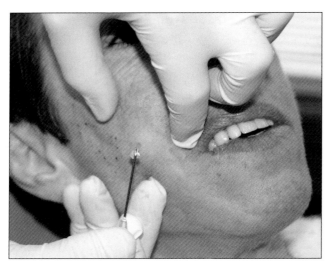

FIGURE 23.1: *Removal of Bio-Alcamid using an 18-gauge needle and bimanual pressure.*

injectable soft tissue filler, Bio-Alcamid is, at least to some degree, removable. Should this be required, a small amount of local anesthesia is infiltrated into the skin overlying a prominent area of product, and the collagen capsule is

pierced using an 18-gauge needle. The product is then easily expressed through the puncture site using firm bimanual pressure (Figure 23.1).

COSMETIC TREATMENTS

The aesthetic applications of Bio-Alcamid include chin and cheek augmentation and softening of the nasolabial folds. In some parts of the world, Bio-Alcamid is also used for lip augmentation; however, in my opinion, the aliquot size required during placement makes this a less than ideal lip filler. The volume used is entirely dependent on the degree of correction required, but a general guideline would be 1–2 mL in each nasolabial fold, 3–5 mL for chin augmentation, and 3–5 mL per side for malar augmentation. The principles of treatment are identical for cosmetic and reconstructive patients. Figure 23.2 demonstrates results for a thirty-four-year-old HIV-positive male who presented with a three-year history of facial lipoatrophy. Facial contour was restored using 6.5 cc of Bio-Alcamid in each cheek. Six months following the initial procedure, 0.5 cc was added to the left suprazygomatic area and 0.5 cc was removed from the left cheek.

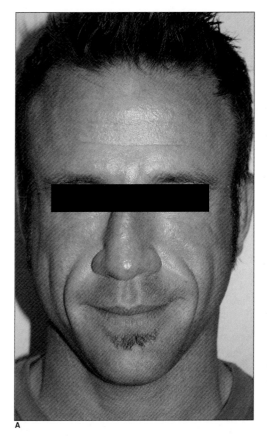
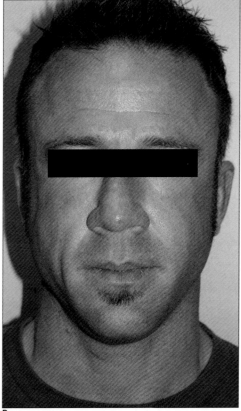

A   B

FIGURE 23.2: *Facial recontouring with Bio-Alcamid,* **A**, *before and,* **B**, *eight months posttreatment.*

COMPLICATIONS

Postoperative infection was reported in twelve of two thousand patients in one series. All cases of infection were caused by *Staphylococcal* species and all required removal of the prosthesis. The author has also observed migration of the implant material over time – typically with gravity – if the initial aliquot volume was too large.

SUGGESTED READING

Pacini S, Ruggiero M, Morucci G, Cammarota N, Protopapa C, Gulisano M. Bio-Alcamid: a novelty for reconstructive and cosmetic surgery. *Ital. J. Anat. Embryol.* 2002;107:209–14.

Protopapa C, Sito G, Caporale D, Cammarota N. Bio-Alcamid in drug-induced lipodystrophy. *J. Cosmet. Laser Ther.* 2003;5: 1–5.

CHAPTER 24

Silicone

David Duffy

Injectable liquid silicone (ILS), used worldwide since the 1940s to elevate scars and wrinkles, is the Jekyll and Hyde of dermal implants. Although capable of producing highly desirable and permanent results in *capable hands*, it is extremely technique-sensitive and easily abused. It has produced highly publicized disfiguring complications, particularly when adulterated and used in large volumes by untrained, nonmedical personnel. The occasional report by credible authors detailing extremely favorable results is overwhelmed by a torrent of lurid accountings of silicone-induced disasters. This disparity has produced rancorous disagreement (largely supported by anecdotal evidence). Advocates of ILS earnestly believe that almost all the horror stories, including death and disfigurement, are due to criminal misuse or media-fanned hysteria often involving agents that are unrelated to silicone. Critics just as earnestly believe that the advocates are lying about the true incidence of complications following proper use.

HOW DOES SILICONE FIT IN TODAY?

If ILS can overcome a reputation tainted by misuse, abuse, adulteration, and substitution of unrelated substances, it may take its place among a variety of agents used in the exponentially growing field of soft tissue augmentation. This process may be facilitated by multiple scientific, regulatory, and product developments, including (1) an exhaustive federal study that could not support an association between silicone and immune-related health conditions[1]; (2) the availability of two types of liquid silicone now approved by the Food and Drug Administration (FDA) for human use as ophthalmologic implant devices; (3) the FDA Modernization Act of 1997, which permits physicians to use drugs and devices for off-label purposes; and (4) proof of concept. The approval of ArteFill (polymethyl-methacrylate/collagen suspension) by the FDA represents

tacit bureaucratic recognition of the underlying principles, safety, and efficacy of at least one device for permanent soft tissue augmentation.

LEGAL TO USE SILICONES

Two forms of liquid silicone can legally be employed off-label for soft tissue augmentation in the United States. Adatosil 5000 (Bausch and Lomb Surgical), approved in 1994, and Silikon 1000 (Alcon Labs), approved in 1997.[2]

Although permissible to use in the United States (with the possible exception of Nevada), the use of all forms of liquid silicone is forbidden in several Western European countries. The long-term legal liabilities and costs associated with bringing a permanent soft tissue implantable agent to market (manufacturers of ArteFill are rumored to have spent over $75 million) have been a powerful deterrent against the reintroduction of silicone for this purpose.

ADVANTAGES

Silicones, which are man-made polymers containing silicon, oxygen, and methane, are used by the ton in a broad variety of medical and nonmedical applications. At the practical level, ILS is as close to an ideal implant as could be devised. It is permanent (although touch-ups may be required with age-induced atrophy); it is unaffected by exposure to air, sunlight, and most chemicals[3]; it does not support bacterial growth; and it is noncarcinogenic and retains its viscosity over a wide range of skin temperatures. In addition, ILS does not require refrigeration or skin testing, and at $60 per cubic centimeter, it is the least expensive

---

[1] Although this study may be flawed by its failure to address implant interactions with infectious and inflammatory processes.

[2] These numbers designate the viscosity of these silicones in centistokes; 100 centistokes is the viscosity of water. Accordingly, Adatosil is 50 times as viscous as water, and silicon is 10 times more viscous.

[3] ILS can be contaminated by prolonged contact with certain types of rubber, from which it absorbs traces of other chemicals. It should not be gas sterilized, for the same reason.

of any currently available filler in the United States. By way of comparison, ArteFill (Artes Medical) costs $750 per cc and requires both skin testing and refrigeration.

LABORATORY INVESTIGATIONS

The notion that all forms of silicone could be considered biologically nonreactive was based on short-term studies carried out at a time when nothing was known at the molecular level about the long-term interaction of implants in the kaleidoscopic milieu that characterizes biological systems. Silicone was considered to be so completely inert that its sole drawback was its tendency to migrate through tissue planes when implanted in large volumes (as much as five quarts). This problem was, it was supposed, solved by the misguided addition of adulterants to stimulate fibroplasia and anchor this material in place. Apparently, no one considered the possibility that additives would nullify the biological inertness of ILS. Horrific complications stemming from the use of large volumes of silicone combined with these adulterants by physicians who, in retrospect, should have known better helped lay the foundation for the disrepute and suspicion that characterize the use of ILS to this day.

SILICONE IMMUNOLOGY AND TOXICOLOGY

Silicones are not inert. Some have clear biological effects. Degradation of ILS to silica has been postulated. ILS can be phagocytized or transported intact and in small volumes incorporated into regional lymph nodes, without adverse effects.[4] This phenomenon has been compared to the benign process that occurs following the injection of tattoo pigments into the skin. Degradation of ILS to silica has been postulated.[5] Recent molecular investigations that study inflammatory events following foreign body implants suggest the following: (1) that inflammatory processes may be triggered not by the implant itself, but by a surface layer of plasma proteins (fibrinogen) which coats the implant and for which there are specific receptors; (2) bacteria may colonize implants in the form of antibiotic-resistant biofilm colonies, producing antibiotic-inaccessible persistent cellulitis; (3) a clinically significant heritable component may exist that predisposes certain individuals to the development of abnormalities in foreign body processing; in the future, these patients may be excluded from treatment by appropriate pharmacogenomic or human leukocyte antigen testing; (4) the presence of phagocytosable particulates in adulterated silicones can produce chronic inflammation,

decreased macrophage function, and bacterial proliferation. With time, a more precise understanding of the biological processes that affect implant integration may make many of the vitriolic debates regarding the risks and benefits of ILS scientifically irrelevant.

IS SILICONE RELEVANT?

In an era that has witnessed an explosion of new choices for all types of fillers, there is every possibility that ILS will remain, as it is now, a therapeutic artifact employed effectively by experts as a boutique modality, or misused criminally by lay shooters in back rooms. There are a host of reasons why ILS may never make it into the approved and respectable mainstream, stemming from mistrust or disapproval by almost every major institution that passes judgment on therapeutic modalities. ILS has few advocates. It is almost universally misunderstood and misrepresented by the media, medical community, malpractice insurance carriers, the FDA, the legal system, and the public at large. Financially, there is no incentive for reputable physicians to use ILS and strong incentives not to. Temporary fillers provide continuous repeat visits, a less stressful source of income, and freedom from character assassination and banish the specter of baseless lawsuits faced without benefit of malpractice insurance. It is also worth remembering that many of the jurors who try these cases are selected on the basis of their scientific unsophistication. For patients who demand permanent fillers, ArteFill is available, although expensive. It would then be a fair question to ask, Why would anybody use ILS? and the answer is surprisingly simple. Those who have had long-term experience using ILS, with serious complications occurring in a fraction of 1% of cases, have been impressed with the ability of this simple, inexpensive agent to achieve extraordinary results and positively and favorably transfigure the lives of the vast majority of treated patients who cannot afford other alternatives. It is unconscionable to deny patients with disfiguring cosmetic defects the opportunity to be treated with an agent that would spare them thousands of dollars, and ceaseless repetition of uncomfortable injections endured to maintain a normal appearance using temporary fillers. If for nothing else, the use of ILS should not be abandoned for such a humane purpose.

PHILOSOPHICAL CONSIDERATIONS

The use of a permanent filler implies a permanent relationship. Physicians who contemplate employing permanent implants should consider carefully whether they want this patient lifelong. They should also have an understanding of the mind-set of individuals who believe that they are exempt from the possibility of complications, and who demand permanent fillers.

---

[4] However, phagocytosis and transport of injected free silicone may occasionally be associated with complications at sites distant from the treated area.

[5] Silica is a known stimulus for granulomata.

Using temporary fillers on a trial basis gives the physician an opportunity to know the patient well and evaluate individual responses to soft tissue augmentation as well as the patient's psychological biases and cognitive ability to understand both advantages and the specific risk factors inherent in permanent fillers. Patients who are stubbornly determined to receive permanent fillers will sometimes be less than truthful about having received ILS or other types of fillers somewhere else, if they think that telling the truth will exclude them from receiving further treatments. Previous treatments by other practitioners who have used silicone (or other agents) of unknown purity or volume carry with them the onus of blame for delayed complications unrelated to later treatment technique.

INCORPORATING SILICONE INTO YOUR PRACTICE

The decision whether to use liquid silicone entails multiple philosophic and practical considerations. The checklist begins with a letter to your malpractice carrier, which may exclude silicone by name. If your carrier will not cover the use of this material, patient arbitration agreements can be employed, although these are not foolproof. Worth remembering is the fact that although ILS is legal to use, its legal status is questioned on a regular basis. Before making the decision to use ILS, experience using semipermanent and more forgiving temporary dermal fillers, such as Radiesse and Sculptra, which are injected at the same depth (and in the case of Sculptra, provide similar scaffolding effects), is a good starting point.[6] Training should be initiated by carefully observing the techniques used by practitioners who employ ILS regularly. The concept of using ultrasmall volumes and undercorrecting takes some getting used to. Small, flexible scars that have responded well to temporary fillers are a good starting target. Ideally, you then begin with a patient who you know well, whose response to other fillers has been frustratingly short.

ASSESSING PATIENT SUITABILITY

A large number of factors are associated with optimal or less than optimal outcomes following permanent fillers. They include lifestyle, patient and family medical history, and the individual characteristics of the defects to be treated. Certain sites and types of defects are more problematic based on volume needed for correction, susceptibility to trauma, infectious processes, insufficient dermal thickness, excessive muscular activity, or the potential for embolic phenomena on the basis of proximity to arteries.

---

[6] Although combinations of silicone and other long-lasting agents may be incompatible.

PRINCIPLES

The use of permanent fillers necessitates planning and an acute awareness of multiple factors that affect technique protocols and implant integration, including depth sensitivity, volume sensitivity, and the physical properties of the dermis or scar (density, stiffness, elasticity, location, and depth). Patients with multiple allergies or chronic infectious processes such as carious teeth or sinus infections and patients who will be subjected to trauma in the course of their daily lives may be at greater risk for complications. Although there appears to be no connection between collagen vascular disease and silicone in any form, malpractice concerns suggest avoidance of patients with a personal or family history of autoimmune disease.

Depth Sensitivity

Injections into subcutaneous fat are ineffective. Mid- or superficial dermal injections of ILS may produce excessive fibroplasia when treating superficial scars or rhytids. For these shallow defects, some authorities advocate so-called tattooing: injecting droplets of silicone less than 0.01 cc into the middermis. Unfortunately, injections at this shallow level in superficial scars may result in hypertrophic scarlike nodules. In the case of shallow crow's feet–type rhytids located in areas of reduced dermal thickness, nodules or visible implants may become apparent long after treatment, as dermal atrophy increases with age.

Volume Sensitivity

Many of the serious problems involving permanent fillers occur when relatively large volumes are employed for the correction of facial hemiatrophy or augmentation of the breast, buttocks, and hips. Large volumes present a much increased potential antigenic burden and substrate for foreign body granulomas or bacterial colonization. Textural abnormalities are also more common following the use of large volumes of ILS.

Physical Properties of Dermal Defects

Dermal thickness, mobility, and elasticity vary greatly from one area to another, resulting in different degrees of suitability for the treatment of defects. Scar response is modified by depth, degree of fibrosis, ratio of width to depth, and type of border (jagged, pitted, smooth, rounded, abrupt, or corrugated). Attempts to inject inflexible scars and wrinkles will result in dispersion of material to the borders of the defect, resulting in doughnutting or beading. Good results following ILS rely on exactly the right balance of elasticity, distensibility, and dermal bulk.

FACIAL AUGMENTATION

Different facial areas exhibit regional-specific profiles of response and complications.

Facial Augmentation and Patient Selection

For facial augmentation, ILS is particularly suitable for the treatment of nasolabial folds, marionette lines, postsurgical and traumatic facial contour depressions, and lipoatrophy associated with HIV, sudden weight loss, trauma, or aging. ILS has also been used for volumetric enhancement of the lips and cheekbones. It is extremely effective for the correction of minor postrhinoplastic defects, groovelike depressions surrounding permanent implants, and areas where osseous atrophy has occurred. Pliable depressed scars caused by acne, excoriation, trauma, varicella, microbial infections, surgery, and skin grafts can also be treated effectively.

Rhytid Orientation

Vertical rhytids are often less fibrotic, more flexible, and easier to correct than those which are oriented horizontally. Ridging, beading, and overcorrection often follow the injection of such horizontal creases on the face as the forehead wrinkles, the mental crease, and the fine horizontal rhytids traversing the philtrum. Scars and rhytids involving the philtrum itself are often impossible to correct using any type of filler.

Glabella

Injection of implantable agents of many different types into lateral glabellar rhytids that overlie supratrochlear and supraorbital arteries has been followed by tissue necrosis, amaurosis fugax, or permanent blindness. At least one case of amaurosis has been reported following silicone injections.[7] Naivety regarding the risk of intravascular ILS injection is evidenced in the statement of one highly experienced authority, who suggests that aspiration is unnecessary when injecting ILS since it does not contain particulates. Because of its proximity to underlying sinuses, the glabella may also be especially susceptible to infectious or allergic inflammatory processes, which may trigger inflammatory granulomas.

Periocular, Rhytids, and Scars

Periocular skin is so thin and distensible that it is almost impossible to inject viscous deep dermal fillers without producing nodules.

---

[7] Reported in 1988, this complication has never been cited in any previous text written on the subject.

Nasolabial Folds

When treating the nasolabial folds, it is important to be aware that their most proximal segments overlie the angular arteries. These can be tortuous and superficial, and prone to embolic phenomena and necrosis if inadvertently injected. Aspiration should be carried out before injecting these areas. Nasolabial folds that are very broad or very deep or adjacent to a fold of redundant skin may require excessive volumes of silicone, which will produce a rubbery texture or an aesthetically unattractive outcome.

Melolabial Folds (Marionette Lines) and Oral Commissures

Marionette lines must be treated cautiously to avoid protrusion of the implanted material into the oral cavity, resulting in a puffy appearance and the sensation of nodularity inside the mouth.

Centrofacial and Malar Augmentation

Low volume correction of mild atrophy in these areas is uniformly successful. High volume applications in this area are often followed by textural changes and gradual unsightly enlargement when observed for many years.

The Lips

The lips may be the least favorable site for permanent soft tissue augmentation. Complications following lip augmentation occur at a disproportionately high rate following any and every type of soft tissue filler. Predisposing factors include muscular activity; proximity to the oral cavity (a vast reservoir of potentially pathogenic bacteria); exposure to ultraviolet light; herpetic infections; trauma, including lip biting; infectious processes (periodontal disease, carious teeth); and bacterial contamination following dental procedures. All of these factors can trigger T-cell activation, granulomatous complications, and excessive fibroplasia, sometimes starting years after treatment. When followed for long periods of time, unsightly, unnaturally firm fibrotic enlargement of the lips can occur. This is most often seen in patients who have received large volumes of ILS and who also have significant chronic dental infections. Patients whose lips have been augmented with liquid silicone might benefit from the prophylactic use of minocycline 100 mg once daily before undergoing dental procedures.

Perioral Rhytids

There are two types of perioral rhytids. The first are U-shaped and broad based, representing muscle diastases. These are easily effaced by gentle stretching and fully correctable with soft tissue augmentation. The second – rigid palpable V-shaped pucker lines – are too superficial or inflexible to be satisfactorily treated using permanent soft tissue augmenting agents. Resurfacing is better therapy. Rhytids that involve the philtrum or bridge the mucocutaneous borders and extend into the vermilion are notoriously difficult to correct.

CONTRAINDICATIONS AND EXCLUSIONARY CRITERIA

Every year, my personal list grows longer. All authoritative publications warn against arterial injections and breast or penile augmentation, and the treatment of bound-down scars or cysts. No legitimate physicians attempt to create feminine contours in the breasts, hips, buttocks, and thighs, which require massive volumes of ILS. This type of backroom treatment is frequently associated with essentially untreatable intermittent episodes of eruptive inflammatory nodules. These may be precipitated long after injection, by exercise or by infectious processes occurring elsewhere in the body. Fluid migration along tissue planes initiated by muscular activity or gravity is particularly problematic following large-volume injections of the lower extremities. Severe pain, nodularity, and hyperpigmentation associated with significant elevations of serum tumor necrosis factor alpha (TNF-α) have also been noted. The transsexual population is at particular risk for these disasters. ILS is safe for pregnant patients, but its use is prudently avoided because of malpractice concerns. Patients who carry out strenuous activity immediately posttreatment may develop vasodilatory-induced nodule formation. Patients with chronic infectious or inflammatory processes may be at greatly increased risk for granulomatous complications. Achauer (1983) reported one of the first documented disfiguring adverse events following the so-called proper use of ILS following the treatment of a patient with Weber-Christian disease.

I exclude from lip augmentation patients with histories of chronic sinus infections, carious teeth, labial herpes simplex, and patients who are routinely subjected to facial trauma (martial arts and various sports). Patients who bite their lips are also excluded from lip augmentation. I also exclude patients with a personal and/or family history of collagen vascular disease (I will most assuredly be blamed if collagen vascular disease ever develops in them). Patients with multiple allergies may be at greater risk for inflammatory complications. Serious complications to ILS resemble sarcoidosis, which has been triggered in susceptible patients by trauma, and foreign bodies. Patients with disease entities associated with T-cell activation or with elevations in TNF-α, including psoriatics and rheumatoid arthritics, may be riskier to treat. I have treated patients who have histories of keloid formation, but this, too, may be riskier.

Although ILS has been employed successfully for the treatment of HIV-associated lipodystrophy, the possibility of delayed granulomatous complications following immune restoration must be considered. The occurrence of delayed granulomatous reactions as a consequence of drug interactions must also be considered. Paradoxically, eruptive granulomas occurred twenty years after successful silicone facial scar treatment following therapy with biologics for psoriasis.[8] Other permanent agents have also been associated with drug-induced granuloma development. One patient treated with ArteFill developed granulomas at the treated sites following treatment with interferons.

TECHNIQUE, PRINCIPLES, AND TRAINING

The first principle involving the use of liquid silicone is the need for hands-on training. Nothing you can read will prepare you to use effectively and safely any form of permanent implant. Experienced practitioners develop both a tactile and a visual sense of appropriate depth and/or contour response to the injected material. This is based partially on the amount of force necessary to inject the material. Injection force is a function of the syringe diameter, syringe volume, and viscosity of material in the syringe; the gauge of the needle; the depth of the injection; and the physical characteristics of the injection site. Visual cues subsume knowledgeable assessment of desired contour changes and the rapidity with which they occur. Silicone works both by adding volume and as a stimulus and scaffolding for the ingrowth of new tissue. Hence full response to soft tissue augmentation with ILS is measured in months to years. Deep rhytids and scars obviously require larger volumes. Men often require substantially larger volumes than women and may respond more slowly. Patients will be dissatisfied if they are not made aware of these facts. Photographs are the only way of documenting positive (or sometimes not so positive) changes. Documentation is mandatory.

The microdroplet technique, established by Norman Orentreich in 1952, is (in my view) the only acceptable method of using ILS. ILS is most effective, safe, and predictable when microscopic quantities (0.01–0.03 cc per injection site) are employed. Injections are given at least 2–3 mm apart, at the dermal-subcutaneous junction. This technique provides maximum surface to volume area for the stimulation of new collagen. It results in stable, delicate fibroplasia. Larger droplets of silicone may induce excess fibroplasia, resulting in palpable thickening around the implanted material. Undercorrection is the rule! Needle injection angle varies with the desired depth of injection. To avoid injection into the middermis, which may be followed by excessive new collagen formation, the thumb is removed from the syringe plunger well before withdrawing the needle. The total amount of silicone injected per

---

[8] Biologics have been used successfully to treat silicone granulomas. This paradox is explained by cytokine pleiotropism.

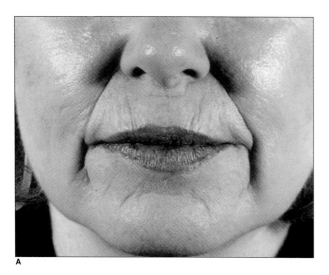 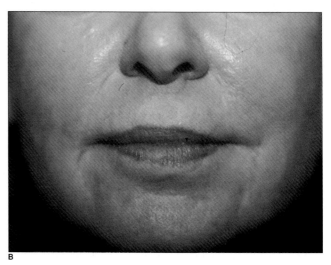

FIGURE 24.1: *Long-lasting efficacy of liquid silicone for nasolabial and melolabial folds:* **A**, *pretreatment;* **B**, *ten years posttreatment (estimated volume 2.5 cc).*

sitting varies with the extent and type of the defects to be injected (Figures 24.1–24.3). In terms of short-term outcomes, cumulative volume is not as important as the volume per injection site. However, larger total volumes of ILS are more likely to cause problems. For treatment of nasolabial or melolabial folds, volumes employed typically vary between 0.25 and 0.75 cc. For facial hemiatrophy, 2 or 3 cc per session has been safely employed. A second pass, injecting more ILS above or below previously treated areas, may lead to droplet coalescence and excessive fibroplasia. Treatments are carried out at one- to two-month intervals

for the first several treatments, and at two- to six-month intervals as the process progresses.

INSTRUMENTATION AND PERSONAL PREFERENCES

Using an 18-gauge needle, 0.4 cc of Silikon is drawn up into a 1-cc leur lock syringe, fitted with an assist device that is ordinarily employed for Zyplast. Injections are carried out using a 26- or 27-gauge, 1/2-inch needle. Two weeks before treatment, anticoagulant drugs, such as aspirin, Coumadin,

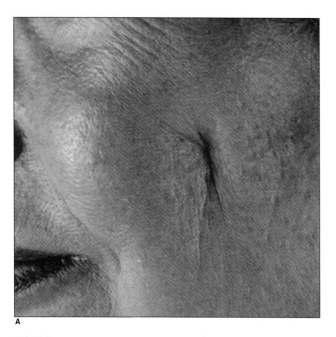 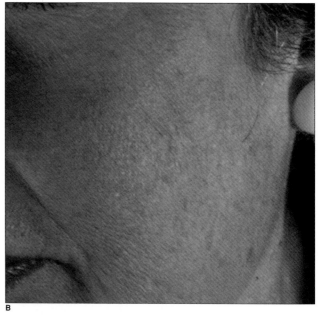

FIGURE 24.2: *Results following the injection of approximately 1 cc of liquid silicone over several months:* **A**, *pretreatment;* **B**, *six months posttreatment.*

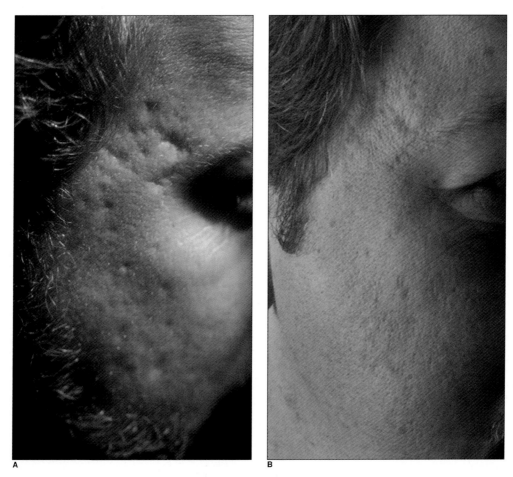

FIGURE 24.3: *Pliable scars located on the temple are an ideal indication for liquid silicone: A, pretreatment; B, two years after implantation of an estimated 4 cc of liquid silicone injected over several months.*

or heparin, are discontinued. Patients are advised not to undergo dental procedures, run marathons, or consume significant amounts of alcohol for at least two weeks after treatment. On the morning of treatment, patients wear no makeup, are carefully cleansed, and are given nerve block anesthesia, which does not distort the areas to be treated. Although topical anesthetics can be employed, their use makes careful marking of the areas to be treated more difficult. With the patient seated under overhead lights, sites to be treated are outlined using an eyebrow pencil. Treatment is administered with the patient in the seated position. Flash and side-lighted pretreatment and posttreatment photographs are taken, using both digital and silver halide photography. Surgical lights, although not color corrected, are used to silhouette the contours of the areas injected.

Some physicians prefer to use insulin syringes (Becton Dickenson). These 0.3-cc syringes must be filled with the plunger out. This type of syringe, with a permanently attached needle, is particularly useful for extremely small volume injections.

COMPLICATIONS

Treatment with ILS can provoke the same spectrum of minor complications and certain major complications associated with other types of soft tissue fillers. Complications can be minor or major, temporary or permanent, immediate or delayed, inflammatory or noninflammatory, and technique or nontechnique related. Most complications specific to ILS are technique related. It is *unforgiving*. Problems often arise when ILS is injected too superficially. These include overcorrection; fibrosis; dyschromia (brown or yellow discoloration of the skin); a peau d'ange appearance sometimes attributed to lymphatic blockage; and bluish discoloration, which follows the treatment of patients with very thin, translucent skin. Telangiectasias occasionally occur. Superficial ILS implants can become visible years after treatment. When small superficial foreign body granulomas occur, they can be treated using dermabrasion, ablative lasers, or electrocautery. Minor overcorrections often flatten with intralesional corticosteroids. There is general agreement that horrific sequelae, including migration, ulceration, fistulation, embolic phenomena, and collagen vascular disease, have not occurred following the use of small volumes of pure liquid silicone by skilled physicians treating properly selected patients.

DISPLACEMENT PHENOMENA

Occasionally, patients who have undergone glabellar or nasolabial augmentation develop excessive, ridgelike fullness adjacent to the injection site. This may be due to muscular movement–induced displacement of ILS or to excessive collagen deposition.

Migration and Drift

Although clinically visible large volume migration has never been reported following the proper use of small volumes of ILS, I have personally observed nodules in areas where silicone had not been injected. This occurred in a patient who also developed widespread inflammatory granulomas involving many sites where silicone had previously been injected.[9] This inflammatory complication was triggered by an infected tooth. In another case, histological proof of silicone presence was noted in a patient who developed sarcoidal nodules several centimeters from the injection site. Cases such as this confirm the presence of free ILS presumably transported via the lymphatics to sites distant from the injections. This phenomenon has been postulated in other publications.

TREATING COMPLICATIONS

For extensive inflammatory complications, oral and intralesional corticosteroids and minocycline, 100–200 mg daily, are my current treatments of choice. An enormous variety of compounds have been tried, with varying degrees of success. Despite what uncritical advocates have written, serious complications (that are very difficult to treat) can and do occur.

NEW TREATMENTS ON THE HORIZON

Disfiguring complications following ILS, a common event following backroom injections, occasionally occur following treatment by experts using meticulous techniques. Fundamental research on diseases that clinically and/or immunologically resemble silicone granulomas will unquestionably provide more precisely targeted therapies for intractable silicone granulomas. They will include the use of anti-TNF-α agents such as Etanercept. These drugs have provided effective treatment for massive intractable granulomas following injection of an unknown agent for

hip and buttock augmentation. Costly research aimed at producing profit-making drugs for diseases such as sarcoidosis and psoriasis will provide both mechanistic insights and a source of effective drugs for the treatment of complications that are, at this time, considered untreatable by any means other than surgical removal. *Thermotherapy*, using focused ultrasound, lasers, or radiofrequency devices designed to stimulate collagen contraction, may ultimately be used to produce direct bactericidal effects and disrupt biofilms and denature fibrotic granulomas by precise temperature elevations at appropriate dermal depths. Bacteriophage may be employed to dissolve biofilms circumventing antibiotic resistance in resident bacteria.

PERSONAL CONSIDERATIONS

As more soft tissue augmenting agents come on the market, I find myself choosing silicone less and less. That is not because I do not think that ILS is superior for many defects. It has more to do with my increasing concern for personal risk exposure using an agent that is so widely misunderstood and calumniated. Assuming that they meet exclusionary criteria, there are four sets of patients who I think are most benefited by the use of ILS:

1. those who need small volume augmentation for the reconstruction of depressed scars and postrhinoplastic defects, or low-volume cutaneous atrophies; this application is associated with minimal risk and maximal benefit

2. patients who I know well and have personally treated with small volumes of silicone in the past, whose risk factors are not altered (although long-term exposure to liquid silicone or other permanent implants may increase risks)

3. patients who have had multiple temporary fillers in appropriate areas, with disappointingly short, temporary improvements

4. elderly patients who cannot afford repeated injections of temporary fillers

I routinely turn away patients who were referred for silicone if they do not meet certain psychological criteria, including realistic expectations. I try to avoid treating patients who have previously received ILS from other practitioners. Reports of synergistic adverse effects involving combinations of silicone and other permanent fillers, such as Bioplastique, Aquamid, and ProFill, are appearing in the European literature. Combinations of ILS and scaffold-inducing fillers, such as Sculptra, may also be contraindicated. The screening process I employ for new patients usually starts with a trial of temporary fillers and the provision of literature describing, in minute detail, every possible complication and the clinical setting in which it occurs as well as published diatribes authored by silicone's most

---

[9] Possibly on the basis of memory T-cell activation.

vociferous critics. I couple this with an extraordinarily detailed consent agreement.

SUMMARY

One can make a good case for or against using permanent implants of any kind. Those who use them cite the benefits. Those who oppose their use cite the risks of rare but untreatable complications. Both arguments are logical. I personally believe that the concept of permanent soft tissue augmentation is too important to ignore, and that ILS is the most versatile, cost-effective permanent filler available. Science does not stand still. Progress in the immunologic understanding of the mechanisms that govern successful or unsuccessful long-term integration of soft tissue implants will continue to accumulate. This will result in further advances and refinements in patient selection, more accurate molecular-based diagnosis, and more precisely targeted therapies for complications. Outcomes will be more predictable and beneficial. The historical record for ILS is a proxy for the generic possibilities, good and bad, associated with any form of permanent implant. Lessons learned from ILS will have important implications for other types of implants, just as the knowledge gained from other types of implants will inevitably modify protocols involving the use of permanent soft tissue implants. ILS has created in my own mind the most extraordinary ambivalence. On one hand, it is the most effective modality I have ever employed for specific types of soft tissue defects. On the other hand, it exposes me to legal liabilities that I find progressively less acceptable, particularly since many less controversial alternatives are becoming available. ILS has been chronicled in anecdotes, and no one knows how many patients have been treated – properly or improperly – with this agent. How many have benefited? How many have developed serious complications, and under what circumstances? Before permanent implant materials of any kind can be comfortably incorporated into the everyday pharmacopoeia of the soft tissue augmentation repertoire, oversight programs similar to those established for silicone breast implants must be created. These programs would address five key issues:

1. the need for mandatory long-term surveillance protocols, specifying the number of patients who have been treated, the parameters employed, and the ratio of benefits to complications (the ArteFill manufacturers have completed a five-year study; that is a very good beginning!)

2. the establishment of valid indications and contraindications

3. the creation of a uniform system for determining the immunopathogenesis of serious complications

4. an agreed-on protocol for the treatment of serious complications

5. the establishment of specific training augmentation programs, with documentation, for physicians wishing to administer permanent implant materials

SUGGESTED READING

Achauer BM. A serious complication following medical grade silicone injection of the face. *Plast. Reconstr. Surg.* 1983;71: 251–4.

Bondurant S, Ernster V, Herdman R, eds. *Safety of Silicone Breast Implants*. Washington, DC: National Academies Press; 2000.

Desai A, et al. Case reports: Etanercept therapy for silicone granuloma. *J. Drugs Dermatol.* 2006;5:894–6.

Duffy DM. Injectable liquid silicone: new perspectives. In: Klein AW, ed., *Tissue Augmentation in Clinical Practice: Procedures and Techniques*. New York: Marcel Dekker; 1998:237–67.

Duffy DM. Silicone conundrum: a battle of anecdotes. *Dermatol. Surg.* 2002;7:590–4.

Duffy DM. Liquid silicone for soft tissue augmentation: histological, clinical, and molecular perspectives. In: Klein A, ed., *Tissue Augmentation in Clinical Practice*. New York: Taylor and Francis; 2006:141–238.

Hu W-J, Eaton JW, Tang L. Molecular basis of biomaterial-mediated foreign body reactions. *Blood* 2001;98:1231–8.

Narins R, Beer K. Liquid injectable silicone: a review of its history, immunology, technical considerations, complications, and potential. *Plast. Reconstr. Surg.* 2006;118(3S):77S–84S.

Orentreich D. Liquid injectable silicone. *Clin. Plast. Surg.* 2000; 27:596–612.

Rapaport M. Silicone injections revisited. *Dermatol. Surg.* 2002; 7:594–5.

Shin H, Lemke BN, Stevens TS, Lim MJ. Posterior ciliary-artery occlusion after subcutaneous silicone-oil injection. *Ann. Ophthalmol.* 1988;20:342–4.

Section 6

AUTOLOGOUS FAT TRANSFER

CHAPTER 25

Autologous Fat Transfer: An Introduction

Sorin Eremia

The use of fat as an autologous filling material dates back at least a century. In the 1970s and early 1980s, many plastic surgeons still used eyelid fat from blepharoplasty to fill in glabellar or even nasolabial fold lines through small slit incisions. The results were uniformly temporary, with full resorption after six to thirteen months. Injectable autologous fat grafting really has its roots closely tied to the introduction of modern liposuction. It is unclear who may have been the first to use fat harvested from liposuction, place it in a syringe, and reinject it back into the tissues. There were certainly many who started about the same time. In the early days of liposuction, contour deformities were quite common, and reinjecting fat was an obvious and, as it turns out, the most practical treatment option.

The idea of harvesting fat with a small cannula, in a relatively small syringe for reinjection, probably occurred to several physicians at about the same time. But it is Pierre Fournier who certainly deserves most of the credit for popularizing this procedure starting around 1984–1985. Fournier used a very simple technique of harvesting the fat with a 5- to 10-cc syringe fitted with a 14-gauge cannula, and after letting the fat settle and discarding the separated serum, he reinjected it as "small strands of spaghetti" through a 14- or 16-gauge needle. He used it primarily for nasolabial folds, glabellar frown lines, and marionette lines and was also beginning to place it in hands. I learned the technique from him in late 2004, and I was so impressed that within a few months, I arranged a special fat harvesting and grafting course at Dr. Fournier's Paris clinic. It was attended by a group of twelve to fifteen interested California physicians, representing various specialties, with a strong contingent of dermatologists.

In U.S. plastic surgery circles, the idea that autologous fat could be used as an effective tissue filler was initially received with great skepticism, as was, initially, liposuction. Dr. Mel Bircoll, from Beverly Hills, was an exception, though eventually, it was Dr. Sydney Coleman who became the chief plastic surgeon advocate for injectable autologous fat. In dermatology, Saul Askin, Rhoda Narrins, Bill Coleman, and Bill Hanke were among early users, while Lisa Donofrio has been one of the chief researchers and advocates for the past dozen years and is currently involved with cutting-edge research on tissue-cultured fat. Among other notable pioneers, Jules Newman, a facial plastic surgeon, and Rick Dolski, a general plastic surgeon, leaders of the American Academy of Cosmetic Surgery, were also at the forefront, followed by Mark Berman and Mel Shiffman, who also made important contributions. In Europe, Fournier continued to be a tireless fat-grafting advocate, and Frank Trepsat and Roger Amar cannot be omitted as major influences on the modern uses of fat grafting.

By the middle to late 1980s, numerous physicians from dermatology, facial and general plastic surgery, and cosmetic surgery were embracing and experimenting with fat grafting. I designed and carried out, together with Dan Gormley, the first side-by-side, split-face study comparing autologous fat grafts to Zyplast collagen, published in 1990. We were able to demonstrate clearly superior results with fat starting at six months, and especially at twelve months. The study results provided impetus for continued work and refinements; however, with my own patients, whom I followed long term, I was getting unpredictable, mostly disappointing results past the twelve-month term, even after repeated touch-ups. I was still using a 3- to 5-cc syringe to reinject the fat through 14- to 16-gauge needles. These disappointing long-term results were eventually published as well.

For most initial enthusiasts, the early fat transfer results were disappointing as well, with unpredictable long-term results, especially for the treatment of wrinkles. Efforts to improve results focused on harvesting methods, processing the fat, storing and even freezing the fat, and reinjection techniques. Studies and controversy continue today as to what are the best methods of processing fat, though the majority lean toward short, low-power centrifugation, or at least gravity separation of the fat from serum. The use of even relatively crudely frozen and simply thawed fat for reinjection has yielded results not much inferior from the use of fresh fat. Very sophisticated methods of freezing and thawing fat have been proposed that document increased fat cell viability, although the clinical significance versus the additional trouble remains to be determined.

The true breakthrough for the use of injectable autologous fat came with the switch to using 1-cc syringes to inject small strands of fat through 17- to 18-gauge needles, and now even much smaller needles are used such as 20- or 22-gauge needles or cannulae. The other major development was the use of fat as a volume filler for more than just the typical folds (nasolabial, glabellar, commissural) treated with the early commercial-type filler. Sydney Coleman deserves much of the credit for popularizing both the use of 1-cc syringes and small harvesting and injection cannulae as well as the use of fat as a volume replacement filler throughout the face. His textbook *Structural Fat Grafting* is a must read. Mark Berman has also been instrumental in promoting volumetric use of fat to restore volume to the aging face. In France, Roger Amar developed a very structured method of injecting small amounts of fat around the sheaths of specific facial expression muscles. Results are impressive, but the technique, fat autograft muscle injection (FAMI), is not easy to master, and most fat users simply incorporate Dr. Amar's concepts as needed. Even more cutting-edge is the technique proposed by Ali Benslimane to reinflate the closed orbital space with injection of autologous fat with 22-gauge cannulae.

I can attest from my own experience that when, in the late 1990s, I personally switched to using a 1-cc syringe and 18-gauge needle to transfer fat to the nasolabial folds, my good long-term results (fifteen to twenty-four months) increased dramatically from the previously reported 5 to 15% of cases to about 40% of cases. For other areas where fat is injected deeper, for example, around the periosteum or thin facial muscles, the percentage of persistent results is even higher.

Today, fat transfer is used in several ways, and this section attempts to present them to the reader in a relatively organized fashion:

1. Fat transfer is used in small volumes, much like a commercial filler, for nasolabial folds, lateral commissural folds, occasionally the lips, and so on. In Chapter 26, "Small-Volume Fat Transfer," Dr. William P. Coleman III, editor in chief of *Dermatologic Surgery*, and one of the early fat-grafting pioneers, discusses his methods, which are still very simple, easy to learn and use, and provide a good starting point for anyone interested in fat grafting.

2. Fat transfer is used in larger volumes, in multiple planes, still in very small quantities at each site, to achieve either regional or even full face and neck volume restoration. Dr. Mark Berman, a facial plastic surgeon and a true pioneer of this approach, presents some outstanding results in Chapter 27, "Larger-Volume Fat Transfer." Dr. Berman's techniques incorporate elements of all the other techniques discussed in this text.

3. Fat transfer is used in larger volumes, but only along the muscles, with the FAMI technique, and in the hands. These methods are discussed by Dr. Kimberly J. Butterwick, the most notable FAMI expert in the United States and a pioneer in the use of fat to restore volume to the aging hand, in Chapter 28.

4. Fat transfer is used in combination with other procedures. The choice of fat as a filler is further discussed by noted European plastic surgeon Dr. Constantin Stan, who, in Chapter 29, critically examines fat as an option versus other methods of dealing with volumetric aging changes. Dr. Stan uses the most modern microlipostructure fat transfer techniques, which are quite popular in Europe and around the world, in spite of the availability of so many commercial fillers.

The interested reader is also referred to Dr. Arturo Prado's chapter on fillers (Chapter 41); in certain situations, his preference for fat versus the fillers available in South America is well discussed.

It is obvious from what is presented by the contributing authors that injected autologous fat is an excellent filler. The questions the reader may ask are, why is it not the predominant filler in use today, and how does fat really compare to commercial fillers?

Harvesting and reinjecting fat is certainly more time consuming than using most commercial fillers. It is also more traumatic and has significantly longer recovery time. It is also less precise for correcting small volumes, and six- to twelve-month results, not to mention longer-term results, are less predictable. Properly freezing and storing fat can also involve significant costs and liabilities. In my practice, for small-volume augmentation (1–2 cc of commercial filler equivalent), fat was an excellent alternative to the old collagen fillers, but it is no longer a competitive method for small-volume augmentation. The new fillers available, especially the hyaluronic acid fillers, are simply a better option for most patients. Even for deeper placement, the commercial fillers are now offering very competitive alternatives. However, for larger-volume augmentation, fat still remains the filler of choice.

It should also be noted that significant complications can occur with fat. These include fat embolization and serious infections, especially with atypical mycobacteria. But most annoying can be persistent overcorrection, which is not easy to fix. It takes great skill and patience to properly perform larger-volume fat transfer, and over the years, I have seen some very unhappy patients with either unnatural appearance or specific small irregularities related to volume overcorrection with fat. And in a few cases, the treatments had been performed by very skilled and experienced fat proponents.

In conclusion, injected autologous fat remains one of the best fillers available today, with many ideal filler attributes. Physicians focusing on cosmetic procedures should be familiar with the use of fat grafting as a tissue augmentation and volume replacement method.

SUGGESTED READING

Berman, M. The aging face: a different perspective on pathology and treatment. *Am. J. Cosmet. Surg.* 1998;15:167–72.

Butterwick KJ. Hand study: lipoaugmentation for the aging hands: a comparison of the longevity and aesthetic results of centrifuged vs. non-centrifuged fat. *Dermatol. Surg.* 2002;28:1184–7.

Butterwick KJ. Fat autograft muscle injection (FAMI): new technique for facial volume. *Dermatol. Surg.* 2005;31:1487–95.

Coleman SR. Facial recontouring with lipostructure. *Clin. Plast. Surg.* 1997;24:347–67.

Coleman SR. Structural fat grafts: the ideal filler? *Clin. Plast. Surg.* 2001;28:111.

Coleman SR. *Structural Fat Grafting.* St. Louis, MO: Quality Medical; 2004.

Donofrio LM. Structural autologous lipoaugmentation: a panfacial technique. *Dermatol. Surg.* 2000;26:1129–34.

Eremia S, Newman N. Long-term follow-up after autologous fat grafting: analysis of results from 116 patients followed at least 12 months after receiving the last of a minimum of two treatments. *Dermatol. Surg.* 2000;26:1148–58.

Fournier PF. Fat grafting: my technique. *Dermatol. Surg.* 2000;26:1117–28.

Gormley DE, Eremia S. Quantitative assessment of augmentation therapy. *J. Dermatol. Surg. Oncol.* 1990;16:1147–51.

Hanke CW. Fat transplantation: indications, techniques, results. *Dermatol. Surg.* 2000;26:1106.

Kaufman MR, Bradley JP, Dickinson B, et al. Autologous Fat Transfer National Consensus Survey: trends in techniques for harvest, preparation, and application, and perception of short- and long-term results. *Plast. Reconstr. Surg.* 2007;119:323–31.

Newman J, Ftaiha Z. The biographical history of fat transplant surgery. *Am. J. Cosmet. Surg.* 1987;4:85.

Shiffman MA, Mirrafatti S. Fat transfer techniques: the effect of harvest and transfer methods on adipocyte viability and review of the literature. *Dermatol. Surg.* 2001;27:819–26.

CHAPTER 26

Small-Volume Fat Transfer

William P. Coleman III
Kyle M. Coleman

Fat transplantation can be used to fill subcutaneous defects ranging in size from major to minor. Today, many patients are interested in ambulatory procedures with minimal downtime. Small-volume fat transplantation can easily be performed under local anesthesia, allowing the patient to return to public life within one or two days. Although the term may mean different things to different surgeons, small-volume fat transplantation might include augmentation of the malar, nasojugal, and nasolabial areas. These minor lipoaugmentation procedures can be repeated monthly or bimonthly, eventually leading to a significant improvement with minimal time dedicated to recovery.

Small-volume fat transplantation can be performed all over the body but is most commonly used for facial atrophy due to trauma and aging or for traumatic fat dents of the thighs resulting from liposuction or accidents. It is also useful for augmentation of aging hands. Since several small-volume procedures are needed to obtain the best results, patients must be forewarned that they will often see minimal improvement after the first procedure. Augmentation of subcutaneous defects also requires many times the volume of augmentation of cutaneous defects. The comparatively dense dermis requires very little filling volume to achieve a visual improvement, compared to subcutaneous tissue, which often seems to act as a black hole, soaking up filling materials. The physician who moves from injecting dermal fillers into using subcutaneous fillers learns this very quickly.

Small-volume fat transplantation can also be used as part of a combination approach. In this application, fat is transferred into the subcutaneous tissue, establishing a platform for injection of dermal fillers above. In some cases, collagen fillers can be used in the upper dermis, hyaluronic acid fillers in the lower dermis, and fat injected below to achieve optimal results.

PLANNING

First, the areas to be augmented are carefully delineated using a waterproof marker. Surgeons should develop a system for identifying deeper versus shallower areas for injection. Fat transplantation is a three-dimensional procedure, and most areas that are treated are shaped like a bowl, with the deepest part of the defect in the center. Marking should be done with the patient upright so that the full effects of gravity are apparent. Depending on the personality of the patient, the surgeon may also wish to involve him or her in the marking process.

A thick layer of topical anesthetic, such as EMLA or Elamax, is then applied. These creams usually fix the markings and make them more difficult to remove. This could be an advantage or a disadvantage, depending on the situation, and the surgeon must learn to apply the markings with a light touch to avoid the necessity of heavy scrubbing at the end of the procedure.

Next, the donor area is selected. If the patient is having liposuction, then no special marking is needed beyond what was employed in designating the areas to be suctioned. If fat transplantation is performed as a stand-alone procedure, the donor area should be selected with an eye to giving the patient some minor cosmetic improvement in the harvest site. Commonly patients are asymmetric, with one hip, for instance, being larger than the other. Choosing the larger hip for the donor area can help to make the patient's shape more symmetric.

There is no strong scientific evidence that one area is more advantageous than another in achieving successful augmentation (Rohrich et al. 2004). In many cases, patients who seek fat transplantation have low total body fat. Their thin faces are often accompanied by correspondingly thin bodies. In these patients, it is very difficult to find enough fat to harvest, and the surgeon must take it from wherever it is available. In many thin individuals, the flanks are a good source of fat when very little can be found in the abdomen, hips, or thighs. Once the appropriate area is selected, it is outlined with a waterproof marker.

HARVESTING

Donor site anesthesia is best accomplished using the tumescent technique. The standard tumescent formula containing 0.05 to 0.1% lidocaine and 1:1 million epinephrine is sufficient for both anesthesia and vasoconstriction in the vast majority of individuals. Some anxious patients may also benefit from the use of preoperative oral diazepam at 5–10 mg, but many patients do quite well with local anesthesia alone. The local anesthesia is infiltrated just as with liposuction, using a peristaltic pump until the tissue is firm. It is then wise to wait at least twenty minutes before beginning the procedure. If harvesting fat is done too quickly after infiltration of the tumescent fluid, most of the extracted material will be tumescent fluid and will contain very little fat. After thirty to forty minutes, nearly pure, bloodless fat can easily be obtained.

Before beginning harvesting, it is convenient to anesthetize the recipient area, previously pretreated with topical anesthetic. Tumescent anesthesia of 0.05 to 0.1% is very effective here as well. Alternatively, stock 1% lidocaine with epinephrine can be employed. Facial nerve blocks are also effective.

Once the recipient area has been anesthetized, donor harvesting can proceed. Large cannulae tend to harvest larger clumps of fat, which are more difficult to inject through smaller injection cannulae. Therefore it is more efficient to harvest using a 14-gauge instrument. Although fat can be harvested using liposuction equipment and an inline sterile sputum container, this is more likely to damage fat cells (Nguyen et al. 1990). Manual liposuction using a 10-cc syringe attached directly to the cannula is preferable. Longer cannulae are more efficient because suction is lost in the syringe once the tip of the cannula is withdrawn close to the insertion site.

Using the same puncture hole previously used to infiltrate the tumescent fluid, the cannula with the syringe attached is pushed forcefully into the fatty layer of the selected donor site. The plunger of the syringe is then withdrawn and held out by the fingers of the surgeon's dominant hand. The cannula is then pushed back and forth through the tissue, while the nondominant hand helps to milk fat into the tip of the instrument. In most cases, 10 cc of pure fat can be harvested in 20–30 s. If the patient is thin, harvesting can be slower and quite tedious. The syringes of extracted fat are capped and allowed to stand upright in a test tube holder. After a few minutes, gravity causes separation of the fat from the injected anesthetic. This clear or slightly pink fluid can then be expelled from the syringe. The role of centrifugation to separate fat from blood and anesthetic fluid has been a source of debate (Rose et al. 2006), but the trend has been to use less and less centrifugation. Empirically, it has always been the author's opinion that if centrifugation cleans the fat a little more thoroughly, it does so at the expense of trauma to the fragile graft. Furthermore, since the material is being injected into an environment of traumatized fat, blood, and anesthetic fluid, a small amount of retained injectate blood or triglycerides should have little effect on the final outcome of the augmentation. The same theory supports not cleaning the fat with saline or other fluids.

INJECTION

Once a sufficient number of syringes have been harvested, the surgeon can turn his or her attention to the recipient area. During the harvesting procedure, the local anesthetic containing the epinephrine has been given time to achieve full effect. If tumescent anesthesia is used, it gives the surgeon a preview of the desired augmentation. On the other hand, the surgeon must visually subtract the swelling from tumescence in determining how much fat to inject in each area. For reimplantation, the fat is transferred to 1-cc luer lock syringes attached to a minicannula, usually 18 gauge in diameter. Using smaller cannulae than this can damage the grafts. A puncture can be made with an 18-gauge needle to allow insertion of the minicannula. These small holes usually disappear entirely without treatment, except in rare individuals who have an inherent tendency to scar poorly. The fat is injected slowly, moving the cannula in and out through the tissue, depositing small aliquots (0.05–0.1 cc) throughout the recipient area. The fat is injected in a crisscross manner from at least two different directions to create a network of small pearls of fat throughout the subcutaneous defect. Aggressive molding of the injected material may further damage the fat and is probably not wise. Enough fat is injected to create mild distortion of the recipient areas. The degree of overcorrection varies according to the defect, but the goal is for most of the swelling to be gone within twenty-four hours.

POSTOPERATIVE CARE

Ice is quite useful in diminishing swelling and relieving the mild discomfort that can accompany this procedure. Most patients do not require postoperative analgesia. The most common postoperative complaint is mild burning in the donor area. Just as with liposuction, compression of the donor area improves healing and leads to better contouring. Therefore a girdle or compression garment is encouraged for the first two or three days after the procedure.

If the fat transplantation is performed on the face, no dressing is required. However, patients are asked to refrain

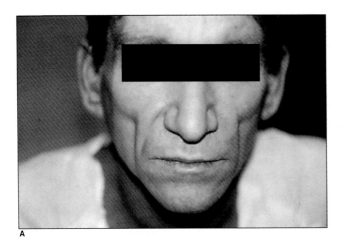
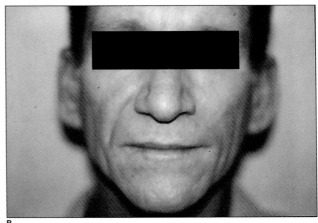

FIGURE 26.1: A, *Pretreatment and,* B, *six months posttreatment with three bimonthly injections of 10 cc of fat into the cheeks.*

from heavy chewing, smiling, talking, or other animation that may displace the injected fat. In other areas of the body, it is useful to splint the area, to hold the fat within the defect into which it has been injected. This splinting can be done with tape applied in four different directions to create 360 degree support around the recipient site. Patients are then cautioned to avoid lying or sitting directly on the augmented area. This can be difficult when the buttocks or outer thighs are treated.

REPEAT AUGMENTATION

Patients undergoing small-volume fat transplantation are instructed not to expect much improvement from the first treatment. The injected fat tends to shrink into a thin plate, which may last for years, but this is often not enough to achieve a visual improvement. After the swelling subsides, many patients are thrilled with their appearance for the first few postoperative weeks and then become disappointed as the fat appears to fade away. Careful preoperative explanation helps to diminish any disappointment. Subsequent augmentations can be performed as soon as one month after the initial one. The surgeon should harvest enough fat at the initial procedure to have material available for several subsequent procedures. Multiple augmentations are problematic for patients who live at great distance from the surgeon's facility. If multiple procedures are impossible, then perhaps these patients should not embark on small-volume fat transplantation in the first place.

When patients return for secondary augmentations, either fresh or frozen fat can be employed. There is a great deal of controversy about the effectiveness of using frozen versus fresh fat for lipoaugmentation (Butterwick et al. 2006); however, Butterwick et al.'s study has shown that frozen fat is an effective material for subcutaneous augmentation. Even if the fat cells do not survive, clinically,

the fibrosis and tissue reaction which occur provide a very real and long-lasting result. Freezing fat means only one harvesting procedure and makes the secondary visits much easier for the patient. When frozen fat is employed, the surgeon should harvest more than he or she thinks will be needed so that plenty of material is available. The syringes that are not used during the initial procedure are allowed to stand up long enough for gravity to thoroughly separate the fat from the triglycerides and injectate fluids. The capped syringes are then frozen immediately. Research indicates that –20 degree centigrade freezers provide more viable fat cells (Moscatello et al. 2005). However, normal residential freezers have been used for over two decades by fat transplantation surgeons with good results. To avoid the potential problem of mixing up patient specimens, the syringes should be double bagged, with the patient's name written on the outside of each. The fat can be safely stored for at least one year. The authors maintain a written log of all the fat stored and notify patients that it will expire shortly to allow them a last chance to use it prior to its disposal.

When the patient returns for reinjection, the procedure is very similar to the initial one, except that there is no harvesting step. The syringes to be used are thawed slowly by suspending them under running water. Immersing the syringes in a warm water bath risks contamination of the material. A few cases of mycobacterium infection have been reported after fat transplantation. This contamination may occur at any point from harvesting to injection, and sterility should be maintained throughout the process.

After the fat has warmed up to room temperature, any residual excess fluid is expressed, and then the fat is transferred from 10-cc to 1-cc luer lock syringes for injection. In some cases, the patient retains significant augmentation from the first procedure and may not require as much fat injection at one or two months post-op. Patients are instructed to return at regular intervals until they

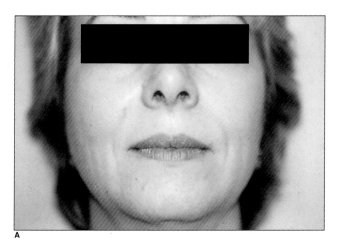
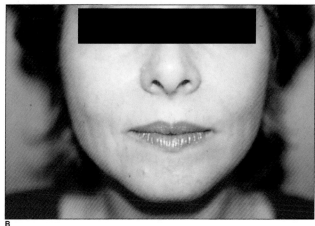

FIGURE 26.2: **A, Pretreatment and, B, one year posttreatment with four bimonthly injections of 5–7 cc of fat into the nasolabial furrows.**

appear to maintain the results from the previous treatments. In most cases, six bimonthly injections will give significant improvement with excellent longevity. The ultimate longevity varies from patient to patient, as with any procedure, but results can persist for many years in some cases. As aging continues and the graft contracts further, additional fat transplantation can be performed if and when needed.

FINAL THOUGHTS

Fat transplantation provides a unique type of soft tissue augmentation. The patient uses his or her own autologous tissue without worries of reaction or rejection. It is the most natural of all soft tissue augmentation options. Small-volume fat transplantation provides an ambulatory approach with minimal recovery and excellent results in most individuals (Figures 26.1 and 26.2).

SUGGESTED READING

Butterwick KJ, Bevin AA, Iyer S. Fat transplantation using fresh versus frozen fat: a side-by-side two-hand comparison pilot study. *Dermatol. Surg.* 2006;32:640–4.

Moscatello DK, Dougherty M, Narins RS, Lawrence N. Cryopreservation of human fat for soft tissue augmentation: viability requires use of cryoprotectant and controlled freezing and storage. *Dermatol. Surg.* 2005;31(11 Pt 2):1506–10.

Nguyen A, Pasyk KA, Bouvier TN, Hassett CA, Argenta LC. Comparative study of survival of autologous adipose tissue taken and transplanted by different techniques. *Plast. Reconstr. Surg.* 1990;85(3):378–86; discussion 387–9.

Rohrich RJ, Sorokin ES, Brown SA. In search of improved fat transfer viability: a quantitative analysis of the role of centrifugation and harvest site. *Plast. Reconstr. Surg.* 2004;113:391–5; discussion 396–7.

Rose JG, Lucarelli MJ, Lemke BN, et al. Histologic comparison of autologous fat processing methods. *Ophthal. Plast. Reconstr. Surg.* 2006;22:195–200.

CHAPTER 27

Larger-Volume Fat Transfer

Mark Berman

Autologous fat transfer, or fat grafting, refers to the removal of one's fat via liposuction and subsequent injection to another location in one's body. The term *space lift* refers to the concept of restoring one's youthful facial appearance by lifting the facial skin away from the skeleton in an anterior vector to restore the natural three-dimensional characteristics of a face. The concept of injecting fat into a face was probably introduced by Dr. Pierre Fournier, also one of the fathers of liposuction, during the first World Congress of Liposuction in Philadelphia in 1986.

When doctors started using fat transfer by injection, they primarily focused on apparent facial defects such as the nasolabial folds, the nasojugal creases (marionette lines), and other obvious facial depressions. According to a recent survey by the American Society of Plastic Surgery, this is still the primary use of the material for most doctors today (Kaufman et al. 2007). However, a better understanding of the aging process reveals a very widespread loss of facial fat (Berman 1998). Over time, the metabolization of facial fat simply causes a global collapse of the skin. Thus, in various positions, the skin hangs to create the appearance of various unattractive folds associated with aging. In deference to popular thought, I contend that gravity does not cause aging, but only affects how we look in different positions. I certainly agree that we also lose elasticity with age; however, we do not increase the amount of skin on our faces. Skin only grows or stretches in response to tension. However, the aging face, by virtue of fat volume decreases, actually exhibits less tension over time – thus there is no force contributing to or causing the skin to actually increase in amount. In youth, our skin's elasticity resembles that of a balloon, while with age, we have less elastic elements, more like a beach ball. A deflating balloon is still round and smooth, while a beach ball simply collapses over itself – our faces behave much the same way.

Also, another interesting, perhaps debatable, observation deals with the rapidity of aging. In youth, when we have maximal amounts of facial fat, the aging process starts out slowly so that from twenty to forty years of age, the changes seem more subtle than they do as we gain in years. This is understandable when you look at the face as a source of fat that does not easily replace its losses. If we always lose a constant, albeit small, amount of fat from the face, then with advancing age, we are losing proportionately larger amounts of fat relative to what we have left. Thus the aging process is no longer purely linear, but almost logarithmic in nature. Logically, putting back optimal amounts of fat would actually reset the aging process, while lifting alone simply camouflages it. Disproportionate fat losses continue, and when the next face lift is performed, there is even greater distortion to the facial features.

The key to correcting the aging face with fat grafts is to fill out the areas in a wide or global fashion and not treat individual creases alone. For example, the nasolabial fold is not a primary crease caused by loss of volume in the fold, but rather a diffuse volume loss in the cheek that allows the skin to fall over the fold when one is erect. To test this, simply place the patient supine and observe the diminution of the fold. By filling the cheek, the skin is lifted and the fold reduced.

So how is the procedure performed? In simple terms, fat is harvested by liposuction and transferred to the areas where needed by injection. There are several techniques available and popularly discussed today. Certainly the reader should be aware of Coleman's (2004) method of harvesting and transferring fat. However, after all of these years (over twenty), I have adopted a simpler method for harvesting fat. Specifically, I now use the Lipivage system, developed by Dermagenesis (no financial involvement). Fat can be harvested from any area on the body where (1) the patient desires it to be removed, (2) it will leave the least noticeable defect, or (3) it can be found. While most patients have abundant stores of fat, often, those who need it the most have very little retrievable subcutaneous fat deposits. Though anecdotal reports have been published, no measurable differences between potential fat harvesting sites or manipulation techniques (centrifugation, washing, etc.) have been demonstrated to be superior in laboratory evaluations (Rohrich et al. 2004). Prior to surgery, the patient is started on prophylactic antibiotics and advised to have any anticipated dental work completed prior to surgery. The patient should be free from any possible infections that could become blood-borne and potentially infect the proposed transplant sites. The patient is photographed and marked prior to coming to the operating room. The marks serve as a guide to where you want to place the volumes of fat to restore the skin to its youthful position away from the skeleton. One must think three-dimensionally in terms of repositioning the skin as opposed to pulling the skin superior and posterior. Those vectors can only lower the anterior vector, which most often needs to be raised. It is advisable for the patient to bring a picture from his or her youth to use as a guide for the new contours you want to achieve.

The patient is given intravenous anesthesia administered by an anesthetist. The fat donor site is generally prepped and injected with local anesthesia. I prefer not to use tumescent anesthesia (thus no need for centrifugation), but rather, I infiltrate directly under the skin with a spinal needle and then infiltrate small amounts of local anesthesia deeper into the fat. I might use 120–180 cc for an abdominal area, using lidocaine 0.5% or 0.2% solution with epinephrine (vasoconstriction) and HCO_3 (neutralize the pH) added. The Lipivage device can be connected to normal suction or to a liposuction machine that is turned down to decrease negative pressure. The Lipivage accepts a luer lock cannula, and the fat that is harvested into the chamber of the Lipivage remains within the filter while fluids (blood, local, grease) pass through. The collection is then transferred to 10-cc syringes and placed on a rack. I recommend that you collect much more fat than intended for use so that the remainder can be frozen (−8 degrees Celsius) for storage and later use. The average patient might use 50 cc of injected fat. Obviously, this can vary from much smaller quantities to over 100 cc.

The face is then anesthetized with local anesthesia – typically 15 cc of lidocaine 1% with epinephrine and HCO_3. Most of the ecchymosis is probably caused by injection of the local anesthesia, so pressure should be applied after injecting each area to try to minimize extravasations from injured vessels. I recommend using Tulip injectors (1.4 mm; no financial interest). The fat is transferred from the 10-cc syringes to 1-cc luer lock syringes with the Tulip injector. A stab wound from an 18-gauge needle provides access for entry of the blunt-tipped injectors. Typically, this is done bilaterally at the medial aspect of the eyebrow, the lateral aspect of the eyebrow, the lateral cheek area, and the corner of the mouth. Occasionally, additional incisions are made at the inferior aspect of the mandible below the point of the mental foramen (Figure 27.1).

Starting at the medial aspect of the eyebrow, the Tulip injector is inserted and passed along the inferior border of the orbital rim. Tiny aliquots of fat are expelled while withdrawing the cannula. The syringe should be held so

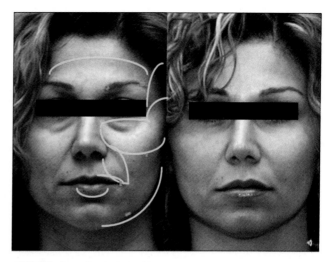

FIGURE 27.1: *Typical injection sites and pattern of injection. Also note how upper and lower lids improved by lifting skin away from the skeleton, while leaving periorbital fat in place.*

that the plunger is secured in the back of the hand for maximum control. Fat is injected in tiny (less than 0.1 cc) quantities over the orbital rim next to the periosteum and then into the bulk of the brow. The idea is to re-create a full, natural brow. An old picture from youth might serve as a good guide.

Fat is then injected around the glabellar area superficially to the corrugator and procerus muscles. It can also be injected into the forehead but should probably be done in the plane under the frontalis muscle to avoid visible lumps. From the lateral brow, fat is feathered out into the temporal area just superficial to the temporalis muscle and can be placed posterior to the hairline. This helps lift the lateral aspect of the brow by restoring natural volume to the depressed temporal area.

From the lateral cheek area, fat is then placed in multiple small aliquots directly over the malar periosteum and then gradually more superficially up toward the skin. If there are prominent lower lid bags, these do not need to be removed; rather, the skin needs to be raised away from the skeletal structures with fat to neutralize the visible defect. Simply, the skin must be tented up away from the underlying structures (examples of results are shown in Figures 27.2–27.4).

From the corner of the mouth, fat can be feathered down around the chin and then all the way across the mandible and into and around the masseter muscle. A lot of fat is lost around the mandible over time, and this adds to the appearance of aging and the blunting of the mandibular angle. In fact, the loss of fat throughout the cheek and mandible is the principal reason for the appearance of platysma bands in the neck. The platysma is a vertical muscle that passes from the clavicle on up to the cheek. As the area around the cheek and mandible collapses, the relative excess of muscle simply translates to the area below

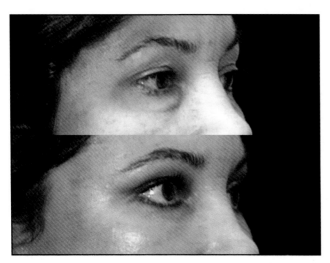

FIGURE 27.2: Mild (or even more significant) upper lid sagging improved by filling, not cutting.

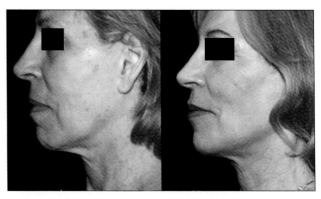

FIGURE 27.4: Fat grafts help restore contour to the mandible, cheeks, and brow (face) following previous traditional face lift and blepharoplasty.

the mandible, resulting in visible bands. Filling the facial structures can thus lift the neck.

Fat is also placed around the upper lip (perioral area), under the nose, and around the nasolabial area. This can actually effect a slight lift to the nasal tip. Combined with the cheek fat grafts, the overall result makes the nose look smaller. This helps us understand the common fallacy that the nose grows with age. The nose just appears to be larger because the facial structures around it are getting smaller. The only exception deals with increases in subcutaneous tissues related to metabolic issues (e.g., alcohol and rhinophyma).

The upper lip is injected along the vermilion border and then deeper into the submucosa tissue and the muscle. The lines of cupid's bow – the phyltrim – can be delineated with fat grafts, too. The lower lip is treated similarly, but the filling is mainly confined to the central two-thirds (Figure 27.5). Doctors who fill the entire lower lip straight across

cause the lip to lose its attractive appearance and instead look artificial – like a sausage and not a well-shaped lip.

Also, if the earlobes appear deflated or shriveled, a small amount of fat can be injected into the lobes to restore a fuller, more youthful appearance.

Patients are all reminded during their consultations that this is not a perfectly predictable procedure. While there will not be any extreme discrepancies, there may be very subtle asymmetries. More important, the patient must be

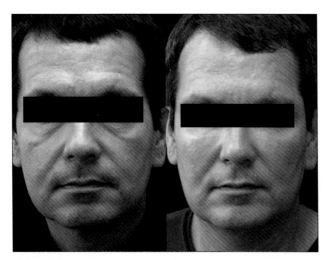

FIGURE 27.3: Facial demarcations softened by filling.

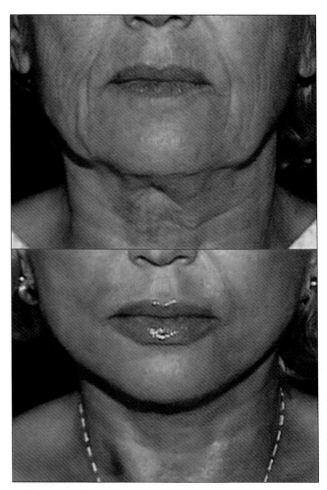

FIGURE 27.5: Lips are enhanced with fat grafting.

advised that additional treatments will likely be necessary to achieve optimal or optimally acceptable results. If a patient is not willing to repeat the operation, then do not do it at all.

Follow-up treatments can be scheduled as soon as one month after surgery. Ultimately, patients reschedule when it is convenient. If the frozen fat remains in good appearing condition, it can be used; otherwise, fresh fat is harvested again. Most patients require one or two follow-up treatments. Once adequate fat has been replaced, then it becomes subject to normal metabolization processes and should last for years, while it slowly dissipates over time.

SUGGESTED READING

Berman, M. The aging face: a different perspective on pathology and treatment. *Am. J. Cosmet. Surg.* 1998;15:167–72.

Coleman SR. *Structural Fat Grafting.* St. Louis, MO: Quality Medical; 2004.

Kaufman MR, Bradley JP, Dickinson B, et al. Autologous Fat Transfer National Consensus Survey: trends in techniques for harvest, preparation, and application, and perception of short- and long-term results. *Plast. Reconstr. Surg.* 2007;119:323–31.

Rohrich RJ, Sorokin ES, Brown SA. In search of improved fat transfer viability: a quantitative analysis of the role of centrifugation and harvest site. *Plast. Reconstr. Surg.* 2004;113:391–5.

CHAPTER 28

FAMI Technique and Fat Transfer for Hand Rejuvenation

Kimberly J. Butterwick

Fat transplantation has endured for decades as one of the optimal methods for restoring volume in the face. There are various techniques of performing fat transplantation, the most recent being fat autograft muscle injection, or FAMI. Initially developed and reported in 1996 by Amar, a French plastic surgeon, FAMI was introduced to the United States in 2001. The distinctive aspect of the FAMI technique is placement of fat parcels in close proximity to, or even within, the muscles of facial expression. The rationale for this placement is that transplanted fat will survive optimally when grafted into the bed of vascular muscle tissue, promoting neovascularization and thus longevity of the transplant. Transplanted fat then will become living tissue, as opposed to a temporary filler. Studies in various fields of surgery regarding fat survival near muscle support this concept, and results as long as five years have been reported.

To learn the FAMI technique, the surgeon must familiarize himself or herself with the muscles of facial expression. Not only is knowledge of the origin and insertion of each muscle critical, but also, awareness of the depth and thickness of each muscle is essential. In addition to establishing a working knowledge of muscle anatomy, the surgeon must gauge the degree of volume depletion in a given patient and develop an artistic sense of where in the face volume replacement is most needed in terms of aesthetic results.

PATIENT ANALYSIS

When patients present for consideration of this technique, their concerns and goals are reviewed. An assessment of their general health is made, and if there are no contraindications to the procedure (i.e., warfarin therapy, debilitating disease), the face is analyzed in detail for volume depletion. The analysis is aided by reference to the patient's earlier photographs, approximately ten to fifteen years prior, and by examining the face by dividing it into thirds. For the superior third, assessment is made of the contour of the forehead and the fullness underlying the eyebrow and glabellar regions. The temples are evaluated for a slanted or hollow appearance. In the middle third, periorbital regions are examined for shadows and hollowness, the presence of the tear-trough deformity, and laxity of the skin. The contours of the malar region are considered with attention to the adequacy of volume both medial and lateral to the zygoma. In the medial cheek, there may be flattening, leading to a tired look. The base of the nose may seem to sink posteriorly, causing an unattractive inferior descent of the tip of the nose. In the inferior third of the face, the perioral area is examined for adequate projection of the lips, lip fullness, elongation of the upper lip, and furrows in the nasolabial fold and marionette regions. Youthful aesthetic features include a smooth, uninterrupted mandibular border and a smooth chin with good height (distance from lower lip to mandibular border). Volume loss will result in depression of the buccal and preauricular regions, which is often more prominent in patients who have previously undergone rhytidectomy. The overall shape and symmetry in the face should be determined and brought to the patient's attention. Classic proportions should be drawn on the patient's photograph for comparison and analysis.

After a thorough assessment and discussion of risks and benefits with the patient, the procedure is scheduled. In our office, a preoperative exam is performed two weeks prior to the procedure to ensure the patient's health. Medications that may promote bleeding are discontinued, preoperative laboratory examination is obtained (CBC, chem panel, PT/PTT), and informed consent is reviewed. Photographs are taken for later use in the operating room. The donor site for fat harvesting is agreed on. The ideal donor site has never been proved, although outer thighs and hips seem to yield dense, relatively avascular fat quickly. Any site may be chosen, depending on the patient's deposits.

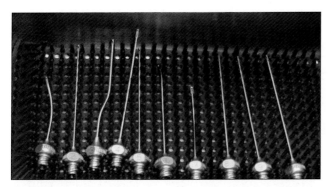

FIGURE 28.1: FAMI injection cannulae: numbers 1–10 appropriately angled for various contours of the face. Fat is transferred to and injected with 1-cc syringes via a female to female transfer hub. Injection through a 1-cc syringe results in smaller fat particles and requires less injection pressure than larger syringes.

SETUP

The cannulae necessary for the FAMI technique are shown in Figure 28.1. The use of the Amar FAMI cannula set is essential for facilitating placement of fat. The bends and curves of these cannulae correspond to the contours in the underlying skeletal structure and muscle anatomy, allowing easy transplantation of fat without trauma to the muscle or vasculature. The numbers on the hub should be visible while injecting because they align with the opening of the cannula tip. The opening is purposely designed to be superficial or deep, depending on the muscle group for which it is intended.

PREPARATION FOR FAMI

Patients are brought to a preoperative area, where the problem areas are reviewed and marked for correction. The operative photos can be drawn on to ensure communication with the patient and staff. It is important to again point out preexisting asymmetries, as the patient may only notice them postoperatively. In the operating room, the face and donor sites are prepped and draped in a sterile fashion. Light sedation may be achieved with oral and IV medication at this point. Appropriate nerve blocks are performed. Supplemental local anesthesia of the face may later be necessary and is readily achieved with direct infusion of tumescent anesthesia. The donor site for harvesting is anesthetized with Klein's tumescent anesthesia, lidocaine 0.1%. Attention is then directed toward obtaining the fat.

HARVESTING AND PROCESSING FAT

Most methods of fat transplantation emphasize gentle harvesting of the adipocytes. Factors such as excess vacuum pressure, blood in the aspirate, and even lidocaine have been shown to affect viability of the fat cell. However, the adipocyte appears to be rather sturdy, so these precautions may be more important in theory than in reality. Nevertheless, in general practice, harvesting cannulae with larger openings attached to 10-cc syringes are usually recommended to avoid shearing of the cells and excess vacuum pressure. During harvesting, the syringe is held with 1–2 cc of negative pressure. The author prefers the 12-Klein finesse cannula for harvesting. Syringes are placed upright in a syringe rack to allow the aspirate to separate into supranatant and infranatant fractions. The syringes are decanted of fluid, completely filled, and centrifuged for three minutes at 3,600 rpm, removing blood and lidocaine, which may impact fat survival. Although debated, centrifugation has been shown in some studies to improve longevity of the fat graft, due in part to the concentration of the number of cells transferred and also to removal of inhibiting factors. Harvested fat is transferred from 10-cc syringes to 1-cc syringes for placement, which require less pressure to inject and result in smaller fat parcels, which are more readily vascularized. It is important to harvest three to four times the fat that one wants to utilize because approximately 40% of the volume is lost during centrifugation. Extra fat may be stored in a medical grade freezer for later use.

TECHNIQUE

The FAMI technique is a systematic approach to fat transfer usually starting from the most cephalad muscle groups to the caudad groups. After anesthetizing the treatment areas and harvesting and processing the fat, 1-cc syringes are prepared for injection. Planning which muscles to inject is considered prior to the procedure, and the appropriate cannulae are determined by the site. Generally, 1–3 mL of centrifuged fat is placed per muscle. Insertion sites are made with an 18-gauge No-Kor needle. The appropriate cannula is advanced, usually starting at the origin of that muscle to the insertion of the skin. Figure 28.2 demonstrates some of the most common injection areas. Once in place, fat is laid down in a retrograde fashion in a quick, smooth motion, as if tracing the muscle path. Usually, two to four retrograde passes along the muscle are required to empty a 1-cc syringe. An immediate contour improvement is visible, which is best viewed from the head of the table looking downward. With experience, the surgeon will enjoy sculpting the face in different areas with varying quantities. A novice to the FAMI technique can safely place 1 cc in all muscle groups without fear of distortion or overcorrection. One caveat is in the infraorbital area (orbicularis oculi), as nodules and cysts may form in this region. No more than 0.5 cc should be placed in each infraorbital region until more experience and skill are gained by the surgeon. Even with experience, it is rare for the author to place more than

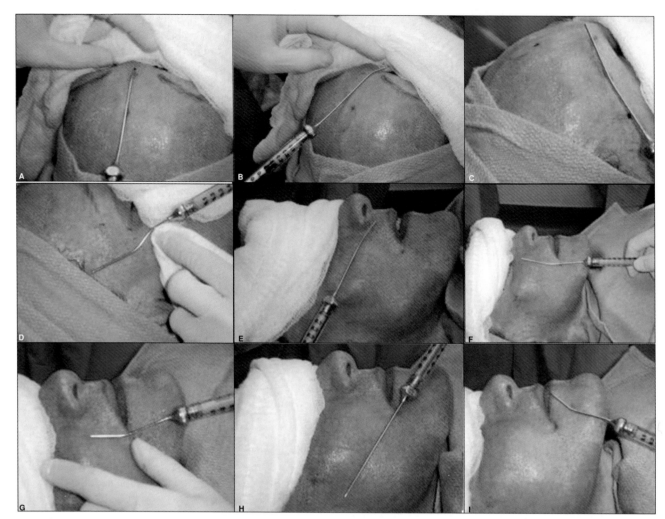

FIGURE 28.2: A, Injection of procerus and, B, corrugator is performed from a midline incision site with the number 6 cannula. C, The hard edges of the bony orbit can be concealed with an injection utilizing the number 2 cannula, under the orbicularis. If needed, fat may be injected up to the upper eyelid crease. D, The temple is one area in which the fat is not placed within the muscle, but rather, is placed in the deep subcutaneous space with the bayonet-shaped cannula number 3. E, Injection of zyomaticus minor starts with the number 4 cannula at the origin of the muscle on the bone and continues to its insertion, interdigitating with the orbicularis and levator muscles of the lip. Note that the injection crosses medial to the nasolabial fold and, in so doing, actually raises the platform of the nose. F, The ori-gin of the levator labii superioris is best reached with the number 5 cannula. The nondominant hand palpates the orbit rim and protects the orbit during injection. G, The levator anguli oris is a deep muscle originating in the canine fossa. Injecting along this muscle with the number 7 cannula minimizes the nasolabial folds and also elevates the base of the nose. H, The injection of the zygomaticus major from the insertion at the commissure to its origin along the malar bone. The injection softens and fills the depression under the cheek bone. I, The depression anguli oris is performed with cannula number 7 from the origin along the mandible to fibers of the insertion within the orbicularis oris. This helps to project the lower lip from a recessed position.

that. An assistant records amounts placed in each muscle and the corresponding cannulae. At times, one side may require more augmentation to compensate for preexisting asymmetries.

A question often asked is, how does the surgeon know that the muscle is injected? Since this technique is anatomically based, it is important to palpate the origin of the muscle on the bone and to follow from that point to the known insert of that muscle. At times, the muscle seems to fill up like an encased sausage, and one can feel the fat within the

facial envelope (i.e., zygomaticus major and depressor anguli oris). At other times, the muscle is so thin (i.e., zygomaticus minor) that one bases placement solely on bony landmarks. The cannulae themselves also assist the surgeon. The opening at the tip is either deep or superficial, depending on the plane of the particular muscle, with engraved numbers on top indicating that one is holding the cannula properly. The tip design is either rounded or somewhat pointed for ease of movement in those areas in which the cannula enters deeply along the bone.

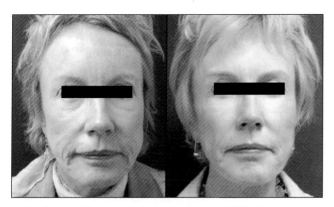

FIGURE 28.3: *Before and four months after FAMI of 34 cc.*

One of the main difficulties in learning FAMI is not technical, but rather, conceptual. Knowing how much and where to place the fat is the art of the procedure. Starting with localized regions, such as perioral or periocular regions, can help the surgeon learn this technique and gain confidence. There is a safety net as well because almost any patient over forty years of age can benefit from the addition of 1 cc of volume per muscle per side. With time, this technique may become a favorite to perform because of the artistry involved. It is recommended that practitioners take a FAMI course or preceptorship for both technique and conceptual development.

POSTOPERATIVE COURSE

Following the procedure, the patient is usually alert and in no pain. A compression dressing or garment is applied to the donor site. Topical antibiotic ointment is applied to the insertion sites. Patients are instructed to sleep with their heads elevated for the first week and to avoid vigorous facial movements and exercise.

Mild purpura usually first appears on the second or third postoperative day and may persist for seven to ten days. Edema may be pronounced, depending on the quantity of fat placed. If 20 cc or less is placed, the edema generally resolves within five days. If larger quantities of 40–50 cc are placed, the patient will usually elect to stay home for seven to ten days. Quantities greater than this are rarely placed, as most patients will not tolerate the prolonged deforming edema that is produced by large volumes.

Patients are seen in the immediate postoperative week and then at eight and sixteen weeks (Figure 28.3). Enhancement procedures, if necessary, are usually carried out at six months and one year with frozen fat.

LONGEVITY

Patients are told that approximately 30 to 40% of the fat will endure. This is an approximation and varies depending on the areas that are injected. In areas that are relatively immobile, such as the forehead and upper face, a greater percentage of the fat tends to survive. In the perioral area, particularly the lips, perhaps only 10 to 20% of the fat survives, most likely due to constant movement, interfering with neovascularization. Therefore touch-up procedures are usually desired at six months and one year. When the patient returns at this time, typically less than 10 cc is injected, and generally in the perioral region, specifically, the depressor anguli oris and the depressor labii inferioris as well as the lips. Often, for enhanced aesthetics, fat is added to the malar areas or brow areas. Once survival of the fat is achieved, however, long-term results are seen for a number of years. Results will vary depending on the patient's weight, health, and level of exercise. Endurance athletes should avoid vigorous exercise for eight weeks. Patients are told that results will endure for three to five years.

COMPLICATIONS

The complication rate is very low with all forms of fat transfer, and FAMI is no exception. Edema and purpura are expected sequelae, but more serious side effects are rarely seen. Potential side effects include bleeding, infection, extrusion, and necrosis. Asymmetries may be seen, but these tend to be very mild. Overcorrection can be a problem, primarily in the periorbital area, and caution is exercised particularly in the lower lid area. More serious potential side effects, such as muscle injury and embolic events, have not been reported with the FAMI technique, using the proper equipment (Table 28.1). The use of blunt-tipped cannulae for injection, withdrawing before injecting, and using a retrograde injection technique all minimize the chance of injecting intravascularly. Blindness and stroke have both been reported with fat transfer, but these cases have occurred in the glabellar region when sharp needles are utilized, rather than blunt-tipped cannulae, and with high injection pressures through 10-cc, rather than 1-cc, syringes.

TABLE 28.1: Equipment for FAMI

Amar cannula set
12-g Klein finesse cannula
10-cc syringes
1-cc syringes
Syringe rack
Klein's tumescent fluid 0.1%
Lidocaine for nerve blocks 1.0%
18-gauge No-Kor needle
Sterile towels and towel clamps
Centrifuge with sterile sleeves

FAT TRANSFER TO THE HANDS

The use of fat transfer is not limited to the face; in fact, the aging hand is an excellent area to fill with fat. As the hand ages, not only are cutaneous manifestations present, such as lentigines, fine wrinkling, and telangiectasia, but there is often a marked atrophy of soft tissue. This typically results in skeletonization of the hand, with the appearance of muscle tendons, deepening of metacarpal spaces, and prominence of veins. Fat and other synthetic fillers can be utilized to camouflage these telltale signs of aging. Fat makes an ideal filler for the hands in that adequate volume can be placed quickly and relatively inexpensively compared to synthetic fillers. Results are also long lasting in the back of the hands, up to three years or longer.

Technique

Utilizing the same technique for harvesting and processing, the fat is also transferred to 1-cc syringes for injection into the back of the hands. Older techniques involved placing a large bolus in the center and then massaging the fat throughout the dorsum of the hand. However, due to crushing of adipocytes, this would not be expected to result in the long-term survival of the graft. When fat is placed in a retrograde manner with 1-cc syringes, the small parcels of fat are crisscrossed throughout the dorsum of the hand, and this produces smooth results with optimal longevity. In this area, a true FAMI procedure is not utilized, as one would not want to inject or injure the muscles of the hand. To minimize injury, the fat in the back of hands is placed only in the subcutaneous space.

With the patient in the supine position, the hands are prepped and draped in a sterile fashion. Anesthesia is easily achieved with a bleb of lidocaine 1.0% at the dorsal wrist crease. Additional anesthesia is given by placing a bolus of 2–4 cc of tumescent lidocaine 0.1% at the dorsal wrist. The patient is instructed to make a fist and the anesthesia is then massaged throughout the back of the hand. A small stab incision is then placed, and a long, straight, 18-gauge blunt-tipped cannula is utilized for placement. The cannula is attached to a 1-cc syringe, and each syringe is emptied with three to four rows of fat placed in a fanlike pattern (Figure 28.4). The strands of fat are crisscrossed and woven throughout the back of the hand until desired aesthetic results are achieved – usually 10 cc per side. Care must be taken to inject between the digits distally to the web space of the dorsum of the hand and to treat the medial and lateral aspects of the dorsum of the hand for an overall smooth appearance. The actual procedure can be performed relatively quickly (five to ten minutes per hand), as one becomes familiar with the steps of the procedure.

Postoperatively, patients are told to elevate their hands for twenty-four to forty-eight hours and to minimize exces-

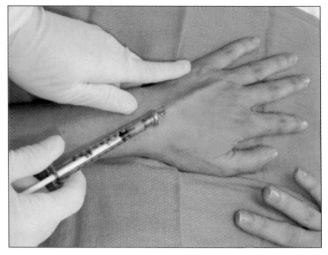

FIGURE 28.4: The dorsum of the hand is injected with the straight number 10 cannula by interweaving strands of fat placed in a retrograde manner.

sive movement for one week. Preoperative antibiotics are given and continued throughout the first postoperative week. Patients often experience significant swelling that does not resolve for two to three weeks. Sometimes a bluish cast is seen on the back of the hands, indicating cyanosis of the graft, until full vascularization is achieved. Patients may experience pain with fat grafting of the hands for the first twenty-four hours. The use of tumescent anesthesia at the time of the injection has served to virtually eliminate this problem. It is important to use centrifuged fat, as stated previously. A side-to-side comparison study in the dorsum of the hands showed a much greater duration and patient satisfaction with the centrifuged fat (Figure 28.5). Not only

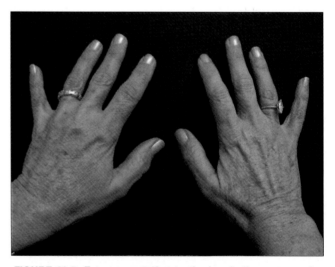

FIGURE 28.5: Fat augmentation to the hands three years after the procedure. Note that the patient's left hand is fuller than the right hand (noncentrifuged fat).

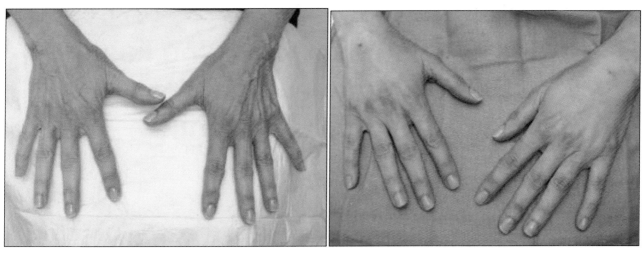

FIGURE 28.6: Before and immediately after fat augmentation of 10 cc to the hand.

does skeletonization of the hand improve, but also, texture, color, and quality of the skin (Figure 28.6).

CONCLUSION

Autologous fat transfer is a very safe and versatile filler and volumizer for the face and hands. Although a number of new subcutaneous synthetic fillers have been introduced to the market, autologous fat will still have a significant role in the cosmetic arena, as it has for over one hundred years. The fact that fat is nonallergenic, is relatively inexpensive when large quantities are needed, and has a long safety history ensures that fat transfer procedures will be useful in one's practice for years to come. The FAMI procedure takes some time and training to learn, but it truly provides high satisfaction for both the patient and surgeon. Fat augmentation to the hands performed concomitantly with FAMI is a quick, safe procedure that will ensure that the patient's face and hands are equally rejuvenated.

SUGGESTED READING

Butterwick KJ. Hand study: lipoaugmentation for the aging hands: a comparison of the longevity and aesthetic results of centrifuged vs. non-centrifuged fat. *Dermatol. Surg.* 2002;28:1184–7.

Butterwick KJ. Fat autograft muscle injection (FAMI): new technique for facial volume. *Dermatol. Surg.* 2005;31:1487–95.

Coleman SR. Facial recontouring with lipostructure. *Clin. Plast. Surg.* 1997;24(Suppl 2):347–67.

Donofrio LM. Structural autologous lipoaugmentation: a panfacial technique. *Dermatol. Surg.* 2000;26:1129–34.

Eremia S, Newman N. Long-term follow-up after autologous fat grafting: analysis of results from 116 patients followed at least 12 months after receiving the last of a minimum of two treatments. *Dermatol. Surg.* 2000;26(Suppl 12):1148–58.

Fournier PF. Fat grafting: my technique. *Dermatol. Surg.* 2000;26(Suppl 12):1117–28.

Fulton JE, Suarez M, Silverton K, Barnes T. Small volume fat transfer. *Dermatol. Surg.* 1998;24:857–65.

Pinski KS. Fat transplantation and autologous collagen: a decade of experience. *Am. J. Cosmet. Surg.* 1999;16(Suppl 3):217–24.

Primalpictures.com. Interactive head and neck. Available at: http://www.primapictures.com. Accessed 10/15/2007.

Primalpictures.com. 3D head and neck anatomy w/ special senses and basic neuroanatomy. Available at: http://www.primapictures.com. Accessed 10/15/2007.

Sommer B, Sattler G. Current concepts of fat graft survival: histology of aspirated adipose tissue and review of the literature. *Dermatol. Surg.* 2000;26(Suppl 12):1159–66.

CHAPTER 29

Adding Volume to the Aging Face: Fat Grafting versus Fillers and Implants in Europe

Constantin Stan

In the course of aging, loss of fat volume generally leads to a hollow-looking face with sunken eyes and flattened cheeks, all considered hallmarks of an aging face. Restoring a more youthful appearance cannot be accomplished simply by lifting sagging soft tissue structures; rather, it has to be complemented with restoration of lost volume. To properly accomplish such a restoration, the physician must think in terms of three-dimensional shape and volume restoration of an aged-looking face. The combination of lost volume due to atrophic changes in fat and, to some extent, muscle and even bone tissue and loss of elasticity of the skin envelope and retaining ligaments of the face results in a typical sunken midface appearance, accented by facial lines, deep wrinkles, and creases. Recontouring the face in a well-planned, three-dimensional way, rather than just filling a line here and there, or haphazardly adding volume, can restore a natural appearance and actually provide a nice lifting effect for sagging skin. Essential to success is selecting the proper (injectable) filler (autologous fat or commercial products), the proper plane of injection (superficial or deep), and the proper amount of filler. Proper injection of filler in the deeper planes restores a naturally round contour. Dermal fillers, on the other hand, are best suited to minimizing superficial skin wrinkles and folds.

As with all aspects of aesthetic facial surgery, facial rejuvenation starts with proper patient evaluation, followed by explanation of the findings and proposed solutions. Photographs and computer models can provide visual information about what can be realistically achieved, based on the patient's past and present appearance.

The aging process impacts not only the position, volume, and tension of soft tissue structures in the central oval of the face, but also structures in the facial periphery and neck region.

Involutional changes in fat structure occur in different regions and layers of the face. The same is true for muscle tissue, which can be simplistically separated into superficial and deep layers. Bone resorbtion and remodeling

obviously represent the deepest layer of volume loss. Contour restoration for the deeper layers requires larger filler volumes, and autologous fat remains an inexpensive and reasonably safe and effective alternative to modern commercial volumetric hyaluronic acid (HA) fillers, such as Restylane Sub-Q (Q Med) or Voluma (Corneal, the manufacturer of the Juvéderm family of products distributed in the United States by Allergan), and even to classic precontoured permanent facial implants made of various relatively inert materials.

Volume restoration for the more superficial layers of the face requires smaller volumes of filler. The anatomic areas best suited for small-volume fat injection are the periorbital region (eyebrow, upper eyelid, lower eyelid), malar region and midcheek junction, nasolabial fold, marionette lines, jowls/jaw-chin junction, and temple region.

The goal of restoring a youthful contour is a smooth, large, full, and uninterrupted unit from the lower lid to the nasolabial fold and a firm jawline, complemented by a three-dimensional, volumetric, anterior fullness of the face.

Volumetric facial restoration involves volume replacing and contouring of the face and neck through filling the significantly affected structures. It can be associated with other surgical or nonsurgical procedures.

Volume restoration can be accomplished in many ways, using both surgical and nonsurgical techniques, and utilizing various filling materials, ranging from autologous tissue, especially fat, to commercial fillers and implants. But apart from the ideal theoretical treatment choices, it is the skill of the treating physician, the availability of particular fillers in the country of treatment, and patient preferences that ultimately determine the pathway to volume restoration. In Europe, we are fortunate to have many product choices. We will review the most commonly used, but the discussion will be focused on the use of autologous fat, which, in the opinion of the author and many other European plastic surgeons, remains an excellent option both alone and in combination with other methods and products.

Volume restoration with hard, shaped implants has its advantages, disadvantages, and limitations. Popular materials include hard silicone, MedPore, or ePTFE. These implants are generally designed for placement over or under the periosteum, under the deepest layer of fatty tissue. They have the advantage of permanency of results, but the disadvantages of an invasive surgical technique, limitations on where they can be placed, and a certain incidence of bone resorbtion and infections. The use of ePTFE more superficially, such as in lips and nasolabial folds, has resulted in many complications and has been largely abandoned around the world.

Volume restoration with resorbable implants can be done with commercial volume-restoring injectable fillers or with autologous fat grafts, each with its advantages and disadvantages.

It cannot be understated that over the past ten years, commercial volume-restoring injectable fillers, available as intermediate-lasting fillers, slowly resorbable (mainly HA-based) fillers, and long-lasting nonresorbable fillers, have been a major driving force in office-based facial rejuvenation. In Europe, the chief controversy with respect to commercial fillers has been which types of filler should be used.

One has to carefully examine the risk to reward ratio of using a very long lasting filler, including those that induce reactive collagen deposition. Currently HA-based fillers, with relatively good safety profiles, are widely favored over nonresorbable-type fillers.

Non-HA, slowly and nonabsorbable fillers that have been used in Europe during the past few years, but have not gained wide popularity, include poly-L-lactic acid (New-Fill/Sculptra), polyacrylamid gels (Aquamid, Evolution, and Eutrophill), hidroxyapatite (Radiesse, Atlean, Beautifill), acrylic hydrogen (Outline, Dermadeep, and Dermalive), alkyl-imide (Bioalcamid), polymethylmethacrylate (PMMA; Artecoll and ArteFill), and dimethylsiloxane. Although these products have received the CE mark mandatory for all injectable products used in Europe, it should be noted that a CE mark can be obtained without the rigorous type of clinical testing and assessment of a filler's efficacy and safety profile that would be required to obtain Food and Drug Administration approval in the United States. This lack of adequate prior testing and timely reporting of complications allowed for the occurrence of many problematic complications from the use of permanent and poly-L-lactic acid fillers. While in theory, these types of filler present great appeal, the difficulty in treating complications such as granulomas, infections, and product migration, or even simple overcorrection, makes their use more difficult to justify. It must be said that through better experience, better injection

technique, and improvements in the products themselves, the rates of complications have decreased. For the future, the process of obtaining the CE mark for fillers in Europe is expected to change in the next few years, to bring it more in line with U.S.-type standards, requiring more comprehensive animal and clinical studies prior to approval and a database for systematic reporting of early and late side effects.

The availability of the newest generation of longer-lasting, volume-restoring HA fillers has even further reduced the rationale or impetus for use of problematic nonresorbable fillers. First, in 2004, came the large particle–sized Restylane SubQ from Q-Med Laboratories; then, in 2005, using a new optimized HA cross-linking technique, came Voluma, from Corneal/Allergan laboratories. Preliminary European clinical studies suggest minimal side effects apart from a few of the usual short-term reactions, which disappear after a few days, and one year or longer persistence of volume restoration for the cheeks and chin areas in more than 70% of patients, but a final determination as to their role has yet to be made.

Advantages of commercial injectable fillers over fat and implants include a less invasive procedure; less and simpler anesthesia requirements; less need for an operating room environment, equipment, and assistants; and, generally, a much shorter and simpler recovery, with minimal, if any, downtime for the patient. Disadvantages are the high cost for larger volumes; variable duration of correction based on product choice; and, when compared to fat, greater chance of an inflammatory reaction and granulomas.

In spite of the availability of a wide choice of commercial fillers, in the opinion of the author, fat grafting, and particularly the technique known as microfat grafting, remains the procedure of choice for volumetric restoration of the aging face, whether performed alone or in combination with other surgical or nonsurgical cosmetic procedures. This technique is reliable, reproducible, and cost-effective, even in a day-surgery facility. Based on experience, the duration of correction with the so-called living implants, once properly placed in the target area, is twelve to thirty-six months. Longevity appears to be site-specific, but is also technique-dependent (donor area, harvesting, and processing and injection techniques, including size and type of harvesting and injection cannulae).

Just as fillers have improved over time, so, too, have fat-grafting techniques. The so-called microlipostructure (MLS) fat-grafting technique preferred and practiced by the author was introduced by Frank Trepsat (Lyon, France) in 1998 and John W. Little (Washington, D.C.) in 2002. Without being a new technique, MLS is a refined method of the classic lipoinjection technique popularized by Pierre Fournier in Europe and refined by Sydney Coleman in the United States, with introduction of smaller harvesting and, especially, reinjection cannulae. Micrografts of fat tissue are now harvested with even smaller cannulae (1 or 2 mm) and reinjected with as small as a 22-gauge cannula (McInthyre). In general, I favor the Benslimane set of cannulae for MLS and the Coleman cannulae sets for lipostructure.

FAT TRANSFER TECHNIQUE

Fat Harvesting

A sterile technique with antiseptic scrubs before surgery and antiseptic preps is mandatory. The donor site is injected with the Coleman variation of the Klein 0.05% lidocaine tumescent liposuction solution formula (1,000 mL ringers lactate, 500 mg lidocaine, and 1 mg epinephrine with 12.5 mg bicarbonate). The fat can be harvested from various areas, such as the abdomen, flanks, medial or lateral thigh, and buttocks, with a blunt-tipped, 1- to 2-mm-diameter cannula, depending on the individual patient's anatomy.

The fat is extracted using 10-mL luer lock syringes and than centrifuged in the same syringes in a sterile manner for one minute at 3,000 rpm with an electric centrifuge (Byron Medical) or a manual centrifuge (Euromi). The supernatant is removed and the fat is transferred to 1- and 3-mL syringes for reinjection.

Fat Injection

While amounts needed vary from patient to patient, on average, the author harvests enough fat to result in about 40 mL of pure yellow fat available for injection. In a review of the author's experience, the mean amount of fat grafted was 25 mL per patient. Most patients required fat injection in the infraorbital regions, malar regions (cheek augmentation), midcheek hollows (the lower aspect of the nasojugal grooves), nasolabial folds, and upper and lower lips. The goal is to re-create the youthful "ogee" line described by Little. The appropriate average fat volumes for grafting per area are depicted in Figure 29.1.

The target area can be anesthetized by a combination of regional nerve blocks and local infiltration of 0.5% lidocaine with 1:200,000 epinephrine. The author avoids infiltration of local anesthetic with epinephrine in the eyelid and tear-trough deformity area in the hope of maximizing fat graft survival because attempts at overcorrection in anticipation of some fat graft loss can lead to problems in these areas.

The prepared fat is injected into the target areas with 1-mL syringes using 22-gauge or 0.6- and 1-mm-diameter blunt cannulae. The most commonly used entry points for the cannulae are the lateral oral commissures and/or the crow's feet area. To distribute 1 mL of injected fat, at least twenty-five to thirty tunnels are made in stacked and cross-stacked, toothpick-shaped layers, with slow movements and

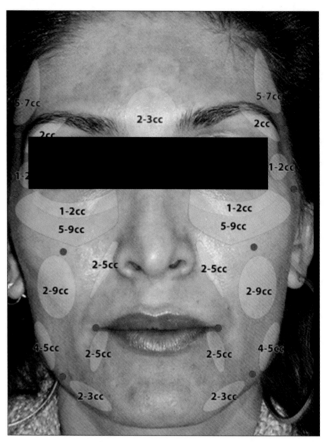

FIGURE 29.1: *Recommended entry sites (red points) and average amount of fat injected per region.*

slow injection to increase adipocyte contact with the vessels and further increase viability. This is the key to the technique and is why this modern fat injection method is called *microlipostructure.*

The average quantities of fat injected per area depend on careful preoperative facial analysis, with the goal of restoring the original degree of fullness present in the patient's youth. Overcorrection should always be avoided.

The injection plane advocated by Coleman is deep, just above bone, but in some areas, such as the upper eyelid region, the first plane of micrografting is superficial into the lid, and the second plane of injection is deep under the septum and toward the superior orbital rim. In the lower eyelid region, the author prefers to remain superficial at all times, either subdermal or within the oricularis muscle, as advocated by Roger Amar. Working with microcannulae, the main precaution is not to apply too much force on the plunger. This is especially true for the upper eyelid, where unnecessary trauma leads to bruising, prolonged edema, and even a risk of blindness. The use of a compression dressing for a few days can help stabilize the fat graft placements.

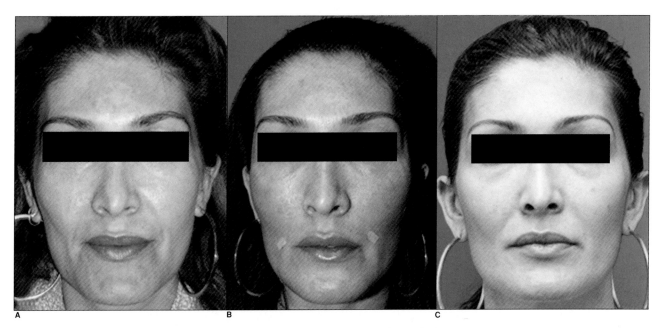

FIGURE 29.2: Face rejuvenation with volumetric fat transfer. A, Preoperative views of a forty-one-year-old female. B, Day 1. C, Two years postoperative. Note persistence of volume in the midface and upper eyelid region, giving a youthful appearance.

The procedure described is a simple and effective technique that can be performed in a well-equipped office or outpatient surgery facility. The results are a natural, youthful appearance, with minimal morbidity. These relatively long-lasting results lead to excellent patient satisfaction (Figures 29.2 and 29.3).

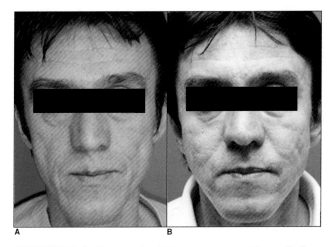

FIGURE 29.3: A, Preoperative thirty-seven-year-old man. B, Four years postoperative after volumetric fat transfer. Note persistence of injected fat in the midface area and anterior mandibular line.

SUGGESTED READING

Benslimane F. Anthropological bases for periorbital rejuvenation. Speech presented at 7th International Congress of Romanian Society of Aestetic Surgery; June 16th 2006; Bucharest, Romania.

Carruthers J, Carruthers A. *Soft Tissue Augmentation*. New York: Elsevier; 2005.

Coleman SR. The technique of periorbital lipoinfiltration. *Oper. Technol. Plast. Reconstr. Surg.* 1994;1:20–6.

Coleman SR. Ideal filler? *Clin. Plast. Surg.* 2001;28:111–19.

Coleman SR. Structural fat graft. *Quality Medical Publishing* 2004; XX:29–53, 293–353.

Lam SM, Glasgold SJ, Glasgold RA. *Complementary Fat Grafting*. Philadelphia, PA: Lippincott, Williams, and Wilkins; 2007.

Shiffman MA, Mirrafatti S. Fat transfer techniques: the effect of harvest and transfer methods on adipocite viability and review of the literature. *Dermatol. Surg.* 2001;27:819–26.

Sommer B, Sattler G. Current concepts of fat graft survival histology of aspirated adipose tissue and review of the literature. *Dermatol. Surg.* 2000;26:1159–66.

Stan C, Ticlea M. Combinacion de procidimientos para embellecimiento y rejuvenicimento en chirugia ambulatoria. Speech presented at: X-as Jornadas Mediterraneas of Spanish Society of Aestetic Medicine; May 6th 2002.

CHOOSING A FILLER

CHAPTER 30

Fillers: How We Do It

Deborshi Roy
Neil S. Sadick

Injectable fillers have become an integral part of nonsurgical enhancement of the face and body. A wide variety of fillers are currently available in the United States, and even more are available worldwide. In the last few years, there has been an explosion in the use of injectable fillers. Due to the specific nature of each filler material, each one has different applications, advantages, and disadvantages. In this chapter, we will be discussing all of the available fillers and the various techniques we employ during treatment of the face and body.

MATERIALS AND MECHANISMS OF ACTION

The mechanism of action that all injectable fillers share is the augmentation of an existing area to a desired target volume. There are permanent and semipermanent fillers. In the nonpermanent group are short-acting, intermediate, and long-acting fillers, depending on the length of duration of the product.

The collagen-based fillers include bovine collagen (Zyplast, Zyderm) and recombinant human collagen (Cosmoplast, Cosmoderm), which are in the short-acting category. The older bovine collagen fillers require a skin test prior to use, whereas the newer human collagen fillers do not. Collagen-based fillers are injected into the dermis, in the superficial and deep planes, depending on which one is being used. These fillers are manufactured with lidocaine, making the injections easier to tolerate. Collagen-based fillers can be used anywhere on the face but are most commonly used in the perioral area, especially the nasolabial folds and lips. Collagen-based fillers are injected through a

30-gauge needle. It is necessary to overcorrect by approximately 50% of the desired target volume.

The hyaluronic acid (HA) derivatives are another group of injectable fillers. The major difference between the products in this group is the origin of the HA: animal (Hylaform) versus nonanimal (Restylane, Juvéderm). In either case, cross-linked HA is injected into the deep dermis or subdermis and traps water within its structure to add volume. Over time, it undergoes isovolemic degradation and gradually dissipates. HAs can be used anywhere on the face but are mostly used in the perioral area, especially in the nasolabial folds and lips. Most of the products can be easily injected through a 30-gauge needle, but some are easier to inject with a 27-gauge needle. With HA-based fillers, the correction is usually 100 to 150% of the desired target volume.

Calcium hydroxyl-apatite (CaHA) in the form of microspheres suspended in a carboxymethylcellulose and glycerin base is an intermediate-acting filler (Radiesse). This is a bulkier injectable, requiring at least a 27-gauge needle for injections. More pressure is needed to deliver this product into the deep dermal/subdermal plane. Deeper injections into the supraperiostial plane can be performed with less resistance. This product is mainly used in the midface and lower face. It can be used to treat individual rhytids and furrows, but can also be used for volumetric filling in cases of lipoatrophy of the face and hands. Postinjection massage and molding of the product are another unique quality of the material. The treatment goal is to approach 100% of the desired target volume.

Poly-L-lactic acid (PLA) is a longer-acting filler that is administered differently than those mentioned above. The product (Sculptra) is a suspension in saline and requires multiple injection sessions over a period of months to achieve the final results. PLA can be used anywhere on the face (depending on the dilution) and is used primarily for volumetric filling in cases of hypoplasia and/or lipoatrophy of the face and hands. PLA is usually best injected through a 26-gauge (or larger) needle to avoid clogging. We prepare the product using lidocaine to increase patient comfort. Postinjection massage is a key component of achieving smooth, natural results. Each treatment should approach 90 to 100% of the desired target volume.

Polymethylmethacrylate (PMMA) spheres covered with bovine collagen (ArteFill) is a permanent filler that has a dual action. The immediate, short-term filling is achieved with the collagen component of the filler. The PMMA spheres are permanent and contribute to the long-term volumetric enhancement. PMMA is used primarily in the lower face and is best injected through a 27-gauge needle. Correction between 90 and 100% of the desired target volume is the goal.

The last three filler materials mentioned (CaHA, PLA, and PMMA), to varying extents, provide a scaffolding for native fibroblast proliferation and collagen ingrowth into the areas injected. Studies have shown that over time, there is a long-term change in the dermis that is related to each product's specific properties.

Injectable liquid silicone is a permanent filler material that has been around for several decades, although concerns with long-term safety were an issue. Newer preparations have been released to the market and have been embraced by many injectors using the microdroplet technique. With both of the permanent fillers available (PMMA and silicone), long-term reactions, such as granuloma formation and migration of the product, are possible.

Autologous fat is a long-acting filler material that is harvested from the lower body and transplanted into the face and hands. Fat transfer requires a minimally invasive harvesting procedure with associated donor-site morbidity as well as extensive recipient site edema and ecchymosis, requiring several days of downtime. The results depend on how much of the free fat graft remains viable, which is usually evident around six months after the initial injection. There are a number of injection techniques, all with variations in harvesting and preparation of the fat, instrumentation used, level of placement, and aftercare.

INJECTION TECHNIQUES

Various injection techniques are employed when performing filler treatments. Most of the techniques are used according to the injector's preference, although in some cases, it is necessary to use a specific technique to achieve a desired goal. These techniques can be used to deliver the filler material to any level of the skin and deeper soft tissues. Thorough knowledge of the anatomy and the specific properties of the injectable filler material are key components of choosing the proper technique:

1. Linear threading: this is one of the most common injection techniques used by injectors. This technique is particularly useful for treating individual rhytids and furrows.
2. Serial puncture: this is another common technique used to treat smaller rhytids and depressions as well as longer rhytids and furrows.
3. Serial threading: this technique is similar to serial puncture but can cover a larger treatment area with more filler material.
4. Cross-hatching and fanning: these techniques are useful for covering a wide area with a larger amount of filler material and are primarily used in volumetric enhancement.
5. Deep depot: this technique is only used in volumetric enhancement and only with certain filler materials because it requires postinjection molding by massage.

AREAS OF USE

Injectable fillers have become one of the most common nonsurgical procedures performed by dermatologists and cosmetic surgeons. Fillers can be used on the entire face, although most products are currently cleared for use in the nasolabial folds only. Off-label use in the dorsum of the hands is becoming more popular. Casual users limit their filler treatments to the nasolabial folds. Advanced users address the upper, mid-, and lower face as well as the hands. Injectable filler treatments may be employed as the primary method of rejuvenation or can be an adjunct to other surgical and nonsurgical modalities.

Upper Face

Use of filler materials in the upper face is limited. In cases of temporal wasting or lipoatrophy, injectable fillers can be used for volumetric rejuvenation. Volumetric rejuvenation of the lateral brow can be performed to achieve a nonsurgical "brow lift." Fillers can also be used in the upper face as an adjunct to botulinum toxin treatments. When there are residual rhytids after maximum muscle relaxation, fillers can be used to minimize these lines in the forehead and glabella. Care should be taken with fillers in these areas because the skin is extremely thin and directly overlies the bone. Deep dermal to subdermal treatments work best here.

Midface

The midface is an area commonly treated with injectable fillers. Nasal defects, whether congenital, traumatic, or iatrogenic, can be treated with fillers. Augmentation of preexisitng contours can also be performed with injectable fillers in the nose. Injections should be performed in the subdermal plane, staying superficial to the perichondrium and periosteum. Using small boluses of material with extensive postinjection molding and massage works best in this area.

The malar and submalar areas are the most commonly treated areas of the midface. Volumetric rejuvenation of hypoplasia and lipoatrophy are best performed with longer-acting fillers using the fanning or deep depot techniques. Treatment of individual rhytids or furrows, such as the upper nasolabial fold, can be performed with any filler material using any of the injection techniques.

Lower Face

Perioral rhytids are another common area treated with injectable fillers. The lower nasolabial folds, marionette lines, and vertical perioral rhytids are all treated with various fillers using different injection techniques.

The lips are a particularly difficult area to treat due to the anatomy of the subcutaneous tissue and the high level of mobility of the areas injected. Lip treatments also require a great deal of delicacy and finesse to achieve natural results. Most injectors stick to filling in the vermilion border of the upper and lower lips. Advanced injectors inject beyond the wet roll and address the philtral columns as well. Most injectors have a particular product that they prefer in the lips.

Off-Face Use

Treatment of the dorsum of the hands is a relatively new area in the use of injectable fillers. Lipoatrophy of the hands along with pigmentary changes are the most common signs of aging. Volumetric replacement, with or without a resurfacing procedure, can be used to rejuvenate the dorsum of the hands. The skin is tented up, and the filler material is injected subcutaneously. Vigorous massage of the injected material is necessary to create a smooth, natural result.

Treatment of the torso and lower extremities is limited to correction of iatrogenic defects. Postliposuction irregularities, where too much volume has been removed, are an ideal area in which to use injectable fillers to restore natural contour. Filler choices depend on the anatomical site and the extent of the volume deficit.

COMPLICATIONS

Complications must be differentiated from expected sequelae of injections. With any injection, especially into the delicate soft tissue of the face, some degree of edema is to be expected. Ecchymosis can occur as well. True complications are not common. Some complications are technique related and usually occur with casual users and novices. Other complications are due to local tissue reaction to the filler material itself.

Technique Related

Asymmetry can occur anywhere and is the most common complication. This can be easily remedied with additional injections to camouflage the asymmetry. In the case of HA-based products, hyaluronidase can be injected into areas where too much filler has been injected to reverse the process. Lumps and bumps, or nodules, are usually due to poor injection technique and can happen with any filler material. When seen immediately after treatment, it is often possible to relieve the situation with vigorous massage. Injection of a small bolus of saline or lidocaine can be performed before massage to facilitate the process. It is not worthwhile to inject the lump with a steroid preparation because this problem does not result from an inflammatory or immune process. Improper depth of placement is most problematic when injections are too superficial. This usually causes nodules of product to form as well as a discoloration of the overlying skin. If massage fails, the best treatment is to wait several weeks (if a nonpermanent product is used) for resolution. Hematomas can occur with any filler material and have to do with injection technique. Knowledge of anatomy and use of short, narrow-gauge needles are the best way to prevent hematomas from occurring.

Material Related

Allergic reactions to the filler material or one of its components are rare, but possible. Skin testing is used for the animal collagen–based products. Migration usually occurs with longer-lasting and permanent fillers. This is a complication that can occur weeks to years after the injection and is most likely related to tissue interaction with the filler material or one of its components. When first noted, massage and intralesional steroid injections can be employed to resolve the problem. If there is a functional or cosmetic concern, surgical excision may be the only solution, although it is extremely difficult to adequately remove the migrated filler material. True granuloma formation is rare but can occur with the permanent filler materials. This is a delayed-type hypersensitivity reaction that can occur months to years after the initial injection. They may be painful, palpable, and visible. Initial treatment consists of intralesional steroids and massage. If these fail, then other modalities may be used, including systemic steroids, certain antibiotics, and immunosuppressive agents. Surgical excision should be used as a final measure because it is difficult to remove the granulomas, and the resultant scars may be disfiguring.

CONCLUSION

Injectable fillers have dramatically changed the way that cosmetic surgeons and dermatologists treat the signs of aging. Nonsurgical methods are gaining in popularity and can be used as a primary treatment or as an adjunct to invasive or ablative treatments. Fillers also accentuate the importance of volumetric rejuvenation as a primary philosophical approach to the aging face and body. By offering a safe, versatile, easy to use, and easy to tolerate modality of treatment, injectable fillers have created an exciting niche to explore and expand the art and science of beauty.

CHAPTER 31

Choosing a Filler

Sorin Eremia

Although our choices of fillers in the United States are still far more limited than for most of the world, with the introduction of several new fillers during the past four years, we now have a variety of different products to meet our patients' needs.

The first step in choosing the correct filler is proper evaluation of the patient and understanding what the patient needs, wants, and also, can afford. The majority of patients who come for a consultation are interested in treatment of the nasolabial folds, treatment of the lateral oral commissural folds (marionette lines), adding volume to the lips, and treatment of the vertical upper and lower lip lines and glabellar frown lines. With increasing public awareness (or after pointing out the possibilities), patients may also be interested in treatment of tear-trough deformities, chin crease and lateral chin depressions, cheek and chin augmentation, and prejowl contours. Finally, some patients lack volume or have undergone age-related volume shifts that need to be addressed and corrected.

In my practice, the vast majority of patients have limited budgets and limited downtime. In general, those patients whose needs cannot be met by 1–2 cc of commercial filler (and/or BOTOX) choose to limit treatment to a limited cosmetic concern. Or, if they can afford it, they may opt for more definitive procedures with longer-lasting and relatively predictable results such as ablative resurfacing and lifts. And while many patients could benefit from volume restoration with fat transfer, given the available choices, only a small percentage of my patients currently opt for it.

At the time of this writing, Restylane and Juvéderm family hyaluronic acid (HA) fillers make up the vast majority of my choices for facial fillers. I virtually abandoned the use of collagen-based fillers (Cosmoderm, Cosmoplast, and Fascian) within a few months of the introduction of Restylane in late 2003, but I am now trying out Evolence, which lasts far longer than previous collagen fillers. In my practice, the use of 2.5:1 magnification loupes, allowing very accurate filler placement, largely eliminates the need for layering two types of fillers. For those rare cases in which layering is desirable, I believe that a less concentrated, shorter-acting HA is preferable to the old collagens. Evolence Breeze might also fill that gap.

I like to use Radiesse in selected patients, though in volume of use, it is a distant second to HA fillers. Its best uses seem to be for deep folds, cheek and chin augmentation, and the hands.

I have used fat for more than twenty-two years and continue to offer it and use it, but it has dropped well into third place. I have used ePTFE, especially the SoftForm and Ultrasoft hollow inserts, but I have long abandoned them due to numerous problems and poor results, worst in the lips. I do not see the need to use Sculptra, especially while routine cosmetic usages remain off-label, nor do I see the need to use ArteFill, given the cost and the potential for problems with both these products.

Looking at each specific anatomic region is the best way to analyze the use of fillers.

THE FOREHEAD

Other than small amounts of HA fillers for deep glabellar frown lines, always in conjunction with the use of neurotoxin, I do not routinely use fillers on the forehead. Particular care must be taken when injecting the glabella to avoid intravascular injections. Neurotoxin alone, or in combination with resurfacing, yields excellent and predictable results on the forehead. Fat can be used very conservatively in the brow area for the most volume-depleted cases. Great care must be taken to prevent placement or migration of the fat under the thin upper lid skin.

UPPER EYELIDS

I think the fillers should be avoided here.

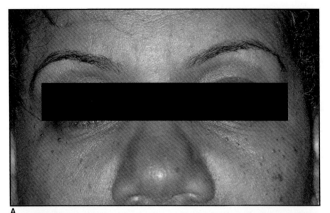

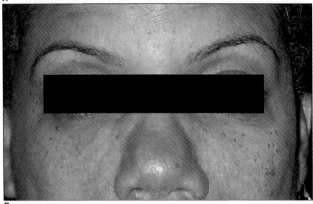

FIGURE 31.1: Tear-trough deformity: A, pretreatment; B, after 0.2 cc Restylane on each side, placed on the periosteum.

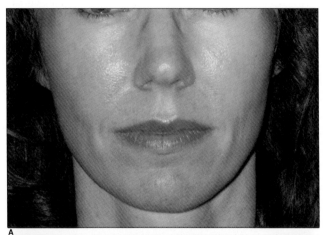

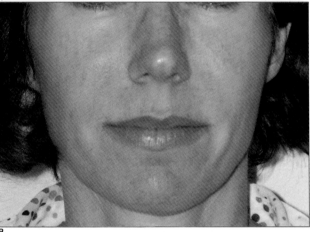

FIGURE 31.2: Cheek augmentation with Radiesse: A, pretreatment; B, after 0.7 cc Radiesse on each side, 0.5 cc to malar area, 0.2 cc to tear-trough area.

LOWER LIDS AND CROW'S FEET

I used to inject Zyderm/Cosmoderm for deep crow's feet, but the use of BOTOX and the availability of fractional resurfacing have largely eliminated the need for fillers in this area.

INFERIOR ORBITAL RIM AND TEAR-TROUGH DEFORMITY

Fillers do very well here. Restylane, Perlane, Juvéderm Ultra (U), Juvéderm UltraPlus (UP), and Radiesse can all be used with excellent results (Figure 31.1). Since ecchymoses can be a problem here, for most patients, I prefer Restylane or Juvéderm-U, which can be injected through a smaller needle. I place the product in the subperiosteal plane or at least under the orbicularis muscle, 0.2–0.4 cc per side. A finger from the noninjecting hand is always kept on the orbital rim margin to protect the eye. Gentle pressure is applied for two to three minutes. Excellent anesthesia, without any distortion of the area, is provided by an infraorbital (IO) nerve block.

THE CHEEKS

Surprisingly little Perlane, Juvéderm-UP, or Radiesse can provide a good degree of malar augmentation. I prefer

Radiesse here, as it lasts the longest of the three. At least 0.5–0.7 cc of product is injected subperiosteally in a criss-cross fashion (Figure 31.2). Fat is also an excellent choice for malar augmentation and would be my choice when larger volumes are needed and multiple other areas are being treated. Again, the IO nerve block can provide good anesthesia for most of the malar area. If I want to go further laterally, I painlessly inject a little lidocaine subperiosteally from a medial injection port, which is already numb from the IO nerve block.

THE NOSE

Radiesse is an excellent filler choice to correct small dorsal nasal contour irregularities.

THE LIPS, NASOLABIAL FOLD, AND PERIORAL AREA

The HA products are great for the lips (Figure 31.3). Radiesse and ArteFill should be avoided due to nodule formation. Fat is tricky for the lip proper. With fat, very small amounts have to be injected, and there is far more downtime

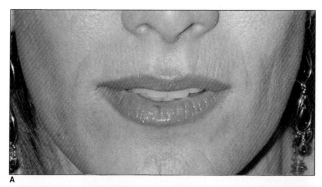

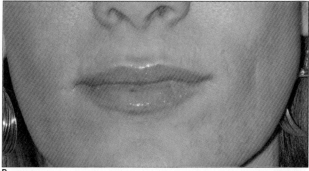

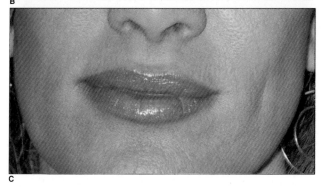

FIGURE 31.3: Lip augmentation with HAs: **A**, *pretreatment;* **B**, *after subtle augmentation of the vermilion border with 0.3 cc Restylane;* **C**, *after additional augmentation of the lip proper to give a full, voluptuous lip look.*

than with HA fillers. On the upper lip, restoring the white roll is essential – 0.2–0.3 cc of HA filler is usually enough (Figure 31.3B). Excessive filler will give the duck lip effect. The vertical lines do not do as well but can be injected with very small amounts. The philtrum lines can also be accentuated. The mucosal surface can be injected to increase overall volume (Figure 31.3C). Care must be taken to maintain good balance between the upper and lower lips. The vertical dimension of the upper lip should be at least 0.6 of the lower lip, preferably more. With age, the upper lip tends to invert, and the lower lip everts. One of the best uses of filler is the triangle that forms when the corner of the mouth sags down. Filling that triangle brings the corners of the mouth up and greatly improves the sad line appearance of the lateral commissural folds (marionette lines). It takes 0.15–0.25 cc of HA filler, on average. Fat is also good here, and I have not had problems with Radiesse either.

The nasolabial folds proper are the bread and butter of filler treatments. My five-year experience with Restylane has been excellent. I inject it in serial puncture fashion, relatively high in the dermis, using 2.5 power loupes. Because I always use IO nerve blocks, there is no distortion whatsoever from anesthetic, and the injections are painless. This allows for very precise placement of the filler and a smooth contour elevation. Since all the HA filler is placed intradermally, I get a lot of filling with relatively small amounts of filler (Figure 31.4). The distension of the dermis appears to trigger new collagen formation.

In my hands, using Restylane, the initial results last eight to ten months. However, with repeated treatments, nasolabial fold correction lasts at least ten to eighteen months. In a retrospective chart review, it was clearly apparent that in a significant number of patients, with repeated treatments at nine- to twelve-month intervals, when the interval between treatments remained relatively constant, the amount of filler used for the nasolabial folds decreased over time. When patients scheduled the appointments for retreatment based on perceived loss of correction in the nasolabial folds only, the interval between treatments increased over time. This effect was largely limited to the nasolabial folds. Interestingly, Radiesse did not seem to induce the same effect, with volume of filler needed or patient-controlled intervals between treatments remaining relatively constant. Juvéderm-U appears equally, but certainly no more, effective or longer lasting than Restylane. Juvéderm flows easier than Restylane, but to me, that is more of a disadvantage as it is harder to control, and easier to overcorrect.

Perlane and Juvéderm-UP are also about equivalent. They must be injected with a 27-gauge needle. If a 30-gauge needle is used for these larger-particle, more viscous products, they break down in the injection process, and the benefits of their use are lost. Occasionally, for patients with very deep folds for which two syringes are needed, it may be advantageous to layer the smaller-particle, less viscous product (e.g., Restylane) over the larger-particle, more viscous product (e.g., Perlane).

Radiesse is a good choice for men and for women with relatively thick skin and deep nasolabial and lateral commissural folds. Many of these ethnic women do not need lip augmentation. I inject Radiesse with a 25- or 27-gauge, 1 1/2 inch needle, using the multiple threading technique as I withdraw the needle. The cost of Radiesse has dropped significantly since it was introduced, and the usual 1.4-cc syringes provide at least as much, if not more, correction than 1.6 cc of Juvéderm, at a lower cost. Initial claims that Radiesse lasted two to three years were grossly exaggerated for these areas; the average is nine to ten months. The incidence of significant ecchymoses is much greater with Radiesse, which is another drawback for its superficial use. Evolence requires a 27-gauge needle. It remains to be seen if the longer initial duration will translate into cumulative longevity increases with repeated use.

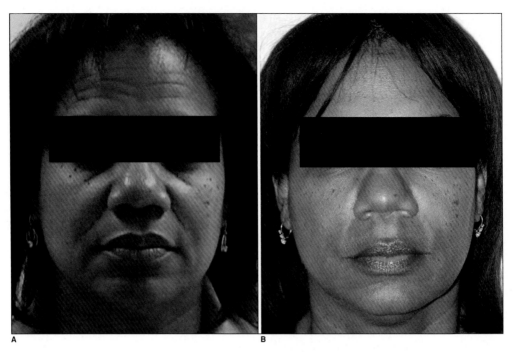

FIGURE 31.4: HA filler for the nasolabial fold, the lateral oral commissural folds, and the tear-trough deformities: A, pretreatment; B, six weeks posttreatment with a total of 1.1 cc Restylane, precisely and efficiently (economically) placed with 2.5 times loupes magnification.

THE CHIN

A small, but for many patients, clinically significant chin augmentation can be achieved with the use of Radiesse (my first choice here), Perlane, or Juvéderm-UP placed subperiosteally. Fat can also be used, but results are less predictable. The chin crease is difficult to correct with fillers, but for some patients, it is of great clinical benefit. What responds very well to small amounts of HA filler are small creases or depressions present in some patients, slightly lateral and superior to the ends of the mental crease.

THE PREJOWL AREA

Definite improvement in this area can be accomplished with Radiesse, Perlane, or Juvéderm-UP, placed over the periosteum, but it takes at least 1 cc per side for good results, which can last upward of one year. The use of Perlane for the prejowl area is also well covered by Dr. Kent Remington in Chapter 9. Fat can also be an excellent choice for this area. This topic as well as total facial volume augmentation with fat are discussed at length in Chapter 27.

SCARS

The use of HA filler for scars is also helpful. Even difficult scars, such as the one shown in Figure 31.5, can respond with careful placement.

THE USE OF NERVE BLOCKS

I perform an IO nerve block for virtually every filler treatment that involves the upper lip and/or the midface (nasolabial folds, tear-trough deformity, and cheeks). I prefer a percutaneous, rather than the classic intraoral, approach. I slowly inject 1–1.5 cc of 2% plain lidocaine on the periosteum about 1 cm below the inferior orbital rim, near the midpupillary line, just lateral to the infraorbital foramen and nerve, and apply pressure to the area for one to two minutes. The block works virtually 100% of the time, and without epinephrine, there is no associated tachycardia. It lasts only fifteen to twenty minutes, which patients really appreciate, compared to their dental experiences. With good technique, the injection is not very painful. For the lower lip and chin, I perform a classic intraoral mental block, but again with 1 cc of 2% plain lidocaine. I find the use of these blocks to be simple and fast, and patients strongly prefer them to topical anesthesia, ice, chilled air, and so on.

Looking forward to 2010, I look to new fillers in the Food and Drug Administration (FDA) pipeline. In the collagen family, based on experience in Canada and Europe, Evolence Breeze, which is better suited for injecting lips and crows feet, should be a nice addition to Evolence (Johnson and Johnson). Evolence, discussed in more detail in Chapter 15, is a novel, ribose cross-linked porcine collagen filler available in the United States since late 2008. So far I have found Evolence to be an useful, competitively priced alternative for the nasolabial folds, where it lasts about

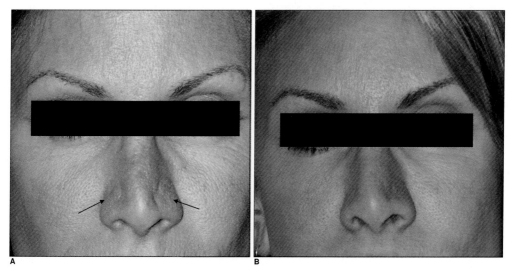

FIGURE 31.5: *HA filler for scars:* **A,** *pretreatment;* **B,** *six months after 0.3 cc Restylane.*

12 months. In the HA family, there is a push to get FDA approval for premixed filler 0.3% lidocaine products, although many physicians now add lidocaine to existing fillers. Prevelle/Puragen, from Mentor, appears to be a little longer lasting than currently available HAs and will also be available premixed with lidocaine. Another HA containing 0.3% lidocaine, Elevess, was supposed to be marketed by Galderma, but that no longer appears to be the case. I am not sure how much help the added lidocaine will be. The old Zyplast/Cosmoplast family of products also contained lidocaine but were plenty painful to inject. I personally prefer nerve blocks anyway, which, when properly performed, are vastly superior.

SUGGESTED READING

Carruthers J, Klein AW, Carruthers A, Glogau RJ, Canfield, D. Safety and efficacy of nonanimal hyloronic acid for improvement of mouth corners. *Dermatol. Surg.* 2005;31: 276–9.

Coleman, SR. *Structural Fat Grafting.* St. Louis, MO: Quality Medical; 2004.

Donofrio LM. Structural autologous lipoaugmentation: a panfacial technique. *Dermatol. Surg.* 2000;26:1129–34.

Eremia S, Newman N. Long-term follow-up after autologous fat grafting: analysis of results from 116 patients followed at least 12 months after receiving the last of a minimum of two treatments. *Dermatol. Surg.* 2000;26:1148–58.

Graivier MH, Bass LS, Buss M, et al. Calcium hydroxylapatite (Radiesse) for correction of the mid and lower face: consensus recommendations. *Plast. Reconstr. Surg.* 2007;120(Suppl):55–66.

Rohrich RJ, Ghavami A, Crosby, MA. The role of hyaluronic fillers (Restylane) in facial cosmetic surgery: review and technical considerations. *Plast. Reconstr. Surg.* 2007;120(Suppl):41–54.

CHAPTER 32

Filler Complications

Michelle Zaniewski Singh

Bernard I. Raskin

Few innovations have changed the face of cosmetic medicine more than the introduction of dermal fillers. Over the last several years, the number of available fillers has increased considerably. As this has happened, surgeons have evolved from the practice of filling lines to the concept of volume correction to restore a youthful appearance to the face.

Along with new fillers, enhanced applications, and areas of the face and body where these fillers are used, there has been a dramatic increase in the number and type of complications reported. How well are these products tested before entering the marketplace? In the United States, fillers approved by the Food and Drug Administration (FDA) undergo rigorous testing prior to approval. However, many fillers are licensed as medical devices, rather than as a drug, and as such, overall safety and efficacy testing is less demanding in the medical device category. The relative assurance of safety offered by FDA approval process does not address off-label cosmetic use of products approved for purposes other than cosmetic soft tissue augmentation. Further safety studies may not address the common cosmetic off-label use of approved fillers for purposes other than those specifically approved, or at least closely related to the FDA-approved uses. Silicone, calcium hydroxyapatite (Radiesse), and poly-L-lactic acid (Sculptra) have been the most glaring recent examples of widespread off-label use of products otherwise approved for narrowly described indications

In Europe, Canada, and much of the rest of the world, fillers are approved with relatively little serious human clinical data studies and woefully little safety data, and the concepts of professional and product liability applicable in the United States are largely nonexistent. It falls on the shoulders of the caring physician, dedicated to the Hippocratic Oath of "first do no harm," to become very familiar with the potential complications of injectable fillers.

Each filler has its own advantages, drawbacks, and complications. Unfortunately, even the most proficient injectors can have complications. Complications can occur with flawless technique. Problems can be early or delayed and may be related or unrelated to patient selection, injection site, or technique. Fortunately, complications following temporary fillers are often temporary, but complications following permanent fillers are sometimes permanent.

GENERAL COMPLICATIONS OF SOFT TISSUE–AUGMENTING FILLERS

Certain complications may be common to all fillers. These include discomfort, bruising, swelling, itching, and a sense of fullness in the injected area. Erythema after injections, lasting days, may occur. Bacterial infections or viral infections, such as herpes simplex, unfortunately can occur. Antiviral prophylaxis can be very useful but is not universally utilized among injectors. Acneiform eruptions have been documented. Headaches may develop. Sterile papulopustular reactions can be seen with any filler and are felt to be related to occlusion of sebaceous or sweat glands. This reaction is usually short-lived and resolves without sequelae and may be facilitated with exfoliation, massage, and topical astringents. Allergic and hypersensitivity reactions can occur with most types of fillers, although the frequency varies with the type of filling agent. Delayed granuloma formation can be an issue primarily with nonhuman collagen semipermanent or permanent fillers. The delayed granulomas may develop months to years later, depending on the type of filler, and may be more problematic in some parts of the face, such as the lips, compared to other areas. Rare reports of visual loss have resulted from medications and fillers injected in the periocular areas.

Patient history, including illnesses, medications, keloid formation, allergies, and bleeding, assists in proper patient and filler selection. Skin testing with certain fillers, such as bovine collagen–containing fillers, can prevent some of these reactions, but allergic reactions occasionally occur in patients with negative skin tests. Avoidance of alcohol, anti-inflammatory drugs, aspirin, vitamin E, antiplatelet agents, and anticoagulants is necessary to diminish the risk of bruising and bleeding. Persistent erythema can be treated by avoidance of alcohol, exercise, sun exposure, and use of ibuprofen and low-dose propranolol (De Boulle 2005). Topical or intralesional steroids may be helpful for localized reactions.

For patients and physicians, hypersensitivity reactions may be distressing reactions to treat. Allergic reactions to bovine collagen and hyaluronic acid have been well described. Patients may be acutely ill. Erythema, induration, pruritis, migratory urticaria, rashes, abscesses, cysts, arthralgias, fevers, and serum sickness–like reactions have occurred. Treatments have included steroids, antihistamines, and cyclosporine.

Granulomas can occur after the injection of any foreign material. They may have a delayed onset, even years after injection of permanent dermal fillers. They may be painful, erythematous, and swollen or may be asymptomatic. For inflamed granulomas, oral or intralesional steroids, oral minocycline, topical steroids, and tacrolimus ointment may be beneficial. Fibrotic uninflamed nodules can be treated by intralesional steroids and 5-fluorouracil, by imiquimod (Bauman and Halem 2003), or by excision.

Changes in pigmentation may occur. Injecting a white filler, such as Radiesse, too superficially can result in linear, whitish colored areas remaining for weeks or months. In thin skin areas, such as the eyelids, hyaluronic acid fillers can produce a Tyndall effect and give the injected area a blue hue. Immediate massage or puncturing and squeeze releasing the excessive product may provide correction. If the bluish hue persists, localized injection of hyaluronidase is beneficial. Transient or persistent post inflammatory hyperpigmentation can occur after use of collagen, hyaluronic acid, Artecoll, or other fillers. Early treatment of pigmentation with topical steroids may be helpful, along with hydroquinone at compounded strengths combined with retinoic acid.

Erythematous papular eruptions are more common with collagen and with semipermanent and permanent fillers containing silicone, poly-L-lactic acid, or ethyl and methylmethacrylate (Narins 2006). Steroid and anti-inflammatory treatments are sometimes unsuccessful. Excision or incision and expression may be necessary in the case of permanent fillers.

Other complications may relate to technique or site placement. These problems are usually noticeable shortly after injection, in contrast to granulomas, which might occur after a prolonged interval. Problems include nodules, visible filler in thin skin, or superficial placement. Other technique or placement issues include palpable filler, irregularity or uneven placement, undercorrection, overcorrection, or migration. Lumps frequently occur in lip augmentation. Early massage can often improve lumpiness. Minor irregularity is often not a cosmetic issue if it is invisible within the lip and not on the vermilion border.

The choice of filler and depth of placement are important issues in tissue augmentation. Restylane and Juvéderm are typically intradermal in the nasolabial region, but subdermal in lip augmentation, and may be above the periosteum in the tear-trough crease of the lower lid to avoid a Tyndall effect. Sculptra is always subdermal and may be used in deeper planes. Cases of vascular occlusion have resulted from Sculptra, although this problem appears to occur less now that more dilute regimens are utilized. Radiesse is injected in the same plane as the hyaluronic acids in the nasolabial areas and is generally well tolerated in this location, but is considered to cause problematic lumps in the lips, and most practitioners avoid Radiesse lip injections as well as not injecting into thin skin. Artecoll must be very carefully injected into the proper plane to avoid problems.

Edema may be due to tissue displacement by the injected implant or due to local tissue reaction, and rarely persists. Ice packs and pressure may prevent or ameliorate edema symptoms.

Injecting forehead lines, crow's feet, or perioral rhytids can result in ridging, beading, or migration of filler, especially in fine lines. After correct placement of the filler, muscle movement can cause migration of filler. Attempts to fill ice pick or depressed scars can instead outline the scars. Subscision of some scars may help to avoid creating the doughnut appearance.

Fillers can cause tissue necrosis. Glabella tissue necrosis is well recognized and was initially described with the original bovine-based collagen. Focal necrosis has been reported for many types of fillers (Narins 2006). The primary areas at risk include the lip and the glabella. Lip necrosis is presumed to be due to the occlusion of the circumoral artery and glabellar necrosis is due to occlusion of the central vein. Postinjection blanching in the glabella can evolve into ulcer formation. Prompt treatment with nitroglycerine paste is indicated, and physicians should keep nitroglycerine paste available for immediate use. A case of lip necrosis was described by Narins (2006). Severe bleeding occurred after initial injection of hyaluronic acid into the lower lip. Injection was continued to receive a full cosmetic correction, and gradual darkening of the mucosa occurred. This progressed to a painful black area over two weeks. The pain decreased and the area sloughed over the next two weeks, while the patient started treatment with antibiotics and oral steroids. There was minimal scarring.

Painless blanching or bruising may be the first indication of injection necrosis. During the subsequent few days, a dusky coloration may occur and progress to a black surface or eschar and ulceration. In the glabella, the needle tip should be kept superficial and medial to avoid injecting the supratrochlear vessels and to avoid overcorrection, which might result in vessel compression.

A protocol for the prevention of injection necrosis of the glabella is described by Glaich (2006), in which immediate massage is performed for any blanching. Rapid vasodilation is facilitated by hot or warm compresses. Nitroglycerine paste should be immediately available for this problem.

One-half to 1 inch should be applied near, but not over, the treatment area, left on for twelve hours, then removed for twelve hours and repeated until clinical improvement. Low-molecular-weight Heparin at a dose of 5,000 IU daily for one week has been reported to be beneficial. For hyaluronic acid–induced incipient necrosis, Glaich reviews that hyaluronidase may be utilized at seventy-five units combined with lidocaine. Because immediate or delayed hypersensitivity to hyaluronidase may occur, the suggestion is made to perform a skin test first.

Deeper injections, as with poly-L-lactic acid, can result in more substantial vascular necrosis if the product is inadvertently injected intravascularly. If immediate white blanching of the skin is seen while injecting poly-L-lactic acid, the injection must be discontinued immediately and the area treated with nitroglycerine paste and massage. Local heat may facilitate the return of adequate blood flow. Poly-L-lactic acid vascular occlusion has been seen more commonly in the temples. The vascular occlusion issue with poly-L-lactic acid appears to be less frequent now that greater product dilution is more commonly utilized.

Retinal artery thrombosis and visual loss have followed glabellar and periocular injection. They have also been reported with other nonfiller medication injections in the region. Fortunately, this is an exceedingly rare occurrence.

Lipoatrophy is a rare complication that has occurred after facial injection of Sculptra in some cases and Restylane in others (Lemperle 2006). Steroid atrophy can occur in patients treated with steroid injections for inflammatory lesions.

COLLAGEN

Injectable bovine collagen was approved by the FDA in 1981. The original products were Zyderm I, Zyderm II, and the more viscous glutaraldehyde, cross-linked Zyplast. Approximately 2 to 5% (Sengelmann 2006) of patients experience hypersensitivity to bovine collagen. Skin testing is required. Two skin tests two weeks apart, with the last at least four weeks prior to treatment, are recommended. Swelling, induration, erythema, or discomfort persisting for more than six hours indicate a positive test. A positive test is also seen with presentation of asymptomatic induration and erythema developing a few weeks after the test. Even after two negative tests, a small number develop localized reactions. These include erythema, induration, and pruritus, which may occur shortly after injection or weeks later. The induration or lumps may not occur in all areas injected but may result only in focal areas. Induration may last for a few weeks or persist for months after the collagen has otherwise clinically disappeared. Lumps may respond to local steroid injections. Alcohol, and sometimes sunlight, can elicit a nonallergic transient or temporary erythema and mild induration, which are addressed by avoiding the offending agents.

Cosmoderm and Cosmoplast eventually replaced the Zyderm line. These are human-type collagens manufactured in a laboratory. Skin tests are not necessary. Cosmoderm is utilized to inject superficial lines, and the glutaraldehyde cross-linked Cosmoplast is designed for deeper rhytids. Both contain lidocaine, so allergy to lidocaine is a contraindication, in addition to the general contraindications listed previously in this chapter. Prolonged induration, erythema, or swelling is rare with these products.

The much longer lasting hyaluronic acid fillers have largely replaced the Zyderm and Cosmoderm lines, but a new, much longer lasting form of cross-linked porcine collagen, Evolence, is now in use in Europe and Canada and is expected to receive FDA approval in the United States shortly. While cross-linked porcine collagen is supposed to cause fewer hypersensitivity reactions than the original bovine collagen, testing should be considered. Evolence has a longer effect than bovine collagen and avoids the mad cow concerns of bovine products. One benefit is that Evolence is colorless.

Autologous collagen is harvested by fat removal and freezing to rupture adipocytes. The liquefied fraction is injected intradermally. The resultant inflammatory response causes deposition of collagen. Theoretically, this process is advantageous because no foreign substances are utilized, but in practice, it has never been particularly popular among practitioners, partly because larger needle sizes seem necessary. Obtaining consistent results has been problematic, in the opinion of one of the authors.

Autologen is a sterile suspension of collagen fibers prepared from the patient's tissue by the Collagenesis Corporation. It requires the harvesting of 3 square inches of skin and careful timing for prompt delivery, and cost may be an issue. Aside from the usual contraindications and complications, surgical complications and scarring can occur in the donor area.

Alloderm and Cymetra are manufactured from acellular, freeze-dried human cadaveric dermis. Alloderm is processed in sheets, and Cymetra is a micronized injectable preparation. Fascian is likewise made from cadaveric acellular human fascia lata, cut into various microsized fragments and then resuspended for injection. Alloderm is placed under general or local anesthesia. Contraindications include gentamicin allergy, collagen vascular disease, and an infected or avascular implantation site. Complications can include swelling, infection, and operative complications. Reconstitution of Cymetra can result in a lumpy or viscous material, making injection difficult. Glabellar injection may result in necrosis or arterial occlusion. Injection around the eyes can cause skin necrosis or retinal artery occlusion. Fascian has been available for several years but has never been particularly popular, partly because it is difficult to inject, although it is inexpensive compared to other fillers. None of the human cadaveric products listed are permanent, although they outlast bovine collagen. To a great extent, these have been superceded by hyaluronic acid and other current fillers. To avoid medical legal problems, physicians must be certain that patients clearly understand and agree to be injected with cadaveric material.

HYALURONIC ACID COMPLICATIONS

Hylaform, Restylane, Juvéderm, Perlane, and Captique are all forms of injectable hyaluronic acid. Minor local injection site reactions or inflammation often resolve without treatment. Delayed reactions are uncommon and may be related to protein contaminants, rather than the hyaluronic acid. Granulomas to hyaluronic acid injections have been documented. Nodularity may be treated with oral cortisone, injectable cortisone, topical tacrolimus, time, or hyaluronidase.

Hyaluronidase (Brody 2005) has been used in the treatment of granulomatous hyaluronic acid reactions and to correct unwanted or excessively superficial hyaluronic acid placement. Preliminary skin tests should be done before the use of hyaluronidase (Brody 2005).

If hyaluronic acid is placed too superficially in the skin, bluish discoloration of the skin can result at the site of placement. This is referred to as the Tyndall effect. Small particles under the skin with a size of about 400 nm scatter blue light with the same wavelength of about 400 nm. Longer wavelengths pass deeper into the skin. The scattering results in partial reflection of blue light back out of the skin, thus giving a blue appearance to the subcutaneous filler. This may be treated by excision and extrusion, watchful waiting, hyaluronidase, and the Q-switched 1,064-nm Nd:YAG laser (Hirsch 2006).

Retinal branch artery occlusion has been reported following the injection of Restylane into the glabellar area (Peter 2006). Generalized hypersensitivity and delayed abscess formation are rare. Systemic reactions have been treated by systemic steroids, minocycline, cyclosporine, and tacrolimus (De Boulle 2005).

Pain on injection is problematic. Infiltrative local anesthesia injection reduces pain but may distort the anatomy, resulting in misplaced injection of the filler. Mixing the product directly with lidocaine, although not recommended by the manufacturers, has become increasingly popular among practitioners.

RADIESSE

Radiesse, formerly Radiance, consists of injectable calcium hydroxyapatite microspheres suspended in an aqueous gel. It was originally FDA approved for vocal cord paralysis and urinary incontinence and has now been approved for aesthetic use. It is often classified as a semipermanent filler, and though it was initially claimed to last at least three years, in reality, when used for skin wrinkles such as nasolabial folds and marionette lines, the duration of correction is more in the range of nine to twelve months. Many physicians prefer Radiesse because it can be considered both a filler and a volume enhancer.

Radiesse can cause lumps, granulomas, and migration. Lump formation may not occur immediately. Complications are less problematic when Radiesse is utilized in deeper folds such as the nasolabial or marionette lines – in these locations, lumps may be palpable but are less likely visually obtrusive. Indurated areas may improve or resolve with injectable steroid; however, granuloma formation may not respond adequately to treatment. Radiesse should be avoided in thin skin areas such as the immediate periocular region due to propensity to develop palpable irregularities. Use in the lips is discouraged as the character of this product predisposes to formation of nodules, which can persist for prolonged periods, and permanent cicatrix has occurred.

An ongoing problem with Radiesse has been pain on injection. Many physicians use a female-to-female syringe coupler to introduce and mix lidocaine (approximately 0.1 cc lidocaine per Radiesse syringe), rendering the injections considerably less uncomfortable. Because this is a particulate product, mixing in lidocaine does not affect outcome.

POLY-L-LACTIC ACID

Sculptra is poly-L-lactic acid (PLA). It received accelerated FDA approval for the treatment of HIV facial lipoatrophy but is used off-label for facial or hand volume enhancement. This product is a volume enhancer, in contrast to the other injectables discussed, which are fillers. Therefore, typically significant volumes are injected into larger areas, such as throughout the central cheeks, or diffusely through the temples. Poly-L-lactic acid can be utilized as a filler in deeper rhytids such as the nasolabial folds. Treatment is performed as a series of injections once monthly, generally utilizing one or two vials per session.

The product is distributed freeze-dried and is reconstituted with sterile water. Previously, vials were diluted with a few cubic centimeters of fluid, but this resulted in difficulty injecting and higher incidence of complications such as nodularity or vascular occlusion. Currently most physicians dilute a vial with about 8 cc of sterile water (range 6–10 cc), with or without additional lidocaine without epinephrine. To mix with volumes greater than about 8 cc, the product is premixed with at least 4–6 cc in advance in the standard fashion. It is then withdrawn from the vial into a syringe, and additional fluid is added by connecting a female-to-female coupling to a larger syringe and mixing the product between the two syringes to develop even distribution throughout the fluid. This renders injections easier and facilitates even distribution of product throughout the treatment area, thus reducing nodularity.

When correction is completed, the results may last up to two years. The poly-L-lactic acid microspheres induce localized inflammation and collagen formation. It is injected into the deep dermis or the junction between the deep dermis and the hypodermis. It should not be used for lip augmentation, although deeper nasolabial and marionette lines do well.

Subcutaneous nodules and granulomas can occur. Massage after injection, higher dilutions as outlined above, advance dilution the night before use, preventing overfilling, avoidance of superficial injections, and avoidance of treating patients with very thin skin are all preventive measures. Agitating the syringe to avoid precipitation is felt to help reduce nodularity by ensuring even distribution of product when injected. One of the authors finds that once the syringe is agitated, the complete injection needs to proceed very quickly in a back-and-forth direction throughout the planned treatment to provide an even distribution. This technique seems to avoid nodular product deposition. When the needle becomes blocked (usually, when injection proceeds too slowly), the needle must be removed from the skin and cleared to avoid having a clump of product injected. The syringe is agitated again, and then injection is continued. Injection technique and dilution therefore seem to make a difference in preventing nodular product accumulations.

Cases of vascular occlusion immediately after injection have occurred. If a white blanch develops during or immediately after injection, immediate massage followed by saline injection and nitropaste application must be initiated.

The subcutaneous nodules can be divided into early- and late-onset types. Early-onset nodules are considered non-inflammatory, and these are usually palpable and rubbery – these were noted in the clinical trials in HIV lipoatrophy patients and are usually not significantly visible. Typically, early-onset nodules occur within one to three months after injection, are typically small – often only 1–2 mm in size – appear gradually without edema, remain stable in size, and respond infrequently or poorly to steroid injections. Pathology shows PLA with a scarce inflammatory reaction. Treatment is by absorption or excision.

Late-onset nodules occur six to thirty-six months after injection. These are considered inflammatory, with pathology generally demonstrating a granulomatous formation with a strong inflammatory cellular reaction. Clinically late-onset nodules present abruptly, may be tender, and are associated with edema and discoloration. The lesions tend to grow with periods of flare-up and temporary remissions. These lesions respond well overall to high-concentration intralesional injections, often 40 mg/cc of triamcinalone or equivalent. Multiple steroid injections over weeks may be necessary. High-strength steroid injection combined with Intense Pulsed Light has also been used, with the Intense Pulsed Light addressing the discoloration or erythema. Mean time for nodule resolution has been reported to be six to eight weeks.

POLYMETHYLMETHACRYLATE

ArteFill is an FDA-approved permanent filler. The product consists of polymethylmethacrylate microspheres suspended in bovine collagen with 0.3% lidocaine. The mixture is injected at the dermal-subdermal junction or the epiperiosteal surface in the face. Overcorrection is to be avoided. The collagen is gradually reabsorbed. Allergy testing to bovine collagen is required. Patients with thin skin may develop permanent visible implants and surface irregularities. Prior keloid formation is a contraindication. Uneven delivery of material can result in palpable or visible irregularities due to clumping of the microspheres. Avoidance of overcorrection is essential. Hypersensitivity may occur to the collagen component. Induration and scarring, or even late granuloma formation, can occur. In the European experience, late granulomas have developed years after injection. The product utilized previously in Europe was composed of variably sized microspheres; however, the current FDA-approved material is more consistently sized and may have less tendency to late granuloma formation since particles less than 20 μm have been removed, thus making the microspheres too large for phagocyte absorption.

All injectable fillers have been reported to induce granulomas, and most have late onset. 50% of patients track the onset to a preceding flu syndrome or facial trauma (similar to silicone). The reported granuloma incidence is 1 to 2%. For granulomas, intralesional steroids have been employed with doses up to 40 mg/cc, and other cases have been reported to respond to combination intralesional steroid and 5 FU. Sometimes excision is necessary. A study of ten granuloma cases from Canada showed eight of ten resolved with treatment and two persistent, although some authors believe that most granulomas slowly resolve without treatment. In the six-month FDA clinical trial, adverse events were similar to Collagen, and no severe events were recorded. In the five-year follow-up of 142 subjects, there was 8.5% mild adverse events (mild sensitivity, mild prominence, slight lumpiness) and 2.1% moderate or severe events (granulomas, enlargement of implant, persistent swelling or redness, lumpiness). In the two cases of granuloma or significant enlargement of the implant, one was a lip and one a nasolabial fold, and one case resolved with injectable steroid, while the other patient had the lump excised. Overall patient satisfaction at five years was determined to be about 90%.

Injection technique is important as the product is three times as viscous as Zyplast. Retrograde tunneling is necessary, and injection must stop before withdrawing the needle to avoid superficial placement at termination. Gentle massage is necessary to help avoid lumpiness. Undertreatment should be the end point with the first treatment, and a second treatment should be planned. Overtreatment must be avoided as the product may induce a continuing buildup of collagen, thus gradually improving the outcome over years.

POLYTETRAFLUOROETHYLENE

With the use of fat transfer or insertion of polytetrafluoro-ethylene (Gore-Tex or Softform), bacterial superinfection or bacterial films may occur. Antibiotic prophylaxis is advisable. In the case of infection, removal is necessary (De Boulle 2005). Late-onset infection can occur. Extrusion of the implant may occur with Gore-Tex enhancement of the lips. Enhancement of the vermilion border may create an unnatural appearance with an exaggerated border and thin lips. This appearance has been likened to a duck's bill. Over time, the product has been known to shrink, resulting in late onset of an unnatural appearance. Augmentation of the rest of the lip is necessary to maintain a natural appearance. These products were popular but are infrequently utilized currently due to the high rate of problems and the improvements achievable with newer injectable fillers.

SILICONE

Silicone is not FDA approved for cosmetic or reconstructive use in the United States. The current product utilized by ophthalmologists is not optimal for cosmetic injection. Injection of liquid silicone can induce fibrosis, hypertrophic scarring, and nodules. Late-onset adverse effects have occurred. Autoimmune syndromes, such as inflammatory myositis, have been reported involving silicone breast implants. Technique is extremely important in avoiding problems. The current recommendation is to inject only a few microdroplets of silicone with each injection session, gradually enhancing the fill over a number of treatments.

CONCLUSION

Soft tissue–augmenting fillers are a very useful tool in cosmetic enhancement. Education and training are essential for avoidance of complications. Complications with soft tissue augmentation may occur early or late and may be related or unrelated to technique. Careful patient selection and technique are of paramount importance. Complications can occur with the best of care. Understanding of complications and their management is important for clinicians who treat patients with dermal fillers.

SUGGESTED READING

Bauman LS, Halem ML. Lip silicon: granulomatous foreign body reaction treated with Aldara (imiquimod 5%). *Dermatol. Surg.* 2003;29:429–32.

Brody HJ. Use of hyaluronidase in the treatment of granulomatous hyaluronic acid reactions or unwanted hyaluronic misplacement. *Dermatol Surg.* 2005;31:893–7.

De Boulle K. Management of complications after implantation of fillers. *J. Cosmet. Dermatol.* 2005;3:2–15.

Duffy DM. Complications of fillers: overview. *Dermatol. Surg.* 2005;31(11 Pt 2):1626–33.

Glaich AS. Injection necrosis of the glabella: protocol for prevention and treatment after the use of dermal fillers. *Dermatol. Surg.* 2006;32:276–84.

Hamilton DG, Gauthier N, Robertson RF. Late-onset, recurrent facial nodules associated with injection of poly-L-lactic acid. *Dermatol. Surg.* 2008;34:123–6.

Hirsch RJ. Management of injected hyaluronic acid induced Tyndall effects. *Lasers Surg. Med.* 2006;38:202–4.

Lemperle G. Avoiding and treating dermal filler complications. *Plast. Reconstr. Surg.* 2006;118(Suppl 3S):92S–107S.

Monheit GD, Coleman KM. Hyaluronic acid fillers. *Dermatol. Ther.* 2006;19:141–50.

Narins RS. Clinical conference: management of rare events following dermal fillers – focal necrosis and angry red bumps. *Dermatol. Surg.* 2006;32:426–34.

Peter S. Retinal branch artery occlusion following the injection of hyaluronic acid (Restylane). *Clin. Exp. Ophthal.* 2006;34:363–4.

Rotunda AM, Narins RS. Poly-L-lactic acid: a new dimension in soft tissue augmentation. *Dermatol. Ther.* 2006;19:151–8.

Sengelmann RD. Dermal fillers. Available at: http://www.eMedicine.com/article/1125066 posted February 7, 2006 and accessed September 30, 2007.

Thaler MP, Ubogy ZI. Artecoll: the Arizona experience and lessons learned. *Dermatol. Surg.* 2005;31:1566–76.

Section 8

NEUROTOXINS

CHAPTER 33

Neurotoxins: Past, Present, and Future

Joseph F. Greco
Jenny Kim

Clostridium botulinum is the Gram-positive soil bacterium most famous in the cosmetic world for its ability to produce the highly sought after neurotoxins. Seven serotypes of *C. botulinum* exist, each giving rise to an antigenically distinct botulinum toxin, botulinum neurotoxin (BoNT) type A, B, C_1, D, E, F, and G (serotype C_2 exists but is cytotoxic and not neurotoxic). All toxins have the ability to bind to motor nerve terminals, become internalized, and block the release of acetylcholine (Ach). However, a complex interplay of several factors, including toxin serotype, potency, duration of action, preparation, volume of dilution, and protein load, creates variation among the neurotoxins. Of the seven distinct neurotoxin serotypes, BoNT type A has been the most scrutinized, studied, and therapeutically successful commercially available form.

The history of how this deadly toxin became available to use as medicine is fascinating and includes work done by many dedicated and astute physicians and scientists. The toxic effect of botulinum toxin was first noted in 1822 by a German physician, Kerner, who described food poisoning caused by ingestion of sausages. It was not until some years later, in 1895, that a Belgian microbiologist, Professor van Ermengen, identified that a bacterium producing a neurotoxin was the cause of botulism in Belgium musicians who became ill after eating sausages. Progress in research was possible after researchers, including Professor Ed Schantz and his colleagues, purified botulinum toxin A in sufficient amount for research. Many researchers contributed to study the activity of botulinum toxin in the 1940s and 1950s, but it was not until the 1960s that it was discovered

that BoNT A inhibited Ach release at the neuromuscular junction to induce its effects.

The first clinical use of botulinum toxin as medicine was pioneered by an ophthalmologist, Alan Scott, who obtained the neurotoxin from Dr. Schantz and injected the toxin to correct strabismus in an experimental model. Dr. Schantz then developed the Hall strain of *C. botulinum* type A toxin, and Dr. Scott successfully used this to treat strabismus and blepharospasm in humans. The original botulinum toxin type A developed by Dr. Schantz was eventually acquired and developed by Allergan Inc. and approved for human use for treatment of strabismus and blepharospasm in 1989. Botulinum toxin A has mainly been used for its effect on skeletal muscle hyperactivity; however, the activity of the toxin appears to be effective against smooth muscle dysfunction as well as some autonomic and pain-related conditions.

In 2002, the Food and Drug Administration's (FDA) landmark approval of BOTOX (Allergan Inc.), the first and only BoNT approved for the temporary cosmetic improvement of rhytids, came over one hundred years after the initial published description of *C. botulinum* and a half century after the pure crystalline form of botulinum type A toxin was isolated. While working with Dr. Alan Scott during the early clinical evaluation of botulinum toxin, Dr. Jean Carruthers observed the aesthetic changes in patients after botulinum toxin treatment. This led to the development of botulinum toxin type A for aesthetic indications, and Carruther's first published their findings on the dramatic cosmetic effects the toxin exerted on periorbital furrows.

Over the past decade, the off-label use of botulinum toxin for the treatment of hyperdynamic lines of the face and neck has risen to a point where BOTOX now reigns in the United States as the undisputed champion of minimally invasive cosmetic procedures in both men and women. A variety of other formulations of botulinum toxin, such as the type A toxin Dysport (Ipsen Ltd.) and the type B toxin Myobloc (Elan Pharmaceuticals) in the United States, are used off-label for cosmetic enhancement in attempts to establish their place in the intoxicating market of *Clostridium botulinum*.

This chapter will serve as an introduction to BoNTs and provide a glimpse of the currently available neurotoxins for use in North America, the European Union, and Asia. Subsequent chapters will expand on this to discuss the details of each available neurotoxin.

NEUROTOXINS

BoNTs are synthesized as single-chain polypeptides, which undergo enzymatic cleavage to yield a 150-kD dichain toxin composed of a 100-kD heavy chain and a 50-kD light chain linked by disulfide bonds (Figure 33.1). The heavy chain functions as the binding and translocation region of the toxin, while the light chain functions as its catalytic domain. Further enzymatic cleavage or nicking

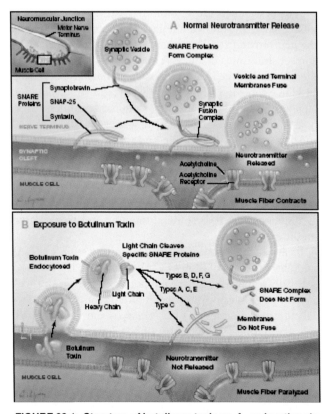

FIGURE 33.1: *Structure of botulinum toxin as, A, an inactive single chain protein (150 kD) and, B, an activated dichain protein (100 kD and 50 kD).*

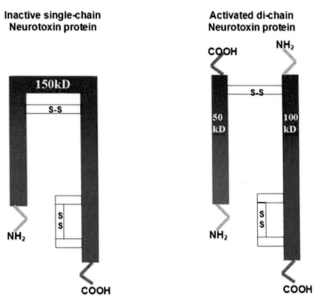

FIGURE 33.2: *Neurotoxin mechanisms of action.*

by proteases converts the toxin to its active form. Once the botulinum toxin is introduced into the body, the presynaptic motor nerve terminal hosts a series of events that lead to paralysis of target muscles. Before understanding this, we must first review the normal sequence of events at the neuromuscular junction (NMJ) and relevant structures responsible for muscle contraction (Figure 33.2).

Ach is synthesized in the motor neuron from acetyl-coenzyme A and choline by the enzyme acetyltransferase. The Ach molecules are then stored in transport vesicles, which aggregate in the presynaptic nerve terminal and await further direction from nerve stimuli. Soluble N-ethyl-maleimide-sensitive factor attachment receptors (SNARE) proteins are a superfamily of proteins that mediate the proper docking and fusion of the Ach-containing vesicles to the plasma membrane. SNARE proteins SNAP-25 and syntaxin-1 bind to the presynaptic neural plasma membrane complex with synaptobrevin (or vesicle-associated membrane protein, VAMP) on the transport vesicles as a prerequisite for the release of the neurotransmitter.

During neuronal stimulation, a motor neuron carries a nerve impulse from its origin in the central nervous system to its final destination, the presynaptic terminal of the NMJ. Terminal depolarization from this action potential causes an increase in intraneuronal calcium concentration through membrane-bound channels. The calcium influx catalyzes the SNARE complex–mediated docking and fusion of Ach-containing synaptic vesicles to the plasma membrane of the nerve terminal. Ach is then released into and diffuses across the synaptic cleft, where the neurotransmitter activates postsynaptic nicotinic cholinergic receptors of muscle fibers. This interaction leads to an influx of sodium and an efflux of potassium from skeletal muscle fibers, causing them to contract.

TABLE 33.1: Mechanisms of Action of Various Neurotoxins

Botulinum Neurotoxin Serotype	Intracellular SNARE Protein Cleaved	Products Currently Available or in Development
A	SNAP-25	BOTOX (U.S.)/Vistabel (EU), Dysport (EU, U.S.), BTX-A (China); PureTox (U.S.); Xeomin (EU), Linurase (Canada); Neuronox/Meditoxin (South Korea)
B	VAMP/synaptobrevin	Myobloc (U.S.)/ Neurobloc (EU)
C$_1$	SNAP-25 and syntaxin	none available
D	VAMP/synaptobrevin	no effect on human nervous system
E	SNAP-25	none available
F	VAMP/synaptobrevin	none available
G	VAMP/synaptobrevin	none available

Through a multistep process of attachment, internalization, and blockade, botulinum toxins derail the normal sequence of events leading to contraction. After injection and diffusion to the target nerve terminal, the toxin binds to presynaptic motor nerve receptors via the 100-kD heavy chain. The toxin-receptor complex is then internalized through receptor-mediated endocytosis into acidic vesicles. The low pH induces a conformational change in the toxin, whereby the heavy chain forms a transmembrane ion channel through which the newly dissociated light chain passes into the neuronal cytosol. At this point, the final and most critical action of the botulinum toxin takes place. The 50-kD light chain functions as a Zn^{2+}-dependent endoprotease, which enzymatically cleaves a specific protein of the SNARE complex (Table 33.1), preventing aggregation, docking, and fusion of the Ach-containing vesicles. Subsequent Ach release is blocked and muscular contraction is prevented.

All serotypes inhibit Ach exocytosis by the inactivation of SNARE proteins. However, each BoNT serotype cleaves a SNARE protein at a different site, yielding distinct truncated substrates, which are degraded and recycled at varying rates. This includes serotypes that cleave the same substrate. Serotypes A, C$_1$, and E cleave SNAP-25, while serotypes B, C, F, and G cleave synaptobrevin/VAMP. Serotype C$_1$ additionally cleaves syntaxin. Additionally, competition among BoNT serotypes for binding to the presynaptic membrane does not exist as no two serotypes share the same receptor.

Transitory collateral sprouting of nerve terminals occurs following neuromuscular paralysis. The smaller axonal sprouts reestablish neurotransmission through functional synaptic communication with the skeletal muscle fibers. After botulinum toxin degradation and SNARE substrate replenishment, the restoration of the parent nerve terminals' exocytotic activity coincides with retraction and elimination of the collateral sprouts. This display of versatility likely fuels the initial recovery of motor activity before the primary intoxicated neuron returns to its original activity state.

DIFFERENCES AMONG NEUROTOXINS

All BoNTs diffuse to the NMJ, share a high affinity for cholinergic neurons, and inhibit the release of Ach. The extent and duration of paralysis induced by botulinum toxins depends on the interplay among numerous factors, including toxin serotype, half-life, and rate of turnover of truncated substrates responsible for effective docking and fusion of Ach-containing vesicles.

Botulinum toxin serotypes share similarity in their 150-kD therapeutically active dichain constitution. However, structural differences exist among the serotypes with respect to their associated nontoxic protein domains, which, together, create a macromolecular progenitor toxin. The molecular weight of the nontoxic domains in botulinum type A toxins is 300 kD and in type B toxins is 150 kD. Commercially available toxin complexes exist as dimers so that the molecular weights of the entire neurotoxin complexes are 900 kD for type A toxins (300 kD neurotoxin dimer + 600 kD nontoxic domain dimer) and 600 kD for type B toxins (300 kD neurotoxin dimer + 300 kD nontoxic domain dimer).

Differences in efficacy of commercially available preparations may be affected by the proportion of active versus inactive forms of the toxin. The 150-kD BoNT must be activated by endogenous or exogenous proteases prior to cleaving SNARE proteins. Protease nicking yields the active heavy and light, dichain complex. Endogenous proteases nick and activate botulinum toxin type A so that the great majority of recovered toxin from cultures is already activated. Commercial preparations of type A toxin therefore have the highest levels of activated toxin. In contrast, botulinum toxin types E and F are recovered from culture primarily in the inactive, nonnicked form. All other serotypes fall somewhere in between. Clinically, this is relevant as competition may exist between the nicked versus nonnicked forms for binding and internalization in presynaptic neurons, where nonnicked forms may simply occupy endosomes without the ability to disrupt Ach exocytosis. Exogenous activation by proteases during commercial preparation of toxins is a less efficient process, with potentially higher levels of inactive competing toxin.

The potency of a neurotoxin can be measured by its overall dose, or the number of units injected per session to achieve effective clinical results in a single patient. Clinically effective doses and durations of action among serotypes, and even within preparations of the same serotype, differ markedly. The doses are not interchangeable, and clearly defined conversion factors are not available. Since BoNT type A has been the most widely studied, dosage comparisons are often made using BOTOX as the reference. Significantly larger doses of botulinum toxin type B are required to achieve a similar clinical efficacy when compared to type A toxins, whereas the dosage of Dysport, an alternative type A toxin, is only slightly higher than that of its competitor, BOTOX. BoNT type F has a similar potency as BoNT type A but has a much shorter duration of action. High doses are most often associated with high protein loads, which may place the patient at risk for neutralizing antibody formation.

Prolonged light chain protease activity, persistence of ineffective truncated SNARE substrate, and speed of substrate replenishment play distinct roles in the different durations of action among serotypes. BoNT type A has been the most effective and ideal BoNT for cosmetic use. It induces neuromuscular paralysis for the greatest duration among serotypes, with BoNT type C_1 and BoNT type B following in descending order. BoNT type F and BoNT type E have the shortest duration of action with the most rapid recovery of neuroexocytotic activity at the NMJ. Rationale for the extended inhibition of the type A toxin is primarily threefold as compared to other serotypes. First, the type A toxin light chain is highly stable and persists at the plasma membrane of the presynaptic terminal for a longer period of time, exerting its proteolytic inhibition. Second, SNAP-25a, the cleaved substrate of the toxin, also persists for long periods of time before slow replenishment to the functional SNAP-25. Last, SNAP-25a itself has antagonistic effects on uncleaved SNAP-25, accentuating the blockage created by the type A toxin.

BoNTs are proteins capable of developing both neutralizing (against the 150-kD toxin complex) and nonneutralizing (against the nontoxin domains) antibodies. Only neutralizing antibodies affect biological activity of the neurotoxin. If the levels are high enough, they may prevent neurotoxin binding to the presynaptic motor nerve membrane receptor and cause a loss of responsiveness to the treatment. Factors that increase the risk for antibody formation include those that expose the immune system to more neurotoxin protein, including higher total doses and more frequent injections. Antibody-mediated resistance to treatment with respect to the cosmetic use of current lots of botulinum toxin does not appear to be an issue. The total doses administered are far less than those reported in the neurological literature to stimulate significant antibody formation. However, if newer preparations with lower potency and shorter durations of action require higher total doses and more frequent injections, the rate of antibody formation could theoretically increase to a level high enough

to affect biological activity. Current batches of BOTOX have a significantly low protein load, and no reports of a loss of responsiveness to treatment from neutralizing antibodies exist. Lack of, or diminished responsiveness to, treatment more likely would result from improper dosing, dilution, or storage; incorrect placement of injections; and changes in the patients' perception of improvement as compared to initial treatment results.

AVAILABLE PRODUCTS

BOTOX and BOTOX Cosmetic (Allergan Inc.; marketed as Vistabel in the United Kingdom) are presently the prototypical and most widely used botulinum toxins for the treatment of cervicofacial rhytids. Each vial contains 100 units (U) of a lyophilized form of botulinum toxin type A purified neurotoxin complex with human albumin and sodium chloride in a sterile, vacuum-dried preparation. Reconstitution is required for use and is recommended by gently introducing a specified volume of nonpreserved 0.9% saline solution so as to not agitate the preparation with bubble formation. BOTOX is currently the only FDA-approved type A botulinum toxin for cosmetic use. A much greater evaluation of its use will follow in subsequent chapters.

Dysport (Ipsen Ltd, also distributed for cosmetic use in the United States by Medicis) is an additional preparation of botulinum type A toxin, which is available in packs of 2 × 2.5 mL vials containing 500 U of lyophilized botulinum toxin type A hemagglutinin complex with human albumin, lactose, and sodium chloride. Reconstitution is required and guidelines are similar to those for BOTOX. An efficacy and dose-finding study suggested that 50 U of Dysport was an optimal and safe dose for treating glabellar lines. A direct head-to-head comparative study with BOTOX found that 20 U of BOTOX injected into the glabellar complex was as effective at four weeks but superior at sixteen weeks to 50 U of Dysport. Another study comparing Dysport and BOTOX at a higher ratio of 4:1 showed similar efficacy; however, patients treated with Dysport had a higher risk for adverse effects. Optimal dose comparisons likely fall somewhere between the 2.5:1 to 4:1 Dysport:BOTOX ratios.

Botulinum type B toxin is available as Myobloc in the United States (Elan Pharmaceuticals; marketed as Neurobloc in Europe) in an acidic (pH = 5.6) aqueous solution containing human albumin and sodium succinate. The aqueous solution permits a longer, stable shelf life and precludes the need for reconstitution. Vials of Myobloc are sold in three different labeled volumes containing 0.5 mL (2,500 U), 1.0 mL (5,000 U), and 2.0 mL (10,000 U) of botulinum type B toxin. However, the vials are overfilled and more accurately contain 0.82 mL (4,100 U), 1.36 mL (6,800 U), and 2.53 mL (12,650 U), respectively. Multiple studies of botulinum toxin type B for off-label use in treatment of forehead, glabellar, and crow's feet facial lines show that the type B toxin is effective in temporarily

TABLE 33.2: FDA Status of Various Yet Unapproved Neurotoxins or Neurotoxin Applications

Product	Company/Country	Approved For	U.S. Stage of Development
BOTOX, BOTOX Cosmetic (Vistabel in Europe)	Allergan Inc., Irvine, CA	cervical dystonia[a,b] strabismus[a] blepharospasm[a,b] hemifacial spasm[b] glabellar lines[a,b] adult focal spasticity associated with stroke[b] pediatric cerebral palsy[b] prim axillary hyperhidrosis[a,b]	phase II–III clinical trials for headache, overactive bladder, adult spasticity; expected approvals in 2010–2012
Dysport	Ipsen Ltd., Berkshire, U.K.; Medicis, Scottsdale, AZ	adult spasticity[b] spasmodic torticollis[b] blepharospasm[b] hemifacial spasm[b] cerebral palsy glabellar lines (Germany)	phase III trials for treatment of cervical dystonia; FDA approved in 2009
PureTox	Mentor Corp., Santa Barbara, CA	no approvals	phase III clinical trials for glabellar lines; expected approval 2010–2011
Myobloc (Neurobloc in Europe)	Solstice, Malvern, PA	cervical dystonia[a]	N/A
Chinese BOTOX A (CBTX-A)	Lanzhou Biological Products Institute, China	no approvals outside of China and select markets in Asia and Latin America	N/A
Xeomin (NT201)	Merz Pharma, Germany	only approved for cervical dystonia and blepharospasm in Germany	phase III trials for cervical dystonia, blepharospasm, and glabellar lines; expected approval 2010–2011
Linurase	Prollenium Inc., Canada	same as CBTX-A, but in Canada	
Neuronox, Meditoxin	Medy-Tox Inc., South Korea	no approvals outside Korea	N/A

[a] Approved by the FDA.
[b] Approved by the Medicines and Healthcare Products Regulatory Authority (MHRA, FDA's equivalent in the United Kingdom) or the European Medicines Agency (EMEA, FDA's equivalent in Europe).

reducing the hyperdynamic lines in these areas. A faster onset of action but shorter duration of action have consistently been shown when comparing Myobloc to similar materials containing the type A toxin. In direct, head-to-head comparative studies with BOTOX, Myobloc has been shown to have a faster onset of action, larger diffusion area, shorter duration of action, and greater pain on injection. The increased pain is attributed to the acidic nature of the solution. It is recommended by some authors that practitioners dilute the aqueous solution with preservative containing saline to reduce the acidity. The short duration of action, pain on injection, and periodic sensation of tightness after injection all contribute to the infrequent use of Myobloc in the United States for cosmetic enhancement.

Additional formulations of botulinum toxins that require more intensive evaluation in the United States include a variety of botulinum type A toxins, including a Chinese type, CBTX-A (Lanzhou Biological Products Institute), Xeomin (Merz Pharma), Linurase (Prollenium Corp.), and Neuronox from South Korea (Medy-Tox Inc.; Table 33.2). A direct comparative study between CBTX-A and BOTOX for the treatment of focal dystonia and muscle spasm showed similar efficacies. The dose of CBTX-A required was much higher than for BOTOX, and a number of patients treated with CBTX-A developed a skin rash a few days after injection.

The past decade has witnessed a remarkable growth in the number of minimally invasive cosmetic procedures performed in the United States. According to the American Society for Aesthetic Plastic Surgery, a total of nearly 11.5 million cosmetic procedures were performed in 2006, with botulinum toxin injections representing 28% of the total, at nearly 3.2 million. This is staggering when compared to the figures just ten years prior, when just over sixty-five thousand botulinum toxin injection procedures were performed out of a total of 2.1 million cosmetic procedures. The overall percentage change in botulinum toxin injections performed in 1997 versus 2006 was a 4,783% increase.

Botulinum toxins ride atop this powerful wave of noninvasive cosmetic procedures flooding doctor's offices across the world. This is in part due to their high effectiveness, consistent results, minimal side effects, and relative ease of use for both patients and physicians. In parallel with this trend, pharmaceutical companies are developing newer preparations of toxins with different properties that will, it is hoped, lead to novel competitive products. On the other hand, the development of newer preparations will also most certainly lead to complications if the injectors are not properly educated about the various characteristics, potencies, durations of action, and diffusion areas of the individual products. The doses of various products are not interchangeable, and no standard conversions exist at this time. With the successful and well-documented off-label use of BOTOX over new areas of the face, including the lateral brow; the infraorbital, nasal, and periorbital lines; and the mentalis and depressor anguli oris muscles, it may seem attractive to some novice users to try newer preparations in these areas. The authors strongly caution against this until well-planned and published studies evaluate and document the proper dosing regimens, diffusion capacity, location, and volumes of injection. The following chapters serve to increase knowledge of the variety of neurotoxins currently available and introduce products in development that may become available in coming years.

SUGGESTED READING

American Society for Aesthetic Plastic Surgery. Cosmetic surgery statistics. Available at: http://www.surgery.org/press/statistics.php. Accessed May 30, 2007.

Aoki KR. Pharmacology and immunology of botulinum toxin serotypes. *J. Neurol.* 2001;248:1/3–1/10.

Aoki KR, Guyer B. Botulinum toxin type A and other botulinum toxin serotypes: a comparative review of biochemical and pharmacological actions. *Eur. J. Neurol.* 2001;8:21–9.

Baumann L, Black L. Botulinum toxin type B (Myobloc). *Dermatol. Surg.* 2003;29:496–500.

Baumann L, Slezinger A, Vujevich J, et al. A double-blinded, randomized, placebo controlled pilot study of the safety and efficacy of Myobloc (botulinum toxin type-B) – purified neurotoxin complex for the treatment of crow's feet: a double-blinded placebo-controlled trial. *Dermatol. Surg.* 2003;29:508–15.

Dolly JO, Aoki KR. The structure and mode of action of different botulinum toxins. *Eur. J. Neurol.* 2006;13:1–9.

Dressler D, Hallett M. Immunological aspects of Botox®, Dysport®, and Myobloc TM/Neurobloc®. *Eur. J. Neurol.* 2006;13:11–15.

Flynn TC. Update on botulinum toxin. *Semin. Cutan. Med. Surg.* 2006;25:115–21.

Flynn TC, Clark RE. Botulinum toxin type B (Myobloc) versus botulinum toxin type A (Botox) frontalis study: rate of onset and radius of diffusion. *Dermatol. Surg.* 2003;29:519–22.

Foran PG, Mohammed N, Lisk GO, et al. Evaluation of the therapeutic usefulness of botulinum neurotoxin B, C1, E, and F compared with the long lasting type A. *J. Biol. Chem.* 2003;10:1363–71.

Huang W, Foster JA, Rogachefsky AS. Pharmacology of botulinum toxin. *J. Am. Acad. Dermatol.* 2000;43:249–59.

Kim EJ, Ramirez AL, Reeck JB, et al. The role of botulinum toxin type B (Myobloc) in the treatment of hyperkinetic facial lines. *Plast. Reconstr. Surg.* 2003;112:88S–93S.

Meunier FA, Schiavo G, Molgo J. Botulinum neurotoxins: from paralysis to recovery of functional neuromuscular transmission. *J. Physiol. (Paris)* 2002;96:105–13.

Rosales RL, Bigalke H, Dressler D. Pharmacology of botulinum toxin: differences between type A preparations. *Eur. J. Neurol.* 2006;13:2–10.

Rzany B, Ascher B, Fratila A, et al. Efficacy and safety of 3- and 5-injection patterns (30 and 50U) of botulinum toxin A (Dysport) for the treatment of wrinkles in the glabella and the central forehead region. *Arch. Dermatol.* 2006;142:320–6.

Scott AB. Botulinum toxin injection into extraocular muscles as an alternative to strabismus surgery. *Ophthalmology* 1980;87:1044–9.

Tang XF, Wan XH. Comparison of Botox with a Chinese type A botulinum toxin. *Chin. Med. J.* 2000;113:794–8.

CHAPTER 34

BOTOX: How We Do It

Deborshi Roy

Neil S. Sadick

Botulinum toxin is a powerful medication that has been used to treat various conditions in humans for several decades. In the last few years, there has been an explosion in the use of this drug for cosmetic purposes. Millions have benefited from the therapeutic effects of botulinum toxin, with very few patients experiencing adverse effects. In this chapter, we will discuss the various techniques and therapeutic uses of botulinum toxin in the field of cosmetic dermatology.

MECHANISMS OF ACTION

The mechanism of action of botulinum toxin (BTX) has been well established (Sakaguchi 1983; Carruthers and Carruthers 1992; Keen et al. 1994; Hambleton 1992). Protein interactions at the neuromuscular junction prevent the release of acetylcholine. There are seven known antigenically distinct serotypes of BTX (A–G). The most widely used and studied is botulinum toxin type A (BTX-A). This protein irreversibly binds and cleaves the SNAP-25 protein. There are currently two available preparations of BTX-A on the U.S. market: Botox and Dysport. Botulinum toxin type B (BTX-B) binds to synaptobrevin. BTX-B is available commercially as Myobloc. The temporary nature of therapeutic BTX therapy is due to axonal sprouting at the motor end plate of the neuromuscular junction as well as the development of extrajunctional acetylcholine receptors (de Paiva et al. 1999). This occurs over several months after BTX therapy.

COSMETIC USE

Cosmetic BTX treatments have become one of the most common nonsurgical procedures performed by dermatologists and plastic surgeons. Cosmetic use of BTX can be performed on the entire face and neck, although current Food and Drug Administration guidelines are for use in the glabella (BOTOX Cosmetic) and in the neck for cervical dystonia (Myobloc). Casual users limit their BTX treatments to the upper face. Advanced users address the midface, lower face, and neck, as well. BTX treatments may be employed as the primary method of facial rejuvenation or can be an adjunct to other surgical and nonsurgical modalities.

Dynamic Rhytids of the Upper Face

Facial wrinkles involving the forehead, glabella, and lateral periorbital regions are a common aesthetic problem (Figure 34.1). These wrinkles are a direct result of hyperactivity of the underlying muscles of expression (Pierard and Lapiere 1989). The horizontal rhytids of the central and lateral forehead are due to contraction of the frontalis muscle. We recommend using an average of 15–30 units of BTX-A for treatment of the frontalis. Vertically oriented rhytids of the glabella are due to contraction of the procerus, depressor supercilii, and medial portions of the orbicularis oculi. We use an average of 15–30 units of BTX-A to treat the glabellar complex. Horizontal rhytids of the lateral periorbital area (crow's feet) are due to contraction of the lateral orbicularis oculi muscle. We use an average of 8–15 units of BTX-A to treat each side of the face.

Dynamic Rhytids of the Midface

The midface is not an area commonly treated with BTX. Dynamic rhytids of the midface are usually centered about the nose, due to the lack of muscles of facial expression laterally.

Subciliary rhytids caused by contraction of the medial portion of the lower orbicularis oculi muscle are treated by advanced BTX users. A few well-placed injections of 2 units of BTX-A each are used to treat this area. It is important to avoid the pretarsal portion of the muscle since it is responsible for blinking.

Perinasal rhytids are due to contraction of several small muscle groups. The most commonly injected area is the upper nasal sidewall, where contraction of the nasalis

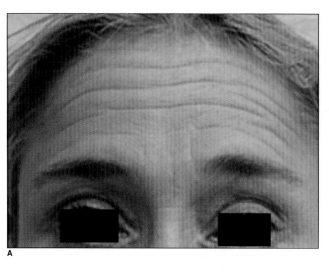
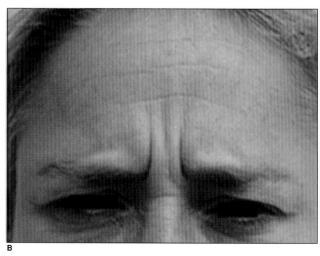
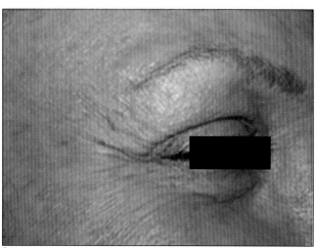
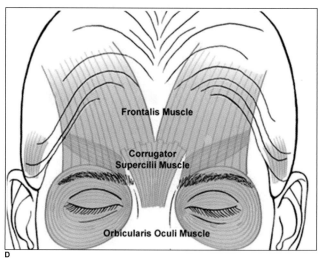

FIGURE 34.1: Dynamic rhytids of three upper facial areas: **A**, *forehead;* **B**, *glabella;* **C**, *lateral periorbital area (crow's feet).* **D**, *Corresponding mimetic muscles of the upper face.*

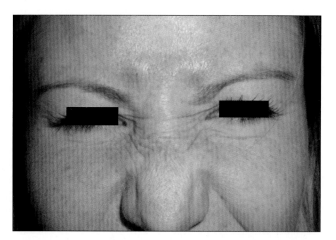

FIGURE 34.2: Bunny lines caused by contraction of the transverse head of the nasalis muscle.

muscle causes so-called bunny lines, the oblique rhytids of the upper nose (Figure 34.2). This usually requires 5–10 units of BTX-A per side. Treatment of the lower nose is usually not directed toward the ablation of rhytids, but toward changing static or dynamic aspects of the nasal tip. BTX treatment can be used to change the rotation of the nasal tip and decrease nasal flaring.

Dynamic Rhytids of the Lower Face

The lower face is not a common area treated with BTX. Dynamic rhytids of this region are in the perioral area. Extreme caution must be used when treating this area with BTX since diffusion of toxin and injection of adjacent musculature can result in functional deficits. The so-called lipstick lines, vertical perioral rhytids caused by contraction

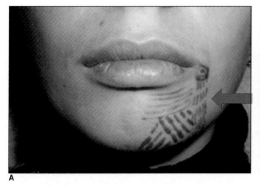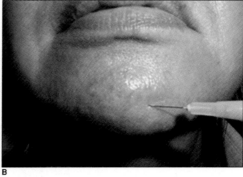

FIGURE 34.3: A, *Red arrow indicates the anatomical location of the depressor anguli oris muscle.* **B**, *Treatment of chin dimpling caused by contraction of the mentalis muscle.*

of the orbicularis oris, are the most commonly treated in the lower face. Several well-placed injections of 2 units of BTX-A along the edge of the upper and lower lips are used to treat this area. A downturned corner of the mouth is treated with injections into the depressor anguli oris muscle. The average dose is between 2 and 8 units of BTX-A per side. Dimpling of the central chin is treated with injection into the mentalis muscle, using 5–10 units of BTX-A in total (Figure 34.3).

Treatment of Neck Rhytids

Cosmetic use of BTX in the neck is primarily for the treatment of platysmal banding. These are vertical bands usually found in the central neck. There are also horizontal rhytids caused by contraction of the platysma muscle, usually seen laterally, which can be treated with BTX injections. The platysma is a thin muscle, and carefully placed injections are crucial to avoid affecting the deeper neck musculature, which can cause dysphagia, hoarseness, and neck weakness. Dosing varies greatly depending on the area treated, but multiple injections of 2–5 units of BTX-A are used.

Other Cosmetic Uses

Hyperhidrosis can also be treated with BTX. The paralytic effect of BTX on the eccrine glands is less studied than the effect on the mimetic muscles of the face. The areas most commonly treated are the axilla, palms, and soles of the feet. In a randomized, double-blinded, placebo-controlled parallel group study, Naumann and Lowe (2001) treated each axilla with 50 units of BTX-A and found that the majority of patients had at least a 50% reduction in sweat production, even eighteen weeks after the initial injection. Lowe et al. (2003) also studied the need for repeat treatments and found that the mean time between treatments was twenty-nine weeks, and that repeated injections were an effective treatment. In a multicenter, randomized, double-blinded trial, Heckmann et al. (2001) demonstrated that the rate of

sweat production responded to BTX treatment in a dose-dependent manner.

INJECTION TECHNIQUE FOR THE FACE

Before any injections are performed, the facial musculature is evaluated thoroughly. Muscle activity is graded as mild, moderate, or severe. This helps to decide how many units of BTX to use to achieve the desired effect. Pretreatment photos are taken and the face is appropriately prepped and marked. Precise delivery of small volumes is the best way to achieve great results with a low incidence of side effects. We prep the face with alcohol swabs prior to injection. We wait a few minutes for all of the alcohol to evaporate before injecting.

We prefer to use the 1-cc Braun Injekt Tuberkulin Solo syringe with a 30-gauge, $\frac{1}{2}$ inch needle. We do not use any anesthesia for the injections, but prefer the Zimmer Cryo 5 cold air device. Firm digital pressure is used after each injection. Occasionally, ice packs are applied for several minutes after the injection. We counsel patients to avoid vigorous massaging of the areas injected, but all other light activity is permitted. We usually perform other facial procedures (such as light, laser, or radiofrequency treatments or superficial peels) prior to injecting with BTX.

The proper amount of toxin to administer should be determined by the injecting physician based on the inherent muscle activity, the amount of wrinkling present, and the desired result. Precisely titrating the correct amount of BTX per injection site is a skill that develops with experience. Provisional dosing guidelines for botulinum toxins A and B used in the upper face, provided by Sadick and Matarasso (2004), suggest the following conversions: when using 20–30 units of BTX-A to treat the glabellar complex, one would need to use 2,000–3,000 units of BTX-B to achieve a similar effect and duration. Their numbers for treatment of the forehead are slightly different: 20–30 units of BTX-A produce a similar effect as 1,000–2,500 units of BTX-B. For the lateral orbicularis (crow's feet), 10–15 units

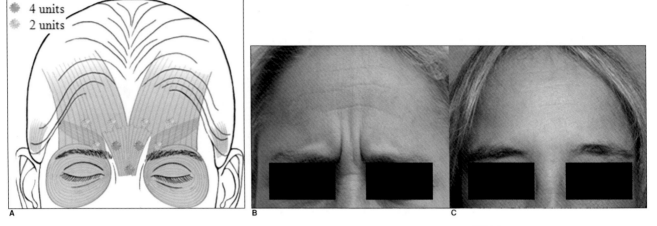

FIGURE 34.4: *Treatment of forehead and glabellar complex:* **A,** *suggested treatment sites and BTX-A doses;* **B,** *patient frowning before treatment; and* **C,** *patient frowning one month after treatment.*

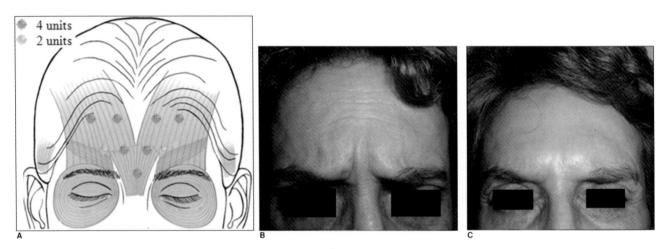

FIGURE 34.5: *Treatment of the forehead and glabellar complex:* **A,** *suggested treatment sites and BTX-A doses;* **B,** *patient frowning before treatment; and* **C,** *patient frowning two months after treatment.*

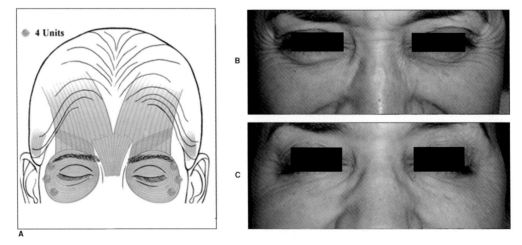

FIGURE 34.6: *Treatment of the crow's feet area:* **A,** *suggested treatment sites and BTX-A doses;* **B,** *patient smiling before treatment; and* **C,** *patient smiling two months after treatment.*

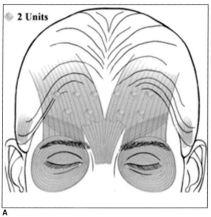
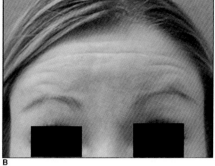
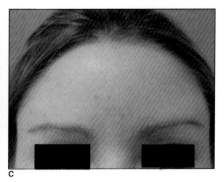

FIGURE 34.7: *Treatment of the forehead:* **A,** *suggested treatment sites and BTX-A doses;* **B,** *patient raising eyebrows before treatment; and* **C,** *patient raising eyebrows three months after treatment.*

of BTX-A are equivalent to 750–1,500 units of BTX-B. Figures 34.4–34.7 outline the suggested areas to inject, the amount of toxin to deliver, and the corresponding results for the most common treatment scenarios.

INJECTION EFFECT

From numerous studies of both botulinum toxin type A and type B, the average length of onset of therapeutic effect and its duration have been determined. These numbers vary slightly from patient to patient and are dose-dependent. In general, a similar therapeutic effect is seen with both products, although the onset of activity of BTX-B seems to be faster. The duration of action seems to be longer for BTX-A, although with larger doses, the duration of BTX-B can be similar to that of BTX-A (Sadick and Matarasso 2004). Sadick and Matarasso also discuss that there is an increased smoothness to the flaccid paralysis obtained with BTX-B when compared to BTX-A. Overall, the two are interchangeable.

COMPLICATIONS

Complications are not common. Some complications are technique related, which usually occur with casual users and novices. Other complications are due to the local and systemic actions of the toxin itself.

Technique Related

Asymmetry can occur anywhere and is the most common complication. This can be easily remedied with additional BTX injections. Improper technique can cause cosmetic as well as functional problems by inadvertently affecting adjacent musculature. In the upper face, arching of the brow, lateral brow ptosis, blepharoptosis, dry eye, and diplopia can result from poor injection technique or diffusion of

toxin. In the lower face, slurred speech and oral incompetence can result. Discussing possible complications prior to the procedure is an important part of obtaining informed consent. After a complication has occurred, it is important that it be identified and treated as soon as possible. Most of these complications resolve on their own in a few weeks, well before the overall effect of the BTX has worn off.

Arching of the brow (Figure 34.8) results from unopposed muscle tone of the lateral brow elevators (lateral frontalis muscle). Correction of this cosmetic problem can be achieved with carefully placed injections of 5 units of BTX-A in the lower lateral frontalis. Care must be taken not to weaken this muscle too much since that will lead to lateral brow ptosis. Lateral brow ptosis (Figure 34.9) occurs with too much weakening of the lateral frontalis muscle. This can occur with erroneous injection placement or aggressive

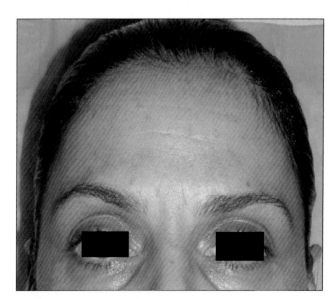

FIGURE 34.8: *Arching of the right lateral brow after BTX treatment.*

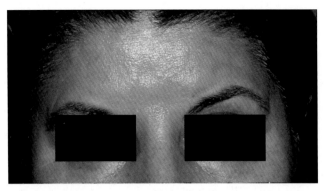

FIGURE 34.9: Ptosis of the right lateral brow after BTX treatment.

treatment of lateral forehead rhytids. Treatment of lateral brow ptosis can be performed with injections of BTX into the lateral brow depressors or the lateral orbicularis oculi muscle. This can raise the lateral brow by a millimeter or two, camouflaging the ptosis.

Blepharoptosis (Figure 34.10) is caused by diffusion of the toxin into the levator palpebrae superioris muscle. This can be treated with naphazoline ophthalmic drops to temporarily raise the eyelid for short periods of time until the BTX effect wears off. For dry eye and diplopia, supportive care can be used and a consultation with an ophthalmologist can ease the patient's concerns while symptoms are present. Supportive care and reassurance are the only treatment of complications occurring in the lower face and neck. Again, most of these will resolve before the overall effect of the BTX wears off.

Toxin Related

A wide range of complaints have been reported after BTX treatments. The most common are headache, nausea, and malaise (BOTOX package insert). Treatment for these complaints usually consists of supportive care. Isolated cases of distal or generalized muscle weakness have been

reported, but these are rare cases and involve patients being treated for neurologic diseases (Bhatia et al. 1999). When BTX is used for cosmetic treatments, immunoresistance and unusual or uncategorized reactions are extremely rare and should be thoroughly investigated and reported.

CONCLUSION

The aforementioned therapeutic uses of botulinum toxin have expanded the ability for cosmetic surgeons and dermatologists to treat the signs of aging. By specifically targeting the dynamic rhytids of the face, BTX has allowed us to address a problem that we could not in the past. Whether used as a primary mode of treatment or as an adjunct to volume replacement or tissue-tightening procedures, BTX is a great addition to the antiaging armamentarium.

SUGGESTED READING

Bhatia KP, et al. Generalised muscular weakness after botulinum toxin injections for dystonia: a report of three cases. *J. Neurol. Neurosurg. Psychiatry* 1999;67:90–3.

BOTOX Cosmetic [package insert]. Irvine, CA: Allergan Inc.; 2005.

Carruthers JDA, Carruthers JA. Treatment of glabellar frown lines with C botulinum-A exotoxin. *J. Dermatol. Surg. Oncol.* 1992;18:17–21.

de Paiva A, Meunier FA, Molgo J, et al. Functional repair of motor endplates after botulinum neurotoxin type A poisoning: biphasic switch of synaptic activity between nerve sprouts and their parent terminals. *Proc. Natl. Acad. Sci. U. S. A.* 1999;96: 3200–5.

Hambleton P. Clostridium botulinum toxins: a general review of involvement in disease, structure, mode of action and preparation for clinical use. *J. Neurol.* 1992;239:16–20.

Heckmann M, Ceballos-Baumann AO, Plewig G. Botulinum toxin A for axillary hyperhidrosis. *N. Engl. J. Med.* 2001;344:488–93.

Keen M, Blitzer A, Aviv J, et al. Botulinum toxin A therapy for hyperkinetic facial lines: results of a double-blind, placebo-controlled study. *Plast. Reconstr. Surg.* 1994;94:94–9.

Lowe PL, Cerdan-Sanz S, Lowe NJ. Botulinum toxin type A in the treatment of bilateral primary axillary hyperhidrosis: efficacy and duration with repeated treatments. *Dermatol. Surg.* 2003;29:545–8.

Naumann M, Lowe NJ. Botulinum toxin type A in treatment of bilateral primary axillary hyperhidrosis: randomised, parallel group, double blind, placebo controlled trial. *Br. Med. J.* 2001;323:596–9.

Pierard GE, Lapiere CM. The microanatomical basis of facial frown lines. *Arch. Dermatol.* 1989;125:1090–2.

Sadick NS, Matarasso SL. Comparison of botulinum toxins A and B in the treatment of facial rhytides. *Dermatol. Clin.* 2004;22:221–6.

Sakaguchi G. Clostridium botulinum toxins. *Pharmacol. Ther.* 1983;19:165–94.

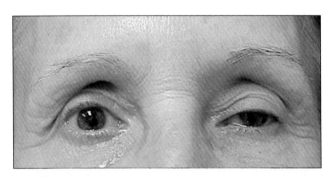

FIGURE 34.10: Ptosis of the left upper eyelid after BTX treatment.

CHAPTER 35

Cosmetic BOTOX: How We Do It

Frederick C. Beddingfield III
David P. Beynet

The most common cosmetic procedure in the United States currently is treatment with botulinum toxin A. It has been proven as a safe and effective treatment for improvement of glabellar lines. It is also commonly used to treat rhytids in the forehead, periocular, perinasal, periorbital, chin, and platysmal areas, among others. Given its extensive safety history and the use of the material in millions of patients for over twenty years, along with its high satisfaction profile and ease of use, knowledge of this treatment is of paramount importance for practicing aesthetic physicians.

Clostridium botulinum toxin type A (BTX-A), developed and marketed as BOTOX Cosmetic by Allergan Inc., is the first type A botulinum toxin approved in the United States and is supplied as a vacuum-dried powder, 100 units per vial. Of note, different botulinum toxins are defined and treated as different products by the Food and Drug Administration (FDA) and other international regulatory agencies. The FDA does not recognize generic biologics (such as botulinum toxins) because the different manufacturing processes alter the final products significantly. Units of BOTOX Cosmetic are not interchangeable with units of other types of botulinum toxin, and there is no recognized conversion factor between different types of botulinum toxin. This is clear since the dose response curves of different toxins are not parallel to each other and the optimal ratio between products appears to be different for different indications. Unreconstituted BOTOX Cosmetic should be stored at 2–8 degrees Celsius. The manufacturer recommendation is to reconstitute the BOTOX with 2.5 mL of 0.9% nonpreserved saline to a final concentration of 4.0 U/0.1 mL. Other dilutions from 1 to 10 mL/100 units have been recommended. Some believe more diffusion may result from diluting with higher volumes. A consensus panel suggested that there is no decrease in efficacy with preserved saline as the diluent and that preserved saline results in less pain with injection (Alam et al. 2002; Kwiat et al. 2004; Carruthers et al. 2004). The dilution can also be modified based on practitioner preference. The manufacturer recommends avoiding agitation or causing foaming with reconstitution. With proper storage at 4 degrees Celsius (never frozen), the reconstituted product can be stored for up to six weeks.

Tuberculin or insulin syringes are commonly used. In general, single-use syringes are preferred and insulin syringes may waste less product as there is no potential space in the hub. Other syringes also have a hub designed to waste less product. The most commonly used needle is 30-gauge; however, some physicians use 32-gauge needles to minimize discomfort. Topical analgesia is not required; however, use of ice may reduce pain and constrict blood vessels, thereby lessening the chance of bruising.

Prior to use, a thorough medical history should be obtained. Medications and foods that inhibit clotting may increase bruising (e.g., aspirin and other platelet inhibitors, nonsteroidal anti-inflammatories, garlic, fish oils, etc.) and should be stopped, if possible, seven to ten days before the procedure. Patients with peripheral motor neuropathic diseases or neuromuscular functional disorders (e.g., myasthenia gravis and Eaton-Lambert syndrome) should not be treated. Patients on aminoglycoside antibiotics may have increased inhibition of neuromuscular transmission, and treatment should be postponed. The presence of inflammatory or infectious skin conditions in the area treated is also a contraindication. Last, pregnancy and lactation are contraindicated, although inadvertent use has not resulted in any known adverse events.

The appropriate use of BTX-A requires an understanding of the art of facial aesthetics and the science of this unique molecule. No two patients are exactly the same, and patients commonly present with baseline asymmetries. Cookbook approaches should be avoided. The mechanism of action of BTX-A is to decrease muscular activity by inhibiting the release of acetylcholine, which is necessary for neuromuscular transmission. To practice the art of facial aesthetic enhancement with BTX-A, knowledge of the facial musculature is essential. This includes the

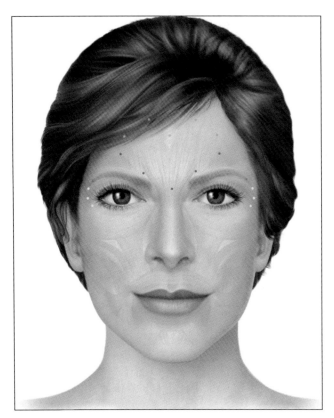

FIGURE 35.1: *Glabella (red dots), forehead (blue dots), brow lift (green dots), crow's feet (yellow dots).*

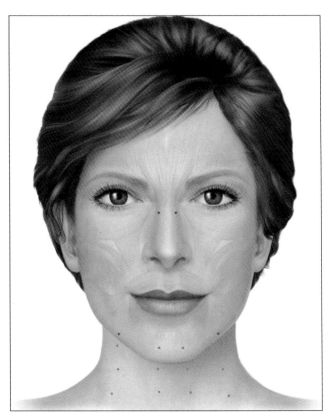

FIGURE 35.2: *Bunny lines (red dots), depressor anguli oris (purple dots), chin (blue dots), platysma (orange dots).*

thickness and pattern of muscle fibers as well as differences in the sex and race of the patient. The basic facial musculature can be seen in Figures 35.1 and 35.2. Men, in general, require higher doses per treatment area. Thin muscles, such as the platysma, require much lower doses than larger muscles, such as the corrugators. Patients should be evaluated for brow and lid ptosis at baseline. Asians and elderly patients may present with brow or lid ptosis at baseline, and the treatment patterns and doses of BTX-A utilized should minimize the chance of exacerbating such underlying conditions. A lower eyelid snap test should be performed to reveal any underlying weakness of eyelid closure and, if present, treatment periorbitally should only proceed with caution, keeping this baseline state in mind.

BOTOX Cosmetic is FDA approved for use in the glabellar area; however, it has now been used in multiple areas, as mentioned earlier. We have included figures to show some of the common and effective uses for BTX-A.

In treating the glabella, BTX-A is utilized to weaken muscles such as the bilateral corrugators, depressor supercilii, and the central procerus, which is responsible, in large part, for the glabellar lines (Figure 35.1, red dots). Often two injections are given per corrugator (which will also treat the modestly important depressor supercilii), with one or two injections in the procerus. It has also been suggested

that BTX-A treatment of the glabella region results in a slight brow lift by weakening the central frontalis effect of brow elevation and thus proportionately increasing the frontalis effect of lateral brow elevation. A more advanced technique is also shown, in which BTX-A is used to weaken the lateral lid depressor muscles, thereby achieving a lateral brow lift (Figure 35.1, green dots).

Also shown in Figure 35.1 is treatment of the forehead (blue dots). To avoid lowering the brow, the forehead, being the primary brow elevator, is most commonly treated in conjunction with the glabellar area, which is composed of primary brow depressors. When treating the forehead for the first time, many physicians will reserve treatment of the forehead area for a two-week follow-up visit after glabellar treatment and utilize a relatively low dose to reduce the possibility of lowering the brow too much. Men particularly have lower set brows, and aggressive treatment of the forehead should be done with caution as lowering of the brow can be an unwanted result.

In Figure 35.1, treatment of crow's feet is shown (yellow dots), which results in partial paralysis of the lateral orbicularis oculi.

In Figure 35.2, treatment of the nasalis, to decrease the presence of bunny lines (red dots); the depressor anguli oris, to release the downward pull on the corners of the mouth (purple dots); the chin, to reduce dimpling (green dots); the masseter, to reduce masseter hypertrophy and help restore mandibular angles (blue dots); and the platysma (orange dots), to reduce neck rhytids, are shown. In summary, although the FDA-approved use of BOTOX Cosmetic is 20 units for the treatment of glabellar lines, there are many new and interesting uses of BTX-A for the treatment of many different facial lines. These uses have been described by astute clinicians, and such advanced techniques allow for facial contouring and the treatment of a variety of rhytids. A proper understanding of anatomy, the individual patient's baseline state, and careful consideration of treatment goals are critical for optimal outcomes.

SUGGESTED READING

Alam M, Dover JS, Arndt KA. Pain associated with injection of botulinum A exotoxin reconstituted using isotonic sodium chloride with and without preservative: a double-blind, randomized controlled trial. *Arch. Dermatol.* 2002;138:510–14.

Carruthers J, Fagien S, Matarasso SL. Consensus recommendations on the use of botulinum toxin type A in facial aesthetics. *Plast. Reconstr. Surg.* 2004;114(6 Suppl):1S–22S.

Kwiat DM, Bersani TA, Bersani A. Increased patient comfort utilizing botulinum toxin type A reconstituted with preserved versus nonpreserved saline. *Ophthal. Plast. Reconstr. Surg.* 2004;20:186–9.

CHAPTER 36

BOTOX: Beyond the Basics

Sorin Eremia

Adapting neurotoxin (NT) to individual patients is the key to natural results. Doing so requires careful evaluation of each patient's anatomy and the position of various key anatomic components, particularly the eyebrows, at rest and at various levels of muscle activity.

As discussed in their own separate chapters by Drs. Beddingfield, Sadick, and Rossi, there are many possible applications of NT on the face and neck.

In my practice, I find that NT is most practical for the upper face. I rarely, if ever, use BOTOX for the perioral area or the chin. I find that fillers are far more practical in these areas as they last much longer and have more predictable results. And for very fine and superficial perioral lines that do not do as well with fillers, resurfacing is a far better choice, especially with availability of the new fractional lasers, ranging from the near-infrared to erbium and CO_2. I do occasionally use BOTOX on the neck. It is very helpful for stubborn platysmal bands postplatysmaplasty procedures and can delay recurrence of bands in patients with a strong platysma muscle combined with thin subcutaneous tissues, but the high cost makes it impractical for most patients. My results with primary treatment of the bands and jowls (Nefertiti neck method) have been variable and too often unimpressive for the cost and duration, and some patients complain of weakness in opening their mouth as a result of weakness of the platysma. Time will tell if prolonged use can improve results. Fine lines on the neck, just as periorally, are best treated with fractional resurfacing, with even better results using the new fractional CO_2 lasers. For these reasons, my use of NTs is focused on the forehead, periorbital area, and proximal nose.

THE FOREHEAD

The forehead presents the greatest challenges and opportunities for truly artistic use of NTs. Various types of cosmetic problems are encountered, which require different approaches, and some of the variations are age and sex related.

The brow position at rest can be flat or arched. The brow itself can have various degrees of ptosis, and the ptosis may be more pronounced in just one area, such as medially or laterally.

The Lateral Brow

Of great importance is how freely the lateral forehead slides up and down, and how much superior excursion of the lateral brow exists. This is determined both by simple manual exam – using a finger to see how easily and how far the lateral brow can be pushed up – and by observing the patient raising the brows. That determines the injection sites on the lateral forehead to achieve the desired lateral brow position and avoid exaggerated lateral brow elevation (Figure 36.1).

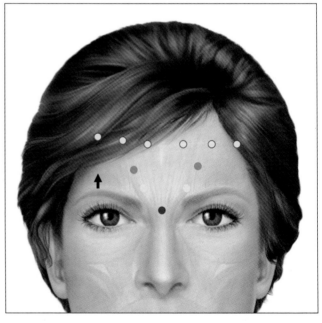

FIGURE 36.1: *Typical forehead: 6.6 units (red dot), 5 units (yellow dots), 3.3 units (green dots), 1.7 units (blue dots). Right side allows, left blunts, reflex lateral brow elevation.*

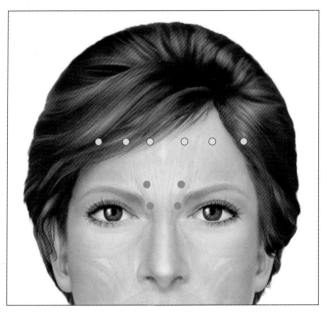

FIGURE 36.2: Alternative forehead: 3.3 units (green dots), 1.7 units (blue dots).

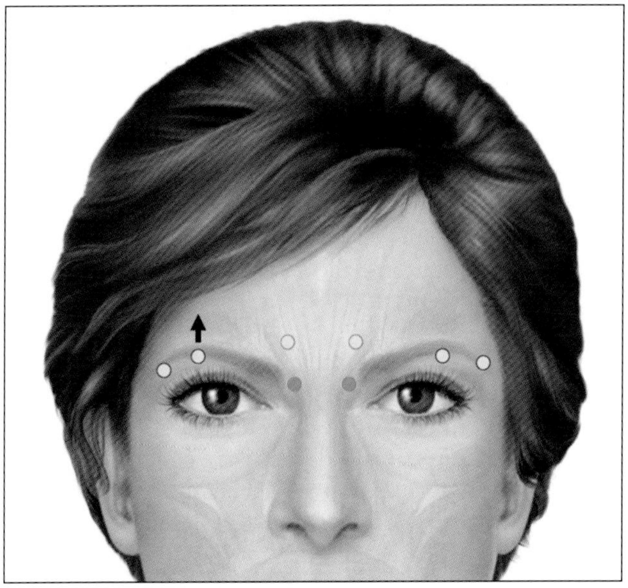

FIGURE 36.3: Frown lines and brow elevation, natural middle and upper forehead: 5 units (yellow dots), 3.3 units (green dots), 1.7 units (blue dots).

The Medial Brow

The position of the medial brow also has to be evaluated. In older women, and in many men, the medial brow sits quite low. Injecting NT on the forehead less than 2–3 cm above the medial one-third of the brow will further drop it down. In such patients, it is better to inject only the medial/inferior aspects of the corrugators and focus more on the depressor supercili by splitting the usual procerrus injection point over the root of the nose into two more laterally based injection points (Figure 36.2). The frontalis is injected at least 3 cm above the brow.

Flat Brows

In some patients, the brow lacks curvature, its position being relatively straight across and, depending on age, more or less ptotic. Subtle but significant elevation of the lateral three-fifths can be achieved by injecting the orbicularis with small amounts of NT (e.g., 1–1.7 units of BOTOX) just below the brow, but above the superior orbital rim (Figure 36.3).

In some relatively young patients without horizontal forehead creases, it may be enough to inject only the glabella and below the lateral brow, as shown in Figure 36.3.

THE PERIORBITAL AREA

The lower lid creases just below the lash line are difficult to treat as NT can readily weaken the pretarsal and preseptal orbicularis just enough to cause problems. But for some Asian patients, judicious placement can be beneficial,

as the resulting lower lid orbicularis weakness can widen the lateral aspect of the eye. In rare cases in which a hypertrophic orbicularis is present, placing 1 unit of BOTOX superficially at two sites, as shown in Figure 36.4, can achieve noticeable improvement. The crow's feet area is relatively straightforward to treat. I generally use 5–6 units of BOTOX divided into two or three injections points (Figure 36.4). Results last about four months, typically less

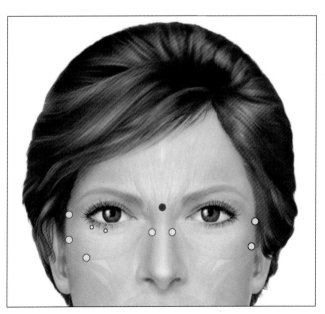

FIGURE 36.4: Crow's feet options, lower lids, nose/glabella bunny lines: 6.6 units (red dot), 2.5 units (large white dots), 1.7 units (blue dots), 1 unit (small white dots).

than on the forehead, where with regular use, most of my patients average four and a half to five and a half months. Larger amounts have been suggested based on scientific studies, but in my experience, patients do not get any better clinical results over time, and marked persistent improvement in crow's feet can be achieved with regular use of smaller amounts of NT. On the forehead, I believe 25–35 units of BOTOX are needed for the entire forehead, with 17–22 units just for the glabellar area.

THE PROXIMAL NOSE

The horizontal creases caused by procerrus activity respond extremely well to NT. I typically use 5–6 units of BOTOX, as shown in Figures 36.3 and 36.4. Rare patients also have significant vertical creases on the sides of the proximal nose, which can be treated with 1–1.7 units of BOTOX, as shown in Figure 36.4. The distal aspect of the nose can also be treated, but I rarely have any such requests from patients. Dr. Rossi's chapter on Dysport covers this area quite well (Chapter 38).

THE NECK

Platysma bands can be injected directly along their course. It is important to start injecting them right at their insertion along the mandibular border. It takes 30–40 units in 2- to 3-unit dosages. Injecting a little further laterally along the mandible can also, in selected patients, release the jowls a bit, with slight to moderate improvement of the jowls.

PATTERNS OF NT USE

Most of the patients I treat fall into one of four categories:

1. The most common group is middle-aged women with a combination of moderate frown lines, moderate horizontal lines, moderate lateral brow ptosis, and variable crow's feet. The forehead is usually treated with 33 units, as shown in Figure 36.1, adapting the lateral forehead injection sites to the lateral brow specifics of the patient. If indicated, the crow's feet are treated with 10 units. If the lateral forehead is relatively immobile, and/or the

patient wants more pronounced lateral brow elevation (some women actually like the Catwoman look), the upper row, or at least the most lateral injection sites on the upper forehead, shown in Figure 36.1, can be omitted.

2. A second group comprises older women, who, in addition to problems mentioned for the first group, also have significant medial brow ptosis. The pattern shown in Figure 36.2 is often better suited. It sacrifices a little on the frown lines but maintains the medial brow as well as possible. It is particularly important in these older patients to preserve good frontalis tonus on the lower forehead. A little filler for deep frown lines can be very effective and long lasting when used together with NTs.

3. I also see relatively young women with one or several of the following: significant squint habit and resulting crow's feet, early frown lines, mild lateral brow ptosis, or flat brows. Isolated crow's feet problems are treated with 10–16 units of BOTOX, as shown in Figure 36.4. The frown lines and lateral brows are treated with 20–23 units, as shown in Figure 36.3.

4. Finally, I see men with deep horizontal lines and variable frown lines. If the horizontal lines predominate, I use 33 units divided into two rows on the middle and upper forehead, at least 3 cm above the brow line. If the frown lines are also prominent, I prefer the pattern shown in Figure 36.2. Crow's feet are treated as necessary. It should be noted that in men, it either takes a little more NT, or the results do not last as long, usually from four to four and a half months, even with regular use. It should be remembered that men have naturally lower and less arched brows than women, and that most men prefer to preserve some expression and really do not like a surprised, or worse, a Spock look.

In conclusion, careful evaluation and planning achieve the best results. I should also note that it was through interaction and observation of some of my European colleagues that I have really refined my personal approach to the use of BOTOX, and I strongly urge my North American colleagues to attend European meetings whenever they can, especially those with good focus on fillers and NTs.

CHAPTER 37

BOTOX for Hyperhidrosis

Frederick C. Beddingfield III

AXILLARY HYPERHIDROSIS

The use of BOTOX for the treatment of severe axillary hyperhidrosis was approved by the Food and Drug Administration in 2004 for patients whose hyperhidrosis is inadequately managed with topical agents.

Prior to administering BOTOX, many clinicians perform a Minor's starch iodine test to document the extent and severity of hyperhidrosis in each axilla. This can then be used to mark the skin with a grid of evenly spaced injection sites (Figure 37.1). The approved dose of BOTOX is 50 U[1] per axilla, injected intradermally in 0.1- to 0.2-mL aliquots per injection site using a 30-gauge needle. In the pivotal trials, 100 U were diluted with 4.0 mL of nonpreserved saline. Discomfort with the axillary injections is minimal, and the placing of ice packs on the axillae prior to treatment generally provides sufficient anesthesia. Vibration and topical anesthetic creams have also been successfully employed to reduce pain.

The largest study reported to date was a fifty-two-week, multicenter, double-blind, randomized, placebo-controlled study involving 322 patients with axillary hyperhidrosis (Lowe et al. 2007). The proportion of treatment responders – those achieving a 2-point reduction on the Hyperhidrosis Disease Severity Scale (HDSS)[2] – was significantly greater four weeks after treatment with BOTOX 75 U or BOTOX 50 U than after treatment with placebo (75% and 75% versus 25%; $p < 0.001$). The median duration of effect of BOTOX treatment was approximately six and a half months. Furthermore, at fifty-two

weeks posttreatment, it was estimated that at least 22% of BOTOX-treated patients had still not returned to having an HDSS score of 3 or 4 (which had been one of the study's key inclusion criteria). Patients whose HDSS scores did increase to this level were eligible for retreatment, and the duration of effect after such retreatment was similar to that after initial treatment, suggesting that efficacy does not decline with repeat treatments. Hyperhidrosis can result in considerable impairment in a patient's quality of life, and importantly, BOTOX treatment was also shown to result in significantly greater improvements in this regard than placebo. Furthermore, BOTOX appears to have an excellent safety profile. Other large studies in the literature, including one with even longer follow-up (sixteen months; Naumann et al. 2003), report similar findings and, in addition, significantly greater patient satisfaction with BOTOX than placebo (Naumann and Lowe 2001).

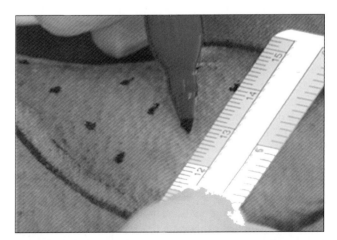

FIGURE 37.1: *Injection grid for axillary hyperhidrosis. After outlining the area of anhidrosis revealed through a Minor's starch iodine test, use a ruler and surgical pen to mark injection points at 1.5- to 2-cm intervals. These should be in a staggered pattern to achieve overlapping areas of anhidrosis. Inject to a depth of 2 mm at a 45 degree angle to the skin with the bevel up. Avoid injecting directly on the ink marks to avoid a permanent tattoo effect on the skin.*

---

[1] Dosing and results reported in this chapter are specific to the formulation of botulinum toxin type A from Allergan Inc. Botulinum toxin products are not interchangeable and cannot be converted by using a dose ratio.

[2] Point scale describing hyperhidrosis as (1) never noticeable and never interferes with daily activities, (2) tolerable but sometimes interferes with daily activities, (3) barely tolerable and frequently interferes with daily activities, or (4) intolerable and always interferes with daily activities.

Reimbursement for BOTOX treatment of hyperhidrosis has become more common subsequent to the recent publication of therapeutic guidelines and treatment algorithms, revisions to the International Classification of Diseases, and the introduction of new current procedural terminology (CPT) codes (e.g., "chemodenervation of eccrine glands; both axillae" for axillary hyperhidrosis).

PALMAR HYPERHIDROSIS

Reports in the literature suggest that BOTOX is highly effective for the treatment of palmar hyperhidrosis, with generally more than 90% of patients reportedly responding to treatment. Typically, first- and second-line treatments for palmar hyperhidrosis are topical antiperspirants and tap water iontophoresis, but many patients find these options lacking in effectiveness, tolerability, or convenience and subsequently find treatment with botulinum toxin type A to be successful and to significantly improve their quality of life.

Anhidrosis has been reported to be sustained for four to nine months, with hypohidrosis continuing for at least one year posttreatment in many patients. As palmar hyperhidrosis tends to affect the entire volar surface of the palms and digits, a Minor's starch iodine test is of limited use. Glaser et al. (2007) emphasize that because of the dense innervation and fine musculature of the hands, skill and precision are required to place each injection optimally and not too deeply (especially over the thenar eminence, where the subcutis is thin; Figure 37.2). They report that the average total dose of BOTOX used is 100 U per palm (range 25–220 U), injected in forty-five to fifty sites spread approximately 1–1.5 cm apart, and with an injection volume of 0.05–0.1 mL. Plastic single-use syringes with a 30-gauge needle are standard, although 31- and 32-gauge needles have been reported to reduce pain. An insulin syringe helps reduce wastage due to the lack of space at the hub.

A variety of approaches have been used successfully to minimize the pain of the injections, including a Bier block; a block of the median, ulnar, and radial nerves; ice; ice plus vibration; topical anesthesia followed by ice; and needle-free anesthesia. Using ice avoids the potential for some clinically significant problems that have been associated with more invasive methods. For example, a nerve block, while very effective and not generally difficult for a physician skilled in the technique, often temporarily affects motor functioning and leaves the patient without full use of his or her hand for a while (e.g., making driving home from the clinic unsafe). In addition, Bier blocks, which are also very effective and safe when performed by experienced physicians, require significant skill and a certain comfort level with the procedure and, rarely, can result in adverse effects as a result of the anesthetic passing into the systemic circulation.

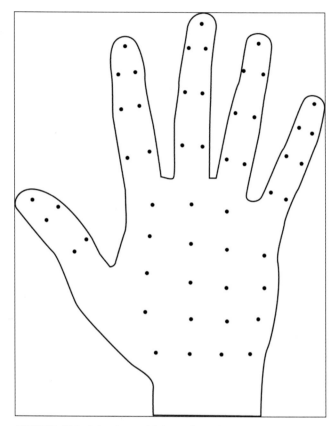

FIGURE 37.2: Injection grid for palmar hyperhidrosis. Ideally, the injections should be placed in the deep dermis, at or near the junction with the subcutaneous tissue (as this is where the sweat glands are located).

There are some reports of patients experiencing minor and transient weakness in the hand muscles for the first few weeks after treatment, but this does not generally impair key activities such as eating, writing, or typing. The incidence of such muscle weakness shows great variability, suggesting that it may depend on the injection pattern, the injection technique, and/or the dilution used. It has been suggested that injecting intradermally rather than subcutaneously can reduce the incidence of muscle weakness; however, intradermal injections have also been reported to be associated with significantly greater pain than subcutaneous injections, at least in axillary hyperhidrosis (Pearson and Cliff 2004).

No specific level of reimbursement is assigned to the new CPT code for palmar hyperhidrosis – "chemodenervation of extremities (eg, hands, feet)" – and reimbursement usually requires supporting medical information. A BOTOX reimbursement hotline (800-530-6680) can offer assistance, if required.

SUGGESTED READING

Glaser DA, Hebert AA, Pariser DM, Solish N. Palmar and plantar hyperhidrosis: best practice recommendations and special considerations. *Cutis* 2007;79(Suppl 5):18–28.

Lowe NJ, Glaser DA, Eadie N, et al. Botulinum toxin type A in the treatment of primary axillary hyperhidrosis: a 52-week multi-center, double-blind, randomized, placebo-controlled study of efficacy and safety. *J. Am. Acad. Dermatol.* 2007;56:604–11.

Naumann M, Lowe NJ. Botulinum toxin type A in treatment of bilateral primary axillary hyperhidrosis: randomised, parallel group, double blind, placebo controlled trial. *Br. Med. J.* 2001;323:1–4.

Naumann M, Lowe NJ, Kumar CR, Hamm H. Botulinum toxin type A is a safe and effective treatment for axillary hyperhidrosis over 16 months. *Arch. Dermatol.* 2003;139:731–6.

Pearson IC, Cliff S. Botulinum toxin type A treatment for axillary hyperhidrosis: a comparison of intradermal and subcutaneous injection techniques. *Br. J. Dermatol.* 2004;151(Suppl 68):95.

Solish N, Bertucci V, Dansereau A, et al. A comprehensive approach to the recognition, diagnosis, and severity-based treatment of focal hyperhidrosis: recommendations of the Canadian Hyperhidrosis Advisory Committee. *Dermatol. Surg.* 2007;33:908–23.

Solomon BA, Hayman R. Botulinum toxin type A therapy for palmar and digital hyperhidrosis. *J. Am. Acad. Dermatol.* 2000;42:1026–9.

CHAPTER 38

Dysport

Bernard Rossi

Following the publication by J. D. A. Carruthers in 1992, botulinum toxin injections started being used for the treatment of wrinkles caused by certain muscle hyperactivity.

The botulinum toxins type A (BtxA), developed by Allergan Inc. in the United States (BOTOX) and by Beaufour Ipsen in Europe (Dysport), have a parallel history, both being initially used for the treatment of muscle spasms. BOTOX was first, being introduced in the United States in 1985, while Dysport started being used in Europe in 1988. (Dysport is also distributed in France by Gallderma under the name AZZALURE.)

They are both very effective and reliable products. Long-term use in large numbers of patients has demonstrated a lack of secondary effects other than those predictable due to diffusion of the toxin to muscles adjacent to those for which treatment was intended. The site of action of botulinum toxins is shown in Figure 38.1. Over time, improved understanding of anatomy, use of appropriate injection volumes, and improved injection techniques have greatly reduced the incidence of these types of complications.

- This empirical knowledge was recently confirmed by results of the scientific studies conducted by Dr. B. Ascher to obtain certification for the product in France. There were nine international well designed clinical studies involving 3,500 patients and up to 6 months of follow-up. Several of these studies have been published: Two Phase II dose-finding studies (Ascher 2004, Monheit 2007)
- One Phase II safety dose1, and one Phase III single-treatment studies (Rzany 2006)
- One Phase III repeat-treatment studies (Ascher 2005)
- One retrospective post-marketing survey (Rzany 2007)
- One prospective repeat-treatment study (Moy 2009)

Regardless of brand name, BtxA is still BtxA, with a molecular weight of its active part, the neurotoxin, of 150 kD. Its effects are summarized in Table 38.1. BtxA is always linked to hemagglutinin, a nontoxic, inactive protein. The

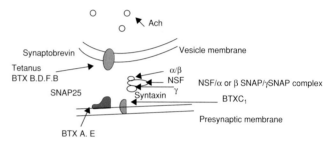

FIGURE 38.1: The site of action of botulinum toxins.

pharmacologic characteristics of Dysport and BOTOX are summarized in Table 38.2.

Although the two are very similar products, manufacturing differences result in some differences in the measurement methods of their respective biological activity, and the products' biologic unit dosages are different. As a result, Dysport and BOTOX are not interchangeable.

The equivalent ratio of units of Dysport to one unit of BOTOX is subject to some controversy and based primarily

TABLE 38.1: Product Comparison: Dysport and BOTOX

Dysport	BOTOX
Early onset of action in a majority of patients	
More significant number of responders at four months	
Action noted at six months in a more significant number of patients	
At the beginning: one injection every four months. After: one injection every six months, according to the perception of clinical efficiency of the patient	At the beginning: one injection every four months. After: one injection every six months, according to the perception of clinical efficiency of the patient.

TABLE 38.2: Pharmacologic Characteristics of Dysport and BOTOX

	Dysport	BOTOX Cosmetic
Clinical onset of action	faster onset (2–4 days)	slower onset (4–7 days?)
Duration of clinical response at comparable dosages and cost	4 months after initial treatment, greater numbers of patients maintain response, cheaper	
Percentage of responders six months after injection	greater	smaller
Treatment session intervals after initial treatment period	every 4 months	every 4 months
Treatment session intervals after several treatments (based on patient perception of duration of results)	5–6 months, a significant number (25%) of patients at every 6 months	5–6 months, somewhat fewer numbers of patients every 6 months

on a few studies published in the neurology literature. It has been claimed to range from 1:1 to 5:1. In his daily practice, the author has been using a dosing ratio of 3 units of Dysport (also defined as "Speywood" units) to 1 unit of BOTOX (also defined as "Allergan" units) to obtain equivalent results. However, the current trend, which is supported by some recent studies, has been to use a dosage ration of 2.5:1 or even lower.

Dysport/Azzalure is available as a lyophilized powder that needs to be refrigerated between 2 and 8 degrees Celsius and reconstituted with preservative-free, normal saline solution. While various studies have shown little change in biological activity if the reconstituted product is kept refrigerated for several days, same day usage is preferable to obtain the most consistent and reproducible results. Universal precautions are taken in terms of needles and syringes used for injection.

The ideal reconstituting volume for Dysport has been subject to much controversy. In effect, the greater the dilution, the greater the diffusion of the product from the injection point. Greater diffusion distance from the injection site can sometimes yield more uniform results but can also shorten the duration of action and lead to unwanted effects on muscles other than those intended. The author always used 2.5 cc of normal saline to reconstitute a vial of 500 units of Dysport. This choice of concentration is supported by a recent study (Kranz 2009).

It is now well established that the size of the proteins associated to BtxA complex does not affect the rate of diffusion, and that the dissociation of the complex is quasi immediate after injection.

TREATMENT TECHNIQUE

The actual injection is always preceded by a consultation, during which the physician analyses the patient's wishes,

explains the risks and benefits, addresses possible unrealistic expectations, looks for counterindications, obtains consent, and completes whatever paperwork is needed in the respective country. There is no need for any tests, premedication, or anesthesia. Treatment technique is illustrated in Figure 38.2.

With the patient sitting up or partially reclined, with all makeup removed and the area cleansed, the patient is evaluated both at rest and contracting the expression muscles. The injection points are then marked. Pretreatment photographs or videos are very useful to document preexisting asymmetries.

The reference point for injecting the forehead in general, and the glabellar area more particularly, is the mid pupillary line (MPL). Proper choice of injection sites reduces the risk of both upper eyelid and of brow ptosis. In Europe, the trend has always been to stay more medial to the MPL, when injecting the lateral end of the corrugators. Now, that technique appears to have also been adopted in the United States. The injection sites must be at least 1 cm away from the orbital rim. The injection site should never be massaged as this will further enhance diffusion of the toxin. In other respects, the injection sites and injection technique are very similar to injecting BOTOX.

The causes for imprecise results are the same as with other neurotoxins:

- poor or obstructed vision when injecting
- poor handling of the syringe, leading to imprecise placement of the product
- variations in the biologic activity of the product, which can vary from batch to batch of toxin produced by as much as 20%, regardless of manufacturer
- The speed and force of injection which increase diffusion
- The reconstituted product concentration (units per cc) or its degree of dilution (cc's of saline used per vial). Lower

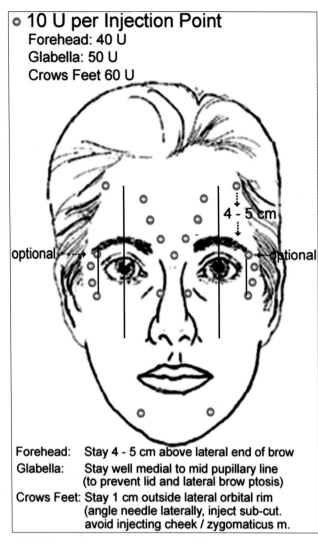

10 U per Injection Point
Forehead: 40 U
Glabella: 50 U
Crows Feet 60 U

4 - 5 cm

optional

optional

Forehead: Stay 4 - 5 cm above lateral end of brow
Glabella: Stay well medial to mid pupillary line
            (to prevent lid and lateral brow ptosis)
Crows Feet: Stay 1 cm outside lateral orbital rim
            (angle needle laterally, inject sub-cut.
            avoid injecting cheek / zygomaticus m.

FIGURE 38.2: Suggested injection sites for Dysport.

concentration/increased dilution increases diffusion and shortens duration of action

The dosages mentioned subsequently are those the author uses in his practice and are based on the author's prior experience as well as previously published studies. The three best indications for Dysport follow.

THE GLABELLA

The procerus and depressor supercili muscles are treated by inserting the injection needle in the central glabellar area, perpendicular to the skin surface, while the opposite hand's thumb protects the orbital rim. The vertical aspects of the corrugators are injected at their medial ends, with the index finger lifting the medial brow to minimize risk of ptosis. Ten units of Dysport are injected at each site. Two to five injection sites may be needed, depending on the patient. 50 units of Dysport is the optimally effective and safe dosing. For comparison with Botox/Vistabel®: 12 to

24 units (and more recently 20 units) is generally considered the optimally effective and safe dosing for the glabellar area (Ascher 2004, 2005, Monheit 2007).

In general, it takes about 50 units of Dysport/Azzalure to effectively treat the frown lines in the glabella. For patients with thicker muscles, an additional 10 units can be injected medially and superiorly. Injecting the glabellar area poses the greatest risk of toxin diffusion toward the upper lid levator muscle and resulting temporary ptosis. For this reason, it is best to stay as medial as possible, and not to inject in the mid-pupillary line (MPL). In two studies (Ascher 2004, 2005) where this "stay medial" rule was followed, the rate of lid ptosis was zero. On the contrary, in studies where Dysport was injected at the MPL (Moy, Brandt, 2009) the ptosis incidence was 2.4 to 2.9%. The injection sites should never be massaged, and having the patient perform frowning movements for a couple of hours postinjection may be helpful to distribute the toxin within the muscle.

The Forehead

The patient is asked to raise his or her brows. The injection is done along a line that runs superolaterally at 30 degrees from the center of the forehead so that it is 3.5–4 cm superior to the orbital rim in the midpupillary line. 40 units of Dysport seems an effective and safe dosing. The range with Dysport is 40 to 60 Spywood units while with BOTOX the range seem to be 16 to 20 Allergan units, with 20 units of BOTOX most often considered the effective and safe dose for the forehead (excluding the glabella).

Four to six injection sites are necessary to distribute at least 40 units of Dysport over the upper forehead. The goal is to maintain frontalis muscle tonus on the lower forehead, which helps maintain the brow in position and prevents brow ptosis. If a small wrinkle persists above the brow, a little more toxin can be injected three weeks later.

Let us not forget that injection dosages should vary according to the size of the targeted muscles, skin thickness, and the effects desired by the patient. In general, women prefer the more youthful look achieved by a more complete erasing of wrinkles, while for men, preserving some expressive movement and less wrinkle erasing may be preferable. That, at least, seems to be the choice of most actors, who also appreciate toxin-induced lack of sweating under the spotlights.

The Crow's Feet Area

The crow's feet form over the lateral orbital rim as a result of orbicularis occuli muscle contractions. Dysport is injected at three to five points following along a line perpendicular to the crow's feet that follows the curvature of the lateral orbital rim but is at least 1 cm lateral to its edge. The most superior injection site is placed just below the lateral corner of the eyebrow, which gives the lateral brow a slight lifting effect.

At least 30 to 60 units of Dysport are needed. Some recent studies (Ascher 2009) suggest the safe and effective dose is 30 units injected at three sites, 10 units each. For comparison, the dosage for BOTOX generally ranges from 12 to 24 "Allergan" units, also equally divided among three injection sites. It is best to avoid injecting too low on the cheek as there is a risk of toxin diffusion toward the smile muscles. Care must be taken to avoid the superficial veins present in this area. The needle is angled a bit and the injection is superficial, just under the skin, since the orbicularis is a thin, superficial muscle.

Other Indications

Treatment of other sites is more recent, less reproducible, less predictable, and more risky:

- The upper eyelid is totally counterindicated.
- The lower eyelid can be carefully treated. The orbicularis is thin and superficial and very sensitive to very small amounts of toxin. Too high a dose will cause pseudobags due to excessive muscle relaxation. If placed too deep, the toxin can diffuse and affect the inferior and lateral oculomotor muscles.

INJECTION TECHNIQUE

First the preseptal orbicularis is injected above the orbital rim, staying well away from the lid margin to decrease the risk of ectropion. Injecting below the inferior orbital rim margin risks diffusion of toxin to the zygomaticus major. The injection is strictly subcutaneous, allowing the toxin to reach the orbicularis from its surface, and very conservative medially. Five units (2.5 per side) of Dysport are distributed over one to four injection sites per side.

USE IN CONJUNCTION WITH OTHER PERIORBITAL PROCEDURES

Neurotoxin use can complement, improve, and maintain results of laser resurfacing, fat injections, and blepharoplasty procedures. The injections can be performed six weeks before or after the procedure and repeated as needed, up to one to two years later.

The Perioral Area

This is a delicate area to treat. Results are less reproducible and there are risks of orbicularis oris dysfunction, leading to various problems, including lip ptosis, lowering or excessive raising of the corners of the mouth, and so on. The author has, in fact, virtually stopped injecting the following sites:

- *levator labialis superioris alaquae nasi.* This can be injected with 3 units, 1 cm superior to the base of the nostril. The goal is to slightly lower the position of the nostril, while lifting the tip of the nose and achieving a little vertical lengthening of the upper lip.
- *dilator nasi muscle.* This is treated by injecting 3 units in the nasolabial fold at the level of the nostril and makes the nostril opening a little smaller.
- *constrictor nasi muscle.* Three units of Dysport can raise the position of the nasal alae slightly.
- *depressor anguli oris muscle.* Injecting this muscle at its midway point can elevate the corner of the mouth. A deeper injection along the linea obliquae mandible will also elevate the corner of the mouth. The effect can be further enhanced by injecting the junction of the platysma muscle with the depressor anguli oris.

The Orbicularis Oris Muscle

Injecting the orbicularis in the area of the lips proper is very delicate, and results are inferior and shorter lasting than using fillers. The vertical upper lip lines can be attenuated by weakening the underlying orbicularis by injecting 1 unit of Dysport divided into three to four injection sites over the central area of the upper lip, well away from the corners of the mouth. However, there are frequent complications such as asymmetry, difficulty pursing the lips, and difficulty sipping liquids.

The Depressor Labialis Inferioris Muscle

Three units of Dysport will lift up the lower lip and give a little forward projection to the chin.

The Mentalis Muscle

Injecting 10 units of Dysport softens the mental crease and projects the chin forward a bit.

The Triangularis Lip Muscles

Dysport injection lifts the lateral commissure but can lead to transient problems with smiling and speech difficulties.

Giving the Face a Softer Appearance

This is accomplished by injecting the mentalis, depressor anguli oris, and levator labialis superioris alaguae nasi.

THE NECK

Horizontal neck lines can be partially treated with multiple superficial injections using Dysport diluted in 4 cc of normal saline. Four horizontal rows of superficial injections are placed, with extra care around the Adam's apple to avoid toxin diffusion to the hyoid muscles.

Treatment of turkey neck deformities is only effective when caused by platysmal bands, rather than skin laxity alone.

When the anterior borders of the platysma muscle are thick and lax, without excessive overlying skin redundancy, especially following face lifts that did not adequately solve platysmal band problems, the use of Dysport can give satisfactory results. Each side of the anterior neck is treated with 40 units of Dysport. Multiple injections of 5–10 units are spaced 2 cm apart along the bands. (80 units for the entire neck.) Dysphagia can occasionally be an unwanted side effect.

The décolleté area at the base of the neck can also be treated with 15 units of Dysport.

In conclusion, Dysport is a highly effective form of BtxA, very comparable to BOTOX but with subtle yet significant differences. Dysport diffuses more readily from the point of injection, which can be both a minor advantage and a disadvantage. The planning of the injection points near the eyebrow has to be done accordingly. It is not advisable to overly dilute Dysport as this further increases diffusion. The author considers the so-called equivalency ratio to be 2.5 units Dysport for 1 unit BOTOX. At this ratio, the effects of Dysport appear, on average, to last a little longer than BOTOX, and in addition, Dysport is less expensive (in Europe, as of the date of this writing).

SUGGESTED READING

Denervation techniques for facial rejuvenation. *Dermatol. Surg.* 1998;24(11). Special issue.

Cosmetic use of botulinum toxin. *Plast. Reconstr. Surg.* 2003; 112(5). Special issue.

Ascher B, Rossi B. PMID: 15518953. Botulinum toxin and wrinkles: few side effects and effective combining procedures with other treatments. *Ann. Chir. Plast. Esthet.* 2004;49:537–52.

Ascher B, et al. A multicentre, randomized, double-blind, placebo-controlled study of efficacy and safety of 3 doses of botulinum toxin A in the treatment of glabellar lines. *J. Am. Acad. Dermatol.* 2004;51:223–33.

Ascher B, Zakine B, Kestemont P, et al. Botulinum Toxin A in the treatment of glabellar lines: scheduling the next injection. *Aesthetic Surg.* 2005;25:365–75.

Ascher B, Rzany B, and the Smile Group. Reproducibility of two four-point clinical severity scores for lateral canthal lines (crow's feet). Presented at European Academy of Dermatology and Venerology Oct. 2006, Rhodes, Greece, and *Dermatol Surg.* In Press 2009.

Kranz G, Haubenberger D, Voller B, et al. Respective potencies of Botox and Dysport in a human skin model: a randomized, double-blind study. *Mov. Disord.* 2009;24(2):231–6.

Lowe NJ, Ascher B, Heckmann M, et al. Btox Facial Aesthetics Study Team. Double-blind, randomized, placebo-controlled, dose-response study of the safety of Botulinum toxin type A in subjects with crow's feet. *Dermatol Surg.* 2005;31:257–62.

Monheit G, Carruthers A, Brandt F, et al. A randomized, double-blind, placebo-controlled study of botulinum toxin type A for the treatment of glabellar lines: determination of optimal dose. *Dermatol Surg.* 2007;33(1):S51–9.

Moy R, Maas C, Monheit G, et al. Reloxin Investigational Group. Long-term safety and efficacy of a new botulinum toxin type A in treating glabellar lines. *Arch Facial Plast Surg.* 2009 Mar-Apr;11(2):77–83.

Pickett A, Caird D. Comparison of type A botulinum toxin products in clinical use. *J Clin Pharm Therapeut.* 2008;33:327–328.

Pickett A. Dysport((R)): Pharmacological properties and factors that influence toxin action. *Toxicon.* 2009.

Pickett A, Dodd S, Rzany B. Confusion about diffusion and the art of misinterpreting data when comparing different botulinum toxins used in aesthetic applications. *J Osmet Laser Ther* 2008; 10(3):181–3.

Ranoux D, Gury C, Fondarai J, et al. Retrospective potencies of Botox and Dysport: a double blind, randomised, crossover study in cervical dystonia. *J. Neurol. Neurosurg.* Psychiatry 2002;72:459–62.

Rzany B, Ascher B, Fratila A, et al. Efficacy and safety of 3- and 5-injection patterns (30 and 50 U) of botulinum toxin A (Dysport) for the treatment of wrinkles in the glabella and the central forehead region. *Arch Dermatol.* 2006;142(3):320–6.

Rzany B, Dill-Mueller D, Grablowitz D, et al. Repeated botulinum toxin A injections for the treatment lines in the upper face: a retrospective study of 103 treatments in 945 patients. *Dermatol Surg.* 2007;33(1):S18–25.

CHAPTER 39

Neurotoxin Alternative: Radiofrequency Corrugator Denervation

James Newman

A new minimally invasive procedure, glabella frown relaxation (GFX), is described to offer an alternative treatment to botulinum toxin A for the reduction of glabellar furrowing. A unique bipolar radiofrequency (RF) device has been developed and used to produce selective denervation of the corrugator muscle by a percutaneous, minimally invasive route that can be performed in an office-based setting. A description of the targeted nerves, procedure, and clinical results to date is given here.

The minimally invasive procedure uses a RF needle and generator specifically designed for peripheral motor nerves (GFX Generator, ACI Inc.). The use of this technology to ablate only the efferent pathway of the distal branch of the frontal facial nerve branch as it enters the corrugator muscle yields a very selective relaxation of the forehead depressor function. This selective efferent nerve ablation provides a nonpharmacologic relaxation of the corrugator muscle by creating a neuroablation of the motor nerve to the corrugator. The application of optimized RF energy has a long history of success in treating various conditions, including cardiology applications such as ablation of tachyarrythmias (Utley and Goode 1999; Hernandez-Zendejas and Guerrero-Santos 1994). Previous studies (Hernandez-Zendejas and Guerrero-Santos 1994; Ellis and Bakala 1998) have demonstrated efficacy of application of RF energy in the human forehead to produce acute and long-term reduction of glabellar furrowing. The GFX generator and handpiece have undergone both animal and human studies to refine the waveform of energy delivery and keep the lesion production process highly reproducible.

TECHNOLOGY

The GFX system is a state-of-the-art technology incorporating the RF generator, nerve stimulator, and associated software. A touch-screen graphical user interface provides for adjustment of controls as well as a display of treatment parameters. The GFX handpiece consists of an ergonomic handle and needle probe, which attaches to the generator.

The needle probe contains the bipolar RF leads, a nerve stimulator, and a thermocouple for the monitoring of tissue temperature during treatment. A foot switch activates RF delivery.

ANATOMY

Detailed information exists regarding peripheral branches of innervation to various facial muscles, including the corrugator, frontalis, procerus, and orbicularis occuli. This information has described for more distal segments of the facial nerve branches as they travel to the specific muscles involved in glabellar furrowing (Ellis and Bakala 1998). The action of these muscles in relation to glabellar furrowing and forehead mimetic movement has also been described (Knize 2000). The lateral body of the corrugator muscle is responsible for the majority of vertical glabellar furrowing. Hence the initial target area for the GFX procedure is the nerve to the corrugator muscle. This nerve is a distal branch of the temporal branch of the facial nerve after it crosses the zygomatic arch. A reliable branch comes off the temporal branch prior to the main branch entering the lateral border of the frontalis muscle (Figure 39.1). The innervation of this muscle can be reliably located around the periocular skin and eyebrow. This specific location makes it amenable to the selective efferent nerve ablation via the GFX procedure. The target nerve caliber can vary with an average caliber of 2 mm based on our anatomic dissections. The number of branches in the lateral approach is one to two.

PROCEDURE

The first target area for the GFX procedure is the nerve to the corrugator muscle as it enters the lateral aspect of the muscle. The procedure begins by assessing the degree of glabellar furrowing. The operator coaches the patient to frown to elicit the proper action of the corrugator, orbicularis occuli, depressor supercilii, and frontalis. Assessment is made using a validated scale (Kim et al. 2005).

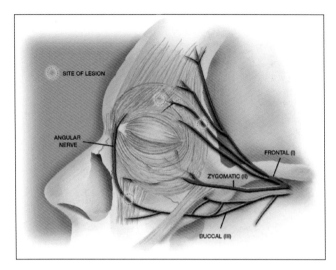

FIGURE 39.1: Motor innervation of the corrugator muscle.

Documentation of the patient's condition is achieved with still photography and digital video of the brow at rest, elevated, and furrowing. This is a good time to establish baseline, note and discuss asymmetries, and allow the patient to see these animations in the mirror.

The forehead area is cleansed and landmarks are noted and marked. A frontal nerve block is performed just deep to the orbital septum, with additional local anesthesia, as needed. Care is taken to avoid overinfiltration so that the motor nerve can be mapped out with the nerve stimulator.

The insertion site is created through the dermis with a 20-gauge needle to facilitate passage of the needle probe beneath the muscle layer. With gentle traction and firm pressure, the needle probe is advanced along a line from the lateral canthal angle past the lateral portion of the eyebrow (Figure 39.2). The probe is then slowly retracted along the insertion path, while continuously delivering electrical stimulation via a switch located on the handpiece. (Stimulation may be delivered within a range of 0.1–10 mA.)

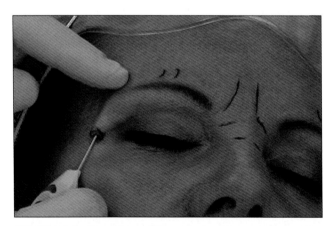

FIGURE 39.2: First, the needle probe is advanced along a line from the lateral canthal angle past the lateral portion of the eyebrow. The probe is then slowly retracted along the insertion path, while continuously delivering electrical stimulation.

The needle probe will cross at an angle over the targeted nerve during retraction. Visual confirmation of muscle contraction is seen as the active probe tip comes in contact with the motor nerve. The frontalis muscle contraction is noted with more superior placement of the probe. As the probe is further retracted and comes in contact with the middle ramus of the temporal nerve branch, corrugator contraction is noted. This corrugator contraction confirms contact of the probe tip with the target nerve and identifies the ablation location. While carefully maintaining probe placement, RF energy is delivered via foot switch activation. A lesion of approximately 2 × 5 mm is created on the nerve at the contact point of the needle probe tip. After delivery of RF energy, while continuing to maintain probe placement, the patient is asked to frown, and corrugator function is again evaluated. Secondary and tertiary lesions are then performed along the course of the mapped out nerve course. The medial limit of ablation is the midpupillary line to avoid heat transference to the sensory supraorbital nerve branches. The plane of ablation should be submuscular, just under the galea, to avoid any subcutaneous heat injury. A similar procedure is then performed on the opposite side.

RESULTS

Safety studies have demonstrated no incidence of skin damage such as depressions, burns, or scars. Recent clinical trial results have been documented regarding the acute efficacy of GFX for the reduction of glabellar furrowing (ACI Inc. 2006). Successful results can be observed immediately, with typical results as shown in Figure 39.3. Patients are able to return to normal activities the same day. The author has performed over two hundred procedures since June 2006, with a success rate of 85%. Patients have had mild discomfort with proper nerve blocks and some selective oral premedication. Patients are able to notice results immediately and maintain their results of a relaxed brow for six months and beyond.

DISCUSSION

GFX will provide the physician with a state-of-the-art device as a treatment option for the reduction of glabellar furrowing. Patients will experience a relaxed, yet natural look, without complete paralysis of muscles. The GFX procedure may be performed in the office setting with local anesthesia as well as during other surgical procedures.

Regarding patient safety, several points must be emphasized: the needle probe tip must be kept at the submuscular level and never activated in the subdermal plane to avoid injury. Also, knowledge of the sensory nerves, particularly the deep branch of the supraorbital nerve, is essential to avoid injury or posttreatment sensitivity. Distinguishing the activity of the frontalis muscle from that of the corrugator muscle is essential to avoid inadvertent injury to the elevating muscle of the brow.

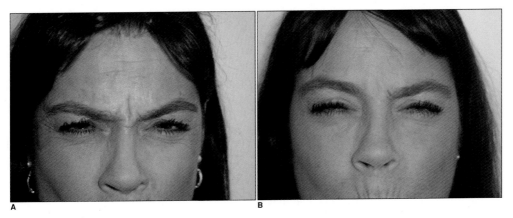

FIGURE 39.3: *A, Pretreatment and, B, three months post-RF corrugator denervation.*

Side effects observed postprocedure have been limited to ecchymosis, edema, and temporary sensitivity. Some patients report discomfort during the eighteen-second application of RF energy. Other patient comfort measures, such as distraction during ablation, ice, and topical anesthesia, have been used successfully.

CONCLUSION

The prospect of a more natural appearance and an increase in the longevity of effect over current chemodenervation therapies are significant. The GFX procedure represents the possibility of a significant advance in the treatment of glabellar furrowing. The results, on clinical evaluation, are very encouraging. Previous research indicates that RF neuroablation of the corrugator nerve has resulted in longevity of effect of up to nine months (Utley and Goode 1999). Clinical trials are currently under way to establish the longevity of the GFX procedure (ACI Inc. 2007b) as well as the possibility of targeting other facial nerves.

SUGGESTED READING

ACI Inc. Safety trial and expanded use. Mumbai, India; ACI; February 2006.

ACI Inc. An efficacy trial of GFX for reduction of glabellar furrowing. Mumbai, India; ACI; February 2007a.

ACI Inc. A multicenter long term trial of the GFX for the reduction of glabellar furrowing. Mumbai, India; ACI; February 2007b.

Ellis DAF, Bakala CD. Anatomy of the motor innervation of the corrugator supercilii muscle: clinical significance and development of a new surgical technique for frowning. *J. Otolaryngol.* 1998;27:222–7.

Hernandez-Zendejas G, Guerrero-Santos J. Percutaneous selective radiofrequency ablation of the facial nerve. *Aesthetic Plast. Surg.* 1994;18:41–8.

Kim EK, Reeck JB, Maas CS. A validated rating scale for hyperkinetic facial lines. *Arch. Facial Plast. Surg.* 2005;6:253–6.

Knize DM. Muscles that act on glabellar skin: a closer look. *Plast. Reconstr. Surg.* 2000;105:350–61.

Utley DS, Goode RL. Radiofrequency ablation of the nerve to the corrugator for elimination of glabellar furrowing. *Arch. Facial Plast. Surg.* 1999;1:46–8.

Section 9

FILLERS AND NEUROTOXINS IN ASIA AND SOUTH AMERICA

CHAPTER 40

Fillers and Neurotoxins in Asia

Taro Kono

Henry H. L. Chan

Ablative laser resurfacing has been considered the most effective treatment option for skin rejuvenation. However, the epidermis is significantly damaged during this process, and this can be associated with potential adverse effects, including transient erythema, pigmentary disturbances, infection, and scarring, especially in Asians (Nanni and Alster 1998). Nonablative skin resurfacing involves selective thermal damage to a subepidermal layer. It is achieved by a combination of laser radiation reaching the dermis and the concurrent use of cooling to protect the epidermis. Although nonablative techniques are associated with less downtime, the degree of improvement appears to be limited (Chan and Kono 2004).

On the other hand, recent advances in fillers and neurotoxins have allowed the use of these agents in Asians, with minimal complications. Both fillers and neurotoxins are effective in producing an optimal cosmetic result. Currently the use of fillers and neurotoxins ranks as the most commonly performed cosmetic procedure in Asia.

PATIENT SELECTION: DIFFERENCES AND SIMILARITIES FROM CAUCASIANS TO ASIANS

The demand for wrinkle reduction is very high, and patient selection is similar to patient selection for Caucasians. The efficacy and complication rate of fillers and neurotoxins in Asians are also similar to those in Caucasians (Nanni

and Alster 1998). However, there are some histologic differences between Asian skin and Caucasian skin, for example, Asian skin tends to have a thicker dermis with more abundant collagen fiber.

With regard to the injection of fillers, certain areas, such as the nasolabial fold and tear trough, can be tricky. Improper injection technique can result in a bumpy feel if the product is injected too superficially. Deeper injection needs a more skillful approach (blindness can occur if material is injected into the vessel). Filler injection into the nose is popular in Asian patients due to their flat nasal features. Asians prefer a conservative approach, especially with regard to lip augmentation.

Neurotoxin injection in Asians is different from Caucasians in various aspects. Wrinkling is less prominent in Asians (platysmal bands, less prominent), and Asian physical features differ in the sense that small eyes and shortened legs (calf hypertrophy) are important (Han et al. 2006). The lower third of the Asian face is wider than that of Caucasians. The average gap between the masticatory muscles of Korean women is 118–125 mm; Korean women have a 12- to 20-mm wider gap than Western women. The use of neurotoxin to reduce masseter muscle volume differs from the use of neurotoxin to ease wrinkles. Wrinkles tend to increase with age, whereas muscular volume decreases over time. The older the patients are, the longer the time required for recovery, with less volume recovered. The

TABLE 40.1: Fillers and Neurotoxins Available in Asian Countries

		Origin	Manufacturer	China	Korea	Thailand	Japan
Neurotoxin	BOTOX	United States	Allergan	not approved (approved in Taiwan and Hong Kong)	not approved	approved	not approved
	Dysport	United Kingdom	Ipsen	not approved	approved	approved	not approved
	BTX-A	China	Lanzhow	approved	approved	not approved	not approved
	Meditoxin	Korea	Pacific Pharma	not approved	approved	not approved	not approved
Collagen	Zyderm 1/2, Zyplast	United States	INAMED	not approved	approved	approved	approved
	Cosmoderm/Cosmoplast	United States	INAMED	not approved	approved	not approved	not approved
	Atero collagen	Japan	KOKEN	not approved	approved	not approved	approved
	Isolagen	United States	Isolagen	not approved	not approved	not approved	not approved
Hyaluronic acid	Restylane/Touch/Perlane/Sub-Q	Sweden	Q-Med	not approved	approved	approved	not approved
	Hylaform/Fine Lines/Plus	United States	INAMED	not approved	approved	not approved	not approved
	Juvéderm-18/24/30/24HV/30HV	France	Coneal Group	not approved	approved	not approved	not approved
	Surgiderm-18/24/30/24XP/30XP/Lips	France	Coneal Group	not approved	not approved	not approved	not approved
	Puragen/Plus/Prevelle	United States	Mentor	not approved	approved	not approved	not approved
Others	Radiesse	United States	BioForm	not approved	approved	not approved	not approved
	MATRIDEX	Germany	BioPolymer	not approved	not approved	not approved	not approved
	Scupltra/New-Fill	United States	Dermic Laboratories	not approved	not approved	not approved	not approved
	Dermalive	France	Dermatech	not approved	approved	not approved	not approved
	ArteFill/Artecoll	United States	Artes Medical	not approved	approved	not approved	not approved
	Aquamid	Denmark	Contura International A/S	not approved	approved	not approved	not approved
	Amaging gel	China	Contura International A/S	not approved	not approved	not approved	not approved

ideal application of neurotoxin is in patients with well-developed masseter muscles, without protrusive bones and without a large amount of fat tissue around the chin (Kim et al. 2005).

In Thailand, Dr. Rojanamatin (personal communication) reports that

regarding wrinkle treatment with neurotoxin, the technique of injection is similar between Caucasians and Orientals. However, lateral brow elevation pattern is not popular among our patients because after treatment, the facial expression sometimes appears unnaturally angry or quizzical. Apart from this, I have noticed that the Oriental nasal bridge is not as high as Caucasian's. If we treat glabellar frown lines with a large volume and too much toxin, we may broaden the area between the brows resulting in a more flattened appearance of nasal bridge. This can be avoided by applying a smaller volume with a higher concentration and using the proper amount of neurotoxin. To get the best result from filler injection, we need to choose good candidates and use proper technique. We also need to choose good quality filler products. We should be very careful about using synthetic or semi-synthetic filler, because delayed complications, such as a granulomatous reaction, may follow. Although uncommon, this is difficult to treat.

In Korea, Dr. Dae Hun Suh (personal communication) reports,

For fillers, Koreans do not think that large lips (for example, Angelina Jolie) is attractive. I concentrate the injection in the middle portion of lower lip. In addition, I inject fillers along the periphery of lip. For nasolabial folds, I avoid over-correction. If it is over-corrected, the use of filler may be noticed by other people when the patient laughs. In the tear trough deformities, we prefer autologous fat transplantation because it frequently needs much amount of fillers so that the expense is too high. Sometimes we use Restylane SUQ. For cheek or chin augmentation, autologous fat transplantation is usually performed. As the second choice, we may use HA's. Hydroxylapatite is used for nose elevation. Plastic surgeons often use Artecoll. It is less frequently used by dermatologists. For neurotoxins, generally, most Koreans like soft appearance. Therefore, I do not prefer lateral brow elevation. If a patient wants lateral brow elevation, I perform it with the same methods as in western countries. Reloxin (Dysport) is also available in Philippines, Malaysia, Thailand and Hong Kong. It is not available in China and Japan. The brand name of Chinese botox is BTX-A which is imported by Hanol Pharmaceutical Company. It had been popular in the past two or three years. Recently,

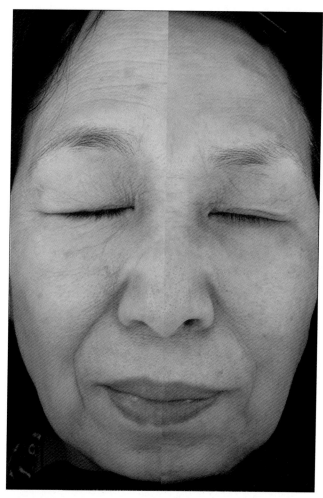

FIGURE 40.1: *Hyaluronic acids (Puragen) combined with neurotoxins (BOTOX) and fractional laser (Fraxel) in a female:* **A**, *pretreatment;* **B**, *six weeks posttreatment.*

its use has been diminished because the price of Botox (by Allergan) was decreased and because it seemed that the side effects of Chinese botox is somewhat greater than Botox (by Allergan).

FILLERS AND NEUROTOXINS IN ASIA

Table 40.1 shows what fillers and neurotoxins are available in Asia (China, Korea, Thailand, and Japan). In general, the most prevalent neurotoxin is BOTOX. Dysport has been very popular in Asia; however, so-called Chinese botox, BTX-A, and Korean botox, Meditoxin, can also be used in Asia. BTX-A is cheaper than the others; however, some doctors indicate that it is less stable and less efficacious. There is still a lack of data in terms of the safety and efficacy of BTX-A. Further large, prospective studies of BTX-A are warranted.

The most prevalent fillers are hyaluronic acids (70% to 90%). Restylane is still the most popular filler used in Asia because many countries approved Restylane first. Recently, many hyaluronic acids have been developed, and the popularity of Restylane seems to be decreasing. Permanent or semipermanent fillers are not as popular as temporary fillers in Asia. Many plastic surgeons have removed silicone, paraffin, and organogen because of poor results with these products. We are very cautious when considering the injection of permanent or semipermanent fillers.

Various fillers and neurotoxins will be approved in Asia within a few years. Table 40.1 could be outdated by the time this chapter is published. Advances and new products come along very quickly in this specialty of medicine. In 2008, short- and long-acting hyaluronic acids, combined with neurotoxins and noninvasive lasers (e.g., fractional lasers), intense pulsed lights, and radiofrequency devices, will continue to increase in popularity (Figure 40.1). Permanent or semipermanent fillers need more time for evaluation in Asia.

SUGGESTED READING

Ahn KY, Park MY, Park DH, Han DG. Botulinum toxin A for the treatment of facial hyperkinetic wrinkle lines in Koreans. *Plast. Reconstr. Surg.* 2000;105:778–84.

Chan H, Kono T. *Laser Treatment of Ethnic Skin*. Philadelphia, PA: Elsevier Saunders; 2004.

Han KH, Joo YH, Moon SE, Kim KH. Botulinum toxin A treatment for contouring of the lower leg. *J. Dermatolog. Treat.* 2006;17:250–4.

Kim NH, Chung JH, Park RH, Park JB. The use of botulinum toxin type A in aesthetic mandibular contouring. *Plast. Reconstr. Surg.* 2005;115:919–30.

Nanni CA, Alster TS. Complications of carbon dioxide laser resurfacing: an evaluation of 500 patients. *Dermatol. Surg.* 1998;24:315–20.

CHAPTER 41

Fillers and Neurotoxins in South America

Arturo Prado

Patricio Andrades

Patricio Leniz

FILLERS

Better fillers will become available for clinical use, and they should accomplish the golden rule of absolute safety (but this corresponds to the perfect filler, which is yet to be discovered). Available products correct wrinkles and provide volume and have the advantage of off-the-shelf use and no donor site morbidity, but their longevity and side effects still cannot be guaranteed. The perfect filler should be safe, autogenous, dynamic, resistant to the aging process, and long lasting or permanent, with no immunologic or toxic effects.

We have classified fillers in the following way:

1. transient, with a duration up to eighteen months

2. long lasting or semipermanent, with a duration up to or more than five years

3. permanent

As to their origin, they can be derived by one of the following means:

1. Fillers can be animal-derived collagen products (Zyderm/ Zyplast, Inamed/Aesthetics) with transient results. These were available for some years in Chile, but surgeons were reluctant to conduct the required allergy tests, by which they feared to lose patients.

2. Fillers can be allogenic human collagen products (Cosmoderm/Cosmoplast, Inamed/Aesthetics; Alloderm as a decellularized dermal allograft, Cymetra, Life-Cell Corp.; preserved-bank fascia lata, Fascian, Fascia Biosystems) with long-lasting results, but these are very expensive, and expense is the most likely reason why they have little popularity in South America.

3. Fillers can be synthetic materials that derive from fermentation of a bacterial strain streptococcus, giving stabilized hyaluronic acid of nonanimal origin (Restylane/Perlane, Q-Med; Captique, Inamed/Aesthetics; Puragen, Mentor; Juvéderm, Leaderm; Teosyal, Belotero, Varioderm, Rofilan, Esthelis, and others). All have only transient results and are extensively used in South America, but our patients think that they could last longer based on the cost-effect concept (their cost being higher than the cost of collagen-based materials).

4. Fillers can make use of hyaluronic acid derived from avian sources (Hyalaform, Inamed/Aesthetics). These have higher risks of hypersensitivity-inflammatory-granulomatous (edema, erythema, pruritus, acneiform lesions) reactions compared to nonanimal sources of hyaluronic acid and also have transient results.

5. Finally, fillers can be alloplastic implants. We will mention four products that have not been approved for cosmetic use by the Food and Drug Administration (FDA) but that do have a long history of use in Europe and South America: Artecoll and Aquamid, with reproducible results and long-term effects; and Bioplastique and medical grade silicone (Adatosil and Silikon), which, because of their results in our community, we do not recommend.

Artecoll (Artes Medical) is a permanent injectable filler composed of polymethylmethacrylate microspheres that are suspended in a transport solution of 3.5% bovine collagen and 0.3% lidocaine. The polymethylmethacrylate microspheres are 20–40 nm in diameter and are packaged in sterile, preloaded syringes. The collagen component dissipates within one to three months, whereas the smooth microspheres become encapsulated forever. Polymethylmethacrylate and collagen are two implant materials that have been reported in human implantation. Skin testing is required, despite a less than 0.1% incidence of sensitivity reactions, to assess for the presence of allergy to bovine collagen. The size of the needle and the viscous nature of the material make dermal implantation impossible. Like all particulate injectable fillers, the risk of clumping and localized foreign body reactions exists. For this reason, and because of the risk of palpability, Artecoll should not be injected into the lips and in areas of thin overlying skin. The small microsphere diameter prevents phagocytosis. Their smooth surface lessens cell adhesion and therefore foreign body reaction, and the collagen vehicle keeps them apart long enough to prevent a mass effect by agglutination. From the ninth day after injection, all the empty spaces around the microspheres are filled with fibroblasts. After two weeks, the first capillary vessels are present, and by the third week, the first collagen fibers can be detected. The early reactions explain why there is no displacement of the product because the microspheres are first embedded in the injected collagen and then, while it is absorbed, by the fibrous reaction of the host tissues. The remaining new connective tissue volume is produced between three and four weeks. After two months, the collagen density increases, with beginning of contraction of the free spaces and reduction of the spaces between the microspheres. By the fourth month, the active fibrosis phase is over, and the implant remains stable. After seven months, there are very few differences between the collagen fibers around the implant and those of the surrounding connective tissue. Histologically, there are few foreign body giant cells, lymphocytes, and loose fibrous tissues. Microspheres are easily recognizable, appearing as extracellular, round, smooth, regular vacuoles.

Aquamid, an acrylic polymer transparent gel (Contura International), is a cross-linked polyacrylamide gel 2.5% in 97.5% pyrogen-free water. It is sold in 1-mL syringes, is kept at room temperature, and is to be injected with a 27-gauge needle. It should be injected deeply, not into the dermis. No allergy test is required, and no overcorrection or undercorrection is required. Histologically, the acrylamide transparent gel causes a fine fibrocellular capsule, without evidence of foreign body reaction. At six and nine months, the fibrous capsule is more pronounced around millions of minidroplets of gel. The capsule is surrounded by fibroblasts and macrophages. The water component of the gel is bound to the polyacrylamide polymer and is not absorbed or biologically degraded. The molecule is not dissolved in water, but looks swollen, like a sponge. The gel is in dynamic equilibrium with the surrounding tissue, but still, the polymer retains its ability to hold water and remains elastic over an extended time. The implant is clinically still palpable at nine months. Aquamid can be removed shortly after the injection, if necessary. If the gel has to be removed at a later stage, a minor surgical procedure might be necessary. Polyacrylamides have been used for many years in the United States and Europe for treatment of drinking water and are also found in soft contact lenses and tissue implant material. Polyacrylamide has a half-life in the human body of longer than twenty years. This may be true for large quantities; however, the injection of 0.1 cc of Aquamid is absorbed into human skin within nine months. Aquamid is approved for use in Europe, Australia, South America, and the Middle East; however, it is not FDA approved. Indications for use include lip augmentation; smoothing of nasolabial folds; filling depressed mouth corners, perioral wrinkles, and glabellar frown lines;

and cheek, chin, nose, and vermilion border contouring. Using a 27-gauge needle in a fine multiline retrograde fashion, Aquamid is injected into the subcutaneous tissue. Aquamid does not migrate. A 1:1 injection to augmentation effect is expected as the product is not absorbable. Fifteen-day intervals are recommended between injection sessions. Cases with hematomas, edema, alteration of skin pigment, itching, tingling, and moderate pain have been reported. Granuloma formation does occur with the use of polyacrylamide gel. Other reported side effects include the following: 1 to 2% of injections experience infection, which is easily treated; temporary reactions typically connected with injection include, for example, reddening, pain, edema, and itching at the site of injection. The most frequent indications for filling purposes are to enhance lips, replace facial volume lost from aging, correct facial deformities, treat depressed scars, and enhance cheekbones and the jawline. Aquamid is not indicated for the treatment of fine wrinkles; it is not to be used in or near anatomic sites with active skin disease or inflammation or during pregnancy or lactation.

Bioplastique is a textured copolymer microparticle filler containing silicone particles. It has a transient carrier (polyvinilpyrrolidone). It was very popular after it was introduced in 1991 in South America. The size of the particles makes them nonphagocytable; however, their irregular shape will induce a strong foreign body reaction as it does increase the total surface area of the implanted particles. The fluid carrier does not allow for the particles to stay apart, which favors cluster formation and increases the potential complication of foreign body reaction. Very active granulomas can be seen, with numerous foreign body giant cells; many phagocytes, with asteroid bodies infiltrating all the spaces, even within the recesses of the particles themselves; and surrounding very thick collagen bundles mixed with fibroblasts and a moderate lymphocytic infiltration. Despite the size of the particles, they can be transported to lymph nodes. Our experience with this product is bad, and we later present a case of a devastating complication.

Medical grade silicone is available in two forms: Adatosil 5000, from Bausch and Lomb Pharmaceuticals Inc., and Silikon 1000, from Alcon Laboratories Inc. Both products are highly purified, injectable, long-chain polydimethylsiloxane oils. The numbers 5,000 and 1,000 refer to centistokes (cS), which is a measure of viscosity (water has a viscosity of 100 cS). Silicone oil can be stored at room temperature (15 to 32 degrees Celsius). After injection, silicone is dispersed into the tissues as millions of microdroplets (1–100 nm in diameter). Lymphocytic infiltration is evidence of transient inflammation, which occurs locally and subsides after two weeks. At one month, the droplets are encapsulated by fibroblasts and collagen. At three to six months, a foamy, translucent, birefringent material is found within macrophages and giant cells. At nine months, granulomatous depots are found in the dermis and subcutaneous tissue, surrounded by fibrous tissue. At fourteen months, an intense fibrosis can be present that clinically gives the impression of soft tissue augmentation. No skin testing is required. Medical grade silicone is FDA approved for intraocular injection as indicated for use as a prolonged retinal tamponade in selected cases of complicated retinal detachment and is used off-label as a soft tissue filler for cosmetic purposes. Areas of injection include filling of facial rhytids and scars, augmentation of facial eminences, and correction of facial asymmetries. Lip augmentation is also an off-label indication. The microdroplet technique is used, with 0.01–0.02 mL of silicone injected subdermally with a tuberculin syringe through a 28- to 30-gauge needle either by means of a linear fanning or a multiple stab technique. In time, the implant can harden through ingrowths of connective tissue, and it may form a granuloma or late siliconoma. Injections of both products should be spaced approximately 2–10 mm apart. The needle is inserted into the skin, which may be tented up as the microdroplet is deposited. Care must be taken to aim the needle medially, away from the bulk of the cheek, when injecting the nasolabial and marionette lines. Many other areas of the face can be treated with microdroplet silicone injections. These include the cheek hollows, midface, glabella, and tear troughs, and the chin, lips, and cheekbones can be enhanced. Application of a topical anesthetic cream provides sufficient analgesia for most patients; however, a regional anesthetic block is generally used before injection of the lips. Overcorrection must be avoided, and injections that are too superficial may result in beading. Injections are typically carried out at one- to two-month intervals. Usually, patients need less than 5 cc for total correction, but total treatment volumes as high as 5–10 cc (1–2 tsp) may sometimes be used, especially for HIV-associated lipoatrophy. This volume of material requires several months to inject. Large volumes of silicone may increase the risk of serious complications by increasing antigenic burden. This is the preferred treatment used in lay clinics of our country and many countries of South America. The lay manipulators call the product biopolymer filler and have caused blindness and irreparable siliconomas in many patients.

Avoiding and Treating Dermal Filler Complications

All fillers have the risk of both early and late complications. Early side effects, such as swelling, redness, and bruising, occur after intradermal or subdermal injections. Adverse events that last longer than two weeks can be due to technical errors (e.g., too superficial implantation of a semipermanent or permanent filler). These adverse events can be treated with intradermal steroid injections, vascular lasers, or intense pulsed light, and later, with dermabrasion or surgery. Late-onset allergy and no allergic foreign body granulomas are also possible due to an immunological reaction. They react well to intralesional steroid injections, which often have to be repeated. Surgical excisions shall remain the last option and are indicated for hard lumps in the lips and visible hard nodules or hard granulomas in the subcutaneous fat. To avoid or treat complications with dermal fillers, knowledge of their composition, physiologic tissue reactions, absorption time, and persistence is indispensable. Most adverse events occurring after the injection of dermal fillers can be prevented by proper injection technique and are of utmost importance if a long-lasting filler is used because it will remain beneath the skin. The treatment of complications should be aggressive and should be initiated as soon as possible after occurrence, either with corticosteroid injections or surgery. It is also important to know the clinical and histological difference between nodules and granulomas because corticosteroids are effective in cellular proliferations but not in nodules of clumped particles or microspheres. Treating complications of dermal fillers effectively, and assuring the patient in the interim before full aesthetic effects are achieved, are key to mastering this so-called noninvasive technique.

Further Thoughts on Fillers

We work in an academic setting, so we must be honest as we teach plastic surgery, and we have always told medical residents that structural fat grafting is the first choice for filling purposes. We also strive for fairness, and we avoid bias in our selection of the best option for the treatment of cosmetic patients, so after scientific evaluation and better understanding of nonfat dermal fillers are reached, we will probably accomplish the premise that no one product should be favored over another, and in this manner, this teaching process could change in the future. At this moment, and in our country, fat is considered to be the ideal filler to correct large and moderate soft tissue defects, with permanence and adequate cosmesis. However, fat grafting does not work equally well for every patient. The execution of the technique and the experience of the surgeon truly affect the outcome. Fat as a free graft does more than just fill the area into which it is placed because when correctly placed and transferred, fat will live. Finding a permanent filler with only some of the properties of fat is among the foremost issues for cosmetic surgeons today.

NEUROTOXINS

Aging and facial animation contribute to the appearance of facial lines and soft tissue malposition. Chemodenervating agents are the answer for these problems and act by the selective and precise focal paralysis of the underlying facial musculature, therefore reducing or eliminating the overlying rhytids. Also, chemodenervation can act as an adjunct for facial rejuvenation because of its influence on

TABLE 41.1: Comparative Neurotoxins in Use in Europe and South America

Brand	BOTOX	Dysport	Xeomin	Prosigne
Manufacturer	Allergan, United States	Ipsen, United Kingdom	Merz, Germany	Lanzhou, China
Preparation	lyophilized	lyophilized	lyophilized	lyophilized
Stabilization	vacuum-drying	freeze-drying	vacuum-drying	vacuum-drying
pH	7.4	7.4	7.4	7.4
Purification process	precipitation chromatography	precipitation chromatography	precipitation chromatography	precipitation chromatography
Serotype	A	A	A	A
Clostridium botulinum strain	HALL A	IPSEN	HALL A	HALL A
Pharmacy form	powder	powder	powder	powder
Storage	Below 8 degrees centigrade	Below 8 degrees centigrade	Below 25 degrees centigrade	Below 5 degrees centigrade
Off-the-shelf life	24 months	15 months	36 months	24 months
Vials	100 U	500 U / 300 U	100 U	100–150 U
Biological activity compared to BOTOX	1	1/3	1	1
Excipients	500 mg/vial of human serum albumin 900 mg/vial NaCl	125 mg/vial of human serum albumin 2,500 mg/vial lactose hemagglutinin	1 mg/vial of human serum albumin 5 mg/vial sucrose	500 mg/vial of human serum albumin 5 mg gelatin 25 mg dextran 25 mg sacarose 900 mg/vial NaCl

facial soft tissue position and shape. A list of neurotoxins used in South America is provided in Table 41.1.

BOTOX (botulinum toxin derived from *Clostridium botulinum*), from Inamed/Allergan, is the most widely used agent and the gold standard product to which we should compare other chemodenervating agents. The bacterium *Clostridium botulinum* is an obligate anaerobe. There are eight different subtypes of botulinum toxin (A, B, C_1, C_2, D, E, F, and G), although only two (types A and B) are currently manufactured for commercial use. All eight subtypes effect muscular paralysis by preventing the release of acetylcholine from the presynaptic neuron at the neuromuscular junction, but they do so at different target sites and with variable effectiveness. Botulinum toxin A is the most potent of all the subtypes and therefore is the one clinically used most frequently. Its effect is through the enzymatically mediated blockade of acetylcholine release from the nerve terminal. Different botulinum toxin serotypes are zinc endopeptidases, each cleaving an intracellular protein important in the translocation of an intact

acetylcholine vesicle from the cytosol to the plasma membrane. Botulinum toxin A and botulinum toxin E cleave the translocation protein SNAP-25 (synaptosome associated protein), and botulinum toxin C acts by cleaving HPC-1 (syntaxin). Botulinum toxin D and botulinum toxin F cleave VAMP (synaptobrevin), and botulinum toxin B acts on the same substrate, but at a different site. At the present time, type A has been studied most intensely and is used most widely. Its effects are both dose-dependent and reversible. Muscle weakness can be appreciated as soon as six hours after exposure. However, full paralysis and obvious clinical effects usually manifest by seven days, and will last between three and six months. Physiologic and clinical effects dissipate as new neuromuscular junctions develop and axonal sprouting takes place.

There are currently three botulinum toxin formulations available, two of the A subtype and one of the B subtype. The two sources of commercially available type A subtypes are BOTOX (Inamed-Allergan) and Dysport (Speywood Pharmaceuticals). BOTOX is 2–4 times as effective in similar-unit doses as Dysport, which is why it is available in smaller vials (100-U vials for BOTOX versus 500-U vials for Dysport). Myobloc (Elan Pharmaceuticals) is derived from the botulinum toxin B subtype and is far less potent per unit dose, in general, than the A subtype (though the bioequivalency formulation has yet to be established). Although all agents have comparable effects, they vary in several ways, including local discomfort with injection, onset of action, and duration of effects. All forms of commercially available botulinum toxin are fragile and should be reconstituted and administered in a specific way to optimize drug potency. The manufacturer of BOTOX (Inamed-Allergan) distributes the vials containing 100 U of freeze-dried crystalline toxin, 0.9 mg of sodium chloride, and 0.5 mg of human albumin in an environment of −5 degrees Celsius. Reconstitution of the dehydrated toxin should be performed with care. When reconstituting the toxin, great care must be taken to avoid turbulence and agitation when adding the saline or when shaking the bottle; both actions can lead to foaming, which can lead to possible denaturation and subsequent clinical ineffectiveness. Using a larger-gauge needle (such as an 18-gauge needle) for reconstitution, or even breaking the vacuum seal by removing the rubber stopper, can help to limit turbulence. Alcohol, used either on the vial cap or on the patient's skin, should be avoided because it can inactivate the toxin. Although the vial can be reconstituted to a dilution of 8 mL/100 U, we prefer a dilution with 4 cc of saline to yield a concentration of 2.5 U/0.1 mL. The reduced volume may limit the potential for possible unwanted diffusion of the toxin to surrounding areas. However, precise application is the most important parameter to reduce side effects.

Prosigne (CBTX-A, Lanzhou Biological Products) or Chinese *Clostridium botulinum* serotype A, arrived in Chile in 2005. It was approved by the Public Health Institute, regulatory organ for medications (similar to the FDA). The lyophilized presentation is 100 U/vial or 50 U/vial of *Clostridium botulinum* toxin, 5 mg of gelatin, 25 mg of dextran, and 25 mg of sacarose.

The product has huge economic implications for our health services, especially in developing countries (the price of BOTOX is 8–10 times higher than that of Prosigne in the same units). Several double-blind, randomized, cross-over clinical studies comparing BOTOX with Prosigne have demonstrated no significant differences between the materials, especially regarding safety and efficacy. Treatment, dose regimen, and titration are the same as for BOTOX, with a ratio of 1:1 (one BOTOX unit is equal to one Prosigne unit), both being diluted with sterile nonbacteriostatic saline as the reconstituting agent, with 5 U/0.1 mL, with a dose for both of 2.5–5 U per injection site. Two differences are important: BOTOX produces 100 U vials of freeze-dried crystalline botulinum serotype A toxin, 0.9 mg of sodium chloride, and 0.5 mg of human albumin in an environment of −5 degrees Celsius. In contrast, Prosigne

has two types of vials: 50 U and 100 U of freeze-dried crystalline botulinum serotype A toxin, with 5 mg of gelatin, 25 mg of dextran and 25 mg of sacarose, and with 0.9 mg of sodium chloride and 0.5 mg of gelatin, respectively, and this last product, used in vaccines, produces more allergic reactions.

APPLICATION

Forehead

Treatment of forehead rhytids can be accomplished by first marking the rhytids during active contraction and subsequently injecting along the lines every 1 or 1.5 cm, for a total of 10 to 20 U. In men with thicker frontalis and more prominent rhytids, an additional 10–15 U may be required. We avoid injecting within 1 cm superior to the eyebrow to reduce the chances of migration and diffusion of the toxin, which may affect the upper eyelid elevators. Superficial injections are preferred in this area because deeper injections (periosteum) will lead to brow ptosis.

Procerus and Corrugators

The procerus, corrugators, and medial orbital orbicularis oculi muscles are responsible for the vertical glabellar rhytids and the horizontal rhytids at the bridge of the nose. The procerus is prominent between the medial margins of each eyebrow, whereas the corrugators lie more laterally. To treat this area, several injection sites are used. We use the hourglass technique, in which the narrowest portion of the hourglass is a single point just inferior to a line joining the medial brow margins. This point receives 2 or 3 U. The inferior (wider) aspect of the hourglass consists of two points just lateral to the dorsal aesthetic lines along a plane just inferior to the medial canthi, and these points receive 2 U per site and are used to treat the proximal nasalis muscle and prevent the bunny look. The superior portion of the hourglass is formed by points just above the medial brow (in line with the medial canthus) that course along the superior orbital rim, where we deposit 4 or 5 U per side.

Orbicularis Oculi

The medial aspect serves as a brow depressor. The lateral fibers are responsible for rhytids that radiate axially away from the lateral canthus (crow's feet). Because this muscle is the underlying etiology for the rhytids, chemodenervation is the optimal treatment, rather than other modalities such as excisional techniques, resurfacing, or soft tissue augmentation. We locate the areas of orbicularis to be treated by having the patient actively squint and then inject in three or four areas. A high concentration (low volume) is injected slowly to prevent diffusion to unwanted areas. The area of injection extends from just inferior to the lateral edge of the eyebrow, down the lateral aspect of the lateral orbital rim, to a point lateral to the infraorbital rim. Two or three units of toxin are injected at each point. If the injection site is too medial, diffusion of the toxin can affect the medial orbital portion of the orbicularis oculi muscle, resulting in lower lid ptosis (retraction and/or ectropion), strabismus, epiphora, and diplopia as well as dry eye symptoms. Injecting more inferiorly can result in unwanted paralysis of the zygomaticus major, with lip ptosis and an asymmetric smile. Injecting more superiorly can result in paralysis of the inferior fibers of the frontalis muscle, resulting in eyebrow ptosis. The orbicularis muscle seems to respond adequately to this more superficial injection.

Eyebrow

Mild to moderate brow ptosis can be managed with chemodenervation of the brow depressors. This technique can also be used as a treatment for inadvertent paralysis of the inferior frontalis fibers. The result is a chemical brow lift. The brow contour can also be reshaped, which can show an apparent improvement of the brow position. For instance, the medial frontalis muscle can be chemodenervated with concurrent treatment to the lateral brow depressor, giving the illusion of a chemical brow lift by affecting the relative positions of the medial and lateral aspects of the brow.

Nose

Nasal flaring results in increased columellar show. When the alar portion of the nasalis muscle has been chemodenervated, it reduces this problem. Approximately 5 U of toxin is injected per side, where the nasalis is visible on active nostril flaring. The nostril geometry itself is not altered with this treatment because its configuration is based more on the lateral crus than on the nasalis.

Nasolabial Fold

The levator labii superioris has the most prominent effect on the medial nasolabial fold, whereas the levator labii superioris has the greatest influence on the middle part of the fold. Chemodenervation of the first acts on the medial part of the nasolabial fold, with some correction for a gummy smile.

Mouth and Lips

Orbicularis oris, depressor anguli oris, and mentalis are the main muscles of this region. The small, vertically oriented rhytids of the upper lip can be treated by chemodenervation of the orbicularis oris. To differentiate functional rhytids from aging changes, the patient actively purses the lips, exacerbating the rhytids if they are functional. To treat this area, the most prominent rhytids are marked and injected in a subcutaneous plane on both sides of the rhytids (0.5–1 U of toxin for each side). The depressors can also be injected with 2 or 3 U. The location of the intramuscular injection should be approximately 1 cm lateral and 1 cm inferior to the angle of the mouth.

Mentalis

Chin irregularities can be seen as a result of a hyperkinetic mentalis muscle. To successfully chemodenervate this area, a total of 10 U is subcutaneously injected, staying at least 1 cm inferior to the mental sulcus. This technique will help avoid oral incompetence due to inadvertent orbicularis oris paralysis from toxin migration.

Neck

The neck requires bigger doses of toxin than the face, and its onset of action is relatively faster. The technique we use is with the patient forcefully grimacing in a sitting position. The platysmal bands are grasped with the nondominant hand and injected with 2.5–5 U into the muscle belly at 1- to 1.5-cm intervals along the band, as far down as where the muscle meets the clavicle.

Gonyautoxin is a paralyzing phytotoxin produced by dinoflagellates (bivalve shellfish). The primary clinical symptom of paralytic shellfish poisoning is acute paralytic illness produced by paralyzing toxins. Paralytic shellfish poison is formed by a mixture of phycotoxins, and their toxicity is due to their reversible binding to a receptor site on the voltage-gated sodium channel on excitable cells, thus blocking neuronal transmission (paralytic shellfish toxin is found on the Pacific Ocean shores of Chile). After the publication of an original study titled "Gonyautoxin: New Treatment for Healing Acute and Chronic Anal Fissures" (Garrido et al. 2005) and done in our clinical hospital, in which doses of 100 U of gonyautoxin in a volume of 1 mL were infiltrated into both sides of the anal fissure in the internal anal sphincter, a total remission of acute and chronic anal fissures was achieved within fifteen and twenty-eight days, respectively. Thus Gonyautoxin was found to break the vicious circle of pain and spasm that leads to anal fissure. This study proposed gonyautoxin anal sphincter infiltration to be a safe and effective alternative therapeutic approach to conservative, surgical, and botulinum toxin therapies for anal fissures.

Based on this idea, we recruited ten cosmetic patients for injection of this diluted toxin into the mimetic muscles of the face. We found three interesting things: (1) the injection was very painful, (2) a moderate paralysis of the injected zones was seen instantly (dose-dependant) but lasted only a few hours (twelve to twenty-four hours), and (3) the patients were able to see the wrinkles being erased and asked for a more definitive treatment.

We need more science to understand what happens with this new neurotoxin injection in the muscles of the face and to compare it to BOTOX, which is, as was said earlier, the gold standard of neurotoxins.

SUGGESTED READING

Fillers

Andre, P. Evaluation of the safety of a non-animal stabilized hyaluronic acid in European countries: a retrospective study from 1997–2001. *J. Eur. Acad. Dermatol. Venereol.* 2004;18:422.

Burke KE, Naughton G, Cassai N. A histological, immunological, and electron microscopic study of bovine collagen implants in the human. *Ann. Plast. Surg.* 1985;14:515.

Cohen SR, Holmes RE. Artecoll: a long-lasting injectable wrinkle filler material. Report of a controlled, randomized, multicenter clinical trial of 251 subjects. *Plast. Reconstr. Surg.* 2004;114:964.

Friedman PM, Mafong EA, Kauvar ANB, Geronemus RG. Safety data of injectable nonanimal stabilized hyaluronic acid gel for soft tissue augmentation. *Dermatol. Surg.* 2002;28:491.

Inamed Corporation. Product information sheet on CosmoDerm and CosmoPlast. Santa Barbara, CA: Inamed Corp; 2003.

Kanchwala SK, Holloway L, Bucky LP. Reliable soft tissue augmentation: a clinical comparison of injectable soft tissue fillers for facial volume augmentation. *Ann. Plast. Surg.* 2005;55:30.

Kane MA. Treatment of tear trough deformity and lower lid bowing with injectable hyaluronic acid. *Aesthetic Plast. Surg.* 2005;29:363.

Lemperle G, Morhenn V, Charrier U. Human histology and persistence of various injectable filler substances for soft tissue augmentation. *Aesthetic Plast. Surg.* 2003;27:354.

Lindqvist C, Treten S, Bondevile BE, Fagrell D. A randomized evaluator, blind, multicenter comparison of the efficacy and tolerability of Perlane versus Zyplast in the correction of nasolabial folds. *Plast. Reconstr. Surg.* 2005;115:282.

Lowe NJ, Maxwell CA, Lowe P, Duick MG, Shah K. Hyaluronic acid skin fillers: adverse reactions and skin testing. *J. Am. Acad. Dermatol.* 2001;45:930.

Manna F, Dentini M, Desideri P, DePita O, Mortilla E, Maras B. Comparative chemical evaluation of two commercially available derivatives of hyaluronic acid used for soft tissue augmentation. *J. Eur. Acad. Dermatol. Venereol.* 1999;13:183.

Monheit GD. Hylaform: a new injectable hyaluronic acid filler. *Facial Plast. Surg.* 2004;20:153.

Narins RS, Bowman PH. Injectable skin fillers. *Clin. Plast. Surg.* 2005;32:151.

Narins RS, Brandt F, Leyden J, Lorenc ZP, Rubin M, Smith S. A randomized, double-blind, multicenter comparison of the efficacy and tolerability of Restylane versus Zyplast for the correction of nasolabial folds. *Dermatol. Surg.* 2003;29:588.

Neurotoxins

Ahn MS, Catten M, Maas CS. Temporal brow lift using botulinum toxin A. *Plast. Reconstr. Surg.* 2000;105:1129.

Becker-Wegerich P, Rauch L, Ruzicka T. Botulinum toxin A in the therapy of mimic facial lines. *Clin. Exp. Dermatol.* 2001;26:619.

Blitzer A, Brin MF, Keen MS, et al. Botulinum toxin for the treatment of hyperfunctional lines of the face. *Arch. Otolaryngol. Head Neck Surg.* 1993;119:1018.

Borodic GE, Cozzolino D, Ferrante R, et al. Innervation zone of orbicularis oculi muscle and implications for botulinum A toxin therapy. *Ophthal. Plast. Reconstr. Surg.* 1991;7:54.

Brandt FS, Bellman B. Cosmetic use of botulinum A exotoxin for the aging neck. *Dermatol. Surg.* 1998;24:1232.

Brin MF. Botulinum toxin: chemistry, pharmacology, toxicity, and immunology. *Muscle Nerve Suppl.* 1997;6:S146.

Carruthers A, Carruthers J. Aesthetic indications for botulinum toxin injections. *Plast. Reconstr. Surg.* 1995;95:427.

Carruthers A, Carruthers J. Clinical indications and injection technique for the cosmetic use of botulinum A exotoxin. *Dermatol. Surg.* 1998;24:1189.

Carruthers JD, Carruthers JA. Treatment of glabellar frown lines with C. botulinum-A exotoxin. *J. Dermatol. Surg. Oncol.* 1992;18:17.

Carruthers J, Carruthers A. Botox use in the mid and lower face and neck. *Semin. Cutan. Med. Surg.* 2001;20:85.

Carruthers J, Carruthers A. Botulinum toxin (Botox) chemodenervation for facial rejuvenation. *Facial Plast. Surg. Clin. North Am.* 2001;9:197.

Edelstein C, Shorr N, Jacobs J, et al. Oculoplastic experience with the cosmetic use of botulinum A exotoxin. *Dermatol. Surg.* 1998;24:1208.

Fagien S. Extended use of botulinum toxin A in facial aesthetic surgery. *Aesthetic Surg. J.* 1998;18:215.

Fagien S. Botox for the treatment of dynamic and hyperkinetic facial lines and furrows: adjunctive use in facial aesthetic surgery. *Plast. Reconstr. Surg.* 1999;103:701.

Fagien S, Brandt FS. Primary and adjunctive use of Botox in facial aesthetic surgery: beyond the glabella. In: Matarasso A, Matarasso SL, eds., *Clinics in Plastic Surgery*. Philadelphia, PA: Saunders; 2000;127–48.

Flynn TC, Carruthers JA. Botulinum-A toxin treatment of the lower eyelid improves infraorbital rhytides and widens the eye. *Dermatol. Surg.* 2001;27:703.

Frankel AS, Kamer FM. Chemical browlift. *Arch. Otolaryngol. Head Neck Surg.* 1998;124:321.

Garcia A, Fulton JE Jr. Cosmetic denervation of the muscles of facial expression with botulinum toxin: a dose-response study. *Dermatol. Surg.* 1996;22:39.

Garrido R, Lagos N, Lattes K, et al. Gonyautoxin: new treatment for healing acute and chronic anal fissures. *Dis. Colon Rectum* 2005;48:335–40; discussion 340–3.

Guyuron B, Huddleston SW. Aesthetic indications for botulinum toxin injection. *Plast. Reconstr. Surg.* 1994;93:913.

Huang W, Foster JA, Rogachefsky AS. Pharmacology of botulinum toxin. *J. Am. Acad. Dermatol.* 2000;43(2 Pt 1):249.

Huang W, Rogachefsky AS, Foster JA. Browlift with botulinum toxin. *Dermatol. Surg.* 2000;26:55.

Jankovic J, Brin MF. Botulinum toxin: historical perspective and potential new indications. *Muscle Nerve Suppl.* 1997;6:S129.

Klein AW. Cosmetic therapy with botulinum toxin: anecdotal memoirs. *Dermatol. Surg.* 1996;22:757.

Koch RJ, Troell RJ, Goode RL. Contemporary management of the aging brow and forehead. *Laryngoscope* 1997;107:710.

Lovice D. Botulinum toxin use in facial plastic surgery. *Otolaryngol. Clin. North Am.* 2002;35:171.

Lowe NJ. Botulinum toxin type A for facial rejuvenation: United States and United Kingdom perspectives. *Dermatol. Surg.* 1998;24:1216.

Matarasso A, Glassman M. Effective use of Botox for lateral canthal rhytides. *Aesthetic Surg. J.* 2001;21:61.

Matarasso A, Matarasso SL, Brandt FS, et al. Botulinum A exotoxin for the management of platysma bands. *Plast. Reconstr. Surg.* 1999;103:645.

Simpson LL. The origin, structure, and pharmacological activity of botulinum toxin. *Pharmacol. Rev.* 1981;33:155.

PART FOUR

COSMETIC APPLICATIONS OF LIGHT, RADIOFREQUENCY, AND ULTRASOUND ENERGY

VASCULAR APPLICATIONS: LASERS AND BROADBAND LIGHT DEVICES

CHAPTER 42

Treatment of Telangiectasia, Poikiloderma, and Face and Leg Veins

Jane G. Khoury

Mitchel P. Goldman

Vascular lesions are one of the most common indications for laser therapy. While first and still commonly used for the treatment of port-wine stains and hemangiomas, this chapter will focus on their use for telangiectasias, facial veins, poikiloderma of Civatte, and leg veins. The most frequently used light devices for vascular lesions are the 532-nm potassium titanyl phosphate (KTP) and, more recently, diode laser; the 595-nm pulsed dye laser (PDL); the 1,064-nm Nd:YAG lasers; and the intense pulsed light (IPL) devices. Table 42.1 outlines the various vascular-specific laser and light-based systems. These systems work through selective photothermolysis with oxyhemoglobin (oxy-hb) as the target chromophore in vascular lesions. The absorption peaks for oxy-hb are 418 nm, 542 nm, and 577 nm. By targeting oxy-hb, pulses of energy are transferred to the surrounding vessel wall to selectively heat and destroy the abnormal blood vessels. The success of vascular lasers depends on their wavelength, pulse duration, and spot size as they relate to vessel depth and diameter:

- The wavelength used needs to have sufficient penetration depth and selectivity for the target vasculature.

- The pulse duration should be less than thermal relaxation time (TRT) to affect the intended target, while sparing surrounding structures. The TRT is the cooling time of the target and is proportional to the square of the vessel diameter. For example, a vessel 0.03 mm in size has a TRT of 0.86 ms, as compared to a 0.1 mm vessel, which has a 9.6-ms TRT. Longer pulse durations allow for slower heating of the target, which prevents rapid temperature spikes, which cause vessel wall rupture and purpura. When pulse durations exceed the TRT of the target structure, more heat diffuses outside the vessels, leading to unwanted thermal damage to surrounding tissue.

- The spot size should match the diameter of the target structure.

The use of epidermal cooling devices is important to minimize the absorption of laser energy by nontargets such as epidermal melanin. Chill tips, air cooling units, contact cooling with quartz or sapphire crystals, cold gel, and pulsed delivery of cryogen spray are among the modalities employed to mitigate epidermal injury and increase the

TABLE 42.1: Vascular Specific Lasers and Intense Pulsed Light

Supplier	Product Name	Device Type	Wavelength (nm)	Energy (J/cm²)	Pulse Duration (ms)	Spot Diameter (mm)	Cooling
American BioCare	OmniLight FPL	fluorescent pulsed light	480, 515, 535, 550, 580–1,200	Up to 90	up to 500		external continuous
Aesthera	Isolaz (PPx)	pulsed light	400–800				
Candela	V-Beam	pulsed dye	595	25	0.45–40	5, 7, 10, 12	DCD
	C-Beam	pulsed dye	585	8–16	0.45	5, 7, 10	DCD
	Gentle Yag		1,064	up to 600	0.25–300		DCD
CoolTouch	Varia	Nd:YAG	1,064	up to 500	0.3–500	2–10	DCD
Cutera	Genesis	Nd:YAG	1,064	up to 300	0.1–300	3, 5, 7, 10	copper contact
	XEOC	pulsed light	600–850	5–20			none
Cynosure	Cynergy	pulsed dye	595, 1,064	up to 40, up to 600	0.5–40, 0.3–300	5, 7, 10, 12	cold air
		Nd:YAG					cold air
	PhotogenicaV/ PhotogenicaV-Star	pulsed dye	585–595				cold air
	SmartEpill II	Nd:YAG	1,064				cold air
	Acclaim 7000	Nd:YAG	1,064				
	PhotoLight	pulsed light	400–1,200				
DermaMed USA	Quadra Q4	pulsed light	510–1,200	10–20	60–200		none
Iridex/ Laserscope	Lyra	Nd:YAG	1,064	5–900	20–100	1–5 cont. adjustable	cooled sapphire crystal
	Aura	KTP	532	1–240	1–50	1–5 cont. adjustable	cooled sapphire crystal
	Gemini	KTP/Nd:YAG	532, 1,064	up to 100	1–100	1–5 cont. adjustable	cooled sapphire crystal
	VariLite		532, 940	up to 990	10–100	1–5 cont. adjustable	cooled sapphire crystal
Lumenis	Lumenis One	pulsed light	515–1,200	10–40	3–100	15 × 35, 8 × 15	cooled sapphire crystal
		Nd:YAG	1,064	10–225	2–20	2 × 4,6,9	cooled sapphire crystal
	Quantum	pulsed light	515–1,200	3–90	1–75	35 × 8	cooled sapphire crystal
	Vasculite Elite	pulsed light	515–1,200	70–150	2–48	6	
		Nd:YAG	1,064				
Med-Surge	Quantel Viridis	diode	532	up to 110	15–150	10 × 20, 20 × 25	none
	Prolitell	pulsed light	550–900	10–50		40 × 16	none
Orion	Harmony	fluorescent pulsed light	540–950	5–20	10, 12, 15		none
		Nd:YAG	1,064	35–145	40–60	6	none
		Nd:YAG	1,064	35–450	10	2	none
Palomar	MediLux	pulsed light	470–1,400	up to 45	10–100	12 × 12	none
	EsteLux	pulsed light	470–1,400	up to 45	10–100	12 × 12	none
	StarLux	pulsed light/Nd:YAG	550–670/ 870–1,400/ 1,065	up to 700	0.5–500		
Sciton	Profile	Nd:YAG	1,064	4–400	0.1–200		contact sapphire crystal
	Profile BBL	pulsed light	400–1,400	up to 30	up to 200		
Syneron	Aurora SR	pulsed light/RR	580–590	10–30/2–25 RF	up to 200	12 × 25	contact sapphire
WaveLight	Mydon	Nd:YAG	1,064	10–450	0.5–90	1.5, 3, 5	contact or air cooling

safety profile of current laser devices used in the treatment of vascular lesions.

VASCULAR-SPECIFIC LASER SYSTEMS

PDL

The PDL was introduced in the late 1980s and transformed the treatment of vascular lesions. While the original PDL emitted light at 577 nm, it was later increased to 585 nm to allow deeper tissue penetration without compromising its ability to target oxyhemoglobin. Currently available PDLs emit wavelengths at 585 nm or 595 nm and are considered by most to be the treatment of choice for facial telangiectasias and vascular birthmarks. Skin cooling protects the epidermis and provides anesthesia, while allowing higher energy to be delivered to target vessels.

Initially, the PDL was limited by smaller spot sizes and pulse durations of 350–450 ms, which resulted in explosive absorption of laser energy, producing seven to fourteen days of posttreatment purpura. Current systems now offer variable pulse durations up to 40 ms, larger spot sizes up to 12 mm, and higher peak fluences that increase depth of penetration, speed of treatment, and treatment efficacy, while minimizing treatment pain. While the risk of purpura increases significantly with pulse durations less than 6 ms, pulse stacking with longer pulse durations can be employed to achieve subpurpuric vessel clearance. This works by incrementally increasing the intravascular temperature and changing the properties of the red blood cells to slow down blood flow so that there is more target for subsequent pulses. The most recent advance in PDL is to deliver a second laser pulse at a different wavelength (1,064 nm), which can take advantage of the shifting of the absorption curve with 595 nm from oxygenated hb to deoxygenated hb, which is better absorbed by 1,064 nm.

KTP and 532-nm Diode Laser

The KTP laser is a frequency-doubled Nd:YAG laser that emits a green light at 532 nm. More recently, 532-nm lasers employ diodes instead of KTP. This laser has good absorption by hemoglobin and has been shown in bilateral comparative studies to be more efficacious in the treatment of facial telangiectasias than the PDL. However, it was also found to have more edema and crusting and has been associated with atrophic scarring from the use of small-diameter pulses and inadequate epidermal cooling. At 532 nm, the shallow depth of penetration limits it usefulness in nonfacial areas, and the affinity for epidermal melanin constitutes a greater risk of dyspigmentation in darker skin types.

Nd:YAG Laser

The Nd:YAG laser, with its wavelength of 1,064 nm, can penetrate to a depth of 4–6 mm and is useful in the treatment of deeper blood vessels often resistant to treatment with the shorter-wavelength lasers such as the PDL and KTP. In addition, it has a lower absorption for melanin, making its use safer in patients with darker skin pigment. However, the longer wavelength has a diminished affinity for oxygenated hemoglobin, and much higher fluences are required for efficacy. In our experience, the 1,064-nm Nd:YAG is the treatment of choice for facial reticular veins, particularly periorbital. As noted previously, sequential exposure to the 1,064-nm wavelength after a 595-nm laser pulse also appears to increase treatment efficacy of vascular lesions.

COMBINATION LASERS

Laser systems that employ a sequential delivery of two different wavelengths convert properties in the blood with the first wavelength that increase absorption of the second wavelength. Hemoglobin is converted into methemoglobin, and microclot formation occurs, increasing absorption 3–5 times more than with oxyhemoglobin. Examples of this are the Cynergy Multiplex at 595 nm and 1,064 nm (Cynosure Inc.). A picture of facial erythema and telangiectasias treated with the Multiplex is shown in Figure 42.1.

IPL System

IPL systems emit noncoherent light in the 515–1,200 nm range, with pulse durations in the millisecond range. Filters are used to block out shorter wavelengths, allowing the IPL to emit blue-green to yellow wavelengths that selectively target cutaneous vessels. A primary advantage of the IPL is its wide range of wavelengths and pulse durations. This facilitates the treatment of vessels of various depths and diameters as well as treating darker skin types. By treating with longer pulse durations or double and triple pulsing, additive heating of larger vessels is achieved, while the chilled crystal provides epidermal protection.

The large surface area of the crystal allows for efficient use of energy, greater depth of penetration, and quicker treatment sessions. The IPL is primarily used for the treatment of facial telangiectasias and is the treatment of choice for poikiloderma of the neck and chest. IPL can also be used to treat telangiectasias of the trunk and lower extremities; however, because of the broad spectral filters and wide range of wavelengths, energy delivery is not as easily controlled as with laser devices. Caution should be employed when using high fluences, pulse stacking, or multiple passes, especially in darkly pigmented or tan patients and in locations other than the face.

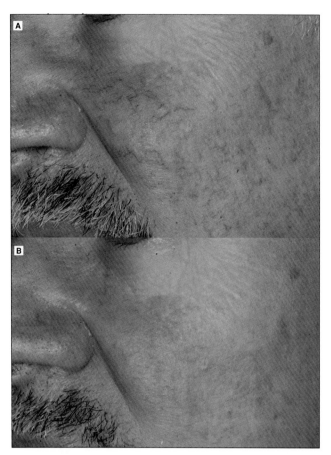

FIGURE 42.1: A, *Before and,* B, *after three treatments with Cynergy Multiplex 7 mm spot size, PDL 7 J/cm², 10 ms short interpulse delay, Nd:YAG 45 J/cm², 15 ms.*

VASCULAR LESION TELANGIECTASIAS

Telangiectasias are superficial cutaneous vessels at a depth of 200–300 μm that measure 0.1–0.5 mm and represent dilated venules, capillaries, or arterioles. Factors such as alcohol, estrogen, corticosteroids, and chronic actinic damage can precipitate their onset. Telangiectasias are also a common feature of rosacea and an increased number of smaller vessels can manifest as facial erythema or flushing. Trauma or tension after surgical procedures, such as excisions, face lifts or rhinoplasty, can promote neovascularization, resulting in telangiectasia.

Telangiectasia that are arteriolar in origin are small in diameter, bright red in color, and do not protrude about the skin surface. Those that arise from venules are wider, blue in color, and often protrude. Telangiectasia arising at the capillary loop are often initially fine, red lesions but become larger and bluish-purple with time because of venous backflow from increasing hydrostatic pressure. Telangiectasia have been subdivided into four classifications based on clinical appearance: (1) simple or linear, (2) arborizing, (3) spider, and (4) papular. Linear and arborizing telangiectasias are very common on the nose, midcheeks, and chin.

These lesions are also seen with frequency on the legs but may often be blue. Spider telangiectasias, also referred to as spider angiomas, are always associated with a central feeding arteriole. They typically appear in young children but can also appear in healthy adults. In the past, these have been treated with electrocautery, which is painful and can lead to punctuate scarring. Papular telangiectasias are frequently part of genetic syndromes, such as Osler-Weber-Rendu, or systemic conditions, such as CREST syndrome, and collagen vascular diseases, such as lupus erythematosus.

Poikiloderma of Civatte is a variant of telangiectasia involving the neck and upper chest and occurring from accumulated ultraviolet exposure. Poikiloderma consists of a combination of telangiectasia, irregular pigmentation, and atrophic skin changes. While PDL and 532-nm KTP have been successful, multiple treatments are often needed, and mottled response may be seen because of the small, circular spot size of the laser and large surface area to be treatment. In addition, as vascular-specific lasers, they may do little to improve hyperpigmentation and textural changes. For this reason, in our opinion, the IPL is the first-line treatment for poikiloderma. The entire neck and chest can be treated in one session without any anesthesia in five to ten minutes. Patients must be aware that footprints representing the shape of the contact crystal may be present, and great care must be taken to avoid skip areas and to not treat tan patients to minimize the appearance of these footprints (Figure 42.2).

Cherry hemangiomas and venous lakes are commonly encountered vascular lesions that represent dilated venules and are amenable to treatment with the same laser systems. Cherry hemangiomas, also known as cherry angiomas, are

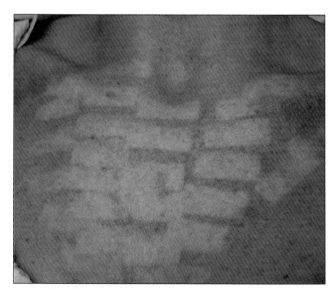

FIGURE 42.2: *IPL footprints representing the shape of the contact crystal may occur. Great care must be taken to avoid skip areas and not to treat tan patients.*

the most common vascular proliferation. They most commonly occur in patients after the third decade and increase in size and number with advancing age. They occur predominantly on the trunk and proximal extremities. They may initially appear as red macules 0.5–2 mm in size and may become dome shaped with time. Unlike angiomas, venous lakes are dark-blue to violaceous, compressible lesions that commonly occur in sun-exposed areas, especially the ear and lower lip, in older patients.

FACIAL VEINS

Facial reticular veins are often seen on the temple and periorbital areas in patients with genetic predisposition or after facial cosmetic surgery. Because of their size and depth, reticular facial veins are better treated with longer wavelengths that provide deeper penetration. The authors have found the variable spot–sized 1,064-nm Nd:YAG to be the laser of choice in the treatment of facial reticular veins. The 1,064-nm Nd:YAG we use for facial reticular veins is the Cool Touch Varia (New Star Lasers). One should always treat the vessel from distal to proximal so that blood flow is not compromised, thereby minimizing the laser target (hb). Remember to always stay outside the orbital rim when treating periorbital veins. It is also important to avoid treating vessels medial to the midpupillary line as veins in this area have a retroorbital flow, unlike veins lateral to the midpupillary line, which flow into the jugular vein. The 3.5-mm spot size is recommended for most vessels with fluences ranging from 180 to 230 J/cm^2, with a 25-ms pulse duration for 1-mm vessels and a 50-ms pulse width for 2- to 3-mm facial reticular veins.

Patient Selection

Because of the competitive absorption of melanin at many of these wavelengths, the easiest patients to treat are those with fair skin (Fitzpatrick I–III). Tan patients and Fitzpatrick skin types IV–VI are more challenging and have a higher risk of complications. They require modifications of IPL filters, wavelength, and laser settings and the use of test spots. Patients must have realistic expectations and should be willing to undergo multiple treatments at four- to six-week intervals to achieve optimal results. Patients' medical history, medications, and previous laser treatments should also be discussed.

Contraindications

Treatments should be avoided in tan patients or phototypes IV–VI, unless the practitioner is very experienced with the laser and light systems and with managing potential complications. Other contraindications include active herpes simplex infection, history of seizures induced by bright lights, active lupus erythematosus, gold therapy, and recent history of isotretinoin use.

Pretreatment Patient Education

Multiples treatment sessions (usually three to five) may be required for improvement of facial telangiectasia, erythema, poikiloderma, and leg veins. Angiomas and venous lakes usually only require one to two treatment sessions for complete resolution. It is important that patients understand that facial erythema and telangiectasia recur over time and that laser treatment does not prevent the development of new vessels. Maintenance treatments are often recommended six to nine months after the initial series. Patients with a significant history of herpes simplex infections should be given a five- to seven-day course of antiviral medication (valacyclovir or famciclovir) starting the day of treatment. The posttreatment course is usually limited to mild erythema and edema, usually lasting less than twenty-four hours. However, always inform patients of the potential for redness, swelling, burning, pain, bruising, crust formation, hyper- and hypopigmentation, blistering, and scarring, which are very rare potential adverse effects of treatment.

Safety Concerns

All individuals in the treatment room should wear wavelength-specific glasses. Patients should have intraocular metal eye shields placed when treating the eyelids or any skin within the orbital rim. Even with appropriate eye protection and closed eyes, patients may still report flashes of light during treatment. Check to make sure the eye shields or goggles are wavelength-specific and appropriately placed, then reassure the patient that this is normal and that his or her eyes are protected. Masks are not necessary. Flammable substances, such as alcohol, acetone, or oxygen, should be removed from the treatment field due to their risk of ignition.

Treatment Technique

Remove all makeup, moisturizers, sunscreen, and lipstick before starting treatment. Dark makeup and lipstick absorb significant amounts of light, which can lead to a burn. Also have the patient remove all sunscreen as it can interfere with absorption of the laser or light source. Pretreatment photographs should always be taken prior to any treatment. Cover the eyebrows and other hair-bearing areas to avoid unintended epilation with the laser and light therapy.

The PDL and 532-nm KTP are very effective in treating telangiectasias. In general, large spot sizes of 10–12 mm with fluences of 6–8 J/cm^2 are used for erythema, whereas smaller spot sizes of 5–7 mm at 8–10 J/cm^2 are used to treat discrete telangiectasias. Table 42.2 provides a guideline for the devices and their parameters; however, treatment settings vary by device and an operator's manual specific to each laser system should be reviewed. The

TABLE 42.2: Laser and Light Devices and Treatment Parameters

System	Wavelength (nm)	Energy (J/cm^2)	Pulse Duration (ms)	Spot Diameter (mm)	Cooling	Vascular Condition	Comments
PDL	585–595						pulse stack or 50% overlap
V-Beam		6.5–9	6–10	7–10	cryogen		
V-Star	595	??	??	??	??		
Cynergy	595	8–12	6–10	7	air cooling	facial erythema, telangiectasias	
KTP	532	12–14	10	3–4	quartz crystal		do not pulse
Aura		10–13	5–8	1–2			stack
IPL	515–1,200					facial	
Lumenis One	560 nm filter	16–18	4.0/4.0		sapphire	erythema,	10–40 ms delay
Vasculight	560 nm filter	30–35	2.4–3.0/4.0–6.0			rosacea,	(depending on
Quantum	560 nm filter	26–35	2.4–3.0/4.0–6.0			telangiectasias,	skin type)
Aurora		16–22				angiomas,	
Estelux		19–30	20			venous lakes	
Sciton BBL	560 nm filter	12–14	10–20				
Nd:YAG	1,064						do not pulse
CoolTouch		180–210	25–50	3.5	cryogen air	facial veins	stack
Varia					cooling		for facial veins
Cynergy							treat distal → proximal 25 ms pulse duration for 1-mm vessels; 50 ms for 2- to 3-mm vessels

clinical end point for telangiectasias is a transient purpura of a few seconds' duration that corresponds with intravascular thrombus formation. While most facial telangiectasias are amenable to treatment, perialar telangiectasias are more difficult to treat. Recurrences occur more easily, and multiple treatments and purpuric settings are often needed to achieve clearance. Small cherry angiomas and venous lakes respond well to long-pulsed 532-nm and 595-nm wavelengths; however, larger, more hypertrophic lesions often require purpuric settings. In addition, port-wine stains and nevus simplex (not discussed in this chapter) require purpuric settings for more effective treatment.

With the PDL, the risk of purpura increases significantly with pulse durations less than 6 ms. Purpura is the result of rapid energy deposition that results in explosive heating and vessel wall rupture. More recently, pulse stacking has been employed as a way to achieve subpurpuric clearance of vessels. In addition, vessel rupture and purpura can be minimized with increased epidermal cooling, longer pulse duration, and the use of longer wavelengths. Different areas of the face have different purpuric thresholds, with the jawline having the highest risk for purpura. Patients may also be on medications or supplements that increase their risk of bruising. NSAIDs (Aspirin, Advil, Motrin, Ibuprofen), Coumadin, Plavix, vitamin E, garlic, ginkgo biloba,

ginseng, and green tea are a few common medications that are frequent offenders. Pretreatment with herbal supplements bromelanin or arnica as well as posttreatment ice for ten minutes every hour for the remainder of the day of treatment can be employed to mitigate this risk.

When there is corresponding photodamage or when treating large surface areas, the IPL is often preferred because of its ability to treat other manifestations of sun damage (i.e., solar lentigo) as well as its treatment efficiency with the large crystal size. In addition, when treating vascular lesions with the IPL, do not press hard on the skin surface with the crystal as this blanches the vessel by squeezing out the target chromophore and decreasing treatment efficacy. When using the IPL to treat skin types III and IV, longer wavelengths, the use of longer and multiple pulse durations (4.0–5.0 ms), and longer delay times are considered safer. If no IPL is available, 20 to 30% overlap of the PDL may minimize a mottled appearance of treated areas.

The Nd:YAG is our preferred laser when treating deeper blood vessels and larger target vessels as this longer wavelength penetrates more deeply into the skin. This longer wavelength also has less absorption by melanin and is commonly used in patients with darker skin types. As mentioned earlier, it is also the treatment of choice in facial reticular veins. This longer wavelength has a diminished affinity for hemoglobin and fluences up to 10 times that of the KTP, and PDL are often required for efficacy. Because of this, this laser tends to be the most painful of the vascular lasers. In addition, there is an increased risk of blistering, scarring, and skin atrophy at these high energy levels; therefore pulse stacking is never used with the 1,064-nm laser.

Compared to the treatment of facial telangiectasias, fluences should be lowered by about 2–3 J/cm² in the treatment of poikiloderma of the chest and neck to avoid adverse effects. A good rule of thumb is to decrease fluence by 10 to 20% when treating nonfacial skin. For example, while a Lumenis One IPL setting of a 3.5/3.5 ms double pulse separated by 20 ms at a fluence of 17 J/cm² may be a modest setting for facial telangiectasias, it may lead to footprints and hypopigmentation if used on a chest with photodamage.

While these devices are usually well tolerated, many practitioners use topical anesthesia to increase patient comfort. If anesthesia is needed, we recommend the use of epidermal cooling devices, such as the Zimmer cooler, as topical anesthetic creams cause local vasoconstriction and minimize target chromophore. Some practitioners recommended skin stimulation, activity, rubbing, or warmth to increase the target and therefore treatment response.

Posttreatment Instructions

The immediate application of ice packs for ten to fifteen minutes is extremely helpful in reducing posttreatment erythema and edema. Prior to leaving the office, SPF 30+ is applied on the patient, with instructions to avoid sunlight until healing is complete. In addition to discussing expected posttreatment sequelae, patients are given written instructions to

- avoid excessive sunlight and wear sunscreen SPF 30+ every day
- if the treated area is red or swollen, apply an ice pack or cold compress for ten to fifteen minutes every hour, as needed
- use only gentle cleansers and moisturizers until healing is complete and avoid use of acne medications, lightening agents, acids, or fragranced products until healing is complete
- if blistering or crusting occurs, apply a topical antibiotic or Aquaphor healing ointment to the area twice daily; do not pick at the area as this increases the risk of scarring, and avoid direct sunlight to the area
- call the physician's office if any problems, questions, or concerns arise

Complications

Current IPL systems have minimal and transient adverse effects such as erythema or burning during treatment.

Graying or blanching of the skin after a pulse is indicative of epidermal damage. This will usually result in a blister and possibly hypopigmentation and textural change. This can be prevented by correctly selecting patient and laser parameters and by the use of appropriate epidermal cooling and good technique. Side effects include mild redness, swelling – particularly in the periorbital region – bruising with occasional blistering, crusting, and rare instances of atrophy.

LEG VEINS

Leg vein therapy is one of the most commonly requested cosmetic procedures. Leg veins are more challenging to treat than facial vessels because of their varied size, hydrostatic pressure, thicker vessel walls, feeding reticular system, and deeper locations. Leg vein changes include spider veins, reticular veins, perforators, tributaries, and varicose veins arising from reversed blood flow in the great and small saphenous vein. Thirty percent of the population by age twenty, and 80% of the population by age eighty, have some type of abnormal leg vein. Symptoms range from heaviness to aches and pains, night cramps and/or restless leg, and ankle edema. An appropriate patient evaluation should be performed before considering treatment options. When larger varicose veins are present, the associated telangiectases cannot be successfully treated without addressing the underlying hydrostatic pressure. In the presence of venous reflux, intravascular laser treatment (ILT) should be performed before considering selective treatment of superficial spider veins.

While laser and IPL sources have become an increasingly popular treatment for leg veins, sclerotherapy still remains the treatment of choice for spider veins and small reticular veins. Efficacy is higher and the side effect profile is lower compared with light- and laser-based treatment. However, many patients are biased toward laser, thinking that new technology supersedes traditional methods of treatment, while others are needle-phobic and have less resistance to laser treatment than sclerotherapy. Physicians may also have their own biases based on comfort level and experience with lasers versus sclerotherapy.

Laser Treatment

While the PDL, KTP, and IPL are very useful for small vessels, they have a limited depth of penetration and may result in dyspigmentation in tan patients or Fitzpatrick skin types IV–VI. Longer-wavelength lasers, such as Nd:YAG, allow for treatment of larger-diameter vessels, deeper vessels, and patients with darker skin types. A higher fluence is needed with the Nd:YAG to compensate for decreased hb absorption, and this can lead to more pain.

To maximize efficacy, it is important to match laser parameters to vessel size, for example, smaller vessels require high fluence with a small spot size, whereas larger,

TABLE 42.3: Optimal Laser and IPL Parameters for Treatment of Lower Extremity Vessels

	Wavelength (nm)	Pulse Duration (ms)	Spot Size (mm)
Diameter of vessels			
100 μm	580	1	–
300 μm	590	10	–
600 μm–1 mm	600	20–100	–
Vessel depth			
Less than 1 mm	>500	–	small (2–6)
Greater than 1 mm	>600	–	large (6–12)

Note: Adapted from Sadick NS, Laser Treatment of Leg Veins. In: Goldman MP, Weiss RA, eds., *Advanced Techniques in Dermatologic Surgery.* 2006.

TABLE 42.4: Summary of Vein Treatment Sequence

- Saphenous incompetence
  - **Endovenous RF or laser**
  - **Ligation ± short stripping**
  - **STS or POL foam**
- Saphenous branches
  - **Ambulatory phlebectomy**
  - **Foam sclerotherapy**
  - **Ambulatory phlebectomy**
  - **Foam sclerotherapy**
- Reticular veins
  - **Foam and glycerin sclerotherapy**
- Telangiectatic spider veins
  - **Glycerin sclerotherapy**
  - **Laser/IPL**

blue vessels require a lower fluence, larger spot size, and longer pulse widths (Table 42.3). Pulse stacking is commonly employed with PDL and IPL to generate more heat for subpurpuric clearance of vessels; however, pulse stacking is not recommended with the Nd:YAG as too much epidermal heat is generated, which can lead to epidermal damage. If necessary, a second pass can be performed after waiting for the skin to cool.

The clinical end point of therapy with lasers of leg veins is immediate vessel contraction and erythema. Prolonged vessel contraction and blanching are signs of overtreatment and can result in epidermal necrosis, pigmentary changes, and scarring. Epidermal cooling, the use of conservative settings, and test spots in darker patients help minimize this risk. There is a higher risk of dyspigmentation in tan and patients with Fitzpatrick skin types IV, V, and VI; therefore strict sun protection is recommended. Posttreatment hyperpigmentation represents melanin and usually resolves in two to six months; however, refractory cases may be treated with a Q-switched ruby laser.

While laser therapy for veins is gaining in popularity, it continues to be more expensive, more painful, and less efficacious than sclerotherapy. Hydrostatic pressure is not addressed with laser therapy of veins. For vessels greater than 1.5 mm in diameter, sclerotherapy remains the gold standard treatment. Vessels greater than 3 mm are not responsive to lasers. In the author's experience, laser and light therapy are best used to treat fine matting postsclerotherapy and isolated telangiectases, especially with very small vessels (less than 0.3 mm), which may be difficult to cannulate. Table 42.4 summarizes the author's treatment algorithm for leg veins.

Sclerotherapy of Telangiectasias and Reticular Veins

Sclerotherapy remains the gold standard for the treatment of telangiectasias and reticular veins. The optimal sclerosing agent is one that induces endothelial destruction

through endosclerosis and fibrosis. If the sclerosant is too weak, inadequate endothelial damage will occur, leading to thrombosis with no fibrosis and resultant recanalization of the vessel.

Too strong a solution may lead to uncontrolled destruction of vascular endothelium, which may result in hyperpigmentation, neoangiogenesis (telangiectatic matting), and ulceration secondary to sclerosant extravasation. Currently the only agents approved by the Food and Drug Administration (FDA) are sodium tetradecyl sulfate (STS) and sodium morrhuate. The use of glycerin and hypertonic saline for sclerotherapy is off-label. While hypertonic saline was commonly utilized in the past, it has fallen out of favor with many due to pain and its side effect profile, especially with the introduction of foam sclerotherapy and glycerin in the late 1990s. Table 42.5 summarizes the different sclerosing agents and their characteristics.

Technique for Treating Telangiectasias and Recticular Veins

With the patient in a standing position, a pretreatment physical examination is done to assess the extent and cause of the leg veins. Any patient with extensive venous insufficiency and bulging varicose veins should receive an ultrasound of the great saphenous vein (GSV) and the saphenofemoral junction. A review of contraindications to sclerotherapy should be performed (Table 42.6).

Choose Sclerosant

The only FDA-approved agents are sodium tetradecyl sulfate and sodium morrhuate; glycerin and hypertonic saline are used off-label (Table 42.4). Our protocol is as follows:

- for telangiectasias of less than 1 mm, glycerin (nonchromated)

    for 1- to 3-mm-diameter varicosities, 0.25% STS foam

    for 3- to 6-mm-diameter varicose veins, 0.5% STS foam

TABLE 42.5: Sclerosing Solutions and Their Characteristics

Sclerosing Solution	Class	Allergenicity	Advantages	Risks
Hypertonic saline (HS) 11.7–23.4%	hyperosmotic	none	no allergenicity FDA approved (off-label)	skin necrosis pain muscle cramping posttreatment hyperpigmentation (esp. in punctuate pattern)
Hypertonic saline and dextrose (Sclerodex)	hyperosmotic	low (reactions to phenethyl alcohol component)	less pain than HS	still painful skin necrosis (<HS) allergic reactions to phenethyl alcohol component
Sodium tetradecyl sulfate (STS) (Sotradecol)	detergent	rare anaphylaxis	**FDA approved**	hyperpigmentation (increases with higher concentrations) skin necrosis (higher concentrations)
Polidocanol (POL) (Aethoxyskerol)	detergent	rare anaphylaxis	painless no risk of necrosis in concentrations <1%	**FDA warning letter sent Nov. 2005** polidocanol is not an active ingredient contained in any FDA-approved drug product and the FDA does not sanction its use and distribution in compounded products
Sodium morrhuate (Scleromate)	detergent	highest risk of anaphylaxis		skin necrosis hyperpigmentation pain
Ethanolamine oleate	detergent	urticaria, anaphylaxis, pulmonary toxicity	FDA approved (primarily used for esophageal varices)	viscous, difficult to inject hemolytic reactions reports of acute renal failure in large doses skin necrosis pigmentation
Polyiodinated iodide (Varigloban)	chemical irritant	iodine hypersensitivity, anaphylaxis		skin necrosis pain on injection brown color makes intravascular placement difficult to confirm
72% glycerin with 8% chromium alum (Chromex)	chemical irritant	rare anaphylaxis	very low risk of hyperpigmentation, no risk of necrosis	high viscosity pain on injection hematuria/ureteral colic w/ large doses (>10 cc) purpura potential to create hyperosmotic state – must be used with caution in diabetic patients
72% glycerin diluted 2:1 with 1% lidocaine with epinephrine	chemical irritant	less than chromated glycerin	FDA approved (off-label for cerebral edema and acute glaucoma) less pigmentation less matting	same high viscosity and pain are mitigated by diluting with lidocaine localized urticaria

TABLE 42.6: Contraindications to Sclerotherapy

- History of deep vein thrombosis or blood clotting disorders
- History of ophthalmic migraines or other visual disturbances (foam sclerotherapy)
- Hypersensitivity to sclerosant
- Patient taking disulfuram should not be treated with polidocanol or sclerodex (hypertonic saline) since they contain ethyl alcohol
- Pregnant or breast-feeding patients; associated with dilation of the entire venous system, which persists for up to three months postpartum
- Patients taking tamoxifen; tamoxifen is responsible for superficial phlebitis in patients treated by sclerotherapy
- Patients taking systemic estrogen preparations; persistent telangiectatic matting is increased in patients on oral contraceptive agents or hormone replacement therapy
- Travel; administering sclerosing injections immediately prior to a long flight or trip
- Inability to ambulate

- for those greater than 6 mm, encourage CTEV (endovenous closure) with phlebectomy

Foam sclerotherapy with STS has many advantages over liquid STS:

- increased volume but decreased total sclerosant injected
- highest concentration contacts vessel wall
- total obliteration of the vessel
- very slow washout
- can be used as contrast agent under Duplex ultrasound
- foam is made with two syringes and a two-way connecter; one syringe with 4 cc air is mixed with one syringe of 1 cc STS to make foam

Injection Technique

Our injection technique is characterized by the following steps:

- Patients lie down (never treat patients who are standing up).
- A 30-gauge, ½-inch needle is bent at a 30 degree angle.
- Nondominant hand traction is used to keep skin taut.
- Alcohol is swabbed on the skin prior to injection to increase the index of refraction, making vessels more visible.
- Brisk injection with low injection pressure prevents vascular distention and optimizes interaction between sclerosant and endothelium.
- A quantity of 0.1–0.4 cc of sclerosant is injected via the *empty vein technique*: as the vessel is injected with the sclerosant, vessel clearance will be seen. Keep slowly injecting until you cannot follow vessel clearance any further (the vessel has gone deep).
- Start from the most proximal point and treat the largest vessel first, working toward smaller vessels (i.e., treatment with foam sclerotherapy of the perforator and reticular

veins before using glycerin for treatment of the spider telangiectasia).

Foam sclerotherapy is only indicated for vessels larger than 1 mm in diameter as its use in smaller vessels can lead to increased pigmentation and matting. One week of a class II (30–40 mm Hg) graduated compression stocking placed immediately following sclerotherapy is critical to treatment success. It has been shown to decrease the extent of thrombosis as well as decrease the risk of recanalization, pigmentation, and telangiectatic matting. Walking for thirty minutes after treatment ensures rapid dilution of the sclerosing solution and minimizes thromboembolic events.

Treatment Interval

Most patients will require two to three treatments per leg with a minimum interval between treatments of six to eight weeks. If telangiectatic matting occurs, allow a rest period of six to nine months as we have found that most resolves on its own in that time (Figure 42.3). If matting persists, confirm that there is no feeding vein and consider laser/IPL treatment. If a poor response to treatment is seen with

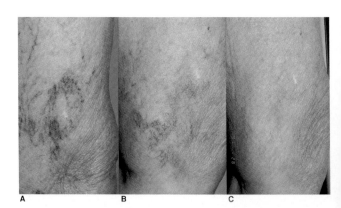

FIGURE 42.3: **A,** *Pretreatment.* **B,** *Telangiectatic matting developed after two sclerotherapy sessions.* **C,** *Clearance one year later.*

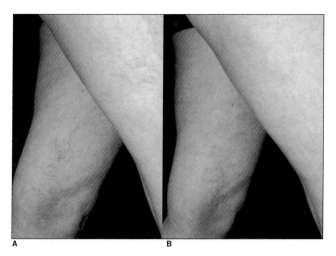

FIGURE 42.4: A, Pretreatment. B, Two months after one treatment with STS 0.25% foam and glycerin.

treatment, (1) reexamine the patient to find a possible source of reflux previously missed, (2) increase the concentration of sclerosant, and (3) consider switching to another sclerosant. Figure 42.4 demonstrates typical results.

VARICOSE VEINS

In any patient with extensive venous insufficiency and bulging varicose veins, an ultrasound of the GSV and the saphenofemoral junction should be performed to evaluate for incompetence. If the GSV is larger than 0.5 cm and if any reflux is seen, the patient will need endovenous intervention of the GSV. FDA approved since 2002, intravascular laser treatment is a minimally invasive in-office treatment alternative to surgical stripping of the GSV.

There are two types of endovenous procedure: ILT and endovenous radiofrequency ablation. Once obtaining percutaneous access to the GSV under tumescent anesthesia, energy is directed from inside the vessel to shrink and seal the targeted vein. Although initially developed by dermatologic surgeons, endovenous ablation has been embraced by many other specialties, including radiology, vascular surgery, and anesthesiology. Initially only performed with bipolar radiofrequency, several lasers are now used for endovenous ablation. They are divided into lasers that target hemoglobin (810, 940, and 980 nm) within the vein and lasers targeting water in the vein wall (1,320 nm). Comparative studies between the 810-nm diode laser, 1,320-nm Nd:YAG laser, and high-frequency radiation showed comparable results for the 1,320-nm Nd:YAG and high-frequency radiation over the 810-nm diode laser.

Endovenous occlusion with ILT is our preferred method to treat GSV-related varicose veins. There is reduced pain and bruising with the 1,320-nm Nd:YAG. Tumescent anesthesia is critical to the safety of the endovenous technique as it provides a heat sink to protect perivascular tissues from the intravascular energy. It also

decreases the size of the treated vein, allowing for better absorption of energy by the target chromophore, and reduces intravascular blood. The tumescent technique provides safe and effective anesthesia for patients with immediate postprocedure ambulation, which is vital to prevent the formation of deep vein thrombosis. Possible complications of endovenous laser treatment include purpura, swelling, pain, thermal skin burns, and transient numbness. Following the procedure, a compression stocking is worn for seven days, and most patients return to work within forty-eight hours.

Treatment Technique

All visible varicose veins are marked out with the patient standing. Still standing, the GSV is located first with Doppler (to avoid putting too much gel on the skin, which will prevent marking the vein). The location is confirmed with Duplex ultrasound, with the patient lying down in the operative position, and the access point for laser entry is marked out.

The lights are turned off, and a Venoscope is placed over the course of the GSV. This transilluminates superficial varicose veins that are 1–2 mm in depth. They are marked with another marking pen color and are removed with microphlebectomy after the ILT procedure is performed. The patient is then taken to the operative suite, surgically prepped in a sterile manner, and placed in a 30 degree Trendelenburg position.

The area surrounding the GSV and distal tributaries to be treated is then infiltrated with 0.1% lidocaine tumescent anesthesia. The amount of fluid averages 800 mL, with a typical systemic lidocaine dose of 8 mg/kg. The GSV is then accessed through a 3-mm incision in the medial midthigh, usually 20 cm inferior to the safeno-femoral junction (SFJ). A 500- to 600-μm laser fiber is inserted into the vein within a protective sheath to allow insertion of the fiber. The sheath is then removed.

Correct placement of the laser fiber tip 2 cm distal to the SFJ is confirmed through catheter length measurement, duplex examination, and viewing the He:Ne aiming beam through the skin. The laser is activated in a continuous firing mode with slow mechanical withdrawal at a rate of 1 mm/s. This technique minimizes pain and maintains efficacy of treatment.

The proximal portion of the GSV is treated with laser closure, and the distal portion, including all varicose tributaries, is removed with a standard ambulatory phlebectomy technique. It is important that treatment with the laser is limited to the GSV segment above the knee to prevent paresthesia to the saphenous nerve.

The treated leg is then wrapped in copious padding to absorb the tumescent fluid with an overlying compression bandage. No incisions are closed to allow for drainage of the anesthetic solution over twenty-four hours.

The patient returns the next day, when the leg is checked for hematoma or other adverse sequelae, and the bandage is changed to a 30- to 40-mm Hg graduated compression stocking. The compression stocking is left on twenty-four hours a day for one week.

SUGGESTED READING

Telangiectasias, Facial Veins, and Poikiloderma

Alam M, Dover JS, Arndt KA. Treatment of facial telangiectasia with variable-pulse high-fluence pulsed-dye laser: comparison of efficacy with fluences immediately above and below the purpura threshold. *Dermatol. Surg.* 2003;29:681–4; discussion 685.

Baumler W, Ulrich H, Hartl A, Landthaler M, Shafirstein G. Optimal parameters for the treatment of leg veins using Nd:YAG lasers at 1064 nm. *Br. J. Dermatol.* 2006;155:364–71.

Bernstein EF, Lee J, Lowery J, et al. Treatment of spider veins with the 595 nm pulsed dye laser. *J. Am. Acad. Dermatol.* 1998;39:746–50.

Goldman MP. Optimal management of facial telangiectasia. *Am. J. Clin. Dermatol.* 2004;5:423–34.

Ross EV, Smirnov M, Pankratov M, Altshuler G. Intense pulsed light and laser treatment of facial telangiectasias and dyspigmentation: some theoretical and practical comparisons. *Dermatol. Surg.* 2005;31(9 Pt 2):1188–98.

Sadick NS. Laser and intense pulsed light therapy for the esthetic treatment of lower extremity veins. *Am. J. Clin. Dermatol.* 2003;4:545–54. Review.

Tanghetti E, Sherr E. Treatment of telangiectasia using the multipass technique with the extended pulse width, pulsed dye laser (Cynosure V-Star). *J. Cosmet. Laser Ther.* 2003;5:71–5.

Uebelhoer NS, Bogle MA, Stewart B, Arndt KA, Dover JS. A split-face comparison study of pulsed 532-nm KTP laser and 595-nm pulsed dye laser in the treatment of facial telangiectasias and diffuse telangiectatic facial erythema. *Dermatol. Surg.* 2007;33:441–8.

Weiss RA, Goldman MP, Weiss MA. Treatment of poikiloderma of Civatte with an intense pulsed light source. *Dermatol. Surg.* 2000;26:823–7; discussion 828.

West TB, Alster TS. Comparison of the long-pulse dye (590–595 nm) and KTP (532 nm) lasers in the treatment of facial and leg telangiectasias. *Dermatol. Surg.* 1998;24:221–6.

Woo SH, Ahn HH, Kim SN, Kye YC. Treatment of vascular skin lesions with the variable-pulse 595 nm pulsed dye laser. *Dermatol. Surg.* 2006;32:41–8.

Leg Veins

Ceulen RP, Bullens-Goessens YI, Pi-Van DE, et al. Outcomes and side effects of duplex-guided sclerotherapy in the treatment of great saphenous veins with 1% versus 3% polidocanol foam: results of a randomized controlled trial with 1-year follow-up. *Dermatol. Surg.* 2007;33:276–81.

Dover JS, Sadick NS, Goldman MP. The role of lasers and light sources in the treatment of leg veins. *Dermatol. Surg.* 1999;25:328–36.

Frullini A, Cavezzi A. Sclerosing foam in the treatment of varicose veins and telangiectases: history and analysis of safety and complications. *Dermatol. Surg.* 2002;28:11–15.

Goldman MP, Weiss RA. Treatment of leg telangiectasias with laser and high-intense pulsed light. *Dermatol. Ther.* 2000; 13:28–49.

Guex JJ, Allaert FA, Gillet JL, Chleir F. Immediate and midterm complications of sclerotherapy: report of a prospective multicenter registry of 12,173. *Dermatol. Surg.* 2005;31:123–8.

Huang Y, Jiang M, Li W, Lu X, Huang X, Lu M. Endovenous laser treatment combined with a surgical strategy for treatment of venous insufficiency in lower extremity: a report of 208 cases. *J. Vasc. Surg.* 2005;42:494–501.

Kauvar ANB. The role of lasers in the treatment of leg veins. *Semin. Cutan. Med. Surg.* 2000;19:245–52.

Leach BC, Goldman MP. Comparative trial between sodium tetradecyl sulfate and glycerin in the treatment of telangiectatic leg veins. *Dermatol. Surg.* 2003;29:612–14.

Lupton JR, Alster TS, Romero P. Clinical comparison of sclerotherapy versus long-pulsed Nd:YAG laser treatment for lower extremity telangiectases. *Dermatol. Surg.* 2002;28:694–7.

Omura N, Dover J, Arndt K, Kauvar A. Treatment of reticular leg veins with a 1064 nm Nd:YAG. *J. Am. Acad. Dermatol.* 2003;48:76–81.

Puggioni A, Kalra M, Carmo M, Mozes G, Gloviczki P. Endovenous laser therapy and radiofrequency ablation of the great saphenous vein: analysis of early efficacy and complications. *J. Vasc. Surg.* 2005;42:488–93.

Rao J, Wildemore JK, Goldman MP. Double-blind prospective comparative trial between foamed and liquid polidocanol and sodium tetradecyl sulfate in the treatment of varicose and telangiectatic leg veins. *Dermatol. Surg.* 2005;31:631–5; discussion 635.

Sadick NS. Advances in the treatment of varicose veins: ambulatory phlebectomy, foam sclerotherapy, endovascular laser, and radiofrequency closure. *Dermatol. Clin.* 2005;23:443–55.

Sadick NS, Wasser S. Combined endovascular laser plus ambulatory phlebectomy for the treatment of superficial venous incompetence: a 4-year perspective. *J. Cosmet. Laser Ther.* 2007;9:9–13.

Weiss RA. Endovenous techniques for elimination of saphenous reflux: a valuable treatment modality. *Dermatol. Surg.* 2001;27:902–5.

Weiss RA, Dover JS. Leg vein management: sclerotherapy, ambulatory phlebectomy, and laser surgery. *Semin. Cutan. Med. Surg.* 2002;21:76–103.

Weiss RA, Sadick NS, Goldman MP, Weiss MA. Post-sclerotherapy compression: controlled comparative study of duration of compression and its effects on clinical outcome. *Dermatol. Surg.* 1999;25:105–8.

Yamaki T, Nozaki M, Iwasaka S. Comparative study of duplex-guided foam sclerotherapy and duplex-guided liquid sclerotherapy for the treatment of superficial venous insufficiency. *Dermatol. Surg.* 2004;30:718–22.

CHAPTER 43

Vascular Lasers

Paul J. Carniol
Abby Meltzer

Laser treatment of vascular lesions requires an understanding of the variety of vascular lesions as well as the available vascular lasers. The more commonly occurring cutaneous vascular lesions can be divided into a few categories: hemangiomas, vascular malformations, telangiectasias, and pyogenic granulomas. The natural history and treatment of these lesions varies, depending on the diagnosis.

Although a minority of hemangiomas are present at birth, the majority usually appear shortly after birth and grow for a limited time (Marler and Mulliken 2001; Mulliken et al. 2000; Mulliken and Glowacki 1982; Bautland 2006). Usually by eighteen to twenty-four months of age, hemangiomas will stop growing. Currently it is believed that hemangiomas develop as a result of in utero implantation of placental cells into the fetus (Phung et al. 2005), and most hemangiomas will subsequently regress spontaneously.

However, it takes years for this to occur. During this time, children can be subject to teasing from their peers. Frequently, even after regression, there will still be visible residual changes in the skin. If treated early, many of these hemangiomas will respond to treatment with a vascular laser such as a pulsed dye laser. In response to the laser treatment, some of the hemangiomas will stop proliferating, and some will regress.

Considering this, when possible, and depending on the particulars of the hemangioma and the patient, the first author recommends initiating treatment during the first few months of age. Typically, patients up to twelve to fifteen months of age can be treated with the laser without using general anesthesia.

As for all patients, care must be taken to maintain all laser safety precautions, especially eye protection. This can be especially challenging in an uncooperative child.

In selecting the laser settings, the authors recommend starting with the lowest fluence laser settings that elicit a mild response. The first author uses the first one or two laser pulses as test spots. After one to two pulses, it is best to stop and observe the effect of the test spots. If there is a mild response, then proceed with the treatment; however, if there is a an excessive response and you are already using a low fluence, stop treatment and have the patient return for reevaluation of the test spots before further treatment.

For some noticeable hemangiomas that have not responded sufficiently to laser therapy, or if, for any variety of reasons, the patient or the lesion are not candidates for laser treatment, surgery can be considered. The decision to use surgical intervention is always complex. When deciding whether to undertake surgery, the risks of surgery should be compared to the potential risks of not performing surgery.

It is possible for a patient to have more than one site involved with hemangiomas. Therefore, in young children, it is important to consider the possibility of involvement of other regions, including the upper airway. Upper airway involvement can cause significant airway obstruction. Often, this can be treated with lasers. In some patients, systemic corticosteroid therapy may be necessary.

Facial hemangiomas can also cause visual obstruction. Due to potential central nervous system effects from this visual field obstruction, even if the hemangioma later regresses, there can be permanent vision loss. As such, early intervention is recommended as soon as there is a risk of visual obstruction. This may consist of systemic therapy or injection of the lesion. Considering the direct associated risks, the first author recommends that injection in this area only be performed by a physician who has experience with this procedure.

Port-wine stains and vascular malformations typically are present at birth. These cutaneous lesions enlarge proportionately as the child grows. Over time, the number of blood vessels usually does not increase, but the vessels can increase in diameter. In association with the increase in vessel diameter, there is usually associated darkening and thickening of the port-wine stain.

These lesions can be associated with intracranial vascular malformations. In one study, 78% of patients with port-wine stains with cutaneous involvement of the V1 dermatone had neurological and/or ocular involvement (Ch'ng and Tan 2007).

In the past several years, the pulse dye laser has been used to treat these lesions. The majority of these lesions will lighten after treatment with the pulse dye laser (i.e., V-Beam, Candela). Typically, complete clearance is not achievable (Lanigan and Taibjee 2004). In one study, a series of treatments with the pulse dye laser at two-week intervals was more efficacious than treatment at six-week intervals (Tomson et al. 2006).

Some of these lesions will not respond to the pulsed dye laser (Lanigan and Taibjee 2004). More recently, a sequential pulse dye and 1,064-nm YAG laser has been developed that can be used to treat resistant lesions (Cynergy). This laser first fires the pulse dye laser, and then, after a minimal delay, it fires the 1,064-nm laser. The fluence of each laser as well as the delay between lasers can be adjusted. Furthermore, if desired, each of the component lasers can be used independently.

In one study of vascular lesions treated with a pulse dye laser, with a ten-year follow-up, it was noted that there was darkening of the residual lesion over time following treatment. However, even though there was some darkening, the lesions were still lighter than before treatment (Koster and De Borgie 2007). In the majority of patients with port-wine stains, complete clearance cannot be achieved (Lanigan and Taibjee 2004). Although, in the first author's experience, the vast majority of these lesions are responsive to laser treatment, it has been noted that a significant portion of the lesions are not responsive to pulse dye lasers (Lanigan and Taibjee 2004).

There is some controversy over the treatment interval for port-wine stains. Depending on the appearance of the skin during the recovery period, the first author usually waits one to three months between treatments. This interval allows time for the tissues to recover from the laser treatment. In contrast to the first author's practice, in one study, port-wine stains treated with a pulsed dye laser at two-week intervals had a greater response than those treated at six-week intervals (Tomson et al. 2006).

Many people are bothered by facial telangiectasias. As could be anticipated, these telangiectasias can be treated with vascular lasers. Most of the telangiectasias will respond to treatment with either a 532-nm laser, 940-nm laser, or 595-nm pulse dye laser. The choice of laser can depend on multiple factors.

Typically, there is no ecchymosis after treatment with a 532-nm or 940-nm laser. Therefore the first author prefers to use these wavelengths for treatment of telangiectasias. The first author has reported that smaller-diameter vessels respond better to a 532-nm laser and that larger-diameter vessels respond better to a 940-nm laser (Carniol et al. 2005).

When it first became available, ecchymosis was associated with treatment with the pulse dye laser. During the past decade, modifications have been made to this laser, including longer pulse durations and using a series of pulses, rather than one short pulse. These modifications have diminished or eliminated the ecchymosis associated with treatment.

Pyogenic granulomas are lobular capillary hemangiomas. Some patients report minor prior trauma preceding the appearance of this neoplasm, while others do not report any preceding trauma. These lesions can be treated either with excision and closure or shave excision with cautery of the base.

The literature has varied on the optimal treatment regimen. Recently, one retrospective study reported that a majority of 128 children treated with shave excision and cautery of the base, over a ten-year period, did not have a recurrence of this neoplasm (Pagliai and Cohen 2004). The first author varies his treatment technique depending on the presentation of the lesion. If the lesion has a narrow base and does not seem to have a significant component below the skin surface, then it is treated with shave excision and cautery of the base; however, if the lesion has a broad base and a significant deep component, then it is treated with excision.

SUGGESTED READING

Bautland CG, et al. The pathogenesis of hemangiomas: a review. *Plast. Reconstr. Surg.* 2006;117:29e–35e.

Carniol PJ, Price J, Olive A. Treatment of telangiectasias with the 532nm and the 940/532nm diode laser. *Facial Plast. Surg.* 2005;21:117–19.

Ch'ng A, Tan ST. Facial port-wine stains – clinical stratification and risks of neuro-ocular involvement. *Plast. Reconstr. Aesthetic Surg.* 2007.

Koster PHL, De Borgie CAJM. Redarkening of port-wine stains 10 years after pulsed-dye laser treatment. *N. Engl. J. Med.* 2007;356:1235–40.

Lanigan SW, Taibjee SM. Recent advances in laser treatment of port-wine stains. *Br. J. Dermatol.* 2004;151:527–33.

Marler J, Mulliken J. Vascular anomalies – classification, diagnosis and natural history. *Facial Plast. Surg. Clin. North Am.* 2001;9:495–504.

Mulliken JB, Fishman SJ, Burrows PE. Vascular anomalies. *Curr. Probl. Surg.* 2000;37:519–84.

Mulliken JB, Glowacki J. Hemangiomas and vascular malformation in infants and children: a classification based on endothelial characteristics. *Plast. Reconstr. Surg.* 1982;69:412–20.

Pagliai KA, Cohen BA. Pyogenic granuloma in children. *Pediatr. Dermatol.* 2004;21(1):10–13.

Phung TL, Hochman M, Mihm M. Current knowledge of the pathogenesis of infantile hemangiomas. *Arch. Facial Plast. Surg.* 2005;7:319–21.

Tomson N, Lim SP, Abdullah A, Lanigan SW. The treatment of port wine stains with the pulse-dye laser at 2-week and 6-week intervals: a comparative study. *Br. J. Dermatol.* 2006;154:676–9.

FULLY ABLATIVE TISSUE REMODELING (CO$_2$, Er:YAG, PLASMA)

CHAPTER 44

Overview of CO$_2$ and Er:YAG Lasers and Plasma Devices

Edgar F. Fincher

Sorin Eremia

Laser skin resurfacing remains the most effective modality for skin rejuvenation. Indications for treatment include dyschromia, photoaging, rhytids, skin laxity, and acneiform scars. Although numerous nonablative laser and light devices have been developed over the years, none of them is able to deliver results equivalent to ablative devices. The effectiveness of ablative lasers results from their ability to accomplish two major effects: first, complete and total vaporization of the epidermis removes unwanted pigment and solar-damaged cells; second, there is deeper penetration and diffusion of thermal energy that heats dermal tissues, causes tissue contraction, and stimulates new collagen production. The net effect of these two processes is that a new, more uniform epidermis is regenerated, without unwanted pigmentation. Additionally, solar elastosis is removed from the superficial dermis, yielding a brighter, more lustrous skin tone, and immediate tissue contraction plus new collagen production lead to the reduction of wrinkles and tighter skin.

The use of ablative lasers for skin resurfacing goes back to the 1980s. Early devices consisted of continuous wave CO$_2$ lasers. These lasers provided adequate ablation of tissue; however, longer dwell times resulted in prolonged and unpredictable thermal heating, charring of the tissue, and a high risk of scarring. The true breakthrough occurred in the early to mid-1990s, when CO$_2$ pulsed lasers with pulse durations in the millisecond domain were introduced for resurfacing. The addition of efficient scanners made these systems even more practical. The new generation of lasers, when used at correct settings, were able to vaporize tissue, with the high heat of vaporization actually providing a cooling effect to the remaining tissue at the base. The thermal dynamics of this tissue vaporization actually provided a cooling effect to the residual tissue at the base of the laser field, yet still provided enough heat to cauterize small vessels and nerve endings to provide a bloodless operative field. Furthermore, the thermal heating was sufficient to stimulate significant tissue tightening, both from an immediate effect on collagen and by activating fibroblasts to produce new collagen and elastic tissue deposition. The laser-resurfacing gold standard for many years was provided by two systems: the Coherent

Ultrapulse device with a computerized pattern generator, and a conceptually very different device, a spiral-scanned, high-power, continuous CO_2 wave system from Sharplan Lasers, which was equally popular. Both systems continue to have many loyal, adept users today, who consider either of these lasers the benchmark for tissue resurfacing. The big difference in treatment parameters with these devices is making a single pass at high power and, if necessary, a second pass for small areas of more severe rhytids such as the upper lip and glabella. This treatment approach allows for vastly faster and safer recovery, with virtually the same dramatic long-term levels of improvement. Delayed hypopigmentation nevertheless remains a problem in a small but significant percentage of patients, especially for types I and II skin. Through various mergers, both these systems are now under the Lumenis brand. Overtreatment with multiple laser passes and inadequate postoperative care (use of deeper ablative resurfacing requires intensive aftercare to induce very rapid reepithelialization, prevention, and, if they occur, prompt and effective treatment of complications) led to many problems and complications and a drop in popularity. An attempt to resolve problems with many weeks of persistent erythema and latent hypopigmentation led to development of very short pulse laser systems with microsecond dwell times. While some believed these CO_2 lasers provided safer and more predictable tissue ablation, and decreased the incidence of side effects, many more passes were necessary, and the results were not as good or as predictable. As a result, these devices never gained much popularity.

As the search for safer alternatives in laser resurfacing continued, the Er:YAG lasers soon followed with the offer of increased water absorption with less collateral tissue heating, and thus a more precise depth of ablation. The first erbium lasers were short-pulsed lasers that provided only minimal depth of ablation with each pass and thus required many passes to achieve complete ablation. Lack of tissue heating provided no hemostasis, which was a major nuisance, and the level of skin tightening achieved was far inferior to the CO_2 laser. Long-pulsed, variable-pulse, and dual-mode erbium lasers then followed with increased depths of ablation and longer dwell times that provided enhanced tissue heating and better hemostasis and tissue tightening compared to the earlier short-pulsed lasers. The addition of computerized pattern generators to CO_2 and erbium systems provided faster, yet more predictable treatments. The scanner allowed the operator to dial in the desired treatment pattern, place down relatively large spot sizes, control the exact amount of tissue overlap, and reduce the possibility of pulse stacking or unwanted pulses to the treatment area.

The newest technique for skin resurfacing is the use of plasma energy. The Portrait (Rhytec Inc.) is not a laser, but rather, a plasma generator. In short, this system utilizes plasma energy derived from excited nitrogen gas to create thermal ablation and deeply penetrating thermal modification for epidermal resurfacing and dermal collagen rearrangement. This chapter will briefly review the technical aspects of each of these resurfacing modalities, along with general treatment protocols for resurfacing.

ABLATIVE RESURFACING: LASER-TISSUE INTERACTIONS

The basic theory behind laser resurfacing relates to the ability of the lasers to remove the epidermis through tissue vaporization. More specifically, the infrared lasers utilize water present in intracellular and extracellular fluid as their target chromophore. The laser energy is absorbed by the keratinocytes, and when sufficient energy is delivered, the cells are vaporized, leaving behind only remnants of desiccated debris. This zone of immediate tissue vaporization is termed the *zone of thermal ablation* (Figure 44.1), and this accounts for the removal of damaged epithelium. Regeneration and healing then occur from skin appendages. A significant portion of residual heat does diffuse beyond the cell and penetrates into the surrounding tissues. A

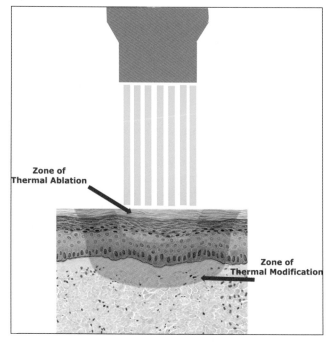

FIGURE 44.1: *This diagram illustrates the tissue effects that occur during ablative laser resurfacing. The zone of immediate laser-tissue interaction is termed the* **zone of thermal ablation.** *This is where the majority of the laser energy is absorbed and results in vaporization of the tissue. Residual heat then diffuses into the surrounding tissue, creating the* **zone of thermal modification.** *This is the area where the thermal energy causes contraction of collagen and stimulates fibroblasts to produce new collagen in the wound.*

significant portion of this energy, known as the *zone of thermal activation*, is responsible for two very important effects regarding wrinkle reduction and tissue tightening. First, the thermal energy is able to cause contraction of dermal collagen. In vitro studies demonstrate that heating collagen fibers to approximately 60 to 62 degrees Celsius causes contraction (shortening) of collagen fibers. It is this shortening that is thought to correlate with what is seen visibly as immediate tissue tightening. Second, thermal activation is responsible for stimulating a wound-healing cascade that includes major inflammatory modifiers such as interleukin-1β, tumor necrosis factor alpha, transforming growth factor beta, and many matrix metalloproteinases. The net result of this cascade is the production of new collagen from dermal fibroblasts. Histologic analysis of postresurfacing skin reveals that the upper dermis is filled with a layer of new collagen fibers with randomly oriented elastin fibrils, in effect creating a controlled or limited scar. These studies further demonstrate that this new collagen production by fibroblasts can continue for six to twelve months and appears to correlate to long-term wrinkle reduction, skin thickening, and tightening.

In summary, thermal ablation vaporizes superficial layers of tissue, removing a damaged and aged epidermis, and promotes regeneration and healing of new epidermal tissue. Thermal activation causes immediate tissue contraction and new collagen production to reduce wrinkles and tighten skin. It is this unique combination of effects that provides the unmatched degree of tissue rejuvenation. Although results are unmatched by less invasive, nonablative lasers, there are potential side effects that must be considered when electing to perform ablative resurfacing. With increasing depths of penetration, the threshold for unwanted side effects (i.e., delayed healing, scarring, hypopigmentation) is lowered. Patient selection and appropriate preoperative planning and postoperative care are essential for successful outcomes.

CARBON DIOXIDE (CO_2) LASER

The CO_2 laser continues to be the industry standard by which all other resurfacing devices, ablative or nonablative, are measured. The reason for this lies in the fact that the CO_2 laser delivers unsurpassed tissue tightening and wrinkle reduction. The CO_2 laser has a wavelength of 10,600 nm, placing it in the infrared domain. With a high specific absorption for water, this laser deposits approximately 80 to 90% of its energy in the first 30–40 μm of tissue, accounting for its highly predictable depth of ablation. When adequate energy is delivered to the tissue, intracellular water absorbs the laser energy and leads to immediate vaporization of the cells. The residual laser energy passes deeper into the tissue and to surrounding tissue to produce a zone of thermal modification (described previously),

leading to contraction of collagen fibers and immediate tissue tightening. Compared to other resurfacing lasers, the CO_2 laser penetrates deeper and provides a larger zone of thermal modification and thus enhanced tissue tightening. Other beneficial effects of the CO_2 laser are its ability to provide coagulation and a bloodless field during treatment. Resurfacing with short-pulsed erbium lasers, by comparison, leads to bleeding from dermal vessels after multiple passes. The presence of blood not only limits visualization, but also blocks penetration of subsequent laser passes into the underlying tissue.

Laser protocols have changed over the years with advances in technology. Early pulsed lasers consisted of single-pulse systems that required careful operator technique to ensure an even treatment and to prevent pulse stacking. Furthermore, early continuous lasers had a higher potential for irreversible thermal injury and scarring. With the advent of spiral-scanned, short–dwell time and short-pulse lasers, some with microsecond-pulse durations, laser energy was now delivered in pulses shorter than the thermal relaxation time of the epidermis (1 ms), creating a much safer operation. The addition of computer-generated scanning systems was the next major advance. These scanning systems enabled the user to select the pattern (circle, square, rectangle, hexagon, etc.), the size of the scan, and the percentage of beam overlap. The addition of these scanners further advanced the safety margin of skin resurfacing, creating a more predictable operation and significantly shortened operative time. Today, short-pulse lasers equipped with scanners are the standard. Treatment with a single pass at high power settings with the classic CO_2 lasers has been shown equally effective over the long term for all but the most severe types of rhytids. The second author (SE) has been using the same 40-W, continuous-wave laser with a spiral-scanned, computerized-pattern-generated laser since 1995. The typical settings are "feather touch" spiral scan mode, 36 W, 11-mm square pattern. For the past ten years, most patients have been treated over the entire face with a single pass at these levels, followed with a second pass only for selected areas of deeper rhytids, especially the upper lip. Most patients can achieve excellent results with this protocol (Figures 44.2–44.4), which greatly decreases recovery time as well as risks of complications, including late hypopigmentation. With full epidermal and superficial dermal ablative lasers, reepithelization occurs primarily from hair follicles and sebaceous glands. A major shortcoming of fully ablative CO_2 lasers is the limitation of their use to the face. Treatment of off-face sites, such as the neck, chest, or extremities, has a higher risk of scarring due to thinner skin in these areas and/or a reduced density of skin appendages from which reepithelialization can occur. The new fractional CO_2 lasers are attempting to overcome this obstacle and are discussed separately in Chapters 58 and 64.

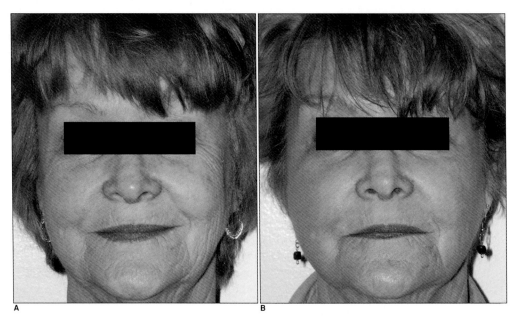

FIGURE 44.2: **A,** *Pretreatment.* **B,** *Twelve months post-full-face, single-pass, high-power CO_2 laser treatment.*

TREATMENT PROTOCOL

The actual treatment settings will vary with the specific device; however, some general guidelines are worth mentioning. Preoperatively, patients are provided with antibiotic prophylaxis beginning the day prior to the operation. Antibiotics include an anti-*staphylococcus* prophylaxis and an antiviral to prevent herpes reactivation and the possibil-

ity of scarring. Some surgeons will also include antifungal coverage with fluconazole to prevent yeast infection. These are continued for one week postoperation. Various types of anesthesia are utilized, depending on the patient and the areas to be treated. In general, focal areas, such as perioral and periorbital regions, can be adequately covered with regional nerve blockades. Full-face resurfacing, on the other hand, usually requires regional nerve blocks

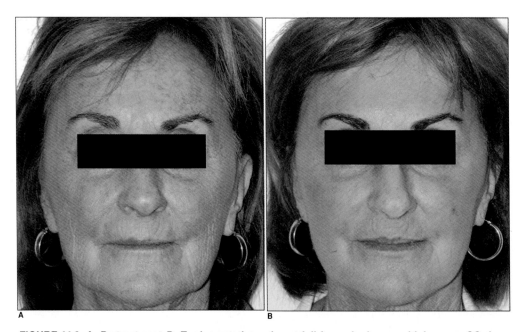

FIGURE 44.3: **A,** *Pretreatment.* **B,** *Twelve months and post-full-face, single-pass, high-power CO_2 laser treatment. Note that more severely wrinkled areas, such as the upper lip, may need an additional pass or retreatment six to twelve months later, as was eventually done for this patient.*

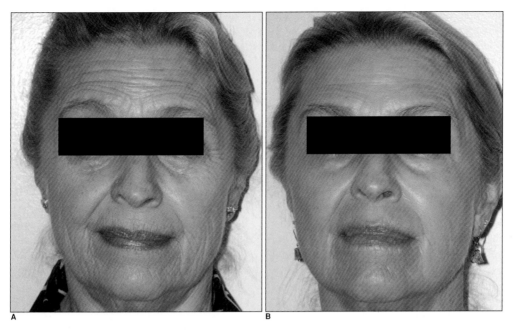

FIGURE 44.4: **A,** *Pretreatment.* **B,** *Twelve months and post-high-power CO_2 laser treatment, full face single pass, with second passes over the glabella, crow's feet, and upper lip.*

plus supplemental local tumescent anesthesia of the sides of the face and variable levels of sedation, ranging from oral benzodiazepines plus analgesics (i.e., IM meperidine, ketorolac, Stadol) to IV sedation. Safety requirements for the procedure include eye protection for patients and operators; the absence of any flammable gases (oxygen, anesthetic inhalants); moist towels around the patient to prevent combustion of surgical drapes; ointment application to eyebrows to prevent charring; and a fire extinguisher, for emergencies.

With high-power, spiral-scanned, continuous-wave lasers, and even with high-powered classic-pulsed lasers, single-pass treatment with an additional pass to selected areas has been the favored approach of most experienced CO_2 enthusiasts for at least the past seven to ten years. Full-face resurfacing with lower-power or ultrashort pulse lasers may require delivering more passes than using longer-pulsed systems, at anywhere from one to three passes to the tissue. In general, two passes are delivered to the crow's feet, forehead, and perioral area. A single pass usually suffices for the lateral cheeks and thin eyelid skin. An optional third pass to the perioral area for deep rhytids, focal deeper rhytids, and deep acne scars can be performed, if necessary. Sterile saline-soaked gauze is used to wipe away char between passes. The skin must then be dried thoroughly before applying the next laser pass; otherwise residual water absorbs laser energy, thus limiting energy to the tissue itself. With multiple passes, no wiping is generally performed after the final pass, as the dessicated tissue can serve as a biological dressing. However, with single-pass treatment, gauze abrasion increases the effectiveness of the single-pass

treatment to a level of maybe one and a half passes, but also prolongs recovery. Why not make a second pass at a lower fluence? That option is limited because lowering the fluence significantly can have the opposite effect, by carbonizing, rather than vaporizing, tissue.

Postoperative wound care consists of either an open dressing of petrolatum-based ointment with repeat application three to four times daily, along with gentle cleansing with a non-detergent-based cleanser, or the use of a modern closed-dressing system. The closed – actually, semipermeable – dressings, which are far superior to petrolatum-type aftercare, consist of flexible bandages that can be left in place for four to five days before removing and transitioning to an open dressing. In reality, at least partial changes of these dressings, if not complete replacement, is often needed after one to two days. Flexan, Diamond Seal, Silon, and Vigilon are some of the more common bandages available. The closed bandages have been shown to reduce patient discomfort and speed reepithelization, and are more manageable for patients. Some have argued, however, that closed dressings may delay the diagnosis of an impending skin infection. It is therefore imperative to see the patients frequently back in follow-up when these dressings are used. The authors combined have more than thirty years' experience with ablative erbium and CO_2 lasers and the postoperative use of dressings such as Vigilon and Flexan. In combination with prophylactic antibiotics and antivirals, infections have been virtually nonexistent with these closed dressing systems that greatly simplify the patient's postoperative wound care regimen.

Healing varies a bit with the depth of resurfacing and the choice of dressings, and is always better and faster in patients with thicker, more sebaceous skin. Generally, by postoperative day 5 or 7, the skin reepithelization is complete, and by day 7 or 8, a new, often intensely erythematous epidermis should be in place. The erythema then gradually subsides over the next five to seven days, and by twelve to fifteen days, makeup can be used. Because the skin barrier is compromised, the risk of contact dermatitis to any products applied to the new skin during the first couple of weeks is quite high, and patients should be cautioned as to this possibility.

On occasion, patients will experience prolonged erythema lasting several weeks, even extending to months. Prolonged erythema responds well to Elidel cream. Very low potency topical steroids, oral minocycline, and even the use of repeat pulsed-dye laser treatments have been advocated for stubborn cases. Localized intense erythema is often an early sign of hypertrophic scarring. Careful follow-up and treatment can usually prevent progression to frank scarring. Postresurfacing, white petrolatum is the best product to use during the first fourteen days after the dressings are removed, but prolonged use can lead to milia and acne outbreaks. Transitioning to hypoallergenic, cream-based moisturizers is recommended after reepithelization has occurred. Sunscreens and makeup are generally safe to use by fourteen days postoperation, although limiting routine use of regular commercial cosmetics for up to three weeks reduces the possibility of allergic contact dermatitis. Strict sun avoidance is mandatory during the preoperative and postoperative phases to ensure a safe and effective outcome. Patients will notice an immediate improvement once edema has resolved and reepithelization has occurred; however, maximal benefits are probably not met until six to eight months postoperation. Studies have demonstrated continued collagen production for months following laser resurfacing, and with appropriate care, results will be maintained for ten years or longer. The use of neurotoxin to minimize muscle movement in the forehead and crow's feet areas, especially during the first year, can further enhance long-term results.

Er:YAG LASER

The Er:YAG laser is another infrared laser with a wavelength of 2,940 nm. This specific wavelength provides it with the highest affinity for water absorption of any of the ablative lasers – approximately 10 to 13 times greater than the CO_2 laser. This high absorption has several clinically important consequences. The high absorption means that the laser is extremely specific to cellular tissue, creating a very safe and predictable ablative treatment with each pass and thus minimal collateral tissue destruction. For example, the threshold for vaporization of an Er:YAG is around 0.5–1.0 J/cm^2, versus 5 J/cm^2 for the CO_2 laser;

thus less energy is required for tissue vaporization, and less energy equates to less collateral damage. The corollary to this, however, is that there is less tissue penetration, thus requiring an increased number of passes to achieve an equivalent depth of dermal remodeling. As water in tissue is so efficiently vaporized, a cooling effect on the underlying tissue occurs, resulting in a smaller zone of thermal modification (10–40 μm, versus 50–120 μm for the CO_2 laser) and decreased tissue tightening with the average Er:YAG laser. However, by using much longer pulse widths, certain dual-mode Er:YAG lasers have countered this shortcoming to a certain degree. A smaller zone of thermal effect also means less heat diffusion, less tissue coagulation, and thus more bleeding at deeper passes compared to a CO_2 laser, requiring ancillary methods for hemostasis with certain procedures. The first erbium lasers were short-pulsed lasers with pulse durations in the microsecond domain. These lasers created extremely predictable, albeit limited depths of ablation per pass, requiring multiple passes to achieve necessary depths of tissue ablation. Later, variable-pulse erbium lasers, and soon after, a dual-pulse Er:YAG, were developed by Sciton Lasers. This dual-mode erbium combines two sequential and separately adjustable pulses, the first a short-pulsed laser (200 μs), followed by a long-pulse millisecond laser. This combination extends the duty time and creates a deeper zone of thermal effect for increased tissue tightening and increased hemostasis.

Treatment protocols with the Er:YAG lasers are similar to the protocols for the CO_2 laser described previously, with the obvious exception of requiring more passes. Preoperative prophylaxis, anesthesia, and postoperative care are identical. During the procedure, the number of passes will, again, be dependent on the specific laser system and the energy settings.

In general, Er:YAG lasers are better suited to younger, less severely wrinkled patients (Figure 44.5). When using the dual-mode laser from Sciton, a typical setting consists of 50 μm ablation (short pulse) with 100 μm coagulation (long pulse). Even with the dual-mode system, multiple passes are performed, usually from four to six, with the char being removed between passes. The end point (maximal depth) is reached when areas of pinpoint bleeding or the appearance of a color change to the dull, yellowish-white characteristics of dermal tissue is noted.

Histologic studies with Sciton's laser have shown that depths of thermal effect of over 100 μm are achievable with this system, making it comparable to CO_2 systems. Clinical results comparable to a CO_2 laser are also possible, albeit only after performing multiple passes. Comparison of side effects have also shown that prolonged erythema can occur with both lasers, as can scarring. Hypopigmentation is claimed to be significantly less likely with the erbium lasers versus CO_2, but according to many, it is just as much of a problem when the erbium lasers are used in a way

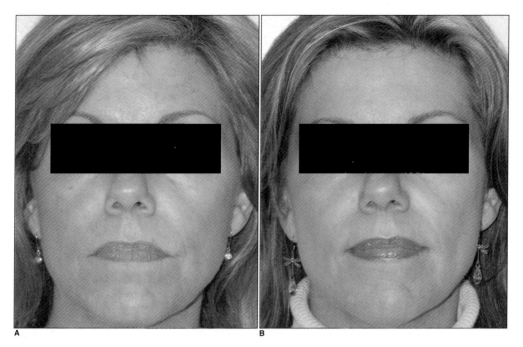

FIGURE 44.5: *Er:YAG lasers are often better suited for younger patients with fine wrinkles and dyschromia:* **A**, *pretreatment;* **B**, *twelve months posttreatment.*

to achieve comparable depths, thermal effects, and comparable long-term results. The exact mechanism of hypopigmentation is still debated, but it is most likely caused by the formation of a thin band of fibrous tissue in the upper dermis. Time will tell if the newer fractional CO$_2$ and erbium lasers will eliminate this problem.

PLASMA SKIN RESURFACING

The latest in ablative skin resurfacing is the use of plasma energy for skin rejuvenation. Plasma technology differs from the previously mentioned technologies in that it is not a laser, but rather, an alternative method of heating and ablating tissues. Plasma is known as the fifth state of matter and is generated by the formation of excited electrons that are then released to generate heat on a target tissue. In this case, an inert gas, nitrogen, is excited by a radiofrequency generator. The radioenergy excites the nitrogen electrons to an activated state and then releases them in a controlled manner through the handpiece onto the target tissue. Each pulse of plasma energy is released onto the target in a Gaussian distribution to provide even tissue heating and a uniform effect.

The Portrait system is currently the only commercially available plasma resurfacing system to date. Previous clinical applications of plasma energy include a process known as *coblation*. Coblation was most often used for the treatment of benign polyps or vocal cord nodules in otolaryngology and in orthopedic procedures. Coblation created an electrical energy field over a film of saline applied to the (skin)

tissue that produced a lower energy heating, which enabled superficial ablation of the target lesions. Trials of coblation for skin resurfacing were examined, but at low settings, with speedy recovery and low risk of complications, it failed to produce significant results. At higher settings, in very experienced hands, results and complications were comparable to CO$_2$ and erbium lasers. Overall, the device was far less precise and more operator-dependent than scanned lasers, and it never really caught on. The newer, nitrogen-based plasma field Portrait system provides both higher energy and deeper tissue penetration, thus creating a deep thermal effect and resultant increased skin tightening and rejuvenation. Finite element modeling predicted depths of tissue penetration of over 400 µm with the high-energy (4 J) settings.

The truly unique feature of plasma resurfacing is that it differs from laser resurfacing by not vaporizing tissue. Plasma energy provides a purely thermal effect that dessicates tissue, leaving behind a layer of intact, but dessicated, epidermis. This tissue layer acts as a biologic dressing, thus promoting rapid wound healing and a faster recovery. This ablated tissue layer sloughs over the ensuing five days, as the new epidermis is formed underneath. The deep thermal effects of the Portrait act in a fashion similar to that of CO$_2$ or erbium lasers: first, immediate tissue contraction is accomplished via thermal coagulation of dermal collagen; second, thermal disruption of solar elastosis and activation of fibroblasts stimulate a wound-healing cascade necessary for neocollagenesis. Histologic studies post–plasma resurfacing have confirmed continued collagen production and

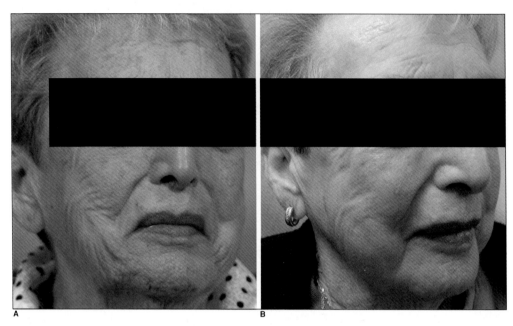

FIGURE 44.6: *High-power plasma resurfacing:* **A**, *before;* **B**, *four weeks after undergoing full-face plasma resurfacing (4J; double pass). Note the significant reduction in both dyschromia and rhytids.*

progressive skin thickening beyond a one-year postoperative time point.

TREATMENT PROTOCOLS

Another feature of the Portrait system is the ability to vary the treatment energies based on the desired effect and healing time. A complete range of effects can be achieved, from a nearly nonablative treatment (0.5 J) to low-energy plasma peels (1.0–2.0 J), to high-energy single or multiple pass treatments for maximum rejuvenation and tissue tightening (3.0–4.0 J). The depth of penetration of plasma energy varies directly with the fluence. At low-energy settings of 1.0–1.5, only the superficial epidermis is included in the zone of thermal ablation, and the remaining epidermis is affected by the zone of thermal modification. A setting of 2.0 J will typically ablate the full thickness of the facial epidermis and create a zone of modification in the upper dermis. It is recommended that settings between 2.0 and 3.0 be avoided because the energy is concentrated at the dermoepidermal junction, increasing the chance of postinflammatory hyperpigmentation. Energies of 3.5–4.0 J provide a zone of thermal ablation that includes the full-thickness epidermis plus papillary dermis, with a zone of modification extending into the upper reticular dermis.

Low-energy peels are typically delivered as a series of three treatments about three to four weeks apart. Following each treatment at 1.5–2.0 J on the face, there are typically four days of erythema and some superficial exfoliation on days 3 and 4. The higher-energy treatments at 3.0–4.0 J are performed as single treatments, with an anticipated healing time of seven to ten days. The typical course following a high-energy (4.0 J), double-pass treatment is bronzing by day 2, followed by epidermal sloughing on days 4 and 5 and resolution of erythema between days 7 and 10 (Figure 44.6). Because the epidermis is retained, there is no need for occlusive dressings in the postoperative period. Even when multiple passes are performed, there is generally no wiping performed between passes to enable the rapid healing possible with the retained epidermis.

Postoperative wound care consists of repeated applications of a petrolatum ointment to maintain an emolliated surface and to encourage epidermal sloughing as the new epidermis regenerates beneath the biologic dressing. As with other laser resurfacing procedures, patients receive perioperative prophylaxis with oral antibiotics and antivirals for one week. It is possible that because of the biologic dressing helping to maintain an intact skin barrier, there is a lessened chance of bacterial infection; however, this has never been studied or proven clinically.

One drawback with the plasma system is that plasma energy is released through repeat pulses, as opposed to the optical scanning technologies available for laser systems that can utilize mirrors and computer tracking. The operator must be exact with the pulse placements to avoid skip areas or pulse stacking. The safety profile of this device does make it safe in the event of pulse stacking, and the newer multiple-pass treatment protocols, combined with the energy distribution profile of the plasma delivery, enable even treatment delivery even if skip areas occur.

The safety profile of the Portrait system is very impressive. No hypopigmentation has been reported to date, and only rare incidences of scarring have occurred – likely the result of pulse stacking at very high fluences. Many of these are correctable with repeat pulsed dye laser treatments. The intact epidermis as a biologic dressing likely helps reduce any bacterial or fungal infections, in addition to assisting in a rapid recovery. One downside is the use of consumable tips, with significant operating costs.

SUMMARY

Advances in technology have provided us with multiple effective methods for laser resurfacing: ultrapulse CO$_2$; Er:YAG; and now, plasma resurfacing. Each of these is an effective means of treating dyschromia, photodamage, and rhytids and providing the much desired skin tightening. In trained hands, each of these devices is extremely safe and predictable. The differences exist in the various energy-tissue physics. With adjustments in energy settings and varying the number of passes, nearly equivalent clinical effects are possible with any of these systems. Despite the advances in technology and the introduction of alternative methods for skin resurfacing, the CO$_2$ laser continues to deliver the most consistently effective improvement in skin tightening and wrinkle reduction; thus it remains the gold standard for skin resurfacing.

SUGGESTED READING

Alster TA, Nanni CA, Williams CM. Comparison of four carbon dioxide resurfacing lasers: a clinical and histopathologic evaluation. *Dermatol. Surg.* 1999;25:153–9.

Duke D, Khatri K, Grevelink LM, Anderson RR. Comparative clinical trial of 2 carbon dioxide resurfacing lasers with varying pulse durations. *Arch. Dermatol.* 1998;134:1240–6.

Zachary CB. Modulating the Er:YAG laser. *Lasers Surg. Med.* 2000;26:223–6.

CHAPTER 45

Contemporary CO₂ Laser Resurfacing

Joseph Niamtu III

Since its introduction, no therapy has been as effective for rhytid effacement as the CO_2 laser. Aggressive CO_2 laser resurfacing remains the gold standard for facial-wrinkle treatment. In addition, the selective removal of epidermis and dermis allows for the simultaneous treatment of dyschromias and a variety of benign lesions. Regardless of the success and drawbacks of aggressive CO_2 laser resurfacing, there remains a popular push for less aggressive therapies. It is somewhat amusing that the media and the industry are heralding a new claim that the public wants more conservative procedures and will not tolerate extended recoveries. In reality, the public has always wanted conservative procedures, and always will. The push for nonablative and minimally invasive procedures has led to some disappointing results for those who expected CO_2-like outcomes. On the other hand, these less invasive procedures have provided patients with increased choices, tailored to their lifestyles and recovery windows. In my practice, laser skin resurfacing remains a popular option. The various choices of treatment include the following:

- CO_2 heavy, characterized by aggressive CO_2 resurfacing, two to four passes, high fluence, high density, reticular dermal injury, twelve to fourteen days' recovery
- CO_2 medium, characterized by a single pass, nondebrided, high fluence, high density, upper dermal injury, eight to ten days' recovery
- CO_2 light, characterized by a single pass, nondebrided, low fluence, high density, basilar and superficial dermal injury, six to eight days' recovery
- CO_2 ultralight (fractional CO_2), characterized by a single pass, nondebrided, low fluence, low density, epidermal injury, four to six days' recovery

CO_2 heavy resurfacing is a moniker for high fluence, multipass resurfacing ($7–8$ J/cm^2 with 30% overlap of the laser pattern). This is the procedure that, when introduced over a decade ago, changed the world of resurfacing forever. This

technique has been modified in my practice in several ways. First of all, many patients can experience similar benefits with less passes – often, two passes are equally effective as three. In addition, I always use simple open wound care consisting only of Vaseline for the first week, and the patient begins washing the face on the second postoperative day. A hypoallergenic moisturizer is begun during the second week. These patients understand that they will experience a protracted recovery, and most are back into makeup in about two weeks. This resurfacing can be performed as a sole procedure or in combination with other surgical procedures, as shown in Figure 45.1.

CO_2 medium resurfacing bridges the gap between aggressive and more conservative laser treatments. This procedure is used for those patients who need more skin rejuvenation than rhytid reduction. Only a single pass of the laser is at a high fluence ($7–8$ J/cm^2 with a 30% overlap), and for that reason, it is imperative not to overlap or "underlap" the treatment area, or a lattice pattern can result. The laser char is not debrided and serves as a wound dressing during the healing period. These patients are treated with the same post-op regimen as CO_2 heavy patients but reepithelialize several days sooner, usually around eight to ten days. This treatment has proven excellent for moderate to severe dyschromias and rhytids on thin skin such as the eyelids.

CO_2 light is the next step down of the less aggressive laser treatments. Patients with or without deep rhytids can obtain improvement of dyschromias and moderate improvement of fine lines and wrinkles with lower-fluence procedures. The CO_2 light procedure is a popular treatment for patients who have less damage or smaller recovery windows. With this procedure, the fluence is $3.0–3.5$ J/cm^2, and the density remains the same (30% overlap). With the CO_2 light treatment, a single pass is made over the entire face, and the char is not debrided, but again serves as a protective dressing for the postlaser period. As mentioned previously, when only a single pass is performed, it is extremely important not to overlap or "underlap" the

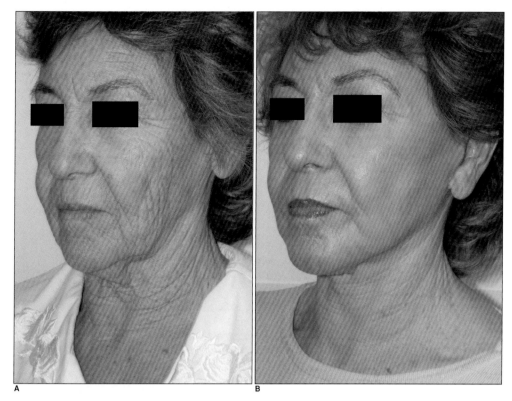

FIGURE 45.1: *Aggressive multipass CO₂ laser resurfacing is still the gold standard for skin rejuvenation. This patient underwent multipass CO₂ laser resurfacing with concomitant face lift, brow lift, blepharoplasty, and cheek implants:* **A**, *pretreatment;* **B**, *posttreatment.*

individual patterns from the computer-generated handpiece. If overlap occurs, tissue is treated to a deeper level, and if the patterns do not touch one another ("underlap"), an untreated area will be visible between the laser patterns. The CO_2 light procedure is similar to a medium-depth chemical peel and usually reepithelializes in a week. This is an attractive option for patients, who can have a procedure with significant results and be back at work in one week. Results generally will self-correct over a period of months but can be disconcerting to the patient. Figure 45.2 shows a before and after photograph of a CO_2 light patient.

The aforementioned techniques all have concentrated, high-density patterns in common. Recently, fractionated resurfacing technology has become a popular option for minimally invasive laser treatment. To answer the call of the contemporary aesthetic patient, fractionated resurfacing provides less tissue destruction and faster recovery. Fractionated resurfacing involves spacing the laser burns in an orderly arrangement, with areas of untreated normal tissue between the laser spots (Figure 45.3). This technology allows preservation of much of the normal tissue so that the patient does not experience a total facial burn and heals faster. Although dedicated lasers are available that perform only fractionated resurfacing, this type of treatment can be

performed with some conventional CO_2 lasers by adjusting the pattern density with the computer pattern generator and the density of the actual laser spot. Ultralight fractionated CO_2 works by applying the CO_2 laser energy in a very narrow scanned beam. This creates very tiny columns of thermal damage that penetrate deep down to the dermis and stimulate the growth of new collagen. The energy is applied in a fractional way; that is, the tiny columns of thermal damage are spaced so that the tissue between each is spared, resulting in a faster healing process. Using the CO_2 laser wavelength for fractionated treatment is advantageous because CO_2 laser energy is considered by many to be the optimal treatment for photoaged and environmentally damaged skin.

Another innovative feature of this ultralight laser technology is how the scanned pattern is laid down. A proprietary process provides a means of making a random pattern of spots within a standard scanner square. The laser burn spots are laid down not adjacent to one another, but randomly over the surface of the pattern; thus there is less heat buildup and less thermal injury because each hit area has time to cool (the thermal relaxation time) before another hit comes close to it. Less thermal injury means less erythema, less pain, and faster healing. Importantly, fractional, nonsequential application of CO_2 energy still results in ablation

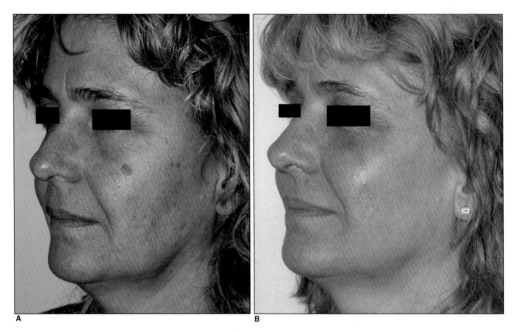

FIGURE 45.2: The CO₂ light procedure consists of a single pass with moderate fluence to provide impressive results for dyschromias and generalized skin health: **A**, pretreatment; **B**, posttreatment.

and the application of heat energy to the epidermis and superficial dermis.

With ultralight fractionated resurfacing, a high fluence is used, just as in aggressive CO_2 laser treatment. A square scanner pattern is also used, but the size is usually smaller. The big difference is that the density setting is 1 and the repeat rate is set at 0.5 s. Using the random pattern, an extremely low density, and a slightly slower repeat rate, the amounts of generated heat and tissue damage can be controlled. Because the treatment is much less ablative, the operator must look closely to see the actual area of laser burn.

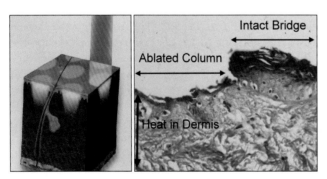

FIGURE 45.3: Basic concept of fractionated resurfacing, in which the laser pulses are separated by distance, which allows normal, unlasered skin between the treated columns, hence less skin damage and faster recovery.

CONCLUSION

CO_2 laser resurfacing entered the cosmetic arena with a big bang and then quieted down for a number of years. This treatment modality still has a prominent place in the armamentarium of cosmetic surgeons, and the versatility of altering the method of CO_2 laser delivery extends treatment options for the surgeon.

SUGGESTED READING

Alster TS, Doshi SN, Hopping SB. Combination surgical lifting with ablative laser skin resurfacing of facial skin: a retrospective analysis. *Dermatol. Surg.* 2004;30:1191–5.

Alster TS, Garg S. Treatment of facial rhytides with a high-energy pulsed carbon dioxide laser. *Plast. Reconstr. Surg.* 1996;98: 791–4.

Niamtu J. Common complications of laser resurfacing and their treatment. *Oral Maxillofac. Surg. Clin. North Am.* 2000;12: 579–93.

Niamtu J III. Digitally processed ultraviolet images: a convenient, affordable, reproducible means of illustrating ultraviolet clinical examination. *Dermatol. Surg.* 2001;27:1039–42.

Niamtu J. Laser treatment of vascular and pigmented lesions. Oral Maxillofac. Surg. Clin. North Am. 2004;16:239–54.

Niamtu J. Non-ablative technologies. *Lasers Surg. Med.* 2004;34: 203–4.

Tanzi EL, Lupton JR, Alster TS. Lasers in dermatology: four decades of progress. *J. Am. Acad. Dermatol.* 2003;49:1–31.

CHAPTER 46

Er:YAG

Joseph F. Greco

Bernard I. Raskin

The Er:YAG laser emits a monochromatic wavelength of infrared light at 2,940 nm, which closely approximates the major peak absorption of water near 3,000 nm. In the water-rich epidermis, laser energy is immediately absorbed, yielding precise tissue ablation with minimal thermal diffusion.

Erbium lasers may be categorized based on their pulse durations, or the time during which cutaneous tissue is exposed to laser energy. Thermal diffusion and collateral spread of laser energy are directly proportional to longer pulse durations.

The short-pulsed erbium laser was initially approved by the Food and Drug Administration in 1996 for skin resurfacing as an alternative to the carbon dioxide laser, with the benefits of a shorter recovery period and fewer side effects. With pulse intervals in the microsecond range, effective tissue ablation with minimal collateral damage is safely achieved. Quality-switched (or Q-switched) erbium lasers were also developed with ultrashort pulse durations in the nanosecond range. As a downside, little to no thermal coagulation or tissue contraction occurs with either the short or ultrashort pulse durations due to minimal spread of thermal energy. However, variable-pulsed erbium lasers were recently developed with longer pulse durations, in the millisecond range, with thermal diffusion of laser energy falling somewhere between the traditional erbium and CO_2 lasers. Longer pulse durations permit a wider spread of thermal energy, resulting in thermal coagulation of collagen and tissue contraction – an advantage when resurfacing beyond the epidermis.

On average, erbium laser light penetrates 4 μm of tissue for every joule per centimeter squared delivered. This direct relationship allows the laser surgeon to efficiently predict a precise depth of ablation. The depth, of course, is determined by the location of the target lesion. Utilizing a variable-pulsed laser, such as the Sciton Contour (Sciton Inc.), a single pass of 5 J/cm^2 delivers a 20-μm depth peel. The average zone of thermal necrosis left behind is between 20 and 50 μm. Stacking of lower energy pulses can serially ablate layers of skin, without increasing the total thermal diffusion. For example, complete epidermal ablation may be achieved through two passes with a 30-μm peel at 7.5 J/cm^2 or through three passes of a 20-μm peel at 5 J/cm^2. Each successive pass ablates the prior zone of thermal damage, instead of broadening it. As the zone of collateral damage is so minimal, manual removal of the ablated tissue is unnecessary between passes. Deeper pathology, as with dermal lesions or extensive photodamage, may require several passes to reach the desired target such as an elastotic papillary dermis. Here the longer-pulsed erbium lasers are more practical as they provide some tissue tightening as well as tissue coagulation to prevent pinpoint bleeding. Most recently, fractional delivery Er:YAG lasers have also been introduced by Alma, Sciton, and Palomar, while other manufacturers are scrambling to jump on the bandwagon of fractional delivery systems. These lasers are discussed elsewhere in the book, specifically, in Section 6 of this part.

CLINICAL BENEFIT

Erbium resurfacing remains a standard therapy in the modern era of minimally invasive cosmetics for photorejuvenation and treatment of various benign and premalignant growths of the skin and mucosa. The patient skin type, underlying pathology, and available downtime dictate the desired depth of ablation. Ideal patients are those with fair skin (Fitzpatrick skin types I–III) with signs of chronic sun damage. Patients such as these typically achieve overall texture and tone improvement with softening of medium to fine rhytids, lightening of brown dyschromia, and reduction of surface irregularities. Contour irregularities from acne and surgical scars may be effectively softened or eliminated by precise sculpting of the defect edges. Postsurgical resurfacing of this type is typically performed at six to ten weeks after surgery or initial insult by stacking two to three passes at 7.5 J/cm^2 (30 μm per pass) over the raised edges. Actinic cheilitis and persistent actinic keratoses may be effectively eliminated through an epidermal and superficial papillary dermal-submucosal ablation.

Cosmetic improvement of various superficial benign growths, such as seborrheic keratoses, syringoma, sebaceous hyperplasia, trichoepithelioma, dermatosis papulosa nigra, and xanthelasma, may be safely performed as well. Effective ablation of the preceding lesions can be achieved through stacking of multiple (two to four) passes at energy levels of 5–7.5 J/cm^2.

PREOPERATIVE CARE AND PROCEDURE

The treatment area is cleansed and topical anesthesia is used for patient comfort. The authors use a compounded topical gel of 7% lidocaine and 7% tetracaine applied for one hour. The topical anesthetic is completely removed with gauze prior to treatment. Alcohol wipes are subsequently applied to the treatment area to ensure complete removal of the anesthetic as any residual water-carrying medium will serve as a competing chromophore for laser absorption. For anxious patients or those with heightened pain sensitivity, clonidine 0.1 mg can be given orally an hour in advance. This drug, which is often utilized by liposuction surgeons, reduces anxiety and pain sensation without mental sequelae and is safe as long as systolic blood pressure is greater than 100.

A long-pulsed Er:YAG laser peel is performed depending on the desired level of ablation; one to several passes with a peel depth of 20 μm (5 J/cm^2) to 30 μm (7.5 J/cm^2) are chosen, with the understanding that the laser energy will penetrate approximately 4 μm of tissue for every joule per square centimeter. For microlaser peels used alone or in conjunction with broadband light for photodamaged skin (see Chapter 51), a single pass with a preset depth of 20 μm is chosen, with a 50% overlap. When complete epidermal ablation is desired, two to three passes with a 30-μm peel or three to four passes with a 20-μm peel are chosen. For dermal lesions and rhytids, three to five passes with a 30-μm peel are used. Certain laser platforms, such as Sciton's Contour, allow the operator to select coagulation levels (preset at 25%, 50%) on the user interface prior to delivering the laser pulse. The authors typically include a 25% coagulation level if the planned ablation involves the dermis.

Feathering along the jawline aids in avoiding clear lines of demarcation between treated and untreated areas. A concomitant smoke evacuator should be used to recover any plume created by the tissue vaporization. Immediate epidermal whitening from proteinaceous debris is noted overlying the treatment area. Postoperatively, the treatment area can be iced for patient comfort. The authors find that a spray with precooled 1:1 mixture of 2% lidocaine and sterile water or saline is beneficial, as well.

Combination therapy with the Er:YAG laser and various minimally invasive cosmetic procedures may synergistically enhance treatment outcome in photodamaged skin. Sequential therapy with a broadband light source followed immediately by a superficial erbium microlaser peel at 20 μm simultaneously targets brown dyschromia, redness, fine lines, and textural irregularities caused by chronic sun damage (see Chapter 51).

Typical areas treated include photodamaged skin of the face, the neck, and the dorsal aspect of the hands in patients with Fitzpatrick skin types I–III. Total treatment time, excluding that required for topical anesthesia, ranges from seven to twenty minutes, depending on the anatomic area being treated and the number of passes desired. Adjustable repetition rate settings on certain laser platforms permit accelerated treatment times, with pulse firing intervals ranging between 0.5 and 2 s. Off-the-face resurfacing, in our experience, has been effective in combination with a broadband light source. Here a single-pass microlaser peel at 20 μm is performed immediately following treatment with a broadband or intense pulsed light source.

PERIOPERATIVE CARE

Aquaphor ointment is applied postoperatively and is continued twice daily, as needed, until the peeling resolves. Strict sun avoidance is emphasized during the immediate posttreatment week, and patients are encouraged to use a broad-spectrum sunscreen thereafter. In general, postoperative pain is minimal and well controlled with over-the-counter preparations. Antiviral prophylaxis with Valtrex 500 mg po twice daily for three to five days beginning one day prior to the procedure is recommended in patients with a history of oral herpes simplex virus outbreaks for epidermal peels and in all patients if the resurfacing involves the dermis. Triamcinalone 0.1% cream can be prescribed one to three days postoperatively for patients who experience significant edema and erythema. Prophylactic oral antibiotic therapy with dicloxacillin (250 mg po four times daily), azithromycin (500 mg po first day loading dose, then 250 mg po daily), or cefazolin (500 mg po twice daily) is reserved for resurfacing procedures involving the dermis. If used, the antibiotics are started one day prior to the resurfacing procedure and continued until reepithelialization is complete.

ADJUNCTIVE TOPICAL AGENTS

Topical retinoids, such as tretinoin and tazarotene, which may enhance reepithelialization after resurfacing procedures, are initiated, if possible, four to six weeks prior to therapy. A topical washout period beginning one week prior and ending one week posttreatment is usually followed. Topical hydroquinone bleaching agents are encouraged in patients with Fitzpatrick skin types IV–VI as well as in those with a history of melasma or postinflammatory hyperpigmentation. In this setting, the authors recommend a single nightly application of Triluma cream or twice daily application of 4% hydroquinone for at least four weeks prior to treatment.

TABLE 46.1: Summary of Available Er:YAG 2,940-nm Laser Platforms

Supplier	Product Name	Energy Output	Pulse Width	Price (US$)[a]
Aerolase	LightPod Era	up to 140 J	0.3 ms	39,500
Aerolase	LightPod Era XL	up to 180 J	0.3 ms	43,500
Harmony		200–1,200 mJ/p	0.5, 1.0 ms	19,900
Candela	SmoothPeel	750 mJ (max)	2,4,6 Hz	39,900
Focus Medical	NaturaLase Erbium	up to 24 J/cm^2 (3 J per pulse)	300 ms	60,000
MedSurge Advances	Asclepion MCL Dermablate	1–100 J/cm^2	500 μs	
Radiancy	Whisper	up to 8 J/cm^2	300 μs	39,900
Sandstone	Whisper-NG	750 mJ	300 ms	35,000
Sciton Inc.	Contour	45 W	0.1–50 ms	23,000
Sciton Inc.	Profile Strata Er:YAG/Nd:YAG/Pulsed Light	up to 400 J	up to 200 ms	148,000
Sybaritic Inc	LaserPeel Soft-MET	5 J/cm^2 at 3-mm spot size	N/A	39,995

[a] Prices as per Aesthetic Buyers Guide (July/August 2007), http://www.miinews.com.

SIDE EFFECTS

Postoperative side effects are minimal with single-pass erbium resurfacing and increase with the number of passes. Overall side effects are similar to carbon dioxide resurfacing; however, they are generally shorter, less intense, and less common. Patients should expect minimal to moderate erythema for two to three days after shallow peels and up to one week or longer with deeper peels. Complete reepithelialization occurs after an average of three to six days, depending on the depth of the peel. Postinflammatory hyperpigmentation is far less common with erbium resurfacing due to the minimal zone of thermal diffusion and subsequent blunted inflammatory response. If it does occur, pigmentation generally fades with time and appropriate sun avoidance strategies. The authors have never observed permanent hypopigmentation or hypertrophic or keloidal cicatrix; however, this risk markedly increases with deeper dermal peels. The authors recommend postponing resurfacing procedures for at least one year from the last day of therapy in patients with a history of isotretinoin use.

CONCLUSION

Patients are seeking maximal effect with minimal downtime in an age when minimally invasive aesthetic procedures dominate the office-based cosmetic practice. Skin resurfacing with the Er:YAG lasers delivers a predictable, precise, and reproducible tissue ablation with minimal surrounding thermal damage. With a single to relatively few passes, multiple aspects of photoaging, including brown dyschromia, surface textural irregularities, and fine to moderate lines, can be effectively softened or eliminated with relatively few side effects. Table 46.1 lists U.S. available fully ablative Er:YAG lasers. Some of these companies now offer fractional Er:YAG systems as well.

SUGGESTED READING

Avram DK, Goldman MP. The safety and effectiveness of single-pass erbium:YAG laser in the treatment of mild to moderate photodamage. *Dermatol. Surg.* 2004;30:1073–6.

Katri KA, Ross V, Grevelink JM, Magro CM, Anderson RR. Comparison of erbium:YAG and carbon dioxide lasers in resurfacing of facial rhytides. *Arch. Dermatol.* 1999;135:391–7.

Pozner JN, Goldber DJ. Superficial erbium:YAG laser resurfacing of photodamaged skin. *J. Cosmet. Laser Ther.* 2006;8:89–91.

Tanzi EL, Alster TS. Single-pass carbon dioxide versus multiple-pass Er:YAG laser skin resurfacing: a comparison of postoperative wound healing and side-effect rates. *Dermatol. Surg.* 2003;29:80–4.

CHAPTER 47

Plasma Skin Rejuvenation of the Hands

Tina S. Alster

Photodamaged skin of the hands occurs as a result of chronic exposure to ultraviolet light and is characterized by roughened surface texture, dyspigmentation, telangiectasias, rhytids, and skin laxity. Although several different noninvasive procedures have been advocated for hand rejuvenation (Table 47.1), many are characterized by an unattainable balance between effectiveness and morbidity. The necessity of epidermal removal during most skin resurfacing treatments leads to significant morbidity during the reepithelialization process, particularly in areas such as the hands, where limited pilosebaceous glands are present.

PLASMA SKIN REGENERATION TECHNOLOGY

Plasma skin regeneration is a novel process that involves the generation of plasma through the use of ionized energy that thermally heats tissue. A pulse of ultrahigh-energy radiofrequency (RF) from the device generator (Portrait plasma skin regeneration) converts nitrogen gas into plasma within the handpiece. The plasma emerges from the distal end of the device handpiece and is directed onto the skin area to be treated. Rapid heating of the skin occurs as the excited gas transfers heat to the skin, resulting in increased fibroblast activity during dermal regeneration. The retained necrotic epidermis effectively serves as a biological dressing for the efficient formation of a new stratum corneum and epidermis.

The essentially instantaneous generation of plasma with controlled application of RF energy produces individual plasma pulses that heat tissue. Adjustment of RF power and pulse width enables control of tissue effects by altering the amount of energy delivered to tissue per pulse. In practice, the energy per pulse is adjustable between 1 and 4 J. The power and duration of each RF pulse are directly proportional to plasma strength.

CLINICAL PROTOCOL

The skin areas to be treated are cleansed with mild soap and water to remove all surface debris. While intralesional lidocaine can be used for anesthesia, application of a topical anesthetic cream (e.g., EMLA or LMX-5) under plastic wrap occlusion for sixty minutes is often adequate. Once the cream has been thoroughly removed and the skin completely dried, the treatment should commence within five to ten minutes. Typical energy settings of 1.5–4 J are applied to the areas, holding the device handpiece perpendicular to the skin at a distance measuring approximately 5 mm from the skin surface. The areas are treated in a single pass with a pulse overlap of 10 to 20%. An additional pass should only be delivered if a low (1.5 J) energy setting is used. Pulse repetition rates of 1–4 Hz are chosen, subject to the discretion of the operator. While skin can be cooled with ice packs or cool water compresses posttreatment, intraoperative cooling of the skin is contraindicated because of its negative impact on the tissue heating necessary to achieve optimal clinical effect.

POSTOPERATIVE COURSE

Immediately posttreatment, a petrolatum-based ointment (e.g., Aquaphor) can be applied to the skin. Patients should be instructed to gently cleanse the treated areas with mild cleanser and water and to reapply the ointment at least three times daily to maintain a moist healing environment. Nonstick gauze dressings can be used to protect the treated areas from ultraviolet light exposure or abrasion due to clothing. Patients should be advised to avoid sun exposure, prolonged water immersion, or exposure to harsh chemicals for as long as the treated skin appears pink in color.

CLINICAL RESULTS

Clinical improvement of 50% is typically observed, with significant reduction in wrinkle severity and hyperpigmentation within one month after a single treatment (Figure 47.1). Most patients also experience increased skin smoothness. Additional treatments can be delivered for

TABLE 47.1: Comparison of Hand Rejuvenation Treatments

Treatment	Advantages	Disadvantages	Take-Home Message
Plasma skin regeneration	one/few sessions needed highly effective	short recovery necessary	best for photodamaged skin (both texture and pigment), but recovery time necessary
Chemical (TCA) peel + pigment-specific laser	requires knowledge of two procedures multiple sessions needed	moderate recovery inadequate for skin laxity	good for dyspigmentation, but limited efficacy for wrinkling
Fractionated laser	minimal to no recovery	multiple sessions needed mild clinical effect	good for those with limited time for recovery

Note: TCA, trichloroacetic acid.

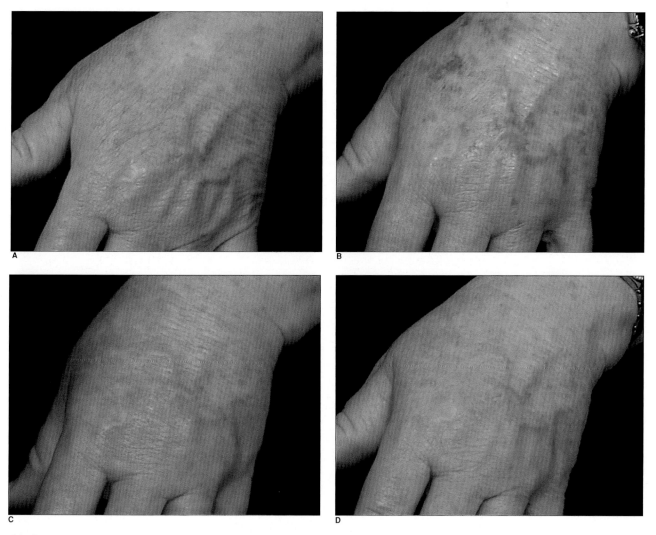

FIGURE 47.1: **A, Photodamaged skin on the dorsal hand of a fifty-four-year-old woman prior to treatment. B, Dorsal hand skin four days after plasma skin regeneration treatment (1.8 J, single pass). C, At two weeks, minimal erythema is noted. D, Improvement of pigmentation and wrinkling are evident three months after treatment.**

further enhancement and maintenance of clinical effect but should be delayed at least one month to assess the results of prior treatment and to give the skin ample time to heal.

SIDE EFFECTS

The use of higher energy settings or multiple passes yields greater clinical benefit, but also prolonged tissue healing (fourteen days versus seven days). Side effects of erythema, edema, and desquamation are uniformly experienced. Epidermal sloughing with clinical evidence of a superficial dermal wound is evident within forty-eight hours of treatment. Reepithelialization with normalization of external skin architecture occurs within a few days. Mild erythema is typical for two to four weeks. While infection, dyspigmentation, and scarring are potential risks of the procedure, the incidence is extraordinarily low when the intraoperative and postoperative protocols outlined previously are followed. No prophylactic antibiotics are recommended;

however, if a postoperative infection is suspected, broad-spectrum antibiotics can be prescribed.

SUMMARY

Plasma skin regeneration is a highly effective rejuvenative skin treatment. Its excellent clinical efficacy and safety profile in cutaneous sites that have notoriously been difficult to treat with ablative laser technology make it my preferred treatment for photodamaged skin of the hands.

SUGGESTED READING

Alster TS, Konda S. Plasma skin resurfacing for regeneration of neck, chest, and hands: investigation of a novel device. *Dermatol. Surg.* 2007;33:1–5.

Bogle MA, Arndt KA, Dover JS. Evaluation of plasma skin regeneration technology in low-energy full-facial rejuvenation. *Arch. Dermatol.* 2007;143:168–74.

Section 3

NONABLATIVE LASER TISSUE REMODELING: 1,064-, 1,320-, 1,450-, AND 1,540-NM LASERS

CHAPTER 48

Nonablative Laser Tissue Remodeling: 1,064-, 1,320-, 1,450-, and 1,540-nm Laser Systems

Bernard I. Raskin

Joseph F. Greco

Sorin Eremia

Lasers utilizing wavelengths of 1,064, 1,320, 1,450, and 1,540 nm were the first nonablative resurfacing modalities. Utilizing technology to cool the surface to protect the epidermis, these lasers effectively heat the dermis selectively, to a limited degree, to stimulate new collagen formation and tightening. The nonablative lasers will be discussed primarily for skin rejuvenation, as other uses, such as for acne scarring and hair removal, are addressed in detail in other chapters. The 1,064-nm wavelength laser reviewed in this section is a long-pulse system, in contrast to the Q-switched units popular for tattoo removal.

The near-infrared lasers induce thermal injury in the dermis, potentially heating and damaging collagen to the point of denaturation. The rate of denaturation is exponentially related to temperature. Because of this relationship, small temperature changes impact denaturation dramatically. The accumulation of denatured material rises exponentially with temperature but proportionally with time, and thus both the amount of energy delivered and

exposure duration are important. At critical temperatures, depending on the tissue type, rapid denaturation occurs. In the dermis, the extracellular collagen protein is the dominant material in coagulation (denaturing) because elastin is extremely thermally stable, even at the temperature of boiling water. The melting point for collagen is between 60 and 70 degrees Celsius, and above these temperatures, dermal scars can result. Thus temperature levels within the collagen are critical to causing mild injury, resulting in production of new collagen versus complete denaturation with resultant scarring. Basically, a critical threshold exists between the temperatures required to cause mild injury with subsequent new collagen production and those temperatures that denature collagen to the point of scar formation. To that end, different manufacturers utilize technology to protect the epidermis, while providing consistent dermal heating without scar-producing heat extremes.

Surface cooling is important in nonablative modalities. These include coolant application, such as a spray, and heat extraction with a solid contact – both methods are effective. More important are the three basic types of skin cooling, precooling, parallel cooling, and postcooling, which define heat extraction before, during, or after the laser pulse. Dynamic cooling devices represent the most aggressive epidermal precooling. Parallel cooling is best accomplished with a sapphire solid contact tip. Postcooling can be provided by either modality.

The 1,064 laser, when utilized in a continuous long-pulse mode, emits an invisible near-infrared beam. Absorption is by protein of any opaque tissue. It is poorly absorbed by hemoglobin and melanin, and thus these chromophores are only impacted with higher energies. At lower energies, the laser can be utilized on darker-complected people. There is a small peak for hemoglobin absorption at 1,064 nm, so blood vessels can effectively be treated, but higher energies are necessary. The main advantage of this laser is the deeper penetration compared to the other near-infrared lasers. In general, depth of penetration is inversely proportional to wavelength, with a longer wavelength providing deeper penetration. However, at about 1,300 nm, water absorption becomes significant, and penetration is reduced from its theoretical levels and therefore reduced compared to the 1,064-nm wavelength.

The other near-infrared lasers are well absorbed by tissue water, thus resulting in bulk dermal heating. Many authors consider the 1,320-, 1,450-, and 1,540-nm wavelengths to be equivalent. In the United States, the 1,540-nm wavelength has never been popular for bulk dermal tissue heating but is now used with fractional resurfacing lasers.

The first-generation devices specifically designed for nonablative skin tightening were lasers delivering light energy in the far-infrared spectrum. Introduced in 1997, CoolTouch (NewStar Lasers) utilized a 1,320-nm Nd:YAG-generated wavelength and a fixed 50-ms pulse width. The availability of cryogen spray pre- and postcooling and the addition of a temperature sensor and a relatively large, 10-mm treatment spot size set CoolTouch apart from the Smooth Beam (Candela Lasers), a smaller, less sophisticated, but less expensive, 1,450-nm diode-generated wavelength laser, and the European-developed Aramis Er:Glass 1,540-nm laser that never quite caught on in the United States. As is too often the case with new devices, the laser manufacturers and some physicians promoting these lasers made unrealistic claims that as few as four treatments could produce significant skin tightening, wrinkle resolution, and improvement in acne scars. In time, it was determined that many treatments (e.g., in the experience of the authors, ten to fourteen monthly treatments with the CoolTouch laser or Smooth Beam) were needed to achieve modest long-term skin tightening or acne scarring improvement. Overaggressive treatments also resulted in dyspigmentation (seen more commonly with the less sophisticated Smooth Beam laser) or rare but annoying scarring thermal injuries. Both the CoolTouch and Smooth Beam lasers

are still available and have proven to be generally reliable, low-operating-cost-type lasers. The latest version of CoolTouch has an option for treatment with sweeping multiple passes, more along the latest Thermage RF treatment protocols. The 1,320 WL is also very effective for endovenous varicose vein ablation, and these lasers can be equipped with an attachment for endovenous laser ablation (EVLA) use. The 1,320-nm wavelength (as well as the 1,064 nm) is now also used for laser fiber-assisted liposuction. Simple attachments for liposuction assisted devices are likely to render these infrared lasers even more multipurposed. Very similar to the CoolTouch, the Sciton 1,319-nm Nd:YAG laser has a variable pulse width, which allows great flexibility as to how the energy is delivered; a fast, large treatment area with a scanned 6-mm spot; and excellent adjustable contact window cooling. One of the chief complaints with the CoolTouch and Smooth Beam lasers is significant patient discomfort. Use of longer pulse widths decreases treatment pain. When compared to the 10-mm CoolTouch spot size, the randomly scanned, smaller, 6-mm Sciton spot also reduces pain. The Sciton unit operates on a platform that can support multiple lasers (such as 1,064-nm Nd:YAG, Er:YAG, and pulsed broadband light units). Of note, the wavelength used by all these lasers has virtually no melanin absorption.

Both the 1,320- and 1,450-nm lasers are commonly utilized for acne treatment. Significant and substantial improvement can be achieved, but results may be inconsistent. Typically, a number of sessions are required; however, prolonged improvement lasting one to two years can result after four or five monthly sessions. Previously, with the Smooth Beam, reliable improvement required high-energy settings, such as a single pass at 12–14 J, which was painful, even with the dynamic cooling system and advance application of anesthesia cream. Patients with inflammatory lesions experienced even more discomfort at these settings. Another problem relatively specific to the Smooth Beam was hyperpigmentation, even in lighter-complected individuals, which was problematic at higher settings, although long-term or permanent postinflammatory pigmentation was rare. However, minimizing pigmentation problems required avoiding settings higher than 8–9 J in Fitzpatrick III individuals. Recently, however, evidence indicates that high settings are no longer required for acne treatment. Utilizing two or more passes at 8 or 9 J provides effective acne improvement, and pigmentation problems are reduced. The first author now treats acne patients at 8 to 9 J with DCD settings of 35–40 ms using a 6-mm spot with two or three passes on a monthly basis. The first author (BR) prefers the Smooth Beam for acne because treatments are standardized, making it easier for physician extenders to perform treatments, and there is no downtime after each session.

Because of differential heat absorption in the tissue, the 1,320- and 1,450-nm lasers are beneficial in reducing sebaceous hyperplasia. Several treatments may be needed, and high-energy settings are required. With the Smooth Beam, settings of 16 J with a 4-mm spot size are recommended, and pulse stacking with two to four pulses is required, depending on the size of the lesion. With CoolTouch, using a preset 50 ms pulse width, settings in the range of 16–18 J were found to be effective for acne. With the Sciton, using longer pulse widths in the range of 100–200 ms, fluences in the 20–24 J range were safely used, even on darker-skinned patients, and treatments were less painful. In a split-face, side-by-side study, the third author (SE) found the 1,319- and 1,320-nm lasers to be essentially equally effective, and both significantly more effective than a variable–pulse width, 1,064-nm laser, for the treatment of acne. None of these systems, however, appeared to provide long-term acne reduction, as seen with Acutane. The authors, however, find this technology to be about equivalent to PDT for the treatment of acne.

These lasers are widely available relatively inexpensively in the secondhand market. The reader is cautioned that some lasers, such as the Smooth Beam, have limited utility life due to critical malfunction of the gas laser tube after a certain number of pulses, and repair can be thousands of dollars. Gradual buildup of dust internally can result in electronic component failures. Although costs can be expensive, manufacturer maintenance agreements may be beneficial on older equipment.

The 1,064-nm Nd:YAG lasers, both millisecond pulse width and Q-switch types, have also been used, usually in a freehand, multiple-pass fashion, to heat the dermis and trigger mild neocollagenesis and slight skin tightening. The 1,064-nm lasers are in wide use for hair removal and, to a lesser extent, for vein treatment, and even mild skin tightening presents a bonus for this application. Results have been variable and often unimpressive in the author's opinions; however, there is a recent report that the Candela 1,064-nm laser provided tissue tightening on the face equivalent to the Thermage monopolar radiofrequency device. The authors have considerable experience in utilizing near-infrared lasers and the more current tissue tightening technologies such as Thermage, Titan, and others. To effect even mild tightening and minimal neocollagenesis with the near-infrared systems typically required multiple treatments over the course of months. In the authors' opinion, only relatively minor improvement occurs in fine lines and wrinkles in the periorbital regions, although variable degrees of tissue tightening and some noticeable acne scar reduction are generally noticeable after nine to twelve sessions. Improvement in active acne is more predictable than wrinkle improvement with these lasers. Improvement also occurs for acne scars, but less impressively than with the newer fractional resurfacing lasers. When compared to the Thermage monopolar radiofrequency device, the current Thermage regimen of multiple passes in one session at lower-energy settings with large (3 cm), fast treatment tips provides more impressive and consistent tightening, including some immediately noticeable tightening. However, the high cost of the Thermage single-use tips is a deterrent to repeated treatments, and IR lasers are excellent, and effective, low-cost options for follow-up or maintenance treatment programs. Other monopolar, bipolar, and light-based systems now exist for skin tightening, and new variations of this technology are being introduced at the time of this writing that reduce patient discomfort or combine technologies for deep heating. In the opinion of the authors, the newer tissue-tightening technologies are superior to the old near-infrared lasers as a primary skin-tightening modality because they perform at least as well in fewer sessions with more reliable, predictable results, and the new fractional resurfacing lasers are significantly better for acne scars. Industry, however, is not abandoning these near-infrared lasers, and Candela is introducing a new 1,310-nm, very long pulsed (1–5 s), large–spot size (12–18 mm) laser for skin tightening. The latest CoolTouch version also has much greater treatment parameter flexibility.

Section 4

BROADBAND LIGHT DEVICES

CHAPTER 49

Overview of Broadband Light Devices

Paul S. Yamauchi

Various techniques have been used for the improvement of cutaneous changes seen with photoaging. These include dermabrasion, chemical peels, and ablative and nonablative lasers. Another option is the use of broadband light devices, which provide a treatment modality for skin rejuvenation with minimal or no downtime. In contrast to ablative rejuvenation laser procedures (CO_2, Er-YAG), which can result in protracted edema and erythema lasting for several weeks as well as pigmentary changes and scarring, broadband light devices induce a dermal healing response without notable injury to the epidermis and also diminish pigmented lesions on the skin such as lentigos. By heating the dermis and dermal vasculature, these broadband devices result in dermal remodeling through fibroblast stimulation and collagen reformation and also allow for reduction of erythema and telangiectasias.

Broadband light devices include a family of light devices known as the intense pulsed light (IPL) systems. The main uses of IPLs as a nonlaser light source include removal of pigmented and vascular lesions, rejuvenation and skin tightening, and removal of unwanted hair. The IPL systems utilize high-intensity pulsed-light sources that emit noncoherent, noncollimated polychromatic light from 515 to 1,200 nm. The mechanism of action of IPL systems is that of selective photothermolysis. Because main chromophores of the epidermis and dermis have specific absorption coefficients, the effective wavelength(s) of light are chosen that would most selectively destroy the target of interest, while sparing surrounding tissue. For instance, hemoglobin absorbs primarily at a wavelength of 580 nm, whereas melanin encompasses the entire visible spectral range.

IPL devices have various filters chosen to selectively block shorter wavelengths. When using IPL systems, cutoff filters (515–755 nm) are employed, which filter out the spectrum of light of wavelengths less than the number designated on the filter. As with laser systems, longer wavelengths in the visible spectral range penetrate more deeply. Choice of an appropriate cutoff filter should be guided by the absorption spectra of the target and surrounding tissue as well as the depth of the target of interest. Keeping the pulse duration (generally between 0.5 and 88.5 ms) lower than the thermal relaxation time of the target structures spares the surrounding tissue from excess heating. In addition, various pulse durations can be delivered over single, double, or triple micropulses with variable delay times. When treating larger target vessels, a higher fluence may be split into multiple pulses with intervening delays of between 1 and 300 ms. The delay allows the nontarget tissues to cool down between pulses, while the heat is retained in the target of interest.

IPL is used to improve diffuse facial erythema seen with rosacea and pigment irregularities and fine rhytids resulting from photodamage. The shorter wavelengths with this device have been shown to improve vascular and epidermal pigmented lesions, and the longer wavelengths are necessary for skin rejuvenation. With a series of treatments spaced every three to five weeks apart, IPL is ideal for the treatment of diffuse erythema in rosacea and photodamaged skin as well as lentigos. Common sites of erythema seen in rosacea include the cheeks, nose, chin, and forehead. In addition, there is a condition known as poikiloderma of Civatte, in which diffuse erythema and lentigines occur on the neck and the V of the chest due to photodamage. IPL is ideal for treating this condition. In addition to erythema, IPL can be used to lessen telangiectasias commonly found on the face, especially on the cheeks, the nose, and the perialar area.

IPL has been investigated for nonablative treatment of isolated cosmetic units as well as full-face rejuvenation. One study reported the use of IPL in improving the cutaneous changes associated with photoaging. Thirty patients received five full-face IPL treatments at three-week intervals. The investigators aimed at using subpurpuric parameters as follows: 550-nm filter, fluences of 30–36 J/cm^2, and double 2.4- to 4.0-ms pulses. Transient erythema lasting a few hours was seen. Fewer than 2% of patients were reported to have purpura or swelling requiring a 1- to 3-day recovery period; no scarring was reported. Clinical results revealed some subjective improvement: 49% of patients reported a 75% or greater overall improvement in the appearance of their skin, 73% of patients reported a 25% or greater improvement of fine wrinkles, and 36% reported a 50% or greater improvement of fine wrinkles. In addition, patients noted improvement of skin smoothness, pore size, and erythema. This early observation demonstrates the potential use of IPL for nonablative rejuvenation with minimal to no patient downtime.

Another study reported mild to moderate improvement of some rhytids without epidermal ablation using the IPL system. The investigators treated thirty subjects with skin types I and II and class I–II facial rhytids. One to four treatments were performed at two-week intervals over a ten-week period. Parameters included a cutoff filter of 645 nm and fluences of 40–50 J/cm^2 delivered over triple pulses of 7 ms with a 50-ms interpulse delay. At six months, nine of twenty-five patients showed substantial improvement of their rhytids. The authors reported that twenty-five subjects showed some improvement in skin quality and facial rhytids. All patients experienced transient posttreatment erythema; no erythema, pigmentary changes, or scarring was seen at six months after treatment.

IPL devices are relatively easy and simple to operate. Typically, they have a push-button screen on the main body of the unit, where various parameters are selected such as the energy setting and pulsed width. Various filters at different wavelength ranges are easily interchanged on the handpiece. Most IPL devices have preprogrammed settings for different applications that allow the user to treat the patient for rejuvenation, rosacea, hair removal, and leg veins. Cooling gel is applied liberally to the areas to be treated to minimize pain discomfort and to protect the epidermis. The patient must be warned that treatment with IPL may be painful and uncomfortable. Goggles are imperative for both the patient and practitioner because the emitting light is very bright. In addition, the skin type of the patient must be taken into account. Caution should be exercised when treating patients of darker skin types. Using high fluences may result in scarring and prolonged hyperpigmentation.

A test spot may be advisable when treating darker-skinned individuals at lower fluences prior to treating the full face.

IPL is a versatile device to treat various aspects of photodamaged skin. In addition, IPL is used to remove unwanted hair and to correct leg veins. There are many other laser devices that perform the same tasks as IPL. Pulsed dye lasers (PDL) emit yellow light at a 577- to 595-nm wavelength, which is well absorbed by hemoglobin. The systems having a pulse duration of 450 μs to 1.5 ms have been used for several years to treat vascular lesions by providing enough energy and short pulse durations to specifically target blood vessels with minimal damage to the epidermis and surrounding tissue. PDL have a low incidence of scarring; however, depending on the parameters used, the PDL can produce cosmetically unacceptable purpura. Newer PDL systems have been developed with longer pulse durations, which decrease the incidence of posttreatment purpura. Both the IPL and PDL correct erythema in rosacea, but PDL are more effective in treating telangiectasias and deeper vascular lesions such as port-wine stains. PDL, for the most part, do not correct lentigines as well as IPL.

Fractional photothermolysis is a recent resurfacing laser technology for treating wrinkles, melanocytic pigmentation, scars, and photodamaged skin. These systems utilize a 1,550-nm erbium-doped fiber laser that emits an array of microscopic spots at variable densities. Treatment creates microzones of injury in the skin that are surrounded by normal intervening skin that rapidly heals the injured tissue. Plasma skin regeneration allows precise and rapid treatment of photodamaged skin, with controlled thermal injury and modification. Radiofrequency energy converts nitrogen gas into plasma, which results in rapid heating of the skin as the plasma rapidly gives up energy to the skin. The technology can be used at varying energies for different depths of effect, from superficial epidermal sloughing to deeper dermal heating. Patients typically develop erythema and edema shortly after treatment, with no immediate epidermal loss or charring. Plasma skin regeneration improves fine lines, textural irregularities, and dyspigmentation. Skin tightening is probably more pronounced with the high-energy treatment. Devices that treat wrinkles through fractional photothermolysis or plasma skin regeneration are probably more effective than IPL in treating fine wrinkles. However, if the clinician has an IPL and a fractionated or plasma regeneration device, then the combination of IPL and one of the two is an ideal treatment modality for rejuvenation of the skin.

Radiofrequency devices employ a 400-W, 6.78-MHz high-frequency generator electrode to disperse radiofrequency energy and create a uniform electric field across the surface of the device tip and into the tissue. Contact cooling is employed to the back surface of the device tip to cool the epidermis and upper dermis. This combination of heating and contact cooling creates a reverse thermal

TABLE 49.1: Summary of Available Pulsed Broadband Light Devices

Manufacturer	Product Name	Device Type	Wavelength (nm)	Energy Output	Pulse Width (ms)
Alma Lasers	Harmony	AFT pulsed light	540–950	5–20 J	10, 12, 15 ms
Cutera	Xeo	Nd:YAG/pulsed light	1,064	6–40 J	0.1–300 ms/ automatic variable
	Solera Opus	intelligent pulsed light	500–635	3–24 J	
Cynosure	Cynergy PL Cynergy III	pulsed light pulsed dye/ Nd:YAG/ pulsed light	400–1,200 585 nm; 1,064 560–950	3–30 J 16–30 J (handpieces)	5–50 ms 5–50 ms
DermaMed	Quadra Q4 Platinum Quadra Q4 Gold	intense pulsed light intense pulsed light	5–1,200 5–1,200	up to 20 J up to 20 J	10–110 ms 10–110 ms
Focus Medical	NaturaLight	pulsed light	510–1,200	35 J	460 ms
Lumenis	Lumenis One	intense pulsed light Nd:YAG light sheer diode Aluma RF	515–1,200 1,064 800 RF	3–100 ms	5–38 ms
McCUE	Ultra VPL	variable pulsed light	530–950 610–1,020	up to 51 J	variable
Novatis	Clareon VR	pulsed light	500–610 740–1,200	up to 35 J	30, 50, 70 ms
	Solarus VR	pulsed light	520–1,200	up to 20 J	20, 40, 60 ms
Palomar	StarLux System	pulsed light/laser	1,064 500–570 870–1,400	up to 700 J	0.5–500 ms
	MediLux System EsteLux	pulsed light pulsed light	470–1,400 470–1,400	up to 45 J up to 40 J	10–100 ms 10–100 ms
Quantel Medical	Prolite II	intense pulsed light	530–1,200	15–44 J	20–72 ms
Radiancy	SkinStation S P R Duet	LHE–light heat energy LHE–light heat energy LHE–light heat energy	400–1,200 400–1,200 400–1,200	up to 65 J up to 65 J up to 65 J total	10 ms 10 ms 10, 35 ms
Sciton	BBL	pulsed light module	410–1,400	up to 30 J	up to 200 1–10 s
	Profile HMV	Nd:YAG/pulsed light	1,064/410–1,400	up to 400 J	0.1–200 ms 1–10 s
	Pro-V	1,319/1,064-nm Nd:YAG pulsed light	410–1,319	up to 400 J	0.1–200 ms 1–10 s
Sybaritic Inc	NannoLight SpectraQuattro	pulsed light pulsed light	410–1,400 410–1,400	up to 45 J up to 40 J	1–30 ms 1–30 ms
Syneron	eLight SR	optical energy/RF electrical energy	580–980	up to 45 J/ up to 25 J	N/A
	eLight SRA	optical energy/RF electrical energy	470–980	up to 45 J/ up to 25 J	N/A

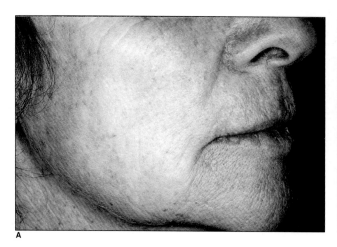 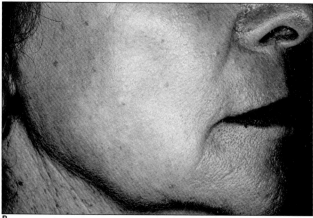

FIGURE 49.1: *Typical BBL treatment results:* **A,** *pretreatment;* **B,** *posttreatment.*

gradient, whereby the greatest heating is deep in the skin, while the outer layer of the skin is cooled, which helps to protect it. Through heating and thermal injury, collagen is heated above 60 degrees Celsius, which denatures and the fibrils immediately contract and also thicken. Dermal remodeling begins with the wound-healing response that produces skin tightening over time. Radiofrequency devices work entirely differently than IPL in that the primary purpose of radiofrequency devices is to produce skin tightening and lifting of the face and neck, without addressing erythema or lentigines. The combination of utilizing IPL and a radiofrequency device is ideal for tightening the skin and lessening erythema and lentigines seen from photodamage.

IPL devices are sold either as a single unit or as a multipurpose device. Multipurpose devices incorporate IPL with a combination of other units such as the 1,064-nm long-pulsed Nd-YAG used for leg veins and hair removal in darker individuals, a fractionated photothermolysis handpiece, Q-switched Nd-YAG device for tattoo removal, and radiofrequency devices. Purchasing a multipurpose device may be less expensive than buying separate devices and would occupy less space in the exam room. The principal disadvantage, however, is should the multipurpose device fail due to a system error, then the clinician would not be able to treat patients for any purpose until the device is fixed, whereas the downtime would be less by having individual devices should one of them fail.

In summary, broadband light devices (Table 49.1) have become available as alternatives in rejuvenating photodamaged skin. Nonablative dermal remodeling techniques have been developed to induce dermal damage without epidermal disruption. This can be achieved when the following requirements are met: first, the wavelength and radiant exposure must be sufficient to create selective dermal wounding and induce collagen remodeling; second,

the epidermis must be protected from thermal damage. Although clinical results may be modest in many instances (Figure 49.1), these nonablative systems offer a reduction in adverse sequelae and recovery time.

SUGGESTED READING

Bitter PJ. Noninvasive rejuvenation of photoaged skin using serial, full-face intense pulsed light treatments. *Dermatol. Surg.* 2000;26:835–43.

Bitter P, Campbell CA, Goldman M. Nonablative skin rejuvenation using intense pulsed light. *Lasers Surg. Med.* 2000;12(Suppl):16–17.

Bogle MA. Plasma skin regeneration technology. *Skin Ther. Lett.* 2006;11:7–9.

Collawn SS. Fraxel skin resurfacing. *Ann. Plast. Surg.* 2007; 58:237–40.

Cotton J, Hood AF, Gonin RM, Beeson WH, Hanke W. Histologic evaluation of preauricular and postauricular human skin after high energy, short-pulse carbon dioxide laser. *Arch. Dermatol.* 1996;132:425–8.

Ditre CM, Griffin TD, Murphy GF, et al. Effects of alpha-hydroxy acids on photoaged skin: a pilot clinical, histologic, and ultrastructural study. *J. Am. Acad. Dermatol.* 1996;34:187–95.

Fisher GJ, Wang ZQ, Datta SC, Varani J, Kang S, Voorhees JJ. Pathophysiology of premature skin aging induced by ultraviolet light. *N. Engl. J. Med.* 1997;337:1419–28.

Fitzpatrick RE. Laser resurfacing of rhytides (review). *Dermatol. Clin.* 1997;15:431–47.

Fitzpatrick RE, Tope WD, Goldman MP, Satur NM. Pulsed carbon dioxide laser, trichloroacetic acid, Baker-Gordon phenol, and dermabrasion: a comparative clinical and histologic study of cutaneous resurfacing in a porcine model. *Arch. Dermatol.* 1996;132:468–71.

Goldberg DJ. Non-ablative subsurface remodeling: clinical and histologic evaluation of a 1320 nm Nd:Yag laser. *J. Cutan. Laser Ther.* 1999;1:153–7.

Griffiths CEM, Russman AN, Majmudar G, Singer RS, Hamilton TA, Voorhees JJ. Restoration of collagen formation in photoaged human skin by tretinoin (retinoic acid). *New. Engl. J. Med.* 1993;329:530–5.

Iyer S, Suthamjariya K. Using a radiofrequency energy device to treat the lower face: a treatment paradigm for a nonsurgical facelift. *Cosmet. Dermatol.* 2003;16:37–40.

Kilmer SL, Chotzen VA. Pulsed dye laser treatment of rhytids. *Lasers Surg. Med.* 1998;19(Suppl 9):194.

Kilmer S, Semchyshyn N, Shah G, Fitzpatrick R. A pilot study on the use of a plasma skin regeneration device (Portrait PSR3) in full facial rejuvenation procedures. *Lasers Med. Sci.* 2007;22:101–109.

Nanni CA, Alster TS. Complications of carbon dioxide laser resurfacing: an evaluation of 500 patients. *Dermatol. Surg.* 1998:24:315–20.

Raulin C, Goldman MP, Weiss MA, Weiss RA. Treatment of adult port-wine stains using intense pulsed light therapy (PhotoDerm CL): brief initial clinical report. *Dermatol. Surg.* 1997;23:594–7.

Raulin C, Werner S, Hartschuh W, Schonermark MP. Effective treatment of hypertrichosis with pulsed light: a report of two cases. *Ann. Plast. Surg.* 1997;39:169–73.

Ross EV, Naseef G, Skrobal M, et al. In vivo dermal collagen shrinkage and remodeling following CO_2 laser resurfacing. *Lasers Surg. Med.* 1996;18:38.

Tanzi EL, Williams CM, Alster TS. Treatment of facial rhytides with a nonablative 1,450-nm diode laser: a controlled clinical and histologic study. *Dermatol. Surg.* 2003;29:124–8.

Trelles MA, Alvarez X, Martin-Vazquez MJ, et al. Assessment of the efficacy of nonablative long-pulsed 1064-nm Nd:YAG laser treatment of wrinkles compared at 2, 4, and 6 months. *Facial Plast. Surg.* 2005;21:145–53.

Wanner M, Tanzi EL, Alster TS. Fractional photothermolysis: treatment of facial and nonfacial cutaneous photodamage with a 1,550-nm erbium-doped fiber laser. *Dermatol. Surg.* 2007;33:23–8.

CHAPTER 50

Titan: Inducing Dermal Contraction

Javier Ruiz-Esparza

Dermal contraction for the purpose of cosmetic improvement can be induced by the application of heat at adequate intensity and for adequate time. The first technology to achieve this was nonablative radiofrequency. Heat was produced by the passage of electrons flowing from an active electrode into the skin and, ultimately, into a passive electrode or grounding plate. This monopolar radiofrequency device spared the epidermis from thermal injury using a concurrent squirt of cryogen fluid applied onto the back side of the treating electrode. The cryogen would be sprayed immediately before, during, and immediately after the emission of radiofrequency. This device had two inherent problems: one was the electrical quality of the energy pulses, which were unpleasant; second, the intensity of those pulses were quite painful. To mitigate such pain, a topical anesthetic was applied for at least an hour prior to the procedure, but even then, the intensity (up to 150 J/cm^2) combined with a short delivery time (1–2 s) made for an experience hard to forget for the patient.

Titan (Altera Inc.) is an alternative device, which uses infrared light (1,100–1,800 nm) as the energy source, and also combines it with cold before, during, and after the energy pulse. This device has been used effectively to achieve skin contraction, but because it uses a multisecond pulse, the energy does not cause the same degree of pain as the radiofrequency device. Furthermore, immediate contraction of collagen can more easily be obtained due to the fact that the energy is delivered in a slow, sustained, and incremental form to the skin and over a period of several seconds, which not only makes contracting the skin much more reliable, but it can also be realized with almost no pain to the patient. Low fluences can be used to produce immediate, almost painless contraction of the skin, and the ability of this device to produce immediate collagen contraction has been confirmed by electron microscopy.

TITAN: CLINICAL USES AND TECHNIQUE

Patient selection is based more on adequate expectations than on age, sex, or skin type. Anyone, at any age, can expect a modest degree of improvement from each treatment. Multiple treatments are desirable when the degree of skin laxity is pronounced. Treatments can be repeated at intervals as short as one month. Basically, any area with unwanted skin flaccidity is, in theory, susceptible to treatment with this device. The energy is applied through a handpiece that has a treatment window of electronically cooled sapphire crystal. The size and shape of the crystal are important with respect of the skin area to be treated. This treatment window is applied directly over the skin to be treated, and the machine is activated with a pedal.

No anesthetic is required. Our patients are asked to wash thoroughly in the office. The skin should be completely free of cosmetics and any substances. A hydrophilic gel can be used for cooling and can be applied onto the skin immediately prior to treatment. I prefer not to use any gels. The treatment window has to be in full contact with the skin during treatment. Gaps will result in burns. We must remember that we are using contact cooling.

Multiple passes will be needed. It is best to treat small areas at a time so that the interval between passes is small. The fluence should be moderate. Even if the patient says that he or she cannot feel anything, heat will accumulate in tissue and subsequent passes will feel increasingly hot. We must refrain from increasing the fluence too much during the first pass because subsequent passes will be intolerable due to heat accumulation in tissue, and the total time of skin heating will be reduced. Edema and nonimmediate contraction will result.

The skin of the cheeks can be treated lateral to the nasolabial fold (Figure 50.1). No overlapping of pulses is needed. How much of the skin of the cheek needs to

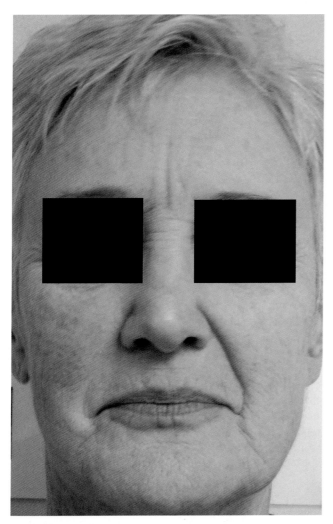

FIGURE 50.1: *Sixty-seven-year-old woman treated with Titan on the right cheek only. Immediate painless contraction was noted. Fifty-five pulses at 34 J/cm².*

be treated depends on the degree of laxity in a particular patient. A young individual with marginal laxity will obtain significant improvement with treatment to only the skin lateral to the nasolabial fold, while treatment of the entire cheek will be best in someone with advanced laxity. Generally, three to four passes will be adequate (fifty to seventy pulses per cheek). A fluence of 34 J/cm² is generally well tolerated. If pain is an issue, the fluence can be dropped as low as 20 J/cm², but more pulses will be needed.

The lateral aspects of the neck should be treated in their entirety, from the mandibular lines to the clavicles (fifty to ninety pulses per side).

Eyebrow lifting can be achieved in some patients – usually in those whose low eyebrows are the result of aging

(B. Novak, personal communication). The skin above the eyebrows is treated best with the V-shaped handpiece. Fluences of 20–25 J/cm² are needed. Extra care should be taken that skin contact is complete before emission of the energy to avoid a burn. The forehead convexity may not align well with the flat surface of the treatment window. Once full contact is established, three to four overlapping pulses are preferred. One should avoid treating too close to the eyebrow itself. I stay 2 cm over the eyebrow line. The shape of the area treated will depend on the part of the eyebrow that needs to be lifted (e.g., lateral for eyebrow tail elevation).

The skin of the lower eyelids can be similarly treated for correction of eyelid bags due to skin laxity. Only skin laxity can be corrected. Fat herniation will remain unchanged. Eye protection is of paramount importance and can be achieved with perfectly fit metal goggles. Three to four overlapping pulses of 20–25 J/cm² will be needed. This is an advanced technique and one-to-one training is essential. A burn in the thin skin of the lower eyelid could lead to scar and ectropion. Clinical improvement becomes apparent one month after the procedure.

Large areas (arms, thighs, and abdomen) are treated best by the glide technique. The machine is set to its maximum output (65 J/cm² for the S-shaped handpiece) and the handpiece is glided over a small area (usually 3–5 cm), while the light is being delivered. This distributes energy in tissue rather evenly if the movement of the operator's hand is steady, and the application of energy is totally painless. Sixty-five pulses per side are adequate. When one finishes, the skin must feel warm to the touch and remain warm for several minutes.

No postoperative care is needed for any of these areas. No complications other than superficial vesicles (in 1% to 3% of cases in my hands), which heal with minimal wound care, have been seen. The patient must be instructed not to manipulate the vesicles.

SUGGESTED READING

Ruiz-Esparza J. Immediate, painless skin contraction at low fluences via a new infrared light device. *Dermatol. Surg.* 2006;32:897–901.

Ruiz-Esparza J, Barba-Gomez J. The medical face-lift: a non-invasive, non-surgical approach to tissue tightening in facial skin using non-ablative radiofrequency. *Dermatol. Surg.* 2003;29:325–32.

Zelickson B, Ross V, Kist D, Counters J, et al. Ultrastructural effects of an infrared handpiece on forehead and abdominal skin. *Dermatol. Surg.* 2006;32:897–901.

CHAPTER 51

Sciton Broadband Light and Er:YAG Micropeel Combination

Joseph F. Greco
David P. Beynet
Teresa Soriano

Nonablative and minimally ablative facial rejuvenation has become increasingly popular over the last several years. Patients desire less invasive cosmetic procedures with maximal effect and minimal downtime. Despite the tremendous effort going into developing novel treatments, currently available nonablative laser and light therapies have demonstrated minimal to moderate improvement in photoaged skin. Recently, the concept of using two different modalities to treat the photoaged skin has been explored. The idea behind this is that two varying mechanisms that target the same downstream event theoretically could lead to an additive and even possibly a synergistic effect to improve the photoaged skin. There is recent evidence for the effectiveness of sequential combined treatment using a broadband light (BBL) therapy followed by an Er:YAG microlaser peel (Profile, Sciton Inc.) for skin rejuvenation.

BACKGROUND

BBL technology utilizes a polychromatic, noncoherent, continuous band of wavelengths to target multiple aspects of photoaging during a single treatment session. As the primary tissue chromophores are melanin and oxyhemoglobin, both pigmented and vascular lesions may be treated simultaneously, while nonspecific bulk heating stimulates dermal remodeling and new collagen formation. Clinically, this correlates with a concomitant reduction and lightening of melanin containing pigmented lesions, telangiectasia, and baseline erythema as well as a mild to modest softening of fine rhytids. Cutoff filters are used to define and limit the lower end of the wavelength spectrum, depending on the clinical lesions to be treated. In treating photoaging with dyschromia and telangiectasias, a 515-nm filter is used to permit increased absorption of lower wavelengths by pigmented lesions. Alternatively, a 590-nm filter may be chosen to protect melanin-containing lesions and allow a more selective treatment of erythema and telangiectasia. The ability to use higher-wavelength cutoff filters permits safer treatments in pigmented skin.

The Er:YAG microlaser peel (MLP) incorporates a dual-pulsed erbium laser, which emits a monochromatic wavelength at 2,940 nm. Water is an ideal chromophore for this laser as its major peak absorption occurs at 3,000 nm. Such a close approximation enables a highly precise superficial epidermal ablation, with immediate absorption of the laser energy and minimal collateral thermal damage. Clinically, this correlates with an improvement in surface texture through a reduction in tactile roughness created by superficial benign and premalignant keratoses. Interestingly, a temporary reduction of surface vellous hairs can occur due to a thermal singing of exposed hair.

PROCEDURE

The photodamaged treatment area is cleansed and topical anesthesia is used for patient comfort. The authors use a compounded topical gel of 7% lidocaine/7% tetracaine applied for one hour. The topical anesthetic is completely removed with a damp washcloth prior to treatment, and a thin layer of a water-based ultrasound gel is applied. Treatment with the BBL source (Profile) is performed using a 515-, 560-, or 590-nm filter with fluences ranging from 8 to 12 J/cm^2, a pulse width of 20 ms, a contact epidermal cooling temperature of 20 degrees Celsius, and a repetition rate of 1 s, using a single pulse with no overlap (Table 51.1). Begin with a preauricular test spot before proceeding medially. Mild erythema and immediate pigment darkening of lentigos typically occur. Caution should be taken to avoid hair-bearing areas, especially the bearded area in males, as it may result in permanent hair loss. A tongue depressor may be used to shield hair-bearing areas, such as the eyebrows, from exposure to the light source.

Immediately following the BBL treatment, the water-based ultrasound gel is thoroughly removed with gauze. Alcohol wipes are subsequently applied to the treatment area to ensure complete removal of the gel, as any residual gel will serve as a competing chromophore for laser absorption. A microlaser peel with the Er:YAG laser (Profile) is

TABLE 51.1: Combination BBL/MLP Treatment Protocol

Preoperative Care	BBL Parameters	MLP Parameters	Postoperative Care
Cleanse treatment area	Fluence: 12 J/cm² (8–12 J/cm² range)	Peel depth: 20 μm (15–20 μm range)	aquaphor ointment BID until peeling resolves
Topical anesthesia	Pulse width: 20 ms Cooling temp.: 20°C	Overlap: 50% single pass	Sun avoidance Broad-spectrum sunblock
Aqueous gel prior to BBL only	Repetition rate: 1 s Single pass, no overlap		TMC 0.1% cream BID 1–3 days PRN significant erythema and edema

performed. Typical settings include the following: a depth of 20 μm (level 2, 5 J/cm²) and an overlap of 50%, with a single pass. Immediate epidermal whitening is typically noted overlying the erythema from the BBL treatment.

Typical areas treated include photodamaged skin of the face, neck, and dorsal aspects of the hands in patients with Fitzpatrick skin types I–III (Figures 51.1 and 51.2).

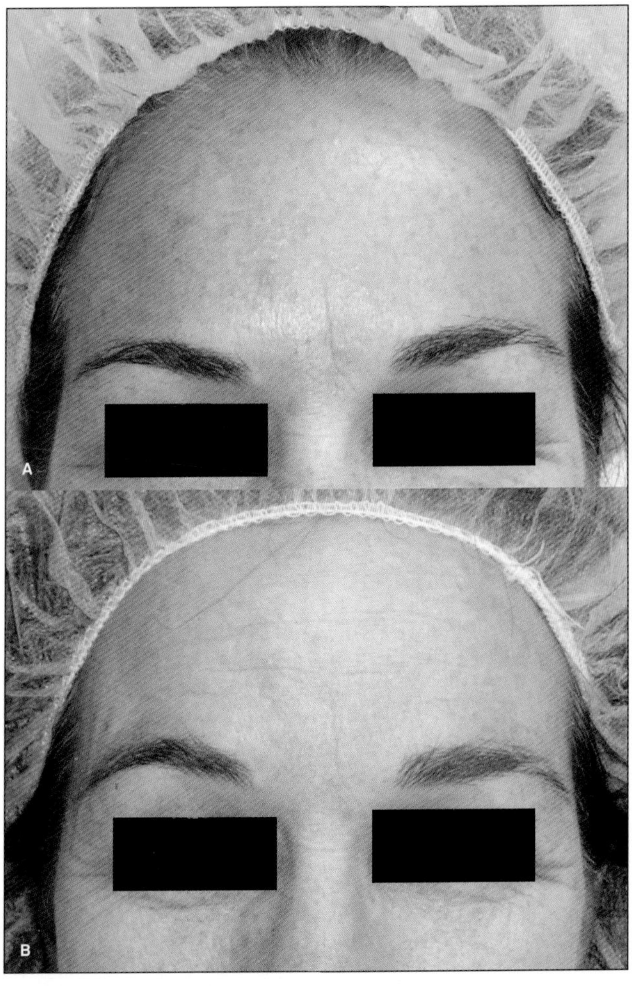

FIGURE 51.1: BBL/Er:YAG micropeel for dyschromia: A, pretreatment; B, posttreatment.

Total treatment time, excluding that required for topical anesthesia, ranges from twelve to twenty minutes, depending on the anatomic area being treated. Adjustable repetition rate settings on both the BBL and MLP platforms permit accelerated treatment times with pulse firing intervals ranging between 0.5 and 2 s.

POSTOPERATIVE CARE

Postoperatively, aquaphor ointment is applied twice daily, and strict sun avoidance is emphasized during the immediate postoperative week. Patients are encouraged to use a broad-spectrum sunscreen thereafter. Antiviral prophylaxis with oral Valtrex 500 milligrams twice daily for five days beginning one day prior to the procedure is recommended in patients with a history of oral herpes simplex virus outbreaks. Triamcinalone 0.1% cream can be prescribed one to three days postoperatively for patients who experience significant edema and erythema.

CLINICAL BENEFITS

Patients with Fitzpatrick skin types I–III and signs of photoaging typically achieve overall improvement of the texture and appearance of their skin with lightening of lentigos, reduction of telangiectasias, and erythema and modest softening of fine rhytids. Additional subjective improvements include the ability to apply makeup more smoothly as well as a decrease in the amount of makeup used per application. This is attributed to a reduction in both surface keratoses and the need to conceal pigmented and vascular lesions.

SIDE EFFECTS

Postoperatively, expected typical side effects include minimal edema, mild to moderate erythema, and peeling. Immediate pigment darkening of lentigos occurs after BBL treatment and typically resolves within five to ten days. Patients usually feel comfortable resuming public appearances anywhere from two days to one week posttreatment. The authors have had two patients who developed

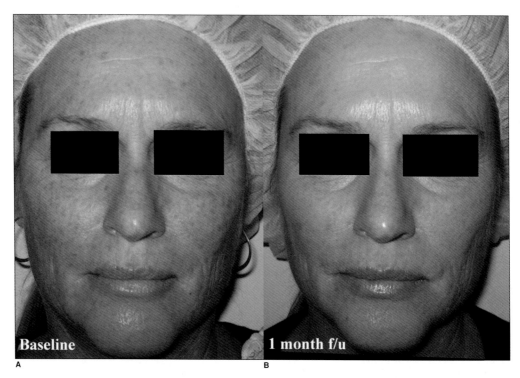

FIGURE 51.2: *Combination BBL/Er:YAG micropeel treatment for dyschromia and fine lines:* **A**, *pretreatment;* **B**, *one month posttreatment.*

acneiform eruptions after the treatment. Although the exact cause of this eruption is unclear, it may be attributed to the occlusive nature of postoperative petrolatum-based ointment.

CONCLUSION

In summary, the combination sequential therapy with BBL and erbium MLP is a safe and effective option to achieve significant improvement of photoaged skin in Fitzpatrick skin types I–III. Their synergistic mechanisms of action target various pathologies of chronic sun damage from the epidermal surface to the reticular dermis, in a safe, reproducible, and relatively quick procedure. Clinically, this translates to improvement in dyschromia, skin texture, and fine rhytides after one to two treatments. Side effects and downtime are minimal. More studies with long-term follow-up will reveal the long-term effects of this combination treatment.

SUGGESTED READING

Alster TS, Lupton JR. Erbium:YAG cutaneous laser resurfacing. *Dermatol. Clin.* 2001;19:453–66.

Ang P, Barlow RJ. Nonablative laser resurfacing: a systematic review of the literature. *Clin. Exp. Dermatol.* 2002;27:630–5.

Avram DK, Goldman MP. The safety and effectiveness of single-pass erbium:YAG laser in the treatment of mild to moderate photodamage. *Dermatol. Surg.* 2004;30:1073–6.

Greco JF, Soriano T, Lask GP, Kim J. Combination treatment with broadband light and erbium-doped yttrium aluminum garnet microlaser peel for photoaged skin: case report of four patients. *Dermatol Surg.* 2008 Nov;34(11):1603–8.

Kim KH, Geronemus RG. Nonablative laser and light therapies for skin rejuvenation. *Arch. Facial Plast. Surg.* 2004;6:398–409.

Ross EV, Smirnov M, Pankratov M, Altshuler G. Intense pulsed light and laser treatment of facial telangiectasias and dyspigmentation: some theoretical and practical comparisons. *Dermatol. Surg.* 2005;31:1188–98.

CHAPTER 52

Aminolevulinic Acid Photodynamic Therapy for Facial Rejuvenation and Acne

Jane G. Khoury

Mitchel P. Goldman

Light therapy is widely used in dermatology. The addition of a photosensitizing medication to the light, collectively known as photodynamic therapy (PDT), can enhance laser and light treatment. PDT has become an increasingly popular therapy for practitioners treating a variety of cosmetic and medical dermatologic conditions. The two commonly used photosensitizers are 20% 5-aminolevuline acid (ALA; Levulan, DUSA Pharmaceuticals) and the methyl ester of 20% 5-ALA (MAL; Metvixia, Galderma). Once ALA or MAL has been applied, it is metabolized into the photosensitizer protoporphyrin PpIX, which is preferentially taken up by rapidly proliferating cells such as tumor cells and sebaceous glands. Irradiation of photosensitized skin with various light and laser sources results in a photooxidation of the target molecules.

A variety of lasers and light sources have been utilized to activate ALA and MAL, including blue light (417 nm), red light (635 nm), pulse dye lasers (585 and 595 nm), and intense pulsed light (420–1200 nm). Table 52.1 demonstrates the absorption spectrum of PpIX and the corresponding PpIX absorbance of various light sources. Depending on the condition being treated, the PDT dose can be customized by controlling the amount of ALA/MAL that enters the skin, the time allowed for PpIX synthesis, the various laser and light sources, and the amount of light that is absorbed. This chapter will focus on the use of ALA-PDT for acne and photodamaged skin. Although currently off-label, its application for photorejuvenation and acne therapy is growing in use and popularity.

PHOTOREJUVENATION

Photorejuvenation is a process in which light energy sources are utilized to reverse the process of sun-induced aging and environmental damage to the skin. While photodamage manifests as wrinkles, pigmentary changes, lentigines, telangiectasias, and textural changes, it can also lead to precancerous conditions such as actinic keratoses and, eventually, basal cell and squamous cell carcinoma.

When Levulan was first approved by the Food and Drug Administration (FDA) in 1999, it was for treatment of nonhyperkeratotic actinic keratoses (AKs) on face and scalp with a drug incubation of fourteen to eighteen hours, followed by blue light activation for sixteen minutes and forty seconds. This was often associated with significant phototoxic side effects, notably burning pain likely due to activation of PpIX in cutaneous nerve endings. In 2004, Touma et al. found that one-, two-, and three-hour ALA application times were as efficacious in clearing AKs as fourteen- to eighteen-hour application times. Avram and Goldman (2004) evaluated the combined use of ALA-IPL for the treatment of photodamage with one treatment

TABLE 52.1: Parameters to Activate Levulan for the Most Popular Light Sources

- Lumenis One: 560-nm filter; 16–18 J/cm^2, 4.0/4.0 with 10–40 ms delay, one pass
- Vasculight: 560-nm filter; 30 J/cm^2; 2.4/4.0 with 10–40 ms delay; one pass or 35 J/cm^2, 3.0–6.0 with 10–20 ms delay
- Quantum: 560-nm filter; 26 J/cm^2; 2.4/4.0 with 10–40 ms delay; one pass; one pass or 35 J/cm^2, 3.0–6.0 with 10–20 ms delay
- Aurora: optical energy of 16–22 J/cm^2 with a radiofrequency of 16–22 J/cm^2; one pass
- Estelux: 19–30 J/cm^2 at 20 ms, one pass
- V-Beam: 10-mm spot size; 7.5 J/cm^2; 6-ms pulse width; two passes with 50% overlap
- V-Star: 10-mm spot size; 7.5 J/cm^2; 40-ms pulse width; two passes with 50% overlap
- Cynergy: 7-mm spot size; 10–12 J/cm^2; 40-ms pulse width; two passes with 50% overlap
- ClearLight: 405–420 nm blue light; 8–10 min under light
- BLU-U: 417 nm ± 5 nm blue light; 8–15 min under light

Note: Adapted from Nootheti PK, Goldman MP, Advances in photorejuvenation and the current status of photodynamic therapy. *Expert Rev. Dermatol.* 2006;1:51–61, with permission of Future Drugs Ltd.

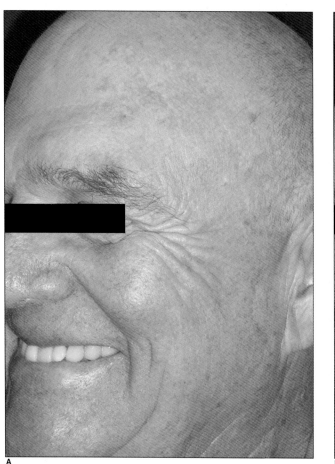
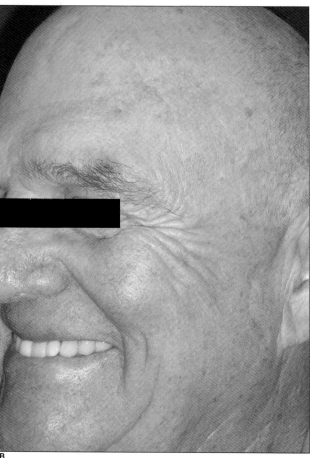

FIGURE 52.1: **A,** *Before treatment and,* **B,** *five years after two treatments. ALA was applied to skin for seventy-five minutes, followed by activation with the Vasculight IPL (Lumenis Ltd.) using a 560-nm filter; 28 J/cm²; 2.4/4.0 pulse duration with 20-ms delay.*

session and found moderate to significant improvement in skin texture, pigment irregularities, and telangiectasias, along with resolution of actinic keratoses. Many other clinical research studies have found similar results, and the reader is encouraged to review the references at the end for further information on these studies. The American Society for Photodynamic Therapy recently published treatment guidelines in January 2006 showing similar efficacy in treating AKs and photorejuvenation with short-contact, full-face treatments. This regimen has now become the standard of care in the United States, though it is still considered off-label (Figure 52.1). Table 52.1 lists several light sources and their parameters for activation of Levulan, while the clinical technique is discussed later in the chapter.

ACNE

Acne vulgaris is one of the most common skin disorders, affecting 80% of the population at some time during life. Acne is a disorder of the sebaceous glands and proliferation of bacteria along with dyskeratinization of the pilo-sebaceous unit. *P. acnes* is a causative factor in acne inflammation within the sebaceous glands. Conventional treatments include topical and oral antibiotics, benzoyl peroxide, retinoids, and hormonal therapy and isotretinoin. Antibiotic resistance, skin irritation, slow onset of efficacy, and systemic toxicity have led many patients and physicians to consider lasers and light sources for the treatment of acne.

Most clinicians are aware that natural and artificial ultraviolet light improves their patient's inflammatory acne lesions. This works by an endogenous PDT mechanism. The presence of *P. acnes* leads to the production of protoporphyrin IX (PpIX) and coproporphyrin III within the sebaceous glands. In the presence of oxygen, exposure to an appropriate light source results in selective destruction of the *P. acnes* and clearance of the inflammatory acne lesions. Long-term effects of ultraviolet light prohibit recommendation of this treatment. However, these

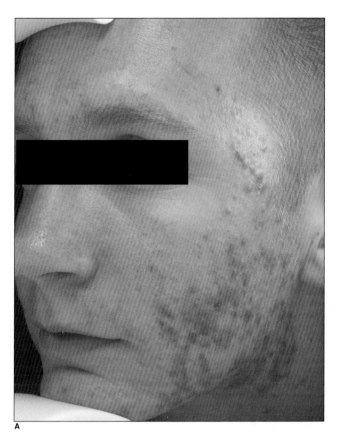 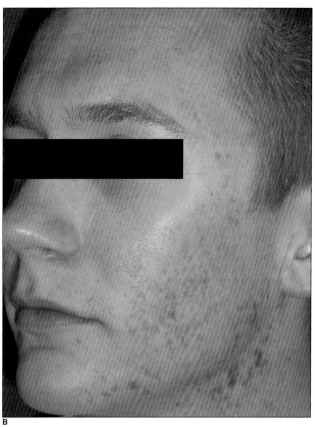

A   B

FIGURE 52.2: A, *Before treatment and,* **B,** *nine months after two treatments. ALA was applied to skin for sixty minutes, followed by activation with Cynergy (Cynosure Inc.) 595-nm PDL with a 7-mm spot size and 40-ms pulse duration at 8 J/cm² and ClearLight (Lumenis Ltd.) for fifteen minutes.*

endogenous porphyrins are the target of the blue and red light sources.

The first clinical trial utilizing ALA-PDT in the treatment of acne was reported by Hongcharu et al. in 2000. Goldman (2003) was the first to report his experience with short-contact (one-hour drug incubation) ALA using IPL or blue light sources in the treatment of acne and sebaceous gland hyperplasia, noting relative clearing without the phototoxic PDT effects reported earlier with longer contact incubation. Gold (2004) also reported his experience with short-contact (thirty- to sixty-minute drug incubation) 5-ALA-PDT with the blue light system. These and other notable studies have been included in the "Suggested Reading" at the end of this chapter. While an off-label use, multiple short-contact ALA-PDT is an efficacious and increasingly popular treatment option for acne vulgaris (Figure 52.2).

PATIENT SELECTION

Good candidates for PDT photorejuvenation have diffuse photodamage and multiple precancerous lesions, are reluc-

tant to undergo ablative laser resurfacing, and hope to avoid the pain and scarring of cryotherapy and surgical excision. Ideal acne patients are those with moderate to severe inflammatory acne vulgaris that has failed to improve with topical medications or patients wishing to avoid oral antibiotics or isotretinoin.

This therapy should not be applied to women who are pregnant or lactating; those with a history of porphyria, lupus, or other conditions that cause photosensitivity; and those taking photosensitizing drugs. In addition, a history of herpes simplex, pigmentation problems, formation of keloid scars, and tanning habits should be evaluated, as should all topical and oral medications, prescriptions, and nonprescription and herbal supplements. Patients with Fitzpatrick skin types IV–V should be treated with caution due to the increased risk of developing postinflammatory hyperpigmentation.

PATIENT EDUCATION

Because of the photosensitizing nature of ALA, patients must plan on remaining strictly indoors for twenty-four hours after the treatment. Not doing so may result in significant phototoxic reactions. Other side effects to be reviewed include redness, skin tenderness, swelling, bruising, scabbing, crusting, dyspigmentation, and possible scarring. Two to four treatments may be necessary to achieve optimal results, especially in acne patients. While the FDA has cleared ALA-PDT for the treatment of AKs of the face and scalp, patients should be aware that all other uses are off-label.

LIGHT SOURCE FOR PDT

The ideal light source in PDT should be well absorbed by the photosensitizer, achieve optimal penetration to reach the target, and have adequate fluence and duration to mediate a photodynamic reaction. Numerous light sources have been documented to treat photodamage and acne with PDT such as blue light, red light, intense pulsed light (IPL), and the pulsed dye laser (PDL).

Blue light uses the maximum absorption peak of PpIX at 410 nm; however, these shorter wavelengths provide less tissue penetration and are ideal for penetration of superficial lesions as photons only reach 1–2 mm deep. The BLU-U is the least expensive light source, with an output at 417 nm, and is strongly absorbed by PpIX (see Table 52.1). While sixteen minutes forty seconds is the set time established to deliver the full 10 J/cm², this is not often necessary, and adequate times can range from ten to fifteen minutes. The ClearLight is a similar system that uses a narrowband light source (405–420 nm), also strongly absorbed by PpIX. The U shape of the BLU-U system is optimal for facial and scalp treatment but may be less practical for trunk and extremities, which may be better treated with the ClearLight system. Other blue light systems are also available, with newer light sources coming to market soon.

Red light uses one of the smaller absorption peaks of PpIX at 630 nm but can penetrate 5–6 mm into the skin and is a desirable light source when deeper lesions are being treated.

Compared to blue light, the long PDL and IPL are less efficient sources for activation of ALA but can provide adequate efficacy if combined with proper skin preparation and ALA application. They are also useful adjuncts to blue light activation and maximize treatment of certain conditions (e.g., IPL for photodamage, PDL for acne or sebaceous hyperplasia). Table 52.1 provides information on several PDL and IPL systems and recommended treatment parameters.

CLINICAL TECHNIQUE

Any review of the literature will reveal that there are many different techniques to achieve successful results with PDT. As described, multiple light sources can be utilized for ALA-PDT. Summarized subsequently are the general guidelines used at our office to maximize PDT of acne and photodamaged skin. Table 52.1 lists the lasers and light sources currently being used for ALA-PDT and the common parameters for the various laser systems. Table 52.2 shows a sample PDT patient guide for acne treatment. Table 52.3 shows home-care instructions for patients following PDT.

- If there is a history of herpes simplex virus infection, it is recommended that the patient begin oral antiviral the day before ALA-PDT therapy.
- Photograph the patient.
- Have the patient wash his or her skin with gentle cleanser and water.
- Skin is prepped with a microdermabrasion procedure to increase the penetration of the ALA as the stratum corneum is an important barrier for ALA penetration.
- An acetone scrub with a 4 × 4 gauze is then performed on the skin.
- Break the two glass ampules in the Levulan Kerastick (DUSA Pharmaceuticals) as per instructions on the stick. Shake the stick for two minutes. While compounded ALA is legal and often less expensive, DUSA Pharmaceuticals has a use patent on ALA and owns exclusive rights to use ALA-PDT on patients. Therefore providers using compounded ALA on their patients are violating DUSA's patent rights.
- The Levulan is painted on the areas of the skin to be treated. Two coats of Levulan are applied and spread uniformly with gloved fingertips. Extra pressure and solution may be used to spot treat particular areas of concern. Care should be taken to get close to the eyes, while avoiding eyelids and mucous membranes.
- Levulan is now allowed to incubate on the skin surface. We recommend an incubation period of sixty minutes, with the patient kept indoors, away from ambient light sources. ALA is unstable at a pH greater than 4.5; therefore topical lidocaine (pH 7.5–9) should not be applied directly to skin after Levulan.
- The face is again washed with cleanser and water. It is imperative that all ALA remaining on the skin surface be removed. Any residual ALA increases the potential for phototoxicity and pain with light and laser irradiation.
- The patient then receives treatment with an appropriate light source.
- Warn the patient to remain out of direct sunlight for twenty-four to forty-eight hours after the procedure.

TABLE 52.2: PDT Patient Guide

What is photodynamic therapy?

Photodynamic therapy (PDT) is a special treatment performed with a topical photosensitizing agent called *Levulan 5-aminolevulinic acid* (ALA), activated with the correct wavelength of light. This is also known as ALA-PDT treatment. These treatments remove sun-damaged precancerous zones and spots called *actinic keratoses*. Sun damage, fine lines, and blotchy pigmentation are also improved because of the positive effect of Levulan and the light treatment. ALA-PDT treatment also has the unique ability to minimize pores and reduce oil glands, effectively treating stubborn acne and rosacea and improving the appearance of some acne scars.

These ALA treatments can be combined with our regular photorejuvenation treatments using IPL, which targets redness and brown spots as well as stimulating formation of more collagen in the skin. There is normally no downtime for IPL treatments without Levulan. However, one can enhance and boost IPL photorejuvenation results by adding Levulan to the treatment process. This is termed an activated *fotofacial*, or *photodynamic skin rejuvenation* when PDT is added to regular IPL photorejuvenation.

How much improvement can I expect?

Patients with severe sun-damaged skin manifested by actinic keratosis and texture and tone changes, including mottled pigmentation and skin laxity, may see excellent results. You may also see improvement of large pores and pitted acne scars. Active acne can improve dramatically.

How many treatments will it take to see the best results?

To achieve maximum improvement of precancerous (actinic keratoses) sun damage, skin tone, and texture, a series of two to three treatments two to four weeks apart is most effective. Some patients with just actinic keratoses are happy with one treatment. Treatment for acne is very similar and also may require two to four treatments every two to four weeks. More treatments can be done at periodic intervals in the future to maintain the rejuvenated appearance of the skin.

What are the disadvantages?

Following PDT, the treated areas can appear red, with some peeling, for two to seven days. Some patients have an exuberant response to PDT and experience marked redness of their skin. Temporary swelling of the lips and around the eyes can occur for a few days. Darker pigmented patches, so-called liver spots, can become temporarily darker and then peel off, leaving normal skin (this usually occurs over seven to ten days). Repeat treatments may be necessary as medicine is not an exact science.

What are the advantages?

- Easier for patients than repeated topical liquid nitrogen, Efudex (5-fluorouracil [FU]), or Aldara because the side effects are minimal, with rapid healing, and only one to three treatments are required.
- The ALA-PDT treatment at our clinic is much less painful then liquid nitrogen, 5-FU, and Aldara.
- Reduced scarring and improved cosmetic outcome compared with cautery, surgery, and Efudex. Liquid nitrogen can leave white spots on the skin.
- Levulan improves the whole facial area treated, creating one color, texture, and tone, rather than just spot treating with liquid nitrogen, cautery, and surgery.

In summary, PDT matches the ideal treatment for actinic damage:
- Well tolerated (essentially painless)
- Easily performed by a specialty clinic environment
- Noninvasive (no needles or surgery required)
- Excellent cosmetic outcome (particularly in cosmetically sensitive areas of the face)

Note: Adapted from Nootheti PK, Goldman MP, Advances in photorejuvenation and the current status of photodynamic therapy. *Expert Rev. Dermatol.* 2006;1:51–61, with permission of Future Drugs Ltd.

- The most common adverse effects include sensations of burning, stinging, or itching in illuminated areas. Erythema and edema are also noted in treated areas and respond well to cold compresses or ice packs. Patients are given La Roche-Posay Thermal Spring Water to apply to their skin four to six times a day. Gentle cleansers and moisturizers (Spa MD Recovery Gel) are also regularly recommended.
- Reevaluate the skin preparation and consider increasing the incubation time if little reaction was noted at follow-up. Repeat the treatment in three to four weeks, if necessary.

TABLE 52.3: Home-Care Instructions for Patients Following PDT

Day of treatment

- If you have any discomfort, begin applying ice packs to the treated areas. This will help keep the area cool and alleviate any discomfort as well as help keep down any swelling. Swelling will be most evident around the eyes and is usually more prominent in the morning.
- Remain indoors and avoid direct sunlight.
- Spray on La Roche Posay Thermal Spring Water.
- Apply Recovery Gel (Spa MD) every two to four hours, as necessary.
- Take pain medication, such as Advil, if necessary.

Days 2–7

- You may begin applying makeup once any crusting has healed. The area may be slightly red for one to two weeks.
- The skin will feel dry and tightened, and moisturizers should be used daily.
- Try to avoid direct sunlight for one week. Use a total zinc oxide–based sunscreen with a minimum SPF 30.

To achieve maximum improvement of precancerous (actinic keratoses) sun damage, skin tone, and texture, a series of two to three treatments two to four weeks apart is most effective. Some patients with just actinic keratoses are happy with one treatment. More treatments can be done at periodic intervals in the future to maintain the rejuvenated appearance of the skin.

Note: Adapted from Nootheti PK, Goldman MP, Advances in photorejuvenation and the current status of photodynamic therapy. *Expert Rev. Dermatol.* 2006;1:51–61, with permission of Future Drugs Ltd.

SUGGESTED READING

Facial Rejuvenation

Alexiades-Armenakas M. Laser-mediated photodynamic therapy. *Clin. Dermatol.* 2006;24:16–25.

Avram D, Goldman MP. Effectiveness and safety of ALA-IPL in treating actinic keratoses and photodamage. *J. Drugs Dermatol.* 2004;3(Suppl):36–9.

Dover J, Bhatia A, Stewart B, Arndt K. Topical 5-aminolevulinic acid combined with intense pulsed light in the treatment of photoaging. *Arch. Dermatol.* 2005;141:1247–52.

Gold MH. A split face comparison study of ALA-PDT with intense pulsed light versus intense pulsed light alone for photodamage/photorejuvenation. *Dermatol. Surg.* 2006;32:795–803.

Goldman MP, Atkin D, Kincad S. PDT/ALA in the treatment of actinic damage: real world experience. *J. Lasers Surg. Med.* 2002;14(Suppl):24.

Katz BE, Truong S, Maiwald DC, Frew KE, George D. Efficacy of microdermabrasion preceding ALA application in reducing the incubation time of ALA in laser PDT. *J. Drugs Dermatol.* 2007;6:140–2.

Marmur ES, Phelps R, Goldberg DJ. Ultrastructural changes seen after ALA-IPL photorejuvenation: a pilot study. *J. Cosmet. Laser Ther.* 2005;7:21–4.

Nestor MS, Gold MH, Kauvar AN, et al. The use of photodynamic therapy in dermatology: results of a consensus conference. *J. Drugs Dermatol.* 2006;5:140–54.

Nootheti PK, Goldman MP. Advances in photorejuvenation and the current status of photodynamic therapy. *Expert Rev. Dermatol.* 2006;1:51–61.

Ruiz-Rodriquez R, Sanz-Sachez T, Cordoba S. Photodynamic photorejuvenation. *Dermatol. Surg.* 2002;28:742–4.

Touma D, Yaar M, Whitehead S, Konnikove N, Gilchrest BA. A trial of short incubation, broad-area photodynamic therapy for facial actinic keratoses and diffuse photodamage. *Arch. Dermatol.* 2004;140:33–40.

Acne

Alexiades-Armenakas MR. Long pulsed dye laser-mediated photodynamic therapy combined with topical therapy for mild-to-severe comedonal inflammatory and cystic acne. *J. Drugs Dermatol.* 2006;5:45–55.

Gold MH, Bradshaw VL, Boring MM, Bridges TM, Biron JA, Carter LN. The use of a novel intense pulsed light and heat source and ALA-PDT in the treatment of moderate to severe inflammatory acne vulgaris. *J. Drugs Dermatol.* 2004; 3(Suppl):15–19.

Goldman MP. Using 5-aminolevulinic acid to treat acne and sebaceous hyperplasia. *Cosmet. Dermatol.* 2003;16:57–8.

Goldman MP, Boyce S. A single-center study of aminolevulinic acid and 417 nm photodynamic therapy in the treatment of moderate to severe acne vulgaris. *J. Drugs Dermatol.* 2003;2:393–6.

Hongcharu W, Taylor CR, Chang Y, Aghassi D, Suthamjariya K, Anderson RR. Topical ALA-photodynamic therapy for the treatment of acne vulgaris. *J. Invest. Dermatol.* 2000;115:183–92.

Itoh Y, Ninomiya Y, Tajima S, Ishibashi A. Photodynamic therapy for acne vulgaris with topical 5-aminolevulinic acid. *Arch. Dermatol.* 2000;136:1093–5.

Orringer JS, Kang S, Hamilton T, et al. Treatment of acne vulgaris with a pulsed dye laser: a randomized controlled trial. *JAMA* 2004;291:2834–9.

Papageorgiou P, Katsambas A, Chu A. Phototherapy with blue (415 nm) and red (660 nm) light in the treatment of acne vulgaris. *Br. J. Dermatol.* 2000;142:973–8.

Pollock B, Turner D, Stringer MR, et al. Topical aminolevulinic acid-photodynamic therapy for the treatment of acne vulgaris: a study of clinical efficacy and mechanism of action. *Br. J. Dermatol.* 2004;151:616–22.

Seaton ED, Charakida A, Mouser PE, Grace I, Clement RM, Chu AC. Pulsed-dye laser treatment for inflammatory acne vulgaris: randomized controlled trial. *Lancet* 2003;362:1342–6.

Taub AF. Photodynamic therapy for the treatment of acne: a pilot study. *J. Drugs Dermatol.* 2004;3(Suppl):10–14.

Section 5

RADIOFREQUENCY

CHAPTER 53

Thermage for Face and Body

Joseph Sedrak
Katrina Wodhal
Abel Torres

Thermage uses monopolar radiofrequency to achieve non-ablative skin tightening. This system employs a patented monopolar capacitive radiofrequency technology called ThermaCool. The ThermaCool device has been approved by the Food and Drug Administration for the noninvasive treatment of rhytids.

This system relies on radiofrequency-derived heat, which promotes skin tightening via two proposed separate mechanisms: first, heat causes immediate collagen denaturation and fibril contraction; second, long-term benefits include progressive dermal remodeling and subsequent tightening from a wound-healing response lasting several months. Thus treatment attempts to provide renewed facial contours without the need for invasive surgery. It has been clinically proven to tighten and gently smooth out wrinkles and requires no downtime from normal activities.

PATIENT SELECTION

Like many cosmetic procedures, patient selection is important. The ideal patient for Thermage has the earliest signs of aging, with mild skin rhytids and substantial laxity but minimal lipodystrophy, and does not desire invasive procedures for rejuvenation. Nonablative skin tightening via radiofrequency is not intended to replace the more dramatic effects of invasive surgical lifts. Results tend to be subtle and are not as reliably produced as those obtained from surgery. The skin contraction reportedly achieved is in the order of 1–3 mm (Sadick 2006). If patient selection is appropriate, these subtle changes are perceptible to

patients, particularly eyebrow position or softening of the nasolabial fold. Educating patients on realistic expectations is paramount to patient satisfaction. In the authors' experience, patients report receiving comments such as, "You look refreshed; what have you been doing differently?"

INITIAL CONSULTATION

During the initial consultation, several key issues should be addressed to avoid confusion and patient dissatisfaction. The Thermage procedure can take anywhere from twenty minutes to two hours, depending on the size of the treatment area. Additional time may be required for premedication pain control, although one must be aware that recent treatment recommendations suggest the practitioner use patient feedback on pain level throughout the procedure to properly adjust treatment settings. Thus current recommendations largely eliminate the need for any pain control medication. First, discuss the length of the procedure and anticipated discomfort during treatment. For example, treating the abdomen can take as long as two hours. It is helpful to adequately manage pain and discomfort for longer treatments using some type of mild sedative. Last, emphasize to the patient that some immediate skin tightening may be evident; however, improved skin tightening may occur subtly over the next six months. A second treatment may be required after three to six months' time. Some practitioners use Thermage more as an adjunct to more invasive procedures such as liposuction. The concept supporting this is that liposuction removes the lipohypertrophy

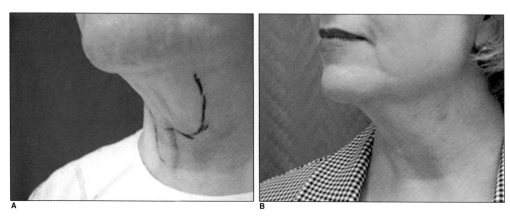

FIGURE 53.1: **A**, *Before and,* **B**, *after liposuction and Thermage.*

and leaves lax skin with residual inflammation making the dermis more likely to respond to thermal remodeling. For example, a study currently in progress by the authors is evaluating the efficacy of Thermage in treating abdominal skin laxity after liposuction. The authors routinely combine Thermage one to two weeks after submental liposuction to enhance skin tightening (Figure 53.1).

EIGHT-STEP TREATMENT ALGORITHM (EIGHT *PS* OF THERMAGE)

1. ***Photos.*** Take standardized pre- and postoperative digital photos to show any changes obtained by the patient. If patients have realistic expectations and adequate photographs are secured, the index of patient satisfaction is much higher. Make a point of identifying a clear anatomic landmark that can be followed (e.g., elevation of eyebrows, increase in eyelid crease prominence; Figure 53.2).

2. ***Pain control.*** Pain medication is not usually necessary; however; if the patient is anxious, a mild anxiolytic medication may be given prior to the procedure (a recent study found no improvement using topical anesthetic agent with pain control; Kushikata et al. 2005).

3. ***Pick tip size.*** Assess the treatment site and select the appropriate tip size and anticipated pulse quantity. The new, smaller "ST" tips are designed for delicate areas around the eyes and hands, as opposed to the larger "TC" tips for use on the face, neck, abdomen, and/or thigh area. The tips differ in their depth of penetration and number of pulses. One tip should suffice for a particular treatment area; however, when dealing with larger areas, such as the abdomen, two tips may be required. This should be taken into account when establishing treatment cost. Make sure to discuss this with the patient during the initial consultation. The tips are sterile and are intended for single use only. One must remember to keep the tip in the package until the patient is completely prepared for the procedure as the tip does begin to time out once attached to the unit. For example, time-out duration is anywhere from 60 to 240 minutes, depending on the tip. Once it has timed out, it is no longer usable. It is also inadvisable to alter the tip so as to prevent the time-out since this may affect efficacy and/or liability.

4. ***Pulse grid application.*** Apply the treatment grid to the skin by moistening inked paper with alcohol. Press firmly to ensure adequate grid placement. The grid helps to ensure even treatment distribution.

5. ***Placement of device.*** Apply a liberal amount of coupling fluid to the skin. Place the tip directly against the skin until a discharge of coolant is heard. Then treatment is ready to begin. Pulses can be delivered via the handheld piece and/or footpad. Always place the tip on the operator's hand to ensure that it is cooling.

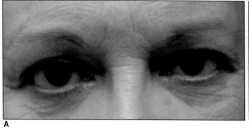
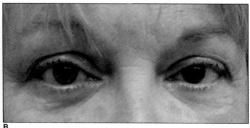

FIGURE 53.2: **A**, *Before and,* **B**, *after Thermage of the eyelids. Notice increase of eyelid platforms.*

TABLE 53.1: Tip Sizes and Recommended Energy Levels

Tip Size	Fluence	Level
0.25 cm² ST (shallow depth)	fluences of 36–72 J/cm²	level of 30.5–35.0
1.0 cm² standard tip	fluences of 81–124 J/cm²	level of 12.5–15
1.0 cm² fast tip	fluences of 62–109 J/cm²	level of 72.0–76.0
1.5 cm² ST (shallow depth) or TC (medium depth)	fluences of 75–130 J/cm²	level of 61.5–65
3.0 cm² STC (medium depth) or TC (medium depth)	fluences of 9–96 J/cm²	level of 360.5–368.5

Note: The setting number *does not* directly correlate to the fluence.

6. ***Pain level setting for optimal treatment.*** Start with a lower setting and titrate treatment based on the patient's pain threshold. The pain scale used to titrate should be from 1 to 4, where 1 represents mild discomfort and 4 represents severe discomfort. With each pulse delivered, ask the patient to rate discomfort until the target pain threshold of 2–3 is reached. The fluence may need to be adjusted during the treatment, based on the treatment site. Expect more discomfort while treating areas over a bony prominence. For example, the jawline is routinely more painful. The treatments should be at a tolerable level, and the authors prefer treatment without medication. The newer treatment paradigm recommends lower fluences (less than 100 J/cm²) with increasing passes (up to five). The average fluence corresponded to a setting of 62 (fluence 83 J/cm²; Bogle et al. 2007). Tip sizes and recommended energy levels are illustrated in Table 53.1, according to the manufacturers' recommendations.

7. ***Plan ahead.*** To ensure symmetric treatment, mentally plan ahead, keeping in mind the total number of pulses available per tip and on each side of treatment area. For example, if two passes are done on one side of the face, it is important to make sure adequate pulses are left to treat the opposite side.

8. ***Posttreatment care.*** Gently remove the grid with mild soap and water. Certain areas may require acetone to completely remove. Apply soothing moisturizer and/or sunblock posttreatment.

TREATMENT TROUBLESHOOTING

Generally speaking, this device is user-friendly; however, following are a few helpful tips. The pulse will not discharge on a concave and/or convex surface. When this occurs, reset the machine and apply the tip to the skin while pulling the skin taught, so as to create a flat surface. In addition,

pulling the adjacent skin helps to diminish the discomfort of treatment. For pain management, make sure to apply ample conductive gel to prevent overheating and burns of the superficial epidermal layer.

Avoid overtreating areas with *high* fluences with the hope of maximizing results. The target temperature for collagen heating to produce maximal remodeling is slightly above 60 degrees Celsius. Excessive treatment may result in contour defects or other injury. If the skin temperature is too hot, the pulse will not be delivered due to the ThermaCool technology, with its built-in temperature sensor.

ADVANTAGES AND DISADVANTAGES

A major advantage of Thermage is the overall safety profile as compared to invasive surgical procedures. In addition, this procedure can be performed on patients of all skin types. Unlike many laser procedures requiring four or more sessions, a single Thermage treatment has produced results in some patients. Recently published studies show that measurable tightening of skin can appear gradually over two to six months after a single treatment session. However, patients have reported seeing an earlier response. Some patients have noted some immediate improvement following a Thermage procedure (Dover and Zelickson 2007).

Disadvantages of Thermage include unpredictable tightening results as compared to surgical procedures. In addition, results are gradual over several months, as opposed to the immediate improvement with surgery. This highlights the importance of establishing patient expectations prior to treatment.

POTENTIAL COMPLICATIONS

In one study, the most frequently reported side effects included swelling, redness, and bumps and blisters on or around the treated area. Most of these side effects subsided

TABLE 53.2: Reported Complications

Complications Reported	Posttreatment Time
Edema, redness, rarely blisters	resolved by 24 hours
Rare persistent edema	Resolved by 1 week
Tenderness, acneiform eruptions,[a] subcutaneous nodules[a]	Resolved by 2–3 weeks
Contour irregularity[a] (subcutaneous atrophy)	Resolved by 6 months

[a] Rare complications <1%.

by twenty-four hours; however, a few patients reported edema lasting for up to one week. Tenderness at treatment sites has been reported to last for up to two to three weeks. Other less common side effects included acneiform eruptions and subcutaneous nodules that spontaneously resolved after two and a half weeks (Table 53.2). There were no permanent side effects noted in this study; however, previous studies have noted a rare (less than 0.08%) but longer-lasting side effect described as a surface irregularity that resolved over a six-month period (Weiss et al. 2006); however, there is a risk that the irregularity could be permanent. When performing Thermage on the eyelids, one must protect the eye with an eye shield. One must be cautious to wipe excessive amounts of ophthalmic ointment from the eyelid as this may conduct heat to the eye. As with any new procedure, patients should be aware that an unforeseeable effect might be possible if the machine malfunctions, and any machine may malfunction. A risk of burn is always possible if the machine malfunctions.

COMBINATION TREATMENTS

Recent studies suggest no change of filler materials (hyaluronic acid gel) post-Thermage when treatments were done the same day (Goldman et al. 2007). However, caution should be exercised when performing filler immediately prior to Thermage therapy. Animal studies noted an increase in foreign body reaction and fibrosis five days, two weeks, and one month after radiofrequency treatment. The long-term sequelae of this phenomenon has yet to be elucidated. Thus, to prevent unnecessary granulomatous and/or foreign body reactions, it is prudent to space out Thermage treatments with filler treatments (Alam et al. 2006). An additional study found no change in inflammatory reaction or filler substance when treatments were spaced two weeks apart (Shumaker et al. 2006). The authors prefer to perform Thermage prior to filler treatments.

No decrease in the efficacy of botulinum toxin denervation was observed when glabellar or perioral areas were treated with radiofrequency within ten minutes of botulinum toxin injection (Semchyshyn and Kilmer 2005). Thus it appears that combining radiofrequency with BOTOX is safe, but the authors prefer to perform Thermage prior to or several weeks after BOTOX treatment. Thermage may be combined with other treatments, as well (Figure 53.3).

COMPARATIVE SKIN TIGHTENING THERAPIES

Modalities for skin tightening include radiofrequency energy, lasers, and combination radiofrequency and diode lasers. The newer generation of products is combining different modalities to achieve greater stimulation of collagen production, while minimizing discomfort (Table 53.3). In addition, studies indicate that the bipolar frequency targets the papillary dermis, in contrast to the dermal-subcutaneous junction for monopolar therapies. Some authors propose that the bipolar units may be safer, with less risk of long-term contour irregularities. Additional comparative clinical studies are needed to determine Thermage's long-term safety and effectiveness and the difference, if any, in efficacy between Thermage and these modalities.

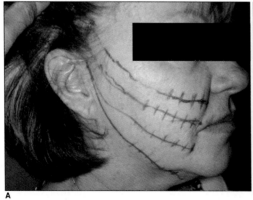 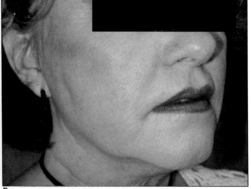

A   B

FIGURE 53.3: **A,** *Before and,* **B,** *after Thermage and Eremia thread lift. Notice softening of the nasolabial fold.*

TABLE 53.3: Modalities for Skin Tightening

Name	Modality
ThermaCool, Thermage	monopolar radiofrequency[a]
Titan, Cutera	BBIRL[b]
ReFirm ST, Syneron	BBIRL + bipolar radiofrequency
Polaris WR, Syneron	diode + bipolar radiofrequency
Accent RF, Alma	bipolar + monopolar radiofrequency

[a] Radiofrequency.
[b] Broadband infrared light, 700–2,000 nm.

SUGGESTED READING

Alam M, Levy R, Pajvany U, et al. Safety of radiofrequency treatment over human skin previously injected with medium-term injectable soft-tissue augmentation materials: a controlled pilot trial. *Lasers Surg. Med.* 2006;38:205–10.

Bogle MA, Ubelhoer N, Weiss RA, et al. Evaluation of the multiple pass, low fluence algorithm for radiofrequency tightening of the lower face. *Lasers Surg. Med.* 2007;39:210–17.

Dover JS, Zelickson B. Results of a survey of 5,700 patient monopolar radiofrequency facial skin tightening treatments: assessment of a low-energy multiple-pass technique leading to a clinical end point algorithm. *Dermatol. Surg.* 2007;33:900–7.

Goldman MP, Alster TS, Weiss R. A randomized trial to determine the influence of laser therapy, monopolar radiofrequency treatment, and intense pulsed light therapy administered immediately after hyaluronic acid gel implantation. *Dermatol. Surg.* 2007;33:535–42.

Kushikata N, Negishi K, Tezuka Y, et al. Is topical anesthesia useful in noninvasive skin tightening using radiofrequency? *Dermatol. Surg.* 2005;31:526–33.

Sadick NS, l. Nonsurgical approaches to skin tightening. *Cosmet. Dermatol.* 2006;19:473–7.

Semchyshyn NL, Kilmer SL. Does laser inactivate botulinum toxin? *Dermatol. Surg.* 2005;31:399–404.

Shumaker PR, England LJ, Dover JS, et al. Effect of monopolar radiofrequency treatment over soft-tissue fillers in an animal model: part 2. *Lasers Surg. Med.* 2006;38:211–17.

Weiss RA, Weiss MA, Munavalli G, et al. Monopolar radiofrequency facial tightening: a retrospective analysis of efficacy and safety in over 600 treatments. *J. Drugs Dermatol.* 2006;5:707–12.

CHAPTER 54

Lumenis Aluma Skin Tightening System

Michael H. Gold

Skin tightening devices have become some of the most popular cosmetic procedures patients are currently asking cosmetic dermatologists to perform in their offices. These devices have been developed to augment many of the other noninvasive cosmetic procedures we are performing on a regular basis in our office settings. They have introduced new terms into our laser vocabulary, which now has to be expanded into the new field of energy-based systems. These energy-based systems utilize terms such as *monopolar, unipolar, bipolar radiofrequency* (RF), and *tripolar*. The RF devices that have been developed for skin tightening, as well as several other devices that rely on the absorption spectrum of water in the infrared range of light, allow sufficient deep dermal heating to produce the desired effects. All the skin tightening devices on the market work via the same basic premise: deep dermal heating, which causes collagen denaturation, followed by collagen repair and ultimate deposition of new collagen and, ultimately, skin tightening. The major skin-tightening devices available on the market at the time of this writing are shown in Table 54.1.

RF energy produces a thermal effect when its high-frequency electrical current moves through the skin. The amount of heat generated in the tissue of the skin can be described by the mathematical formula known as Joule's law: $H = j2/\sigma$, where j is the density of the electrical current and σ is the specific electrical conductivity. The tissue impedance, or resistance, is inversely proportional to the electrical conductivity. From Joule's law, heat is generated as the RF current flows through the skin and encounters resistance in the tissues. Several other variables need to be added to the equation when dealing with the complex nature of the skin such as the magnitude and frequency of the electrical current and the physical characteristics of the skin being treated, including the electrolyte content of the skin, the hydration level of the skin, and the temperature of the skin. Also important is the distribution of the current applied to the tissue, which then takes into account the location of the electrodes used to deliver the energy and the skin's geometry.

In a typical monopolar RF setting, one electrode emits RF energy as the second electrode serves as a grounding pad. The main characteristics of this type of setup are the need for high power densities on and close to the electrode's surface and the deep power penetration. Unipolar RF puts the grounding electrode in the same handpiece that houses the active electrode. With the monopolar RF devices, high energy densities are usually required, which, early on, led to pain during treatment and some safety concerns. These adverse effects associated with the early RF skin-tightening devices have been alleviated thanks to new treatment protocols and better designed treatment tips used for these systems.

Bipolar RF may have the advantage of less pain and a decreased risk of adverse effects by utilizing two electrodes set at a fixed distance. This allows for the precise transfer

TABLE 54.1: Collagen Remodeling and Skin Tightening Devices

Monopolar	Thermage ThermaCoolNXT
Bipolar radiofrequency with diode	Syneron ReFirme™, eMatrix™,
IPL at 1,100–1,800 nm range	Palomar LuxIR™, Cutera Titan® Sciton BBL-SkinTyte
Bipolar radiofrequency with vacuum	Lumenis Aluma
Unipolar and bipolar together	Alma Lasers Accent®XL™
Tripolar	Pollogen Apollo™

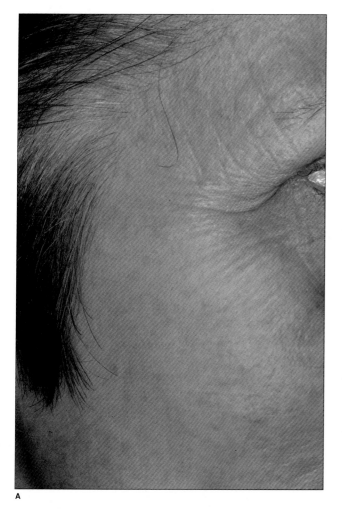
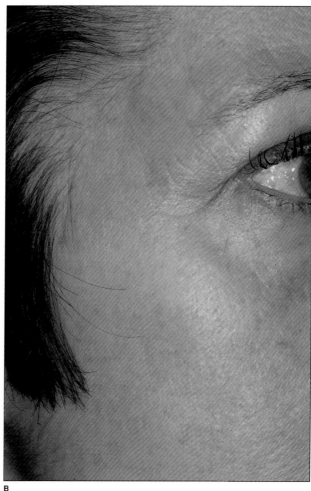

A

B

FIGURE 54.1: **A, Before treatment. B, After six Aluma treatments.**

of energy into the tissue. However, early designs of bipolar RF had limitations related to the depth of penetration, which is limited to approximately half the distance between the electrodes. Thus insufficient energy densities reach the deeper layers of the skin, where collagen denaturation and collagen regeneration need to reach to occur.

A recently designed parallel bipolar RF with an associated vacuum apparatus was thus developed to utilize the premise of increased safety with the bipolar RF design. The, vacuum apparatus increases the depth of penetration of the RF energy and the specificity of energy into the deep dermal tissues, where collagen denaturation and remodeling can successfully occur. Clinical studies performed with this bipolar RF device with a vacuum apparatus, known commercially as the Aluma skin-tightening system (Lumenis Inc.), use the acronym FACES to drive the message to users. FACES stands for "functional aspiration controlled electrothermal stimulation," and clinical results have supported its concept as well as its safety and efficacy.

The first clinical trial performed was a safety and efficacy analysis looking at the reduction of rhytids and skin tightening in the perioral and periorbital regions of the face. The results from this trial showed an improvement in the elastosis score from a value of 4.5 before treatment (on average) to a level of 2.5 at six months (on average). Wrinkle score class improvement was seen in almost all patients, with a mean improvement of 1 point in the patients treated eight times over a two-month period. Pain was virtually nonexistent, and the patients all had positive satisfaction scores. No significant adverse events were seen in the original clinical trial, which led to its Food and Drug Administration clearance in 2004. A second clinical trial confirmed these results in a larger multicenter clinical trial, with improvements demonstrated both clinically and histologically and via several skin topographical analyses. A third clinical trial also confirmed the early findings of improved skin texture, reduction of wrinkles, and skin tightening. Further observations from many clinicians have shown the versatility of the Aluma device, with successful treatments being performed on different parts of the body, from the face to the neck, upper arms, abdomen, and knee areas. Clinical examples are shown in Figures 54.1 and 54.2.

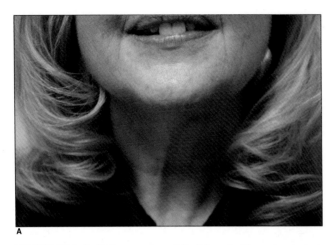
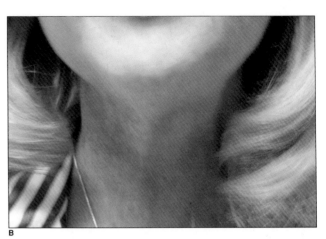

FIGURE 54.2: **A,** *Before treatment.* **B,** *After six Aluma treatments.*

PATIENT SELECTION

Successful candidates for Aluma therapy are any patients considering skin-tightening treatments in the areas described previously. Any skin type may be treated safely. There are no absolute contraindications to performing the Aluma treatments, but caution should be taken with any of these devices in those patients with a history of keloid formation or those on anticoagulant medications.

HOW TO PERFORM THE PROCEDURE

An informed consent should be signed prior to any cosmetic procedure, including Aluma, and pretreatment photographs should also be taken of the treatment areas. Patients undergoing Aluma treatments should have their faces thoroughly cleaned before the therapy is to begin. Once these steps have been performed, a conductive lotion is applied to the treatment areas, and the applicator tip is applied to a treatment area. The device has preset default settings that determine the amount of energy to be given, the power of the vacuum to be given and the time frame for delivery of the energy. The RF energy can be delivered from 2 to 10 W (presented as 1–5 energy levels); the vacuum levels range from 8 to 28 inches of mercury (presented as "1–5" vacuum levels), and the time duration ranges from 1 to 5 s. This allows for the delivery of 2–60 J to the tissue in a single pulse.

Once the treatment parameters are determined and set, the energy is delivered to the skin by pressing the treatment button located on the handpiece. One will see the skin being taken up by the vacuum apparatus, and once the skin is in the vacuum, the energy will be safely delivered. The vacuum then releases the tissue and the treatment is finished. Pain is minimal with these treatments, and the majority of patients find the treatment sessions comfortable. If needed, forced air cooling can be used in conjunction with these treatments.

At the time of this writing, all the parameters for the optimal use of the Aluma device are still being evaluated. What investigators are becoming clearer with at this time is that three passes in the treatment area usually provides the best clinical results. The time frame between treatments and the number of treatments needed for each patient are variable and are being further elucidated at this time. At the time of this writing, most clinicians favor treatments every two to three weeks, and at least four to six treatments are required for optimal results. However, the majority of patients do see clinical results as early as the second treatment, and these treatments should be individualized from patient to patient.

AFTERCARE

The aftercare of patients is relatively simple. Patients are instructed to use a mild skin moisturizer and to avoid sun exposure for several days following the therapy. This is to avoid any potential melanin regeneration, which could possibly occur after any RF treatment.

COMPLICATIONS

As with any energy-based system, complications can occur with improper training and use. Blistering, burning, and scarring are all potential adverse events associated with all the RF devices and other skin-tightening devices. These devices should be used under the supervision of a physician who is knowledgeable in dealing with any potential untoward event. At the time of this writing, no serious adverse events have been associated with the Aluma skin-tightening system. The Aluma has proven to be a versatile device that has become a useful modality in many clinics for successful skin tightening. It is safe and painless, and many patients have experienced successful skin tightening with the Aluma.

SUGGESTED READING

Gabriel S, Lau RW, Gabriel C. The dielectric properties of biological tissues. III. Parametric models for the dielectric spectrum of tissues. *Phys. Med. Biol.* 1996;41:2271–93.

Gold MH, Goldman MP. Use of a novel vacuum-assisted bipolar radiofrequency device for wrinkle reduction. *Lasers Surg.* 2005;17:24(s).

Gold MH, Rao J, Zelickson B. Bipolar radiofrequency with vacuum apparatus – results of a multi-center study. *J. Am. Acad. Dermatol.* 2007;AB207.

Montesi G, Calvieri S, Balzani A, Gold MH. Bipolar radiofrequency in the treatment of dermatological imperfections: clinical-pathological and immunohistochemical aspects. *J. Drugs in Dermatol.* 2007;6(9):890–6.

CHAPTER 55

Ellman Radiofrequency Device for Skin Tightening

Antonio Rusciani Scorza

Giuseppe Curinga

Skin laxity is a common cosmetic complaint of aging patients. Improvement in skin laxity can be difficult to achieve without invasive surgical lifting procedures. The radiofrequency (RF) system is based on an entirely different treatment principle than the photothermal reaction created by most dermatologic lasers. Unlike a laser, which uses light energy to generate heat in targeted chromophores, based on the theory of selective photothermolysis (Anderson and Parrish 1983), RF technology produces an electric current that generates heat through resistance in the dermis and subcutaneous tissue.

Radiorefresce uses Surgitron Dual Frequency RF (Radiowave Technology, Ellman International), which develops a proprietary capacitive coupling method to transfer higher-energy fluences through the skin to a greater volume of dermal tissue than nonablative lasers, while protecting the epidermis (Hardaway and Ross 2002).

The components of the device include (1) an RF generator producing a 4-MHz alternating-current RF signal, the energy level of which is set by the clinician, and (2) a handpiece for directing the RF energy to the skin. The neutral plate of the apparatus is placed approximately 15–20 cm from the patient. Spherical handpieces (5, 10, 15, and 20 mm in diameter) are used. The application of RF energy has been carried out in ambulatory settings, with no need for skin sterilization.

The Surgitron 4.0 Dual Frequency RF has various operative modes. For ideal treatment, the manufacturer recommends a setting of 4.0 Mhz. Patients should be informed that for maximum benefit, the sensation should feel as if the skin is heating just to the brink of pain, but then subsiding. Settings are adjusted based on each individual patient's comfort level. Settings may vary for each anatomic region (forehead cut, 5–7; cheek and other surface cut, 6–10). Before beginning treatment, we apply a restoring cream or gel to reduce side effects. The handpiece traces out spiral vectors against ptosis with a diameter of approximately 1 cm. Based on the patient's characteristics (subcutaneous fat distribution), greater pressure can be applied to cheeks and other body areas, but should be practically absent on the forehead. The handpiece's effectiveness is proportional to the pressure applied. Treatment time varies according to the area (fifteen to twenty minutes average). The burning sensation may vary per area as well (a more intense pain is perceived on the forehead). To diminish side effects (i.e., small abrasions, which heal in three to four days), it is important that the patient remains still during treatment. After treatment, an antidystrophic and restoring cream is applied. Patients are typically able to return to work and social activities immediately after treatment.

RF energy is approved for various surgical procedures for electrocoagulation and hemostasis (ocular dermatologic and general surgery). There are two different kinds of energy diffusion: monopolar and bipolar. The diffusion is basically represented by an electrode's localization. The high frequency (4.0 Mhz) of the electric current converts the latter into a simple radiowave. This wave, emitted by the active electrode, naturally goes toward the passive one. Between the two electrodes, the organic tissue hinders the radiowave flow. At a molecular level, this resistance turns into an intracellular oscillation, leading to a break in links among the water molecules contained in the organic tissue and to the related linking energy release. The thermal effect depends on the characteristics of the treated tissue's conductivity. Therefore tissues with a higher impedance (i.e., the adipose ones) produce greater heat and, consequently, a greater thermal effect. In this way, the energy produced by RF can develop heat that is determined and controlled according to the superficial and deep dermis as well as the adipose tissue up to the muscle border. Studies indicate that tissue tightening occurs through a mechanism of immediate collagen contraction, supplemented by new collagen synthesis during a longer-term wound-healing process. Ultrastructural analysis of human tissues immediately after treatment revealed isolated, scattered areas of denatured collagen fibrils with increased diameter and loss of distinct borders (Zelickson et al. 2004).

The contraction determines a reorganization of the cutaneous tension lines in a physiological way, with a reduction in cutaneous laxity caused by a tightening effect similar

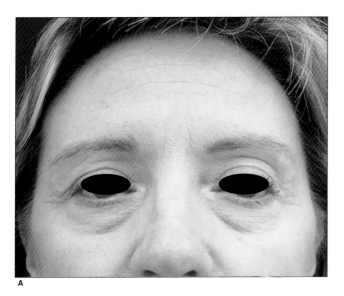 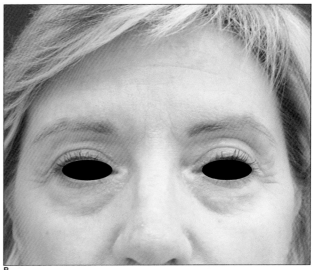

FIGURE 55.1: **A,** *Pretreatment.* **B,** *Three months posttreatment with Ellman Radiage.*

to a microlift (Figure 55.1). In contrast to the literature on Thermage's RF device, which was the first bipolar radiofrequency mechanism, we report additional information on the efficacy and adaptability of Surgitron Dual Frequency RF. The innovations in our study show that it is possible to treat new areas of the body with RF energy without any anesthesia and in ambulatory settings. Furthermore, the equipment does not require any external cooling of the cutaneous surface.

The Surgitron Dual Frequency RF handpiece is extremely versatile, allowing application and adjustment of the RF energy according to antigravitational factors. The Thermage, Aluma, and Syneron tools have rectangular or square electrodes with larger dimensions, which can cause a contraction of the treated area's perimeter, making the contraction itself appear in the geometric shape of the handpiece. The typical pain reported by patients is actually due to the greater dimensions of these handpieces. The larger handpiece dimensions of the Thermage device can cause side effects such as burns and other untoward results (Ruiz-Esparza and Gomez 2003). The larger the treated area, the deeper the effects. The smaller Surgitron Dual Frequency RF, with a specially designed RF electrode tip (variable 5–20 mm), combined with rapid hand movements, greatly reduces deep side effects.

The parameters to be taken into account for an ideal treatment are still disputable, just as the ideal level of energy needed to achieve the best result is still unknown. The energy and treatment mode should be carefully adjusted so as to produce a level of heat that will not cause epidermic damage or excessive pain in the area treated. Moreover, applying the tip of a 0.5-mm electrode with circular movements seems to help evenly disperse the RF electricity. If anesthetics are not used, patients are able to perceive any exceeding electrothermal effect, thus preventing complications.

It is interesting to note that patients not showing a clear improvement did achieve better skin quality and a reduction in cutaneous laxity, as can be seen in the before and after photos, even though the improvement was subtle and therefore not always noticeable by the patients themselves. For this reason, it is important to consider the patient's expectations and to explain chances for real improvement as well as the perception appraisal. Before and after photos are helpful. Of course, an informed consent should also be obtained.

Radiorefresce treatments can safely be used in combination with intense pulsed light, nonablative lasers, biorevitalizers, botulinum toxin, autologus cell rejuvenation (ACR), and fillers. The majority of patients were satisfied with the procedure itself and liked the ability to return to daily routines after leaving the office. We determined that for in-office rejuvenation of the skin, the Dual Surgitron RF device provides a measurable improvement in the majority of patients treated (Rusciani et al. 2007).

SUGGESTED READING

Anderson RR, Parrish JA. Selective photothermolysis: precise microsurgery by selective absorption of pulsed radiation. *Science.* 1983;220:524–7.

Hardaway CA, Ross EV. Nonablative laser skin remodeling. *Dermatol. Clin.* 2002;20:97–111.

Ruiz-Esparza J, Gomez JB. The medical face lift: a noninvasive, nonsurgical approach to tissue tightening in facial skin using nonablative radiofrequency. *Dermatol. Surg.* 2003;29:325.

Rusciani A, Curinga G, Menichini G, et al. Nonsurgical tightening of skin laxity: a new radiofrequency approach. *J. Drugs Dermatol.* 2007;6:381–6.

Zelickson BD, Kist D, Bernstein E, et al. Histological and ultrastructural evaluation of the effects of a radiofrequency based nonablative dermal remodeling device: a pilot study. *Arch. Dermatol.* 2004;140:204–9.

CHAPTER 56

Alma Accent Dual Radiofrequency Device for Tissue Contouring

Gregory S. Keller

Grigoriy Mashkevich

Alma Lasers's Accent is a 200-W, 40.68-MHz, high-frequency radiofrequency (RF) generator. Accent is designed for contact operation using a unipolar probe and a bipolar probe for volumetric and surface heating, respectively.

The unipolar treatment tip handpiece (antenna) creates an electromagnetic field deep within the dermal tissue, which changes polarity 40 million times per second. That polarity change generates heat based on water molecules' movement and their friction between themselves and other tissues.

The unipolar probe delivers the RF energy to tissue from the ball-like extremity of the coupling tip. Delivery of RF energy is to the deep dermis and beyond.

The bipolar probe is designed for surface heating from 2–6 mm in depth, depending on tissue properties. There is a coaxial-grounded electrode that surrounds an RF tip.

The initial effect of treatment is twofold: an immediate three-dimensional collagen contraction (horizontal and vertical fibers), producing a dermal contraction for tightening, and a fibrous septae contraction for contouring. The tissue heating during treatment also produces a secondary wound-healing response, with further collagen deposition and remodeling, resulting in additional tightening over time.

As of the date of this publication, Accent is approved by the Food and Drug Administration for skin tightening and wrinkle reduction in the face and body. Off-label and experimental studies have documented its efficacy for cellulite reduction, collagen deposition, contraction of the fat in the abdomen and arms, and reduction of arm and abdominal circumference (Figure 56.1). Preliminary studies have noted the device to be equivalent to or better than other RF devices in the face, neck, and body.

In clinical use, 3×3 inch squares are drawn on the areas of the body, face, and head and neck that are to be treated (Figure 56.2). Using 15- to 30-s doses of approximately 100 W of unipolar RF energy, the energy is applied with a constant circular contact motion of the probe. Energy is increased until the skin temperature reaches 40 to 42 degrees Celsius. If there is excessive pain in a spot in the treatment area, the probe is passed more quickly over this area. Once the threshold temperature of 40 to 42 degrees Celsius is reached, three passes of 15–30 s are delivered to the treatment area. The bipolar probe is often used in an additional finishing pass. If a more superficial treatment is desired, the bipolar probe alone is used. Titration with this probe is begun at 50 W, seeking 40 to 42 degrees Celsius temperature end points.

In a recent study of the thighs and buttocks, approximately 70% of patients experienced circumference reduction that averaged 0.5 cm. Measurements were performed fifteen days after the second Accent treatment. The two treatments were performed two weeks apart. A similar study of Accent treatment to the arms has confirmed the circumference reduction and volumetric skin tightening. Objective diagnostic ultrasound confirmation of results was also an integral part of this study.

Our clinical results have demonstrated a feeling of skin tightening in almost all our patients. Results in the head and neck appear equivalent to our other RF treatment modalities, with one exception: the submental fat deposits and resulting waddles were volumetrically diminished utilizing Accent, and patients with these deposits experienced

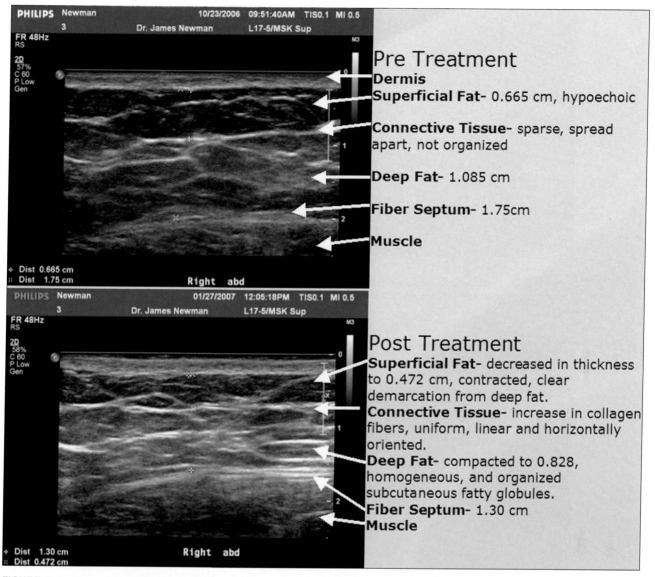

FIGURE 56.1: *Diagnostic ultrasound showing evidence of fat contraction and deposition of collagen following Accent treatment of the abdomen. Images courtesy of Alma Lasers and James Newman, MD.*

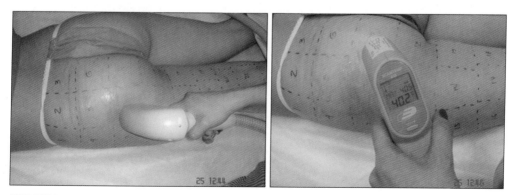

FIGURE 56.2: *Continuous motion Accent treatment with thermal monitoring in 3 × 3 cm grids.*

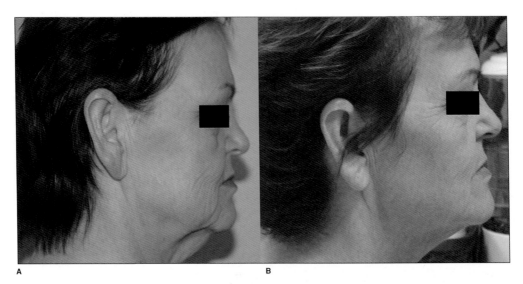

FIGURE 56.3: *Skin tightening and wrinkle reduction with Accent:* **A**, *before and,* **B**, *after treatment. Photos courtesy of Alma Lasers and Dana Kramer, RNFA.*

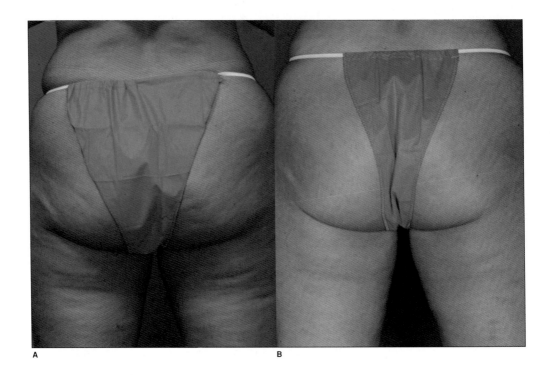

FIGURE 56.4: *Volumetric skin tightening with Accent:* **A**, *before and,* **B**, *after treatment. Photos courtesy of Alma Lasers and David McDaniel, MD.*

a result that was superior to other RF devices (Figure 56.3). Body skin tightening was also enhanced by the volume reduction that is a unique feature of the Accent device. Cellulite reduction was also observed in most of the patients with this problem (Figure 56.4).

SUGGESTED READING

Del Pino E, Rosado RH, Azuela A, et al. Effect of controlled volumetric tissue healing with radiofrequency on cellulite and the subcutaneous tissue of the buttocks and thighs. *J. Drugs Dermatol.* 2006;5:714–22.

CHAPTER 57

Combined Light and Bipolar Radiofrequency

Neil S. Sadick

Patients are frequently seeking efficacious yet little or no downtime procedures. These procedures, however, do require a series of treatments to achieve optimal cosmetic results.

In the author's practice, the use of devices employing a combination of optical energy and bipolar radiofrequency (RF; Syneron Medical Ltd.) has proven successful in meeting patient expectations and patient concerns as well as treating a wide range of conditions and reducing side effects experienced from the use of RF alone. The combination of optical energy and bipolar RF is believed to result in a synergistic effect, resulting in a more effective treatment, while using decreased energy levels to treat a range of skin types. Unlike unipolar RF devices, the energy in a bipolar RF device passes between two electrodes at a set distance, regulating the energy that is delivered (Sadick and Makino 2004).

There is a wide range of devices available that employ optical energy and bipolar RF that can be used for a wide variety of conditions. However, this chapter will cover the FotoFacialRF (intense pulsed light [IPL] plus RF), ReFirme WR (diode laser plus RF), and ReFirme ST (broadband infrared [IR] plus RF) devices alone and in combination with one another as well as the VelaSmooth (IR plus RF) device (Figures 57.1 and 57.2).

Determining the most appropriate treatment is based on a three-step process used in our practice to achieve patient satisfaction, while providing the patient with optimal rejuvenation results. In an initial meeting with the patient, the following approach is employed:

1. Determine goals for rejuvenation and patient concerns (wrinkle reduction, tightening, dyschromia, etc.).

2. Classify the patient using the Sadick Aging Classification System (Table 57.1).

3. Assign the patient to the appropriate rejuvenation program.

During this consultation, we review the expected outcomes of the procedure(s), patient concerns, and the approximate number of treatments that are involved in the patient's personalized rejuvenation program. Concerns that are commonly stated by patients include downtime, discomfort, and lifestyle restrictions. All these concerns are addressed prior to any procedure performed. We cannot say definitively how many treatments will be

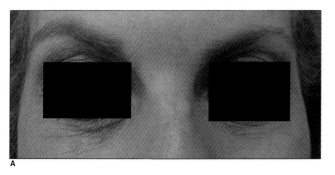
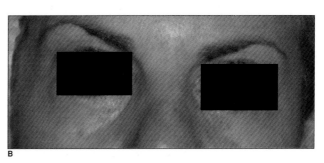

A   B

FIGURE 57.1: *Fifty-nine-year-old female received periorbital treatment ReFirme ST (settings: 120 J/cm^3 and normal) and ReFirme WR (settings: optical energy, 40 J/cm^2; RF, 90 J/cm^3): A, pretreatment; B, one month after second treatment.*

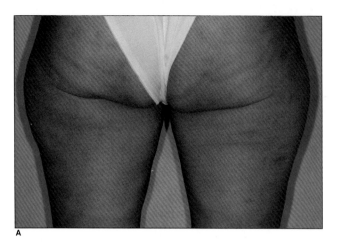 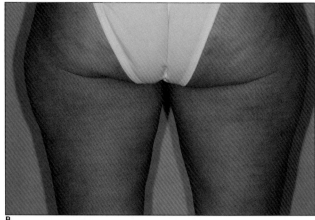

A   B

FIGURE 57.2: *Fifty-eight-year-old female received twelve treatments performed over a six-week period with the VelaSmooth device (settings: optical energy, 3 RF:3; vacuum, 3): A, pretreatment; B, eight weeks after final treatment.*

involved; however, we can provide a range. For the patient interested in treating dyschromia, it is important to discuss with the patient that sun exposure can reverse the effects of treatment.

TYPE I

For the type I patient, the rejuvenation program is, in our practice, generally limited to treatment with the combination IPL (500–1,200 nm) and bipolar RF. IPL with bipolar RF has proven efficacious in treating dyschromia, hyperpigmentation, erythema, telangiectasia, and large pores and rhytids (Sadick et al. 2005). The recommended treatment program includes a series of five to six treatments spaced one month apart. A topical anesthetic is applied and then removed after thirty minutes. A coupling gel and protective eye shields are subsequently applied. The patient is started at an optical energy of 20 J/cm^2 and a RF energy of 20 J/cm^3. Both the optical and RF energies are increased by 2 J/cm^2 or J/cm^3 at each subsequent visit, or as toler-

ated by the patient. After each treatment, the coupling gel is removed and a sunscreen is applied. Follow-up for the next treatment is scheduled for four weeks.

TYPE II

The recommended rejuvenation program for a patient with type II photoaging often includes a series of treatments, depending on the patient's needs and concerns. For a patient with pigmentary alterations and rhytid formation, a series of treatments using combination diode laser plus bipolar RF and IPL plus RF would be employed. The ability to perform these treatments in the same visit is preferred as it reduces the number of visits required to achieve desired results. A patient with laxity and periorbital rhytids would benefit from broadband IR with RF plus diode laser combined with RF. Three to five treatments for each, the broadband IR (700–2,000 nm) plus RF and the combination diode laser and RF, are recommended for each patient.

The use of a diode laser plus RF has demonstrated clinical efficacy for the treatment of rhytids, skin laxity, and skin texture (Sadick and Trelles 2005; Doshi and Alster 2005). As with the combination IPL plus RF, patients are numbed for thirty minutes prior to treatment with the combination diode laser plus RF, and a coupling gel is applied, along with eye protection, after the numbing agent has been thoroughly removed. The levels used to treat the patient remain constant at an optical energy of 40 J/cm^2 and a RF energy of 90 J/cm^3, with an optimal end point of mild erythema and mild edema. Once the treatment is completed and the cooling gel has been removed, a sunblock is applied, and the patient is advised to return for the next treatment in four weeks.

While there are limited publications demonstrating the efficacy of the synergistic effect of the combination of broadband IR plus RF, the author has had successful clinical

TABLE 57.1: Sadick Photoaging Classification Scale

Grade	Components
Type I – Epidermal/superficial dermal	pigmentary skin alterations vascular lesions pilosebaceous changes sebaceous hyperplasia wide pores
Type II – Deep dermal	rhytid formation
Type III – Fat/muscle/bone	lipoatrophy severe rhytids muscle atrophy bone atrophy

experiences. Unlike the previously discussed devices, no numbing preparation is required for the broadband IR plus RF. However, a cooling gel is applied and eye protection is provided for the patient. Settings administered are 120 J/cm^3 and normal. These settings remain constant throughout the series of treatments received by the patient. It is recommended at the initial visit that the patient have three to five treatments spaced four weeks apart to achieve the maximum benefit. Ongoing research projects are in progress.

TYPE III

For subjects with type III photoaging, the main focus is skin tightening and volumetric filling. The filler procedure and skin-tightening treatment can be performed on the same day with thirty minutes of topical anesthesia applied prior to filler treatment. In this setting, the patient would be treated with the combination of broadband IR plus RF (120 J/cm^3 and normal), followed by injection with the appropriate filler. Most commonly, the author uses poly-L-lactic acid or calcium hydroxylapatite for the patient with type III photoaging.

When employing these treatments in combination, the skin is prepped with a numbing cream, and the same pre-procedure skin preparation as previously discussed is followed. The order in which the procedures are performed is not relevant, and the settings used are consistent with those previously mentioned. In the author's experience, the combination of the procedures is beneficial in many ways for the patient as multiple concerns can be addressed with no downtime and no extra office visits required.

While the settings discussed are commonly employed in our practice for the previously mentioned procedures, conservative settings should be employed for thin-skinned individuals for the first treatment session as they can be sensitive to RF treatments. Additionally, the author recommends that retinoids be discontinued five to seven days prior to the procedure for individuals with this characteristic.

Noninvasive treatments for reduction in the appearance of cellulite have gained popularity, and the types of non-invasive treatments have increased significantly. Currently available treatments include topical preparations, endermologie, lasers, lasers plus vacuum/massage, and RF. New devices are continually introduced.

Previous reports have demonstrated the efficacy of the combination treatment that combines broadband IR light (700–2,000 nm) and RF for reduction in the appearance of cellulite (Sadick and Mullholland 2004; Alster and Tanzi 2005; Sadick and Magro 2007). In our experience, the ideal candidate for this type of procedure is a person who maintains a steady weight and leads an active lifestyle and is looking to treat cellulite. It is important to advise patients that this is not a substitute for weight loss, and while a significant reduction in the appearance of cellulite can be achieved, 100% clearance of cellulite is unlikely. It is recommended that a patient have twelve to sixteen treatments, twice weekly, for initial results, with maintenance sessions recommended every three to four months. As with other devices that combine optical energy and bipolar RF, the optimal end point is mild erythema with each treatment. Treatment energy levels for the IR plus RF device range from 1 to 3 for RF, optical energy, and vacuum. If tolerated by the patient, we begin treatment at the maximum treatment level, 3, for RF, optical energy, and vacuum; however, if the patient experiences discomfort associated with the treatment, the vacuum is decreased to 2. By decreasing the vacuum, patient discomfort greatly decreases, and at subsequent treatments, the vacuum may be increased to 3 based on patient tolerance. Biopsies have shown no histopathologic changes.

CONCLUSION

The combination of laser and RF technologies appears to have synergistic effects in terms of whole-body rejuvenation. Studies documenting the additive qualities of the two modalities have not been performed to date; however, lower optical fluence used in combination with RF energy lessens the severity of side effects associated with higher-intensity, light-based technologies. Such multimodality technologies represent a novel approach to whole-body rejuvenation.

SUGGESTED READING

Alster TA, Tanzi EL. Cellulite treatment using a novel combination radiofrequency, infrared light, and mechanical tissue manipulation device. *J. Cosmet. Laser Ther.* 2005;7:81–5.

Doshi SN, Alster TS. Combination radiofrequency and diode laser for treatment of facial rhytides and skin laxity. *J. Cosmet. Laser Ther.* 2005;7:11–15.

Sadick NS, Alexiades-Armenakas M, Bitter P Jr, Hruza G, Mulholland S. Enhanced full-face skin rejuvenation using synchronous intense pulsed optical and conducted bipolar radiofrequency energy (elōs): introducing selective radio-photothermolysis. *J. Drugs Dermatol.* 2005;2:181–6.

Sadick NS, Magro C. A study evaluating the safety and efficacy of the Velasmooth^{TM} system in the treatment of cellulite. *J. Cosmet. Laser Ther.* 2007;9:15–20.

Sadick NS, Makino Y. Selective electro-thermolysis in aesthetic medicine: a review. *Laser Surg. Med.* 2004;34:91–7.

Sadick NS, Mullholland RS. A prospective clinical study to evaluate the efficacy and safety of cellulite treatment using the combination of optical and RF energies for subcutaneous tissue heating. *J. Cosmet. Laser Ther.* 2004;6:187–90.

Sadick NS, Trelles MA. Nonablative wrinkle treatment of the face and neck using a combined diode laser and radiofrequency technology. *Dermatol. Surg.* 2005;31:1695–9.

Section 6

FRACTIONAL LASERS

CHAPTER 58

Fractional Lasers: General Concepts

Sorin Eremia
Zeina Tannous

Ablative CO_2 laser resurfacing using computerized scanners became widely used in 1995. Results were great, but so were challenges with healing and complications. Soon thereafter, ablative scanned Er:YAG lasers were also introduced as a less aggressive method, but even after significant technological improvements, skin tightening results with Er:YAG lasers, in the opinion of many users, were never of the level achieved by the CO_2 lasers. For the past dozen years, ablative resurfacing, particularly with CO_2 lasers, has remained the gold standard for treatment of age- and actinic-related rhytids of the facial skin. The combination of technological improvements with the lasers, experience in how to use these lasers, and know-how in managing the treated areas has dramatically reduced the problems that were initially encountered with these modalities. Nevertheless, prolonged healing time, need for intensive follow-up, significant complication risks, a high incidence of residual hypopigmentation, unimpressive results for acne scars, counterindication of use for darker skin types, and limitations of use for the face only have been major stimulants in the search for better alternatives. For a while, it was felt that nonablative resurfacing and skin tightening with lasers, broadband light, or radiofrequency devices would provide the searched for alternative. In spite of significant and ongoing improvements with nonablative technology, including such innovative ideas as the use of skin suction devices to better position the tissues for energy delivery, results of nonablative resurfacing have lagged far behind ablative techniques.

A revolutionary new concept started to change the future of resurfacing: the development of fractional photothermolysis technology, which may eventually lead to the ideal type of treatment, with relatively low risks, little downtime, and excellent results in most areas of the body and for most skin types. The concept may have its origins in reports of the use of a simple needle-studded rolling pin to treat fine wrinkles and acne scars. The resulting myriad of small puncture wounds heals very rapidly and induces some degree of new collagen deposition. By adding the thermal effect of a laser energy beam, tissue response can be enhanced. So rather than treating the entire skin surface uniformly, fractional photothermolysis treats only a portion of the skin; small islands of skin are treated with surrounding intact tissue. If the column of tissue destruction is very narrow, in the order of 0.1–0.2 mm, healing is very rapid. Thus the original fractional resurfacing concept utilized narrow beams of energy, 100–250 μm in diameter, to treat a fraction (20 to 25%) of the skin surface, leaving intact, normal surrounding tissue around each narrow cylindrical tissue injury zone (Figure 58.1). Thus laser microbeams create microscopic-sized thermal injury zones (MTZ), while sparing the areas surrounding these zones. The trick is to deliver sufficiently high fluence of the properly selected wavelength over a very small surface area to allow beam penetration to the desired depth without too much lateral diffusion of the energy. This would limit thermal damage to a narrow MTZ, leaving a surrounding area of unaffected, healthy tissue.

The result of this type of injury is a type of tissue response that, on one hand, leads to very rapid visible recovery and, on the other hand, to a prolonged thermal injury response of new collagen deposition. In effect, the body is

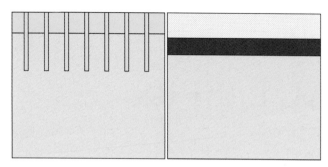

FIGURE 58.1: *Fractional vs ablative resurfacing: laser microbeams create microscopic-sized thermal injury zones (MTZ), while sparing the areas surrounding these zones.*

able to eliminate very rapidly the small plugs of necrotic tissue created, so with very narrow MTZs, within twenty-four hours, the epidermal surface appears intact. The true healing and tissue injury response processes continue, however, deeper in the dermis for several weeks, resulting in variable degrees of collagen deposition and thus improvement in skin texture and tightness. Conceptually, this type of treatment is ideal for acne-type scars, and in practice, the results have been excellent.

Initially, the concept of fractional MTZs was applied with infrared-wavelength lasers in the 1,540–1,550 nm range, and the Reliant Fraxel 750 laser was the first such device. This wavelength had good tissue penetration and could generate very narrow and moderately deep MTZs. The concept, not surprisingly, was quickly applied to 2,940-nm Er:YAG and 10,600-nm CO_2 lasers, as well. The 2,940 WL has the advantage and disadvantage of very high water absorption and generation of little thermal injury. Pinpoint bleeding can be a problem, just as it can be with ablative Er:YAG lasers. Long dwell times need to be used with these Er:YAG lasers to control bleeding and achieve sufficient thermal effect to improve wrinkles.

FRACTIONAL CO_2 LASERS

The CO_2 laser 10,600 wavelength, on the other hand, generates a lot of thermal damage, and care must be taken to avoid excessive lateral diffusion of the heat. To achieve a narrow, deep MTZ with a CO_2 laser, it is necessary to use high power (watts) with a narrow spot size (0.1–0.2 mm) and a relatively short pulse width in the range of 0.1–1 ms. Unfortunately, the parameters used to create a relatively deep (0.5–1.5 mm), narrow wound do not generate sufficient lateral thermal effect to achieve ideal hemostasis. And when enough heat is generated to achieve a balance between hemostasis, depths of injury, and thermal effect for wrinkle improvement, the treatment can be painful, and healing is no longer so fast, taking up to a week. There is controversy as to what type of tissue injury generated by a CO_2 laser is ideal to achieve the best results for wrinkles with the shortest possible recovery time. It should be

remembered that classic, fully ablative CO_2 laser resurfacing only ablates in the range of 0.2 mm into the papillary dermis to achieve outstanding skin-tightening results. Likewise, deep chemical peels and dermabrasion only penetrate in the 0.2–0.3 mm range. Acne scars, which can be 1–2 mm deep, present their own challenge. As of late 2008, fractional CO_2 lasers available in the United States provide a fair amount of versatility. They can be used at relatively low settings, resulting in very short patient downtime, but requiring multiple treatment sessions to provide modest results, comparable to the 1,440- to 1,550-nm fractional lasers. They can also be used at more aggressive treatment settings to achieve more impressive results, but with five to seven days of downtime. However, the recovery is much faster and easier than with ablative CO_2 or even long-pulsed Er:YAG lasers, and while the results might not quite reach the level of a fully ablative CO_2 laser treatment, they are good enough to render most patients quite happy.

In summary, the result to risk and result to recovery ratios are very patient-friendly. With scanned CO_2 laser technology widely available, there are many competing laser systems available, some of them being relatively inexpensive and having no per use cost. Initially, some of the major CO_2 laser manufacturers took widely different approaches to spot size, pulse width, and scanning patterns. Some systems already have, or will have by 2009, the ability to treat patients with more than one spot size and a wide range of pulse widths and scan coverage patterns. This will provide great flexibility in selecting the most appropriate parameters for the type of wrinkle or scar being treated, for various body areas being treated, and for the individual patient's wishes as to results versus recovery time.

FRACTIONAL 1,550-NM LASERS

Much excitement can be created over a new treatment modality, but only time tells how safe and effective it really is. That being said, we now have significant experience with the first fractional laser, Fraxel (Reliant Technologies). Although the Fraxel laser is also discussed by Dr. Narurkar in Chapter 60, we felt a short additional discussion of this original fractional laser, its evolution over the past three years, and what it can do is worthwhile, particularly since both authors are highly experienced with this device.

This 1,550-nm, doped Er:Glass laser works by creating a pattern of either 125 or 250 MTZs per square centimeter. As discussed previously, each MTZ is a cylindrical area of tissue destruction caused by the narrow energy beam of the laser. The depth and width of the MTZ is totally dependent on the total amount of energy delivered by the laser's beam on the spot it hits. The total amount of energy delivered by one pulse is measured in joules. For each pulse, that amount is relatively small, in the order of millijoules. This amount of energy delivered over a fixed surface is known as *fluence* and is measured in joules per square centimeter.

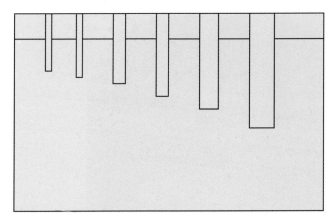

FIGURE 58.2: *Increasing the amount of energy delivered by each pulse not only increases the depth of the column we call the MTZ, but also its width.*

Because, with this type of laser, the spot is very small, the actual fluence is quite higher when measured in joules per square centimeter. When comparing the power of a fractional laser, it is thus important to understand both the concept of maximum energy per pulse and the width of the beam, or its spot size at skin surface level. The maximum amount of energy delivered in one pulse is an absolute number. The fluence will vary with the spot size on which it is delivered. As the fluence is increased, so is the depth of penetration and tissue injury. However, as the laser energy beam burns through the epidermis and dermis in depth, heat is also transmitted laterally, and with increasing depth, there is an increase in the width of the column of tissue injury. Increasing the amount of energy delivered by each pulse thus not only increases the depth of the column we call the MTZ, but also its width (Figure 58.2). The Fraxel 750 was able to deliver pulses of up to 40 mJ. It was shown histologically that the depth and width of the MTZ

increased roughly linearly to the increase in energy. At the maximum setting of 40 mJ, the MTZ reached a maximum depth of 1 mm and a column width of 200 μm. Ideally, with a nonablative, no downtime fractional resurfacing concept, only 15 to 25% of the skin surface should be injured. As the width of the MTZ increases, if the density of MTZs per square centimeter is too high, the resurfacing will take on more of an ablative aspect, and thus complications can develop. The width of the MTZ for a given power setting is also dependent on the temperature of the dermis when the energy passes through and is absorbed by the tissues. If the baseline temperature is raised, such as by heat buildup, the same amount of energy will cause a wider area of injury, and thus the width of the MTZ is also increased. It is therefore important to allow sufficient time between passes, and skin cooling can also be of help. The second-generation Fraxel 1500, now called the Fraxel Re:store, can deliver up to 70 mJ/cm² and the density of MTZs is not fixed to just two settings, but rather, can be varied. This not only allows for deeper penetration, which is potentially important for treatment of scars – particularly acne scars – but it can allow for less painful treatment.

The Fraxel 750 was originally touted as a resurfacing tool for fine facial wrinkles. A series of four monthly treatments, with virtually no downtime and very little risk, was supposed to achieve significant improvement in fine wrinkles. In fact, results for fine facial wrinkles were a bit disappointing, but it turned out to be an excellent tool for treating dyschromia, particularly melasma type, and acne scars, including for dark-skinned patients. It was also found to be a safe and effective device for treatment, with virtually no downtime, of nonfacial areas, such as the neck, chest, arms, and hands, where the combination of dyschromia and very fine wrinkles predominates. In the authors' opinion, fractional resurfacing is a superior

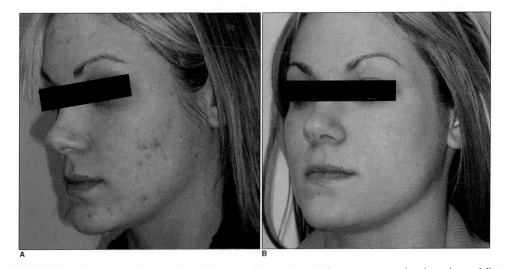

FIGURE 58.3: *Representative results of four monthly treatments for acne scars, dyschromia, and fine lines, with the Fraxel 1,550-nm laser:* **A**, *pretreatment;* **B**, *posttreatment.*

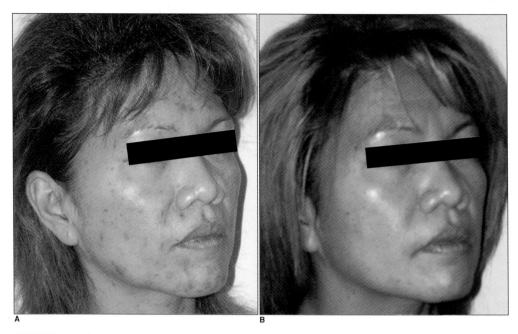

FIGURE 58.4: *Representative results of four monthly treatments for acne scars, dyschromia, and fine lines, with the Fraxel 1,550-nm laser: A, pretreatment; B, posttreatment.*

alternative to peels, nonfractional Er:YAG, or a nitrogen plasma device.

The Fraxel 1500 Re:store is a significant improvement over the 750 model. It is much easier to operate; there is significantly less pain, to the point that using a chilled air skin-cooling device suffices as anesthesia for many patients; and results for facial fine lines have been improved but are still well inferior to a single treatment with fractional CO_2 lasers. Also, results for acne scars, which were already good with the 750 model, appear to be even better, and logically so, due to deeper dermal penetration at maximum pulse energy level. Figures 58.3–58.5 show representative results of four monthly treatments for acne scars, dyschromia, and fine lines with the Fraxel 1,550-nm laser.

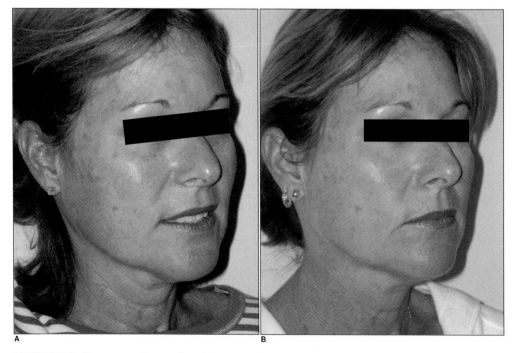

FIGURE 58.5: *Representative results of four monthly treatments for acne scars, dyschromia, and fine lines, with the Fraxel 1,550-nm laser: A, pretreatment; B, posttreatment.*

TABLE 58.1: Fractional Lasers by Category: 1,440–1,550-nm Near-Infrared, 2,940-nm Er:YAG, CO_2s

Wavelength (nm)	Laser/Manufacturer	Features	Comments
1,540 Er:Glass Fiber	Lux1540 Fract/Palomar	fixed pattern, 70 mJ max	low per use cost
1,540	Mosaic/Lutronic	static + dynamic modes	relatively low
1,540		random scan, 70 mJ max	per use cost
1,550	Fraxel Re:store/Reliant	gold std 1,550 fractional 70 mJ max, adjustable parameters	low pain, no downtime, expensive to buy/operate
1,440	Lux1 440 Fract/Palomar	15-mm tip, 10 mJ/beam	320 spots/cm^2
1,440	Affirm/Cyanosure	relatively low power nonablative	used in combination with 1,320 laser
2,940	NaturalLase/Focus Med.	scanned, variable settings	Er:YAG + fractional
2,940 Er:YAG	ProFractional/Sciton	scanned spot, variable patterns, pulse width, and fluence	many features, main problem is bleeding
2,940	Pixel 2,940/Alma	fixed pattern, low power	new model improved
2,940	Lux 2,940/Palomar	scanned spot, variable	competitive to Sciton
10,600 CO_2	Fraxel	40 W, 0.14-mm spot, roller delivery, self-adjust p.w. and density patterns	good, expensive, high per use cost, relatively painful, long recovery
10,600	MiXto/Lasering USA	30 W, 0.3-mm and 0.18-mm spot, 2.5–7.5 ms p.w. variable density pattern	large scan size, lower price, good both for wrinkles and acne scars
10,600	Active/Deep FX/Lumenis	60 W, 1.3 mm (activeFx) 0.12 mm (deepFx) 0.1–1.0 ms p.w. (self-adjust) variable density patterns	expensive, need use both modes, narrow spot/short p.w. = bleeds, moderate per use cost
10,600	X-side Dot-Eclipsemed/ Deka Lasers	30 W, 0.35-mm spot 0.1–2.0 ms p.w., variable density patterns	user-friendly, reasonable price, large spot limits deep scars
10,600	Cyanosure/Deka (Italy)	30 W, 0.35 mm, 0.1–2.0 ms variable density	same laser as Eclipse DOT, but more pricy
10,600	Juvia/Ellipse	15 W flex-fiber delivery scanned 0.5-mm spot, 2.0–7.0 ms p.w.	insufficient power, potential problematic fiber delivery system
10,600	Pixel CO_2/Alma	fixed stamp pattern	relatively low power
10,600	e-CO^2/Lutronic	30 W, 0.12/0.3/1.0 mm spot, 0.1–1.0 ms p.w. (self-adjust) variable density, patterns	user-friendly, three spots reasonable price, problem contact tip
10,600	Exelo/Quantel	30 W, 2–100 ms p.w.	relative unknown

Nevertheless, the improvement in facial rhytids and the level of skin tightening are inferior to results with fractional CO_2 lasers and far inferior to the level achieved with even single-pass, high-power ablative CO_2 lasers. For acne scars, the results following four to five treatment sessions are competitive with single-treatment fractional CO_2. Based on early experience with these lasers, the advantage of the Fraxel and other infrared fractional lasers, such as the Palomar, is the lack of downtime. The disadvantage is the requirement of typically four treatment sessions, and particularly for the Fraxel, the significant per treatment cost of the consumable treatment tip, which, incidentally, is also an issue with the CO_2 Fraxel Re:pair, but not with most other fractional CO_2 lasers.

SELECTING A FRACTIONAL CO₂ LASER

Because fractional CO_2 lasers appear to be, currently, the most versatile and cost-effective resurfacing lasers on the market, a few words on what features to look for in choosing such a unit are suitable. Power is relatively important, especially for speed of treatment and tissue penetration at larger spot sizes and longer pulse widths. Thirty to forty watts is largely sufficient; less than 30 W is questionable. Spot size is important for depth of penetration. Spot sizes in the 0.12–0.1.8 mm range penetrate deeper and are better for deep acne scars. But deeper penetration also hurts more, and to allow deeper penetration, the pulse width is often made very short, which provides less coagulation, and thus more pinpoint bleeding and crusting occurs. A narrow spot size and short pulse width also generate less thermal effect and thus may be less effective for skin tightening and superficial lines. Spot sizes in the 0.3–0.35 mm range are well suited for wrinkles. Look for a laser that offers both a narrow and a larger spot size. Pulse width or dwell time is also critical. Less than 1 ms is often insufficient to provide good coagulation. The 1–3 ms range seems most suited for skin tightening. With shorter pulse widths, higher settings (watts) are needed to deliver the same amount of energy. Total energy delivered per spot (with these lasers measuring in millijoules) equals power (W) × pulse width (ms). Fluence is calculated in joules per square centimeter by dividing the power delivered by the surface area of the spot size. Look for a laser that allows the operator to set the pulse width. This asks for more thought process but gives far more flexibility than lasers that automatically set a pulse width for a given power and spot size. On the other hand, self-adjustment makes the instruments more goof-proof. The ability to select density (what percentage of the skin surface is treated with one pass of the laser) is also a nice feature, as for different body areas, skin types, and types of wrinkles or acne scars, densities may vary from 10 to 40%. Scan size and the shape of scanned areas are also important. Large scan areas (1.5–2 cm) make treatment of large areas faster and easier, with less risk of overlap. Small scan sizes are needed for oddly shaped areas of the face and to fill in any areas missed on the initial pass. In summary, an ideal fractional CO_2 laser should be at least 30 W, offer both a smaller and a larger spot size, offer operator-adjusted pulse widths up to at least 2 ms, and offer adjustable treatment densities with variable scan pattern sizes.

As of the time of this writing, there are already at least several major competitors in each of the three fractional laser categories: the 1,440- to 1,550-nm near-infrared, the 2,940 Er:YAG, and the CO_2 (Table 58.1). Several of each type of these lasers are discussed in greater detail in the subsequent chapters of this text. It would not be surprising if several more are available since the publication of this text. The concepts, however, will remain the same.

The reader should be careful when selecting a fractional laser. First decide what type, and then select among the various devices in that specific category. Before making any final decision, it is wise to try to talk to someone trustworthy who has experience with the laser being considered for purchase.

CHAPTER 59

Palomar Lux 1,540-nm Fractional Laser

Vic A. Narurkar

The fundamental concept of modern-day laser- and light-based therapies relies on the principles of selective photothermolysis. As we learn more about skin and light interactions, it has become evident that additional factors can influence the safety and efficacy of the delivery of photons to desired targets. This is particularly evident in the treatment of darker skin types. Selective photothermolysis can be further enhanced with a novel approach: fractional photothermolysis. Fractional photothermolysis enhances the safety of traditional ablative resurfacing and can be accomplished with nonablative and ablative modalities. The following two chapters will discuss true nonablative fractional resurfacing (TNFSR) with the Lux 1,540-nm laser and the 1,550-nm Fraxel laser.

TNFSR

Fractional photothermolysis is rapidly gaining momentum as a safe and effective modality for facial and nonfacial resurfacing. Fractional resurfacing can be performed by nonablative and ablative methods. There is much confusion about true versus pseudofractional resurfacing, with the latter merely tweaking existing ablative devices with modifications. True nonablative fractional resurfacing has three criteria: (1) creation of microthermal zones of damage, (2) preservation of the majority of the stratum corneum with rapid reepithelialization, and (3) a resurfacing with epidermal extrusion. If all three of these criteria are not met, the device is merely a traditional ablative or nonablative device with modifications, and the risk of bulk heating is still significant, thereby also promoting greater risks of scarring and pigmentary anomalies. The first commercially launched TNFSR device was the 1,550-nm erbium-doped Fraxel laser (Reliant Technologies). The other TNFSR device is the Lux 1,540-nm laser (Starlux, Palomar Medical Technologies).

PATIENT SELECTION AND PREPARATION FOR TNFSR

Skin types I–VI can be treated safely with TNFSR. Pretreatment with hydroquinone preparations of 4% is recommended for all skin type IV to VI patients for at least two weeks and should be continued between treatments and after treatments for at least one month. If topical retinoids are included in the regimen, they need to be discontinued five to seven days before TNFSR treatment. Antiviral prophylaxis is recommended for all patients, and those patients with a documented history of herpes simplex should be maintained on oral antivirals for one week. With higher settings, a variety of transient episodes, including acne flares and edema, are common. Posttreatment guidelines include using topical agents, such as Biafine, for accelerated recovery and the use of oral and/or topical acne medications for patients with a predisposition to acne flares. The author does not advocate the use of topical, intramuscular, or oral steroids post-TNFSR as the inflammatory response is probably integral to efficacy. For reduction of edema, hydration and sleeping at an elevation can assist recovery, as can the use of cool compresses and biorestorative creams. Clinical indications of TNFSR include periorbital and perioral rhytids, full-face mild to moderate photodamage, off-face photodamage and dyschromia, acne scars, surgical scars, striae, and therapy-resistant melasma.

LUX 1,540-NM LASER

The Lux 1,540-nm laser is a stamped fractional laser that is a component of the Starlux infinity platform device. The infinity platform device affords the use of multiple handpieces, which consist of pulsed light devices with contact cooling, dichroic filters, and photon recycling and various laser handpieces. The selectivity of the dichroic filters, in

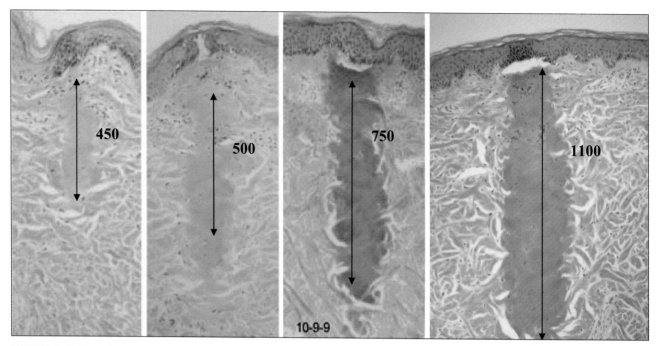

FIGURE 59.1: *Note the cylindrical shape of the dermal effect produced by 1,540- to 1,550-nm fractional lasers. The depth, and to some extent, the width, of penetration increases as the fluence is increased. Deep penetration is important for treatment of deep acne scars. The epidermis recovers almost immediately, while a longer-term remodeling process continues in the dermis.*

addition to the contact cooling, enable these pulsed light devices to be more specific and behave as individual lasers, a trend that is common in the newer generation of pulsed light sources.

The Lux 1,540-nm handpiece employs true nonablative fractional resurfacing using a stamped pattern on delivery. Spot sizes of 10 mm and 15 mm with fluencies up to 100 mJ and depths of penetration up to 1.2 mm are available (Figure 59.1). It is evident that depth of penetration is correlated to fluence and that deeper penetration is particularly necessary for entities such as acne scars and rhytids. Clinical indications for Lux 1,540-nm treatment include acne scars,

resurfacing of the face and nonfacial skin for photoaging, mild to moderate rhytids (Figure 59.2), surgical and traumatic scars, striae, and melasma. Three to five treatments spaced four to six weeks apart are necessary. Recovery is relatively rapid, with the main transient side effects being edema, which can last twenty-four to seventy-two hours; petechiae; and erythema of less than seventy-two hours' duration. Suggested parameters for the Lux 1,540-nm laser are outlined in Table 59.1. Recently, a second-generation Lux 1,540-nm laser handpiece using a zoom lens has been introduced. The spot size is square and allows for variation in the sizes and spacing of the microthermal zones.

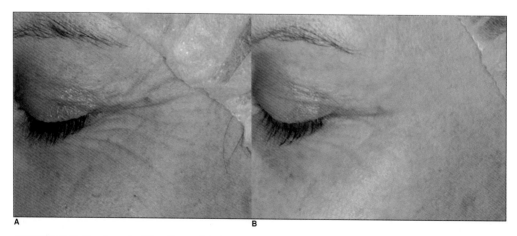

FIGURE 59.2: *Treatment of fine lines with the Lux 1540:* **A,** *before;* **B,** *after a series of three treatments.*

TABLE 59.1: Suggested Parameters for Lux 1,540-nm Fractional Resurfacing

Skin Type	Indication	Spot Size (mm)	Fluence (mJ)	No. of Passes
I–III	melasma	15	10–15	3–5
	periorbital rhytids	10	25–40	3–7
	perioral rhytids	10	50–65	3–7
	off-face resurfacing	10	25–35	3–5
	acne scars	10	40–70	5–7
	surgical scars	10	40–70	5–7
IV–VI	melasma	15	10–15	3–5
	dyschromia	10	25–35	3–5
	acne scars	10	30–50	3–7
	surgical scars	10	30–50	3–7

The Lux 1,540-nm laser is often used in combination with the Lux G and Lux IR handpieces as part of Trilux photorejuvenation. The Lux G is used for the treatment of vascular and pigmented lesions and the Lux IR for skin tightening through soft tissue coagulation. The Starlux device is an example of a platform model for light-based therapies, whereby a power supply stays constant and different handpieces are utilized, which can be pulsed light or laser devices and can be modified as new clinical applications become established. The Lux G is a pulsed light handpiece with absorption spectra that peak in the 532–900 nm range, allowing for selective photothermolysis of vascular and pigmented lesions. The Lux IR employs a fractional delivery of an infrared light source, reducing the risks of bulk heating in the deep dermis and subcutaneous tissue. The platform model allows for easy interchange of the various handpieces. A popular treatment called Trilux is gaining momentum, in which the Lux 1,540-nm laser is utilized for improvement of skin tone and texture, the Lux G handpiece is utilized for the treatment of facial telangiectasias and lentigines (photofacial), and the Lux IR handpiece is utilized to treat skin laxity. Segmental areas can also be treated, where often, cheeks are treated with the Lux G and the periorbital and perioral rhytids with the Lux 1,540-nm laser handpiece. Unlike traditional ablative technologies, there is no reported risk of segmental areas of hypopigmentation or hyperpigmentation.

SUGGESTED READING

Kono T, Chan HH, Groff WF, et al. Prospective direct comparison study of fractional resurfacing using different fluencies and densities for skin rejuvenation in Asians. *Lasers Surg. Med.* 2007;39:311–14.

Manstein D, Herron GS, Sink RK, Tanner H, Anderson RR. Fractional photothermolysis: a new concept for cutaneous remodeling using microscopic patterns of thermal injury. *Lasers Surg. Med.* 2004;34:426–38.

Mezzana P, Valeriani M. Rejuvenation of the aging face using fractional photothermolysis and intense pulsed light: a new technique. *Acta Chir. Plast.* 2007;49:47–50.

Narurkar VA. Skin rejuvenation with microthermal fractional photothermolysis. *Dermatol. Ther.* 2007;1(Suppl):S10–S13. Review.

Rokhsar C, Fitzpatrick RE. The treatment of melasma with fractional photothermolysis: a pilot study. *Dermatol. Surg.* 2005;31:1645–50.

Tannous Z. Fractional resurfacing. *Clin. Dermatol.* 2007;25:480–6.

CHAPTER 60

Fraxel 1,550-nm Laser (Fraxel Re:store)

Vic A. Narurkar

As discussed in Chapter 59, the first commercially launched true nonablative fractional resurfacing (TNFSR) device was the 1,550-nm erbium-doped Fraxel laser (Reliant Technologies). It is the most widely studied device for this indication with the largest series of peer-reviewed publications and clinical experience. The Fraxel laser produces random patterns of microthermal zones (MTZs) with precise dosimetry to accomplish true nonablative fractional resurfacing. The first-generation Fraxel laser (Fraxel 750) employed two settings of microthermal zones (125 MTZ and 250 MTZ). The second-generation Fraxel laser (Fraxel Re:store) employs a variety of MTZ settings and is able to deliver fluences up to 70 mJ. Treatment levels (1–R3) reflect the density of MTZs, allowing for greater flexibility in delivery of energy. This is particularly critical in patients with darker skin types, for whom higher fluencies are required for indications such as acne scars, and variation of MTZs to lower levels allow for significant reduction in postinflammatory hyperpigmentation. Conversely, for indications that require more shallow penetration, such as melasma, both lower fluencies and lower treatment levels can be delivered. It is also possible to vary both treatment levels and fluencies on the same patient for differ-ent anatomic areas, allowing for very precise delivery of energy with the highest safety profile. Each Fraxel laser treatment delivers over a million MTZs. Ultrastructural analysis of Fraxel-induced wounds shows epidermal and dermal necrosis confined to the MTZs of submillimeter size. Epidermal repair is evident at twenty-four hours, and these ultrastructural observations correlate well with clinical findings, as also noted in Chapter 59 (see Figure 60.1). Unlike ablative procedures, there are no open wounds, weeping, or prolonged erythema. With the highest settings, erythema and edema are usually limited to seventy-two hours or less, with the term *social downtime* being utilized for the recovery process. Occasional isolated blistering has been reported, which resolves with proper wound care. Patient treatment involves the use of a topical anesthetic, such as Pliaglis (Galderma Laboratories), applied sixty minutes prior to treatment. Treatment is performed with roller tips of 7 mm and 15 mm, and a Zimmer cooler is essential for patient comfort.

Clinical indications for Fraxel 750 and Fraxel Re:store treatments include facial and nonfacial resurfacing for photodamage, rhytids, acne scars, surgical scars, traumatic scars, melasma, and striae. Safety and efficacy have been

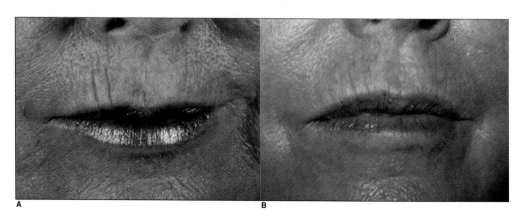

A   B

FIGURE 60.1: *Epidermal repair is evident at twenty-four hours after 1,550-nm Fraxel laser resurfacing.*

TABLE 60.1: Suggested Parameters for 1,550-nm Fraxel Laser Resurfacing

Skin Type	Indication	Fluence (mJ)	MTZ Setting
I–III	facial resurfacing	40	L6–L9
	deep rhytids	40	L9–R3
	eyelid resurfacing	40	L6–L9
	nonfacial resurfacing	30	L5–L9
	acne scars	40–70	L6–R3
	surgical scars	70	L9–R3
	melasma	8–12	L3–L6
IV–V	facial resurfacing	40	L3–L6
	deep rhytids	40	L5–L9
	eyelid resurfacing	40	L5–L9
	nonfacial resurfacing	30	L3–L5
	acne scars	40	L4–L6
	surgical scars	70	L4–L6
	melasma	6–8	L3–L6
VI	acne scars	40	L2–L4
	surgical scars	70	L2–L4

studied for over two years, and there have been no reports of hypopigmentation or permanent scars. Transient hyperpigmentation has been reported and was more evident with the older settings, for which MTZ adjustments were limited. Clinical results have been exceptional (Figure 60.1) and have set TNFSR as the gold standard for skin resurfacing in all skin types. Table 60.1 summarizes guidelines for Fraxel Re:store treatments. Improvements are noted even after a single treatment and continue to be enhanced, with optimal results seen at six to nine months following the final treatment.

CONCLUSIONS

Laser- and light-based devices can be made safer and more effective by modifying the devices, as with true nonablative fractional resurfacing. These technologies are rapidly gaining momentum as the preferred treatment of a variety of indications. TNFSR devices, such as the Lux 1,540-nm laser and the Fraxel 1,550-nm laser, are indicated for facial and nonfacial resurfacing, acne scar treatments, melasma reduction, and scar reduction in all skin types.

SUGGESTED READING

Kono T, Chan HH, Groff WF, et al. Prospective direct comparison study of fractional resurfacing using different fluencies and densities for skin rejuvenation in Asians. *Lasers Surg. Med.* 2007;39:311–14.

Manstein D, Herron GS, Sink RK, Tanner H, Anderson RR. Fractional photothermolysis: a new concept for cutaneous remodeling using microscopic patterns of thermal injury. *Lasers Surg. Med.* 2004;34:426–38.

Narurkar VA. Skin rejuvenation with microthermal fractional photothermolysis. *Dermatol. Ther.* 2007;1(Suppl):S10–S13. Review.

Rokhsar C, Fitzpatrick RE. The treatment of melasma with fractional photothermolysis: a pilot study. *Dermatol. Surg.* 2005;31:1645–50.

Tannous Z. Fractional resurfacing. *Clin. Dermatol.* 2007;25:480–6.

CHAPTER 61

1,440-nm Fractional Laser: Cynosure Affirm

Andrew A. Nelson
Zeina Tannous

Efficacy in laser treatment has always necessitated a balance between the increased therapeutic effect associated with the use of higher-energy fluences and the associated increased risk of adverse events, particularly the risk of scarring. The development of fractional photothermolysis technologies has greatly shifted this balance, allowing for efficacy with decreased risks of adverse events.

Rather than treating the entire skin surface in a uniform pattern, fractional photothermolysis utilizes very small microbeams of diameter 100–200 μm to create microscopic thermal wounds, while sparing tissue surrounding these wounds. The microthermal zones are subjected to high-energy fluences, which result in homogenization of the dermis as well as damage to the overlying epidermis, with the formation and extrusion of necrotic epidermal debris. The intervening areas between the microthermal zones are not subjected to this high fluence but are gently heated by the diffusion of energy. This technology allows for the use of high-energy fluences with potentially greater clinical efficacy. As only a portion of the surface is subjected to the high-energy fluences, there is less downtime associated with the treatment as well as a potentially decreased risk of adverse events.

The Affirm laser (Cynosure Inc.) is a new microrejuvenation technology that incorporates the concepts of fractional photothermolysis and Cynosure's new Combined Apex Pulse array (CAP). The Affirm laser is a 1,440-nm Nd:YAG laser coupled with a special lens that incorporates approximately one thousand diffractive elements, called the CAP array. Originally, the Affirm device was developed with a single 1,440-nm-wavelength laser output device. The 1,440-nm wavelength is absorbed by water, though the Nd:YAG laser is thought to exert its clinical effect primarily through heating and stimulation of collagen. Although the Affirm can be utilized with this single wavelength, it is also available incorporating multiple wavelengths and light sources to improve the treatment efficacy. The Affirm device now also incorporates a 1,320-nm Nd:YAG wavelength as well as a Xenon Pulsed Light (XPL) source. The 1,320-nm Nd:YAG is thought to further stimulate deep collagen through a heating effect. Finally, the XPL allows for treatment of superficial erythema and dyspigmentation.

CAP technology delivers approximately one thousand high-energy apex fluences in a stamped pattern with a 10-mm spot size, surrounded by low-level background heating of the remainder of the skin surface (Figure 61.1). The incorporation of the CAP array diffracts the output of the laser, resulting in a greater treatment surface per single laser pulse as well as a more uniform treatment effect; approximately 20 to 50% of the total energy is delivered to the surface between the microthermal zones. The CAP technology requires full cutaneous contact as well as the use of a cold-air cooling device to protect the epidermis, typically the SmartCool cold air system by Cynosure. No topical anesthesia or tracking dye is required with the Affirm laser, although some patients may prefer the use of topical anesthesia to reduce the mild discomfort associated with the treatment.

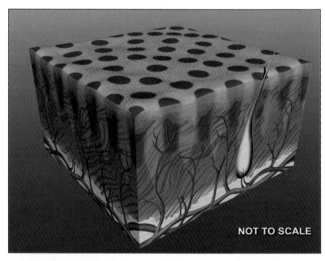

FIGURE 61.1: CAP array output. Photo courtesy of Bruce Katz, MD, and Cynosure Inc.

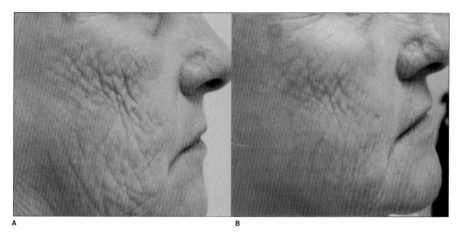

FIGURE 61.2: **A,** *Before and,* **B,** *one month after six treatments at 4.0–7.6 J/cm². Photo courtesy of Bruce Katz, MD, and Cynosure Inc.*

The high-energy apexes, or microthermal zones, treated with the Affirm laser are subjected to sufficiently high fluences to result in coagulation of the collagen. In contrast to other fractional systems, the high-energy apexes associated with the Affirm laser are relatively superficial, reaching approximately 300 µm in depth on histologic specimens; other fractional lasers achieve histologic changes at depths of up to 1,500 µm. The majority of changes associated with photoaging are confined to the epidermis and superficial dermis, 200–250 µm in depth; thus, although the Affirm laser treats relatively superficially, it specifically treats the areas most damaged from photoaging. Additionally, there is only limited damage to the epidermis in the high-energy apexes treated with the Affirm laser, rather than the epidermal necrosis and extrusion of denuded skin associated with other fractional lasers; this may decrease the pain and downtime associated with the procedure. Finally, the skin surrounding the high-energy apexes is subjected to more significant heating due to the incorporation of the CAP, which may potentially result in more improvement of the tone and texture of the skin following several treatments. On the other hand, the shallow penetration and the limited damage to the epidermis resulting from the Affirm laser might, in turn, reduce the efficacy of this laser as compared to other nonablative fractional devices.

In clinical practice, the Affirm laser has been reported to improve superficial aging, fines lines, and wrinkles (Figure 61.2) as well as superficial scars and pigmentary irregularities. Recently, a series of forty patients were treated with the Affirm laser. Patients received three treatments with the Affirm laser, each spaced four weeks apart, with energy fluences ranging between 3 and 7 J/cm², with a 3-ms pulse duration and a 1- to 2-Hz pulse repetition rate. Either one or three treatment passes were performed at each treatment, with significant wrinkles or scars receiving three treatment passes. Overall, 94% of patients developed some improvement in skin texture, pigment, skin vascularity, or

appearance of a scar following the three treatments. However, the majority of these patients (67% of total patients) experienced only mild improvement following the three treatments. Patients' clinical outcomes improved with further treatment sessions, as more patients noted improvement following the third treatment session compared to the first treatment session; when offered the opportunity to undergo additional treatment sessions, 90% of patients elected to continue treatment with the Affirm laser. However, long-term data with a greater number of treatments and the associated outcomes are not currently available to determine the ideal number of treatments. The Affirm device was well tolerated by the patients in this study; the most common side effects of treatment were transient erythema, urticaria, and edema, which resolved in hours to two days. No scars or hypopigmentation was observed as a result of treatment.

The development of fractional photothermolysis may well represent the next leap forward in laser therapies. Fractionated therapies allow for the use of higher-energy fluences, thereby achieving greater efficacy, while limiting the potential for adverse reactions. The Affirm laser not only incorporates this fractional technology, but also utilizes the CAP array to further increase the efficacy of this device. The result may be a microrejuvenation therapy that is efficacious and safe in the treatment of superficial aging, fine lines, wrinkles, superficial scars, and pigmentary irregularities. However, more well-designed studies, longer follow-up periods, and more experience are needed to validate the efficacy and safety of this laser.

SUGGESTED READING

Bene NI, Weiss MA, Beasley KL, et al. Comparison of histological features of 1550 nm fractional resurfacing and microlens array scattering of 1440 nm. *Lasers Surg. Med.* 2006;38:26–31.

Huzaira M, Anderson RR, Sink K, et al. Intradermal focusing of near-infrared optical pulses: a new approach for non-ablative laser therapy. *Lasers Surg. Med.* 2003;32:405–412.

Manstein D, Herron GS, Sink RK, et al. Fractional photothermolysis: a new concept for cutaneous remodeling using microscopic patterns of thermal injury. *Lasers Surg. Med.* 2004;34:426–38.

Wanner M, Tanzi EL, Alster TS. Fractional photothermolysis: treatment of facial and nonfacial cutaneous photodamage with a 1,550-nm erbium-doped fiber laser. *Dermatol. Surg.* 2007;33:23–8.

Weiss RA, Gold M, Bene N, et al. Prospective clinical evaluation of 1440-nm laser delivered by microarray for treatment of photoaging and scars. *J. Drugs Dermatol.* 2006;5:740–4.

CHAPTER 62

Sciton Er:YAG 2,940-nm Fractional Laser

Andrew A. Nelson

Zeina Tannous

Ablative laser treatments have long been considered the gold standard for the treatment of photoaging, scars, and wrinkles. However, the high efficacy of ablative treatments does not come without a price; the healing and downtime, up to two weeks, associated with complete cutaneous ablation and reepithelization are often prohibitive to patients. Thus patients and physicians have increasingly turned to nonablative therapies to achieve clinical improvement. These nonablative therapies have minimal associated downtime and limited side effects; however, they typically require multiple treatments to achieve clinical improvement. Thus physicians seek a device that combines the increased clinical efficacy of ablative resurfacing with the safety and minimal recovery associated with nonablative resurfacing. The development of fractional photothermolysis technology may ultimately allow for this ideal treatment.

Rather than treating the entire cutaneous surface uniformly, the overlying concept of fractional photothermolysis is treatment of the cutaneous surface in microbeams of diameter 100–250 μm; these microbeams create microscopic thermal zones of high energy fluences, while sparing the areas surrounding these zones. Thus the fractional therapies may achieve high efficacy due to the high energy in the microthermal zones, while limiting the potential for adverse reactions by decreasing the amount of skin subjected to these high-energy fluences.

Initially, fractional photothermolysis technology was applied to nonablative lasers. The microthermal zones treated with nonablative fractional devices result in homogenization and coagulation of the collagen in the dermis; additionally, the overlying epidermis is damaged with the formation and extrusion of necrotic epidermal debris. As these microthermal zones heal, clinical improvement develops in the texture, tone, and appearance of the skin. Further efficacy is achieved by heating of the skin between the microthermal zones as a result of diffusion. In contrast to nonablative fractional devices, ablative fractional technologies instantly ablate and eliminate the epidermis and superficial dermis in the microthermal zones. There is reported to be less heating of the skin between the microthermal zones, potentially decreasing the healing time and pain associated with the procedure. As the microthermal zones are completely ablated, it is thought that the healing process will result in more significant clinical improvement compared to nonablative treatments.

The ProFractional laser (Sciton Inc.), a new module that can be added to the Sciton Profile laser platform, offers physicians the opportunity to utilize ablative laser therapy, while incorporating fractional technology. The ProFractional utilizes a 2,940-nm Er:YAG laser; this laser is coupled with a large area pattern generator, a computer-generated high-speed scanner that generates the pattern of ablative channels. The Er:YAG laser targets water as its chromophore. As a unique feature, the ProFractional device can be adjusted to achieve precise, uniform ablative columns to depths of between 25 and 1,500 μm; these microchannels are reported to heal rapidly for a faster recovery than with nonablative fractional therapies. Additionally, the ProFractional device can be adjusted to control the skin surface area subjected to the ablative columns, with an adjustable coverage area between 1.5 and 60% of the total surface area. Finally, the pattern size of the treatment area can be adjusted from a minimum size of 6 × 6 mm to a maximum size of 20 × 20 mm. No topical anesthesia, tracking dye, or cold air cooling device is necessary with the ProFractional system. However, topical anesthesia may be utilized to reduce the mild discomfort associated with the treatment.

The ProFractional laser has been reported to be efficacious in the treatment of scars (specifically acne scars), rhytids, skin tone, and pigmentary irregularities in clinical practice. As a result of its ablative technology, only a single treatment pass per treatment session is necessary with the ProFractional. Substantial clinical efficacy has been reported following a single treatment session with

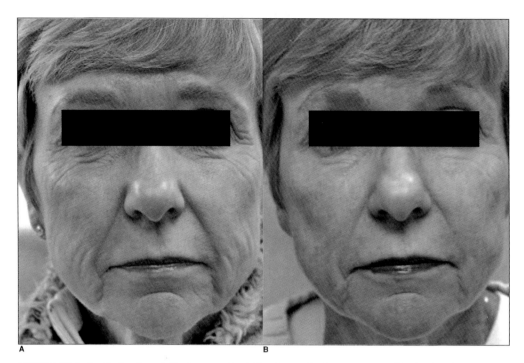

FIGURE 62.1: A, *Pretreatment.* **B,** *Four weeks following a single treatment with the ProFractional, at settings of 150 μm and 1.9% coverage area. Photos courtesy of Michael Gold, MD, and Sciton Inc.*

the ProFractional (Figure 62.1). Although improvement is noted after a single treatment, many patients return for multiple treatments to further increase their improvement; these sessions are typically spaced every four weeks apart to allow for healing and collagen remodeling. ProFractional treatments can be rapidly performed; the perioral and periocular areas take only five and three minutes, respectively, to treat. Finally, as ProFractional is a fractionated device, patients have reported a less significant side effect profile following treatment; the most common side effect reported by patients is mild transient erythema, which resolves in one to two days. Patients can often return to their normal activities immediately following the treatment. The ProFractional device has been used to safely treat all Fitzpatrick skin types without scarring or dyspigmentation, although experience with darker skin types (V and VI) is limited at this time. Long-term side effects as well as efficacy need to be determined and verified with well-designed, controlled studies, which are unfortunately lacking at this time.

Recently, ProFractional treatment has been combined with a MicroLaserPeel (MLP), which uniformly ablates the superficial epidermis up to a maximum depth of 50 μm. This uniform superficial ablation is thought to reduce the appearance of fine lines and superficial photodamage in a synergistic manner when utilized in conjunction with the ProFractional device for treatment of deeper skin tone and texture. Patients treated with this combination might achieve greater clinical efficacy, while only developing a mild transient erythema similar to a sunburn, which

resolves in a few days. Ultimately, multimodality treatment, such as ProFractional plus MLP, may represent a promising treatment option for our cosmetic patients.

Ablative laser resurfacing remains the gold standard therapy for the treatment of photoaging, scars, and rhytids. Unfortunately, the vast majority of patients are either unable or unwilling to tolerate the healing time associated with full ablation of the cutaneous surface. The incorporation of fractional technology completely alters our concept of ablative laser resurfacing. The ProFractional device allows patients some of the benefits of traditional Er:YAG resurfacing, while minimizing the side effects and healing time associated with the procedure. The adjustability of the ProFractional allows physicians the added flexibility to select the ideal treatment depth and density to help patients achieve their ideal cosmetic outcomes. It is important to remember that while the initial clinical results with the ProFractional device appear to be promising, the technology is still in the initial stages of development; significantly more clinical cases and greater physician experience are necessary to determine the exact role of this device. Ultimately, fractional ablative photothermolysis may well become the new gold standard for laser skin resurfacing.

SUGGESTED READING

Huzaira M, Anderson RR, Sink K, et al. Intradermal focusing of near-infrared optical pulses: a new approach for non-ablative laser therapy. *Lasers Surg. Med.* 2003;32:405–12.

Lask GL. Looking ahead to the future of fractional technologies. *Pract. Dermatol.* 2007;4:52–5.

Manstein D, Herron GS, Sink RK, et al. Fractional photothermolysis: a new concept for cutaneous remodeling using microscopic patterns of thermal injury. *Lasers Surg. Med.* 2004;34:426–38.

Owens LG. Sciton's ProFractional offers dramatic results and quick healing. *Aesthetic Buyer's Guide*. March/April 2007:1–8.

Wanner M, Tanzi EL, Alster TS. Fractional photothermolysis: treatment of facial and nonfacial cutaneous photodamage with a 1,550-nm erbium-doped fiber laser. *Dermatol. Surg.* 2007;33:23–8.

CHAPTER 63

Alma Pixel Er:YAG Fractional Laser

Gregory S. Keller

Grigoriy Mashkevich

The Pixel laser is a plug-in device to Alma Lasers's Harmony modular platform. Since the laser unit is situated inside the handpiece itself, a physician can add on a Pixel module to the Harmony without the purchase of an additional machine.

A digital photograph is composed of thousands or millions of individual squares, called *pixels*. Alma Lasers utilizes a so-called pixel mosaic of topographical skin treatment that places dots of erbium laser (2,940 nm) microthermal injury pixels that are interspersed with pixels of untreated skin. Using tight beam focusing, high local laser irradiance is produced in each microthermal column, while keeping average irradiance to low levels that avoid bulk heating of the skin.

These zones of ablative fractional photothermolysis (AFPT) produce tiny thermal wounds, while sparing the tissue that surrounds the tiny columns of tissue injury. The thermal ablative areas of treatment stimulate a wound-healing response that tightens the skin and smoothes wrinkles. Most or much of the treatment area remains intact and becomes a reservoir for rapid wound healing (Figure 63.1).

Approximately 15 to 20% of an 11 × 11 mm spot is treated. Rapid reepithelization and fast epidermal repair result due to the short migration path for new viable cells such as epidermal stem cells and transient amplifying cell populations.

The erbium laser is an excellent modality for AFPT. Micromanagement of the thermal ablative effect is achieved by altering the pixel pattern, the laser energy, the pulse duration, the number of passes, and the number of stacks. While this sounds complex, the treatment is easy to learn and titrate to each patient. The titrational techniques are easy to master by both physicians and medical staff (such as registered nurses and physician assistants in California).

Each 11 × 11 mm spot contains either a 7 × 7 (49) pixel pattern or a 9 × 9 (81) pixel pattern. The 49-pixel pattern provides greater energy (approximately 25 mJ/pixel at a pulse energy of 1,100 mJ) of thermal damage than the 81-pixel pattern (approximately 13 mJ/pixel at a pulse energy

of 1,100 mJ) because the same energy is delivered in fewer zones of injury.

The delivered laser energy is also variable. Recently, the available pulse energy was increased to 1,400 mJ/pulse of 2,940-nm energy.

The erbium laser (2,940 nm) ablates more tissue with less thermal zone of destruction than the carbon dioxide laser. Because of this, it provides excellent control of the delivered energy to tissue. Unlike the carbon dioxide laser, multiple passes and the stacking of pulses allow the physician to titrate both the energy delivery and the thermal damage that he or she wishes to create. Because of the rapidity of pulse delivery, multiple passes can be delivered quickly, with diminished gain per pass (Figures 63.1 and 63.2).

The thermal effect can also be varied by altering the pulse width. A short pulse (0.5 ms) produces less thermal effect than a long pulse (2 ms).

In clinical use, we will usually begin treatment with a short pulse and an 81-pixel grid, using a pulse energy of

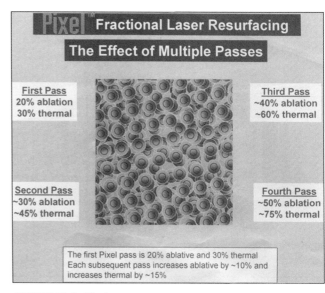

FIGURE 63.1: Pixel patterns.

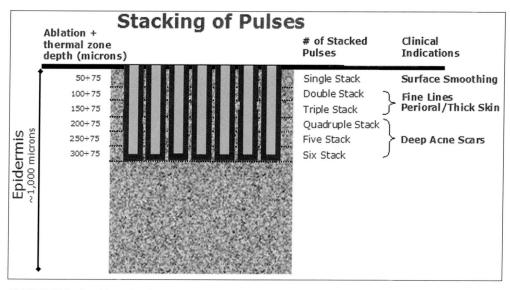

FIGURE 63.2: Stacking of pulses.

1,000 mJ for a patient with Fitzpatrick skin type I. For Fitzpatrick types I and II patients without dermographia, the treatment can be increased by using greater energies, a long pulse, or a 49-pixel spot. For Fitzpatrick types IV and V patients, less energy is used and/or laser energy is titrated with a series of test spots.

Generally, we use a "one-two-three" treatment method: one pass is used for the arms and chest; two passes are used for the neck; and three passes are used for the face. Additional stacks are used for problem areas such as the circumoral and circumocular regions.

Usually, the patient will have sunburn pain for about a day. This can be mostly alleviated with topical sunburn preparations that contain aloe and/or benzocaine (if the patient is not sensitive). There is a sunburn that progresses to a bronzed area, which eventually flakes. The whole process takes about four days but can last six days. Most patients return to work the next day, excusing their appearance as a sunburn.

Treatment parameters are discussed with the patient. If the patient requests a minimal treatment to assess the effects, desires little or no downtime, has extremely sensitive skin, has skin type IV or up, or can tolerate little or no discomfort, the treatment can be reduced by using an 81-pixel spot and 600–800 mJ of energy.

If the patient desires the maximum response with the minimal number of treatments, the treatment can be increased, depending on skin type. Generally, three to five treatments are performed about four weeks apart.

With each treatment, the delivered energy is increased, depending on the result of the previous treatment. If little response is seen from the first treatment, the parameters are adjusted to increase the treatment intensity greatly. A 49-spot pattern with 1,400 mJ and a long pulse will produce a maximum treatment. An 81-spot pattern with 600–800 mJ of energy will produce a minimum treatment.

Pixel treatment may be used in combination with other modalities, including microdermabrasion (to remove the stratum corneum) and radiofrequency skin tightening. We also alternate intense pulsed light treatments for patients with rosacea and telangiectasias.

Our practice primarily consists of patients with sun damage, and Pixel is an excellent modality for treatment (Figures 63.3 and 63.4). We also utilize Pixel for acne scars, hyperpigmentation, wrinkles, rhytids, and skin tightening. Deeper rhytids respond to higher energies and stacked pulses. Pixel is effective, especially in concert with other noninvasive modalities, so that classic chemical or laser resurfacing is a rare choice of treatment in our office.

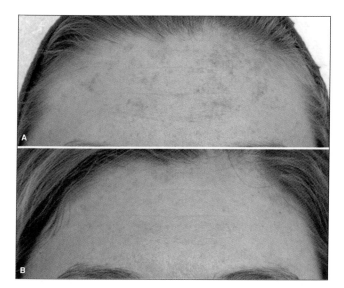

FIGURE 63.3: Pixel treatment of sun-damaged forehead: A, before; B, after one treatment. Photos courtesy of Guilherme Olsen de Almeida, MD, Hospital Sirio-Libanes, São Paulo, Brazil.

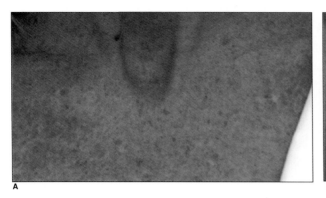
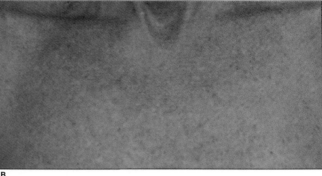

FIGURE 63.4: *Pixel treatment of sun-damaged chest:* **A,** *before;* **B,** *thirty days after a series of three treatments, one month apart each. Photos courtesy of Guilherme Olsen de Almeida, MD, Hospital Sirio-Libanes, São Paulo, Brazil.*

To date, we have observed no serious complications. In particular, no patients have experienced delayed or immediate hypopigmentation.

Unlike other treatments, Pixel treatment is not limited to the face. To date, we have treated the arms, hands, neck, chest, and face with good results and an absence of complications.

SUGGESTED READING

Keller GS, Lacombe VG, Lee PK, Watson JP, eds. *Lasers in Aesthetic Surgery.* New York: Thieme; 2001:131–8.

Khatri KA, Ross V, Grevelink JM, et al. Comparison of erbium:YAG and carbon dioxide lasers in resurfacing of facial rhytides. *Arch. Dermatol.* 1999;135:391–7.

CHAPTER 64

Fractionated CO$_2$ Laser

Joshua A. Tournas
Christopher B. Zachary

The treatment of facial photoaging has spurned many an innovation in dermatology and plastic surgery over the past twenty years. Among these are topical treatments; chemical peels; mechanical treatments such as dermabrasion; and most aggressively, surgical lifts and ablative laser treatments. For such laser treatments, the 10,600-nm CO$_2$ laser has been the gold standard since the early 1990s. The lengthy period of time during which the CO$_2$ laser has been the predominant choice certainly speaks to its clinical efficacy.

However, this efficacy does not come without cost. Providing full-thickness epidermal ablation down to depths of 150 μm with multiple passes, the CO$_2$ laser also provides significant morbidity and downtime in the postoperative period, often lasting three weeks or more. More important, CO$_2$ laser treatment results in persistent erythema in a majority of patients, lasting much longer than the immediate recovery period – in some patients, this can be six months or more. Other side effects include delayed-onset posttreatment hypopigmentation and scarring, which can be especially devastating for both patient and treating physician, given the aesthetic nature of the procedure itself.

While the ablative laser remains a very useful tool in capable hands, patient and physician dissatisfaction with the previously mentioned issues caused a trend among most aesthetic physicians in the early 2000s toward nonablative skin rejuvenation. Like the high-energy, short-pulse CO$_2$ laser, these devices employed the concept of selective photothermolysis, as described by Anderson and Parrish in 1983. Specifically, near-infrared wavelengths, such as 1,064 nm, 1,320 nm, and 1,450 nm, were employed to selectively target tissue water as their chromophore, while using cooling mechanisms to protect the epidermis from superficial damage, allowing higher fluences to reach the deeper dermal structures. In addition to these devices, radiofrequency and combined radiofrequency–intense pulsed light devices

were also developed, which were intended to deliver tissue tightening and improvement in the signs of photoaging. Treatments with these devices are typically less painful than ablative laser treatments; in addition, they require little to no downtime postprocedure. Unfortunately, this lack of side effects was often coupled with a lack of clinical effect, and use of these devices has declined considerably in recent years.

Faced with the potential side effects of the ablative lasers, and the relatively disappointing lack of effect with the nonablative lasers, physicians and researchers sought a middle ground, where measurable clinical effect would be met with a reasonable side effect profile in capable hands. In an attempt to fill this void, in 2004, the concept of fractional photothermolysis was described, whereby a nonablative infrared wavelength of light would be delivered in a series of many very narrow microbeams." Via a scanning mechanism, the first of these devices (Fraxel SR750, Reliant Technologies) could deliver very high fluence pulses of 1,550-nm laser light over a very narrow beam to the tissues with very rapid healing. The pattern of epidermal damage created has been termed *microthermal zones* (MTZs). The fluence of each spot and the density of spots per unit area of skin were adjustable for various applications. The results of such treatments have been fairly promising to date, offering measurable improvements in skin texture, fine lines, and dyschromia.

Even with these improvements, there still existed a gap between the nonablative and fractional devices and the traditional ablative lasers. Around 2006, attempts were made to combine the fractional method of laser delivery with the ablative-wavelength lasers, seeking to provide similar results to fully ablative treatments with shorter recovery times. The results were a variety of fractional CO$_2$ and Er:YAG devices that are new to the marketplace, the discussion of which will form the basis of the rest of this chapter.

CO_2 LASER-BASED SYSTEMS

Reliant Re:pair

The Reliant Fraxel Re:pair laser (Reliant Technologies) is a recently approved device that combines the concepts behind their nonablative Fraxel line of lasers at the 1,550-nm wavelength, discussed previously, with a traditional ablative 10,600-nm CO_2 laser wavelength. Similar to the original Fraxel device (now named Fraxel Re:store), the Re:pair uses a scanned handpiece that employs a movement-sensing mechanism to detect handpiece motion and subsequently deliver a scanned pattern of 120- to 150-μm microbeams that penetrate up to 1,200 μm or more below the skin's surface. Fluence of each laser microbeam and the density of beams or MTZs can be user adjusted to cover 10 to 70% of the surface of the skin. Unlike the devices described subsequently, which use a stamp method, in which the user delivers numerous pulses within a single field before lifting the handpiece and repeating the process in an adjacent area, the Re:pair uses a scanning method of delivery. This method allows a continuous and constant band of MTZs to be laid down in a linear fashion. Typically, each subsequent strip overlaps the previous by 50%, and then the process is repeated in a perpendicular fashion to achieve the desired treatment density and to avoid skip areas.

The Fraxel Re:pair has recently been approved for ablation and resurfacing of soft tissue after preliminary studies proving its safety and efficacy. In these studies, patients were treated with pulse energies of 10–40 mJ with densities of 200–400 MTZ/cm^2 per pass. Treatments were tolerated well, although topical anesthetics and oral analgesics/anxiolytics were routinely employed, in some cases supplemented with nerve blocks – mainly with the higher-energy treatments. Patient results were favorable, with most patients seeing substantial improvement in rhytids, dyschromia, and skin texture. The side effect profile was good, with no permanent scarring seen in any of the treated patients. Following these initial studies, multiple groups have investigated this device for the treatment of acne scars. One study used treatment energies ranging from 20 to 100 mJ with densities of 600–1,600 MTZ/cm^2. Thirty patients received one to three treatments and were evaluated on a quartile scale for improvement in surface texture, atrophy, and overall acne scarring at one and three months posttreatment. Average improvement was noted to be mild (1 to 25%) to moderate (26 to 50%) in all categories. A second study detailed another series of thirteen patients who received two to three higher-energy treatments and had their improvement graded by both clinical assessment on a quartile scale and by skin profilometry (Primos). Similar to the former study, an average of 26 to 50% improvement was noted on the quartile scale. The Primos measurements, however, showed a mean level of improvement of 66.8% in acne scarring.

Lumenis Bridge Therapy

The Lumenis UltraPulse CO_2 laser platform (Lumenis Inc.) has recently been expanded to include both new scanning patterns for the standard handpiece, called PigmentFX and ActiveFX, and a new fractional handpiece called DeepFX. These procedures as a whole are called *bridge therapy*, referring to the intact bridges of skin left between treated laser spots. The PigmentFX procedure is a subablative procedure with a 1.25-mm spot size spaced relatively close together to treat dyschromia. The ActiveFX procedure is similar, with the same 1.25-mm spot size, but with deeper penetration of approximately 200–300 μm. While not fractional in the sense that the standard handpiece is not capable of producing submillimeter spot sizes (although the minimum spot size in the most recent Lumenis device is smaller than previous iterations), the ActiveFX procedure provides an option to physicians who already have a capable CO_2 laser in their offices. The ActiveFX procedure also uses a randomly scanning method of pulse delivery – the pulses are not laid down in a distinct, repeatable pattern, but rather, in a random fashion, designed to avoid bulk heating due to adjacent pulses.

In addition to the PigmentFX and ActiveFX procedures, the DeepFX handpiece was introduced in late 2007 and provides a true fractional CO_2 spot size of approximately 120 μm at depths ranging from 180 to 1,400 μm. Deeper depths are accomplished by a combination of increased energy and pulse stacking. Work with this device has only just begun at the time of this writing, both with the DeepFX alone and as part of the TotalFX protocol, which will combine the fractional resurfacing and dermal remodeling potential of the DeepFX handpiece with the wider treatment area and potential improvement in dyschromia offered by the ActiveFX procedure, using the standard computer pattern generator handpiece.

The main advantages to this group of procedures are that many offices will already have the necessary device present in their practices, and that there is certainly less downtime than with fully ablative CO_2 laser resurfacing. Given that the UltraPulse is also capable of full-surface resurfacing, one could use this device in fully ablative mode over particularly problematic areas and in a fractional fashion over lesser-damaged areas.

To date, there have been no prospective studies using the UltraPulse device with the ActiveFX procedure or with the new handpiece. According to available white papers, this procedure is offering patients appreciable results with single treatments, but most patients are being treated in multiple sessions spaced two to three months apart.

Lasering Mixto SX

Similar to the preceding system, a recently introduced 10,600-nm continuous-wave laser (Slim Evolution, Lasering Inc.) has been fitted with a novel scanning handpiece (Mixto SX), allowing for a scanned pattern of 300-μm spots to be laid down in an area ranging from 6 × 6 mm to 20 × 20 mm. According to white papers, the depth of the spots varies from 20 to 500 μm, treating from 20 to 100% of the treatment area. The user of the device controls the depth of penetration through the manipulation of two factors: the output wattage of the continuous wave (CW) laser and the SX index, which represents the dwell time (range 2.5-16 ms) of the CW laser at each treatment spot, with a longer dwell time resulting in a deeper depth of injury. Patients reportedly tolerate treatments without the anesthesia, though this would likely indicate that the device was used to deliver more superficial treatments than some of the other devices. The histologic correlation between the SX index and lesional depth has not been elucidated but, once available, will make the results with this device much more predictable.

As with the Lumenis device, the Mixto SX device is built on a standard CO₂ platform, which allows for the flexibility of using a fully ablative mode, when required, as well as fractional treatment.

Lutronic eCO₂

The eCO₂ device (Lutronic Inc.) is another fractionally delivered CO₂ laser built on a standard platform. Using a 30-W, continuous-wave laser as its power source, this device is capable of delivering spots in a variety of sizes, akin to the Lumenis device described previously. The sizes available are a truly fractional 120 μm, a midrange 300 μm, and a 1,000-μm spot, as well. Pulse energies vary from 2 to 240 mJ, and this device can deliver anywhere from 25 to 400 spots/cm². Using the 120-μm spot size, the manufacturer claims that its initial internal studies have shown possible treatment depths up to 2.4 mm into the dermis. Unique to this device is the ability to change the pattern of spot delivery from a uniform grid pattern to a random pattern within the 14 × 14 mm treatment zone. This feature is termed *controlled chaos technology* and is purported to reduce bulk heating of the dermal tissue.

SmartXide Dermal Optical Thermolysis Therapy

The SmartXide Dermal Optical Thermolysis (DOT) laser (Eclipsemed Inc.) is again based on a 30-W, continuous-wave CO₂ laser, which delivers laser energy into the tissue in middle-width 350-μm spots. The treatment pattern is 15 × 15 mm, and rather than varying the energy per pulse or the density of spots, with this device, the user-controlled parameters are the dwell time of the laser at each position (from 0.2 to 2.0 ms) and the pitch between spots (0.2–1.0 mm). Per the manufacturer's literature, the maximal energy per pulse is 60 mJ. This device is reported by the manufacturer to be effective in improving skin texture, fine and deep wrinkles, and acne scars. This device

is marketed as a minimal-downtime device at the parameters outlined, which is in line with the relatively low energy pulses utilized. As with many of the other devices built on continuous-wave CO₂ platforms, the DOT laser offers a full range of both standard and fractional handpieces.

ER:YAG LASER-BASED SYSTEMS

Sciton ProFractional

The Sciton ProFractional laser system (Sciton Inc.) is a new fractional handpiece designed to operate on their 2,940-nm Er:YAG Profile platform. This device has a scanning-type handpiece with a 2 × 2 cm window within which the user can control the amount of skin surface treated with 250-μm spots, from 1.5 to 60% of the total treatment field. The treatment area is selectable between 6 mm² and 2 cm². In theory, the ProFractional handpiece should be capable of delivering ablative columns to depths over 1 mm. As this is a modification of an already existing device, controlled trials were not required before the ProFractional was released to market. However, early white papers detailing clinical experience with this device show that most patients are being treated with energies resulting in depths of penetration from 100 to 200 μm and approximately 10% coverage of the skin. Patients generally receive one to two treatments at these settings.

One of the unique aspects of this device is that the user can select the desired depth of penetration for the intended treatment, and the device will then select the appropriate fluence to be delivered to the skin. Most of the early experience with the device is for general photorejuvenation of the skin, but research on its use for acne scarring at higher energies and depths of penetration is in progress. As most of the treatments with this device are more superficial in nature, physicians employing the ProFractional have noted that topical anesthesia with or without adjunctive cold air cooling has been adequate for pain control. For 100- to 200-μm treatment depths, downtime estimates are reported to be on the order of one to two days of mild erythema, which can be covered with makeup after approximately twenty-four hours. Ongoing research is also being conducted using a combination treatment with the MicroLaserPeel procedure, whereby a fully ablative Er:YAG laser is used to ablate the uppermost 50 μm of epidermis, followed by ProFractional treatment at approximately 100- to 200-μm depth; reports have shown promising results in treating dyschromia and fine lines with minimal discomfort and downtime, although the dual treatment is sure to prolong healing.

Palomar Lux2940 Fractional

The Palomar Lux2940 handpiece (Palomar Medical Technologies) is a modular device that mounts on the manufacturer's StarLux platform. This allows a single unit to house intense pulsed light, fractional nonablative, and now fractional ablative devices. The Lux2940 has both 10×10 mm and 6×6 mm treatment areas and can deliver up to 1,000 microbeams/cm². One of the things that makes this device unique is that it is capable of delivering pulses in a variety of methods: there is a short-pulsed, purely ablative mode; a longer-pulsed, coagulative mode; and a combined mode with blended effects. Early white papers have detailed treatments up to 300 μm in depth, but the theoretical maximum depth is over 1 mm. A recent pilot study showed repeatable 1- to 2-point improvements in rhytids on a decile scale.

Alma Pixel

The Alma Pixel device (Alma Lasers) is a 2,940-nm Er:YAG handpiece that operates on the company's Harmony platform. The Pixel is designed to deliver 49–81 (7×7 or 9×9) pixels, or small laser spots, within a single 11×11 mm² treatment field. The maximum pulse energy is 1,300 mJ/pulse, which is spread among the available laser microbeams, allowing for a less dense, higher-fluence (per spot) treatment with the 49-dot pattern or a more dense but lower-fluence treatment with the 81-dot pattern. The width of each pixel is approximately 50 μm, and the depth of penetration for this device is on the order of 20–50 μm, resulting in a superficial peeling effect. The 49-pixel matrix will deliver fewer deeper spots, while the 81-pixel matrix will divide the same amount of laser energy into more numerous but consequently more shallow spots. Given the superficial nature of this procedure, it is not surprising that the treatment would be minimally painful and result in little to no downtime, mainly just erythema lasting approximately one day. The Pixel device is currently in use for treatment of fine lines, pigment irregularities, skin laxity, and scars.

DISCUSSION

While all the devices mentioned in this chapter are fairly new to the market, their increasing prevalence informs us that there certainly is a gap to fill in the photorejuvenation armamentarium. Physicians who were quite comfortable using nonablative rejuvenating devices but who were not willing to move to fully ablative CO_2 or erbium laser treatments (and even those already using these lasers) will likely find that there are devices within this novel fractionally ablative category that will suit them and their patients. Even within this category there already exists a spectrum, from the low-energy and superficial Alma Pixel device, with effects and morbidity closer to the nonablative

devices, to the higher-energy, more deeply treating Fraxel Re:pair device, the results of which more closely resemble results obtained with the fully ablative lasers. Both superficial and deep treatments are available at both common ablative wavelengths, and future research with many more patients will make the ideal depth of treatment more clear as well as whether the ablative and coagulative effects of the fractional CO_2 lasers or the purely ablative fractional Er:YAG lasers will provide the best effect at a given depth of treatment. Much more experience is needed with these devices to fully elucidate where each will fall in the aesthetic realm, but clinical benefit to many patients will likely be the result.

SUGGESTED READING

Anderson RR, Parrish JA. Selective photothermolysis: precise microsurgery by selective absorption of pulsed radiation. *Science.* 1983;220:524–7.

Chapas AM, Brightman L, Sukal S, et al. Successful treatment of acneiform scarring with CO_2 ablative fractional resurfacing. *Lasers Surg. Med.* 2008;40:381–6.

Dierickx CC, Khatri KA, Tannous ZS, et al. Micro-fractional ablative skin resurfacing with two novel erbium laser systems. *Lasers Surg. Med.* 2008;40:113–23.

Goldman MP. CO_2 laser resurfacing of the face and neck. *Facial Plast. Surg. Clin. North Am.* 2001;9:283–90.

Hantash BM, Bedi VP, Chan KF, Zachary CB. Ex vivo histological characterization of a novel ablative fractional resurfacing device. *Lasers Surg. Med.* 2007a;39:87–95.

Hantash BM, Bedi VP, Kapadia B, et al. In vivo histological evaluation of a novel ablative fractional resurfacing device. *Lasers Surg. Med.* 2007b;39:96–107.

Hantash BM, Mahmood MB. Fractional photothermolysis: a novel aesthetic laser surgery modality. *Dermatol. Surg.* 2007; 33:525–34.

Manstein D, Herron GS, Sink RK, Tanner H, Anderson RR. Fractional photothermolysis: a new concept for cutaneous remodeling using microscopic patterns of thermal injury. *Lasers Surg. Med.* 2004;34:426–38.

Rahman Z, Tanner H, Jiang K, et al. Fractional deep dermal ablation induces tissue tightening. *Lasers Surg. Med.* 2009 Feb;41(2):78–86.

Tournas JA, Soriano TT, Lask GP. Nonablative skin rejuvenation as an adjunct to tissue fillers. In: Klein AW, ed., *Tissue Augmentation in Clinical Practice.* New York: Taylor and Francis; 2006:251–65.

Waldorf HA, Kauvar AN, Geronemus RG. Skin resurfacing of fine to deep rhytides using a char-free carbon dioxide laser in 47 patients. *Dermatol. Surg.* 1995;21:940–6.

Walgrave SE, Ortiz A, Elkeeb L, Truitt A, Tournas JA, Zachary CB. Evaluation of a novel fractional resurfacing device for treatment of acne scarring. *Lasers Surg. Med.* 2009 Feb;41:122–27.

OTHER PHOTOREJUVENATION DEVICES

CHAPTER 65

LED Photorejuvenation Devices

Jean Francois Tremblay

Photodamaged skin displays distinct clinical and histological features affecting the epidermis and dermis. Clinical features of photoaging include rhytids, skin textural irregularities, dyschromia and lentigines, and dilated capillaries. Histological features of photoaging include actinic dyskeratosis and thinning of the epidermis, dermal collagen degradation, and increased numbers of abnormal elastic fibers.

These changes in dermal and epidermal integrity associated with photoaging are thought to result from four main mechanisms: (1) the altered proliferative capacity of keratinocytes and fibroblasts, (2) the decreased biosynthetic capacities of fibroblasts, (3) the impaired intrinsic repair mechanisms of skin-derived cells, and (4) the increased production of metalloproteinases and other degrading enzymes.

Traditional ablative modalities used for photorejuvenation, including CO_2 laser, erbium laser, and chemical peels, result in skin repair via direct tissue ablation and wound healing. Although very effective, these therapeutic modalities are associated with significant downtime and potentially serious complications, including skin infections, scarring, and permanent dyspigmentation. These limitations have motivated researchers to look for noninvasive alternatives that would modulate skin biology and promote tissue repair without injury. LED technologies fall under this category of photomodulating devices.

Different wavelengths have been studied and found to have beneficial photomodulating effects at the cellular level. Red light (633 nm) irradiation has been shown to increase fibroblastic activity and collagen production in vitro. Red light was also shown to increase fibroblastic growth factor production by macrophages and to diminish activity and viability of mast cells. Near-infrared light (830 nm) has also been shown to activate fibroblasts and myofibroblasts as well as activating chemotaxis and phagocytic activity of inflammatory cells. Near-infrared light (850–890 nm) has been documented as accelerating healing of ischemic wounds, including nonhealing chronic ischemic leg wounds. Near-infrared light was found to enhance blood and lymphatic flow in the wound tissue through the release of nitric oxide from the blood vessels, causing relaxation and dilatation of vessel walls. Blue light activates endogenous porphyrins in the skin derived from the activity of *Propionibacterium acnes* and has been shown to be beneficial in the treatment of acne vulgaris. High-intensity blue light has also been shown to have anti-inflammatory effects, down-regulating the production of cytokines by keratinocytes. Combination of wavelengths have also been studied (blue and infrared) and were suggested to have synergistic effects and anti-inflammatory and pro-healing properties. Yellow light (590 nm) has been studied and shown to target mitochondrial cytochromes and induce collagen type 1 production and to reduce significantly metalloproteinase type 1.

Commercially available LED devices for the purpose of photorejuvenation include Omnilux Red by Phototherapeutics Ltd. (633 nm) and Omnilux Revive (830 nm/80 J/cm²), both of which provide continuous light energy delivery as interchangeable panels on unique platforms.

Regen, by Energist, has a large, 630-nm head with adjustable light intensity. The Gentlewave device produces pulsed yellow light (590 nm) with on and off times that are thought to be more optimal for mitochondrial targeting and fibroblastic stimulation.

Various clinical studies (see the "Suggested Reading" section) have reported the use and beneficial effects of LED light photomodulation in the treatment of acne vulgaris; photoaging, including dyschromia; fine lines; skin pore size; acceleration of healing following incisional surgeries; and laser resurfacing. Different protocols have been proposed, with no consensus on optimal treatment parameters for best clinical outcome. The jury is still out, as well, on what might be an optimal wavelength or wavelength combination. The spectacular results obtained when combining aminolevulinic acid with LED light are not generally observed when treating patients with LED photobiomodulation alone. Best use and patient satisfaction might be achieved when combining LED therapy with other rejuvenating modalities to optimize results or diminish the side effects of the latter.

SUGGESTED READING

Lask G, Fournier N, Trelles M, et al. The utilization of non-thermal blue (405–425 nm) and near infrared (850–890 nm) light in aesthetic dermatology and surgery – a multicenter study. *J. Cosmet. Laser Ther.* 2005;7:163–70.

Russells BA, Kellett N, Reilly LR. A study to determine the efficacy of combination LED light therapy (633 nm and 830 nm) in facial skin rejuvenation. *J. Cosmet. Laser Ther.* 2005;7:196–200.

Trelles M, Allones I. Red light-emitting diode therapy accelerates wound healing post-blepharoplasty and periocular ablative laser resurfacing. *J. Cosmet. Laser Ther.* 2006;8:39–42.

Trelles M, Mordon S, Calderhead RG. Facial rejuvenation and light: our personal experience. *Lasers Med. Sci.* 2006.

Weiss RA, McDaniel DH, Geronemus R, et al. Clinical experience with light emitting diode (LED) photomodulation. *Dermatol. Surg.* 2005;31:1199–1205.

CHAPTER 66

Photopneumatic Therapy

Vic A. Narurkar

The fundamental concept of modern-day laser- and light-based therapies relies on the principles of selective photothermolysis. As we learn more about skin and light interactions, it has become evident that additional factors can influence the safety and efficacy of the delivery of photons to desired targets. This is particularly evident in the treatment of darker skin types. Selective photothermolysis can be further enhanced with a novel approach. Photopneumatic therapy manipulates the optical characteristics of the skin by applying pneumatic energy at the time of delivery of light, thereby enhancing the delivery of photons to desired dermal targets. This chapter will discuss the Isolaz device for photopneumatic therapy.

While fractional devices modify the laser for greater safety and efficacy, photopneumatic therapy is the first approach to modify the optics of the skin. When the skin is stretched using upward pressure, blue and green photons, which are otherwise very superficially transmitted, are now able to reach deeper dermal targets. These blue and green photons often have the greatest affinity for a variety of chromophores but are ineffective because of limited depth of penetration. Moreover, because of their greater affinity to melanin, with traditional light and laser devices, they can produce a greater risk of epidermal injury. When a positive pressure of 3 PSI is applied, water evaporates at 60 degrees Fahrenheit and cooling occurs naturally. With photopneumatic therapy, a thin mist of water is applied, allowing for natural cooling of the skin.

The first clinical application of photopneumatic therapy was for hair reduction. When pneumatic energy is applied to the skin, the hair follicle is closer to the surface, thereby requiring less energy for destruction and theoretically greater efficacy. During the Food and Drug Administration (FDA) clinical trials for hair reduction using photopneumatic therapy, several patients noticed an acne flare when the treatments were stopped for obtaining clearance by the FDA for long-term hair reduction. This led the investigators to initiate clinical trials to study the safety and efficacy of the Isolaz for acne vulgaris.

Evacuation of sebum was seen, along with mechanical cleansing of pores. A multicenter study demonstrated the safety and efficacy of the Isolaz for all types of acne: comedonal, pustular, and popular. A second clinical trial is under way to assess the safety and efficacy of the Isolaz device for severe acne. Advantages of the Isolaz over traditional light devices include an immediate effect as well as a delayed effect on acne lesions, lack of discomfort, and simultaneous improvement of dyschromia and skin texture as the device utilizes a pulsed light source. The term *porofacial* has been coined to describe the effects of the Isolaz, with which simultaneous improvement of acne vulgaris and photorejuvenation can be accomplished. A series of three to five treatments, spaced two to four weeks apart, is recommended.

In conclusion, photopneumatic therapy with the Isolaz is indicated for hair reduction, photorejuvenation, and the treatment of all types of acne.

SUGGESTED READING

Narurkar V. Novel photopneumatic therapy delivers high efficiency photons to dermal targets. *Cosmet. Dermatol.* 2005;18: 115–20.

Shamban A, Enokibiri M, Narurkar V, Wilson D. Photopneumatic technology for the treatment of acne vulgaris. *J. Drugs Dermatol.* In press.

HAIR REMOVAL AND ACNE: LASER AND LIGHT TREATMENTS

CHAPTER 67

Hair Removal: Laser and Broadband Light Devices

Doug Fife

Thomas Rohrer

The first laser for hair removal was approved in 1996, and since that time, light energy has been proven superior to any other hair removal therapy for treating large surface areas. Effective hair removal by light energy requires three elements: a chromophore in the follicle (in this case, melanin), a light source or laser with a wavelength that selectively targets the chromophore, and the appropriate parameters to heat sufficiently the follicle, without damaging the surrounding structures. A laser generates a monochromatic beam of light (a specific wavelength of light energy). Broadband light devices, also known as intense pulsed lights (IPLs), use filters to narrow down the light energy they deliver to a limited range of the spectrum. As with other laser- or light-based therapies, laser hair removal is based on the principle of selective photothermolysis, in which selective thermal damage of a pigmented target occurs when the target absorbs a wavelength of light energy delivered during a time less than or equal to the thermal relaxation time of the target. Long-term or permanent hair removal occurs with damage or destruction of the follicular stem cells, which are thought to reside in both the hair bulb and the outer root sheath of the bulge area, near the attachment of the arrector pili muscle. Light is absorbed by the melanin in the hair shaft and converted to heat, and the heat spreads out to the stem cells in the outer root sheath and damages the follicle. Melanin in the epidermis represents

an inherent obstacle in effectively delivering the required quantity of energy to the follicle, as the same wavelengths will be absorbed by epidermal melanin as melanin in the follicle. If too much energy is absorbed by melanin in the epidermis, temporary or permanent pigmentary changes can occur. Advances in epidermal cooling have minimized this side effect. Cooling the epidermis before or during the laser pulse allows much higher energies to be used safely. This is especially important for patients with darker skin.

PATIENT SELECTION

The ideal patient for laser hair removal is a fair-skinned patient with dark, coarse, terminal hair who has realistic expectations and no hormonal imbalances. With the recent advances in epidermal cooling and laser technology (longer wavelengths and pulse durations), patients with darker skin types (types IV–VI) with dark terminal hair can also be effectively treated. Hair that is blonde, red, or white is unlikely to be permanently removed by laser treatment. Light hair can be treated with shorter-wavelength lasers (ruby, alexandrite) and will often temporarily disappear for up to three months, but will usually regrow with the same density, thickness, and color.

In very rare cases, the treatment of fine, dark hairs on the lateral face and jawline has been reported to create hypertrichosis, especially in young, Mediterranean females with types III–IV skin. While this paradoxical hypertrichosis is extremely rare, patients should be warned ahead of time of this potential complication. Although there is no evidence of fetal harm from laser hair removal, it is best to postpone treatment in pregnant or lactating patients in our litigious society.

PREOPERATIVE EVALUATION

A preoperative consultation with a thorough history and examination of the skin is essential prior to any laser treatment for hair removal. During this visit, the patient is screened for treatment eligibility; the patient's and physician's expectations are clearly defined; and treatment risks and benefits are thoroughly explained, understood, and given to the patient in writing.

The pertinent patient history that should be obtained includes the following:

previous treatments (method, response, frequency, date of last treatment)

patient's expectations

presence of other conditions may cause hypertrichosis:

- hormonal
- drugs (corticosteroids, hormones, immunosuppressives, minoxodil)
- tumor

history of koebnerizing skin disorder (i.e., psoriasis, lichen planus, vitiligo)

history of keloids or hypertrophic scars

history of postinflammatory hyperpigmentation

history of herpes simplex infection (oral or genital)

history of recurrent skin infections

recent tan (natural or tanning booth)

tattoos or nevi present within the treatment area

drugs that may affect therapy

isotretinoin therapy within the past six months

prior gold therapy

current use of photosensitizing medications

Prior laser treatment should be documented, including the type of laser, settings used, efficacy, frequency of treatment, any side effects, and date of the last treatment. The patient should be questioned about any hormonal abnormalities that may be causing hypertrichosis, and hirsutism should be worked up prior to laser treatment, if present. A history of a koebnerizing skin disorder, such as vitiligo, psoriasis, or lichen planus, may be a contraindication for treatment, as is a history of a photosensitizing dermatosis (i.e., lupus erythematosus). In addition, patients with a history of hypertrophic or keloidal scarring should be avoided. A history of orolabial or genital herpes simplex (HSV) infection near the treatment area warrants prophylactic oral antiviral therapy starting twenty-four hours before laser therapy and continuing for seven days.

A recent suntan or exposure to tanning booths is an absolute contraindication for laser hair removal as such patients are at high risk for dyspigmentation following treatment. Individuals with a tan should be instructed to postpone therapy for six weeks, apply bleaching creams, and use vigilant sun protection measures. Patients should be warned that nevi, lentigines, or tattoos in the treatment area may lighten or disappear after therapy. Therapy should be avoided or postponed in patients taking isotretinoin within the past six months, gold therapy at any time, or photosensitizing medications currently. Patients with a history of postinflammatory hyperpigmentation should be warned that this may occur with laser hair removal.

During the preoperative evaluation, patient and physician expectations should be defined in detail. Patients with fair skin and dark hairs can expect 20 to 30% hair loss with each treatment. The number of treatments required is variable, but studies show that significant reduction requires anywhere from three to seven treatments. The exact number of treatments required is unknown for each patient and treatment site. Patients often require more treatments in areas such as the central face and fewer in areas such as the axilla and bikini.

Some experts have suggested the terms *hair reduction* or *hair maintenance* as more appropriate than laser *hair removal*. Permanent hair reduction is defined as a significant reduction in anagen hairs that persists beyond the duration of the normal complete hair cycle in a certain location. In addition to a reduction in the absolute number of hairs, other signs of clinical improvement include slower regrowth, finer hairs, and lighter hairs. All patients treated with appropriate settings have temporary hair loss that usually lasts up to three months; patients with red, blonde, or white hair can have hair loss maintained by having treatments around every three months.

During the preoperative evaluation, the risks of laser hair removal should be described in detail. The most common adverse reaction is temporary pigmentary change. Other risks include permanent hyper- or hypopigmentation, blistering, ulceration, scarring, infection, paradoxical hypertrichosis, poor or no response, recurrence, folliculitis, and acne flaring. Temporary leukotrichia has been described following IPL or laser therapy and may be permanent in older individuals.

PREPARATION FOR TREATMENT

Six Weeks before Treatment

Patients should be counseled to avoid plucking, waxing, threading, or electrolysis to maintain an intact hair shaft and achieve optimal results. Patients may shave, bleach, or use depilatory creams to manage hair in the preoperative period. Patients should avoid the sun and use a broad-spectrum sunscreen for four to six weeks prior to treatment and during the entire treatment course if a sun-exposed site is being treated. Patients with darker skin types (IV or greater) can use 4% hydroquinone or a combination of hydroquinone/retinoic acid/hydrocortisone cream in an attempt to decrease the risk of pigmentary side effects.

Day before Laser Treatment

Patients are instructed to clip or shave the treatment site one day before treatment. Alternatively, shaving may be performed by the staff immediately before treatment, if the patient prefers. Hairs should be cut to around 1 mm in length to prevent hair char, which may burn the epidermis, and to eliminate the plume of smoke that may be noxious to the patient and operator. Patients with a history of HSV infection in or near the treatment area should initiate oral antiviral medications twenty-four hours prior to the procedure.

Day of Treatment

Topical anesthetic cream may be applied to reduce discomfort. The cream should be applied after shaving the hairs and should be removed completely prior to laser treatment. Available effective anesthetic preparations include LMX4 (4% lidocaine) and LMX5 (5% lidocaine), both manufactured by Ferndale Laboratories. LMX should be applied thirty to sixty minutes prior to the procedure as thickly as possible, without occlusion. Alternatively, EMLA (a eutectic mixture of 2.5% lidocaine and 2.5% prilocaine; Astra Pharmaceuticals) is applied sixty to ninety minutes prior to the procedure under plastic wrap occlusion. Since there is some absorption of topical anesthetic creams, large areas, such as the back, cannot be covered without a risk of toxic levels of absorption. There have been reported cases of death occurring from absorption of topical anesthetic cream under occlusion for laser hair removal.

Before each treatment, the risks of the procedure should be reviewed and informed consent documentation should be obtained. Preoperative photographs are helpful to assess treatment response.

TREATMENT

Selection of Laser

The lasers and light sources with proven efficacy for permanently removing hair are the long-pulsed ruby laser (694 nm), the long-pulsed alexandrite laser (755 nm), the diode laser (800 nm), the long-pulsed Nd:YAG laser

(1,064 nm), and the IPL device (590–1,200 nm). In general, laser hair removal is most effective when the highest tolerated fluence and largest spot size are used. Longer pulse widths may decrease the risks of pigment alteration. The exact settings vary from device to device, and the best results for each device are determined by a combination of consultation with the product manual and personal experience. See Tables 67.1 and 67.2 for a complete listing of devices currently available.

Ruby Laser (694 nm)

The ruby was the first laser used for hair removal. It is most appropriate and effective for light-skinned patients (skin types I or II) with dark hairs but is also more effective than other lasers at treating lighter-colored hair. High epidermal melanin absorption at 694 nm precludes its use in tanned skin or skin type III or greater, as dose-related side effects, such as vesiculation, crusting, and pigment change, can occur. These side effects can happen with any laser system but are more common with the ruby laser. Common pulse widths are 3 or 4 ms, and fluences of greater than $40\,J/cm^2$ are more effective than fluences of less than $40\,J/cm^2$. Devices with integrated active cooling include the E2000 (Palomar) and the RubyStar (Aesclepion-Meditec) lasers. The Sinon (Wavelight) laser includes cooling by forced cold air.

Alexandrite (755 nm)

The longer wavelength of the alexandrite laser allows for greater depth of penetration than the ruby laser. More important, this wavelength is less well absorbed by melanin, allowing more safe and effective treatment of patients with somewhat darker skin types, although anything darker than a light type IV should probably be treated with a longer-wavelength laser such as one at 1,064 nm. The same is true when any kind of tan is present in type III, and even type II, patients. As with other wavelengths, using longer pulse durations provides more epidermal protection. Alexandrite devices now available are equipped with multiple spot sizes, variable pulse widths, and cooling devices utilizing cryogen spray or forced cold air. Using the largest spot size available generally gives the most effective treatment. Larger spot sizes give slightly greater depth of penetration at the same fluence and therefore yield safer, more effective treatment. A typical setting for types II–III skin with no suntan might be $20\,J/cm^2$ with an 18-mm spot size, $30\,J/cm^2$ with a 15-mm spot size, and $40\,J/cm^2$ with a 12-mm spot size, all at a 3-ms pulse duration with a cryogen cooling spray. With 755-nm alexandrite lasers, spot sizes less than 12 mm are ineffective at achieving permanent hair reduction due to scatter of the beam, resulting in failure to reach effective fluences at the required depth.

TABLE 67.1: Hair Removal Laser Comparison Chart (Ruby 694 nm, Alexandrite 755 nm, Diode 800–810 nm, Nd:YAG 1064 nm)

Wavelength (nm)	Device Name (manufacturer)	Fluence (J/cm^2)	Pulse Duration (ms)	Spot Size (mm)	Repetition Rate (Hz)	Features
694	E2000 (Palomar)	10–40	3–100, 3 or 100	10, 20	1	Epiwand sapphire handpiece with active contact cooling; photon recycling; fiber delivery of light
	RubyStar (Asclepion)	up to 35	4	up to 14	1	dual-mode (Q-switched mode for tattoos or pigmented lesions); actively cooled handpiece
	Epitouch (Sharplan)	10–40	1.2	3–6	1.2	triple-pulse technology; dual mode (may also be Q-switched)
	Sinon (Wavelight)	up to 30	4	5, 7, 9	0.5–2	dual mode (may also be Q-switched); cold air unit cooling
	Chromos (Mehl Biophile)	10–25	800	7	0.4–0.6	
755	Apogee (Cynosure)	up to 50	0.5–300	5, 10, 12, 15	up to 3	cold air or integrated handpiece; available in combined platform with Nd:YAG
	Epicare (Light Age)	25–40	3–300	7, 9, 12, 15	1–3	cold air cooling option; Smartscreen software package assists with recordkeeping, protocols, and practice management
	Epitouch ALEX (Lumenis)	up to 50	2–40	5, 7, 10	up to 5	optional scanner covers 4 × 4 cm area within 6 s
	GentleLase (Candela)	10–100	3	6, 8, 10, 12, 15, 18	up to 1.5	dynamic active cooling with cryogen spray
	Ultrawave II–III (Alept Medical)	5–55	5–50	8, 10, 12	1–2	available with 532- and/or 1064-nm Nd:YAG
	Arion (Wavelight)	up to 40	1–50	6, 8, 10, 12, 14	up to 5	cold air cooling unit
800–810	LightSheer (Lumenis)	10–60	5–400	9 × 9 and 12 × 12	up to 2	patented contact cooling device (ChillTip); also available in platform with IPL and Nd:YAG
800	Apex-800 (Iridex)	5–60 (600 W)	5–100	1–5, 10	up to 4	cooling handpiece; adjustable handpiece
800	LightSheer ET, ST, XC (Lumenis)	10–100	5–400	9 × 9, 12 × 12	up to 2	ChillTip cooling handpiece; only XC has 12 × 12 handpiece
	F1 diode (Opus Medical)	10–40	10–100	5, 7, 10	4	air cooling
808	MedioStar XT (Asclepion)	up to 90	5–500	4, 6, 10, 12, 14	up to 4	integrated cooling; integrated scanner
	SLP1000 (Palomar)	up to 575	5–1,000	12	up to 3	SheerCool triple contact cooling; photon recycling

Wavelength (nm)	Device Name (manufacturer)	Fluence (J/cm²)	Pulse Duration (ms)	Spot Size (mm)	Repetition Rate (Hz)	Features
810	Soprano XL (Alma Lasers)	up to 120	10–1,350	12 × 10	up to 10	sapphire DualChill technique + integrated adaptor for Zimmer Cryo 5
808	Velure S800 (Lasering USA)	10–600	10–1,000	2.5, 4, 8, 12		interchangeable inserts for spot size; ADS (automatic detection system) safety system
1064	CoolGlide (Cutera)	up to 300	0.1–300	3, 5, 7, 10	up to 2	contact precooling
	Acclaim (Cynosure)	up to 300	0.40–300	3, 5, 7, 10, 12, 15	up to 5	forced cold air or integrated cooling; available in combined platform with alexandrite
	Lyra/Gemini (Laserscope)	5–900	20–100	10		contact cooling; photon recycling
	Gentle Yag (Candela)	up to 600	0 or 25–300	1.5, 3, 6.15, 18	up to 10	cryogen spray (optional)
	Athos (Quantel)	up to 80	3–5	4	up to 3	
	Ultrawave (Adept Medical)	5–500	5–100	2, 4, 6, 8, 10, 12	1–2	available with 532 and/or 755 nm
	Varia (CoolTouch)	up to 500	300–500	3–10		pulsed cryogen cooling; thermal quenching
	Dualis (Fotona)	up to 400	0 or 1–200			
	Luminis One (Lumenis)	70–150	2–16	4, 6, 9	up to 1	platform can accommodate IPL and diode laser
	Profile (Sciton)	up to 400	0.1–200	3, 6, 8	up to 15	combined platform with erbium/IPL; sapphire plate cooling; 30 × 30 mm scanner allows fast treatment of large areas
	Mydon (Wavelight)	10–480	5–90	1.5, 3, 5, 7, 10	1–10	air or contact cooling

Diode Laser (800–810 nm)

Diode laser systems are also popular and have many advantages, including being reliable and compact in size. The diode laser is also effective, with some studies demonstrating it to be as effective as the long-pulsed ruby laser in removing dark, terminal hair. Like the alexandrite laser, the longer wavelength of the diode laser allows for treatment of patients with skin types III–VI due to lower melanin absorption than 694-nm ruby light. Multiple diode lasers with large spot sizes up to 12 or 14 mm are available with active contact or forced air cooling. As with other wavelengths, utilizing a longer pulse duration will yield greater epidermal protection. In general, fluences of 25–40 J/cm² are used, and the 800- to 810-nm lasers are used at very similar settings to the 755-nm lasers and yield very comparable results. They offer a slight advantage of being a little safer for darker and tanned skin if very long pulse widths, in the order of 100 ms, are used, and because of less beam scatter, they can be effective with a spot size as small as 10 mm. A significant disadvantage, due to the longer wavelength and deeper penetration, is that treatment is significantly more painful than with a 755-nm wavelength laser.

TABLE 67.2: Intense Pulsed Broadband Light Devices (IPLs, BBLs) for Hair Removal: Comparison Chart

Wavelength (nm)	Device Name (manufacturer)	Fluence (J/cm²)	Pulse Duration (ms)	Spot Size (mm)	Repetition Rate (Hz)	Features
590–1,200	EpiLight (Lumenis)	up to 45	15–100 ms	10 × 45 and 8 × 35	0.5	multiple pulsing; contact cooling
695–1,200	Quantum HR (Lumenis)	25–45	15–100 μs	34 × 8	0.5	
400–950	Ellipse (DDD)	up to 21	0.2–500 ms	10 × 48	0.25	dual-mode filtering technique
400–1,200	PhotoLight (Cynosure)	up to 16	5–50 ms	18 × 46		xenon pulsed lamp
525–1,200	Starlux (Palomar) Medilux (Palomar) Estelux (Palomar)	up to 70 up to 30 4–40	1–500 ms 10–100 ms 10–100 ms	16 × 46 16 × 46 16 × 46	up to 1 1 1	contact cooling; fast coverage rate; four handpieces with variable spot sizes (12 × 28 or 14 × 46) and wavelengths (650–1,200 or 525–1,200); fluences vary with device and with handpiece
550–900	ProLite (Alderm)	10–50		10 × 20 and 20 × 250.5		fluorescent pulsed light
400–1,200	Spatouch (Radiancy)	up to 7	35 ms	22 × 55	0.25	light heat energy
510–1,200	Quadra Q4 (Derma Med USA)	10–20	48 ms	15 × 33		quad-pulsed light system
510–1,200	SpectraPulse (Primary Technology)	10–20	3 × 12 pulse delay: 4 and 5 resp 15 × 33			light energy recycling

Nd:YAG (Long Pulsed 1,064 nm)

The 1,064-nm wavelength of the Nd:YAG laser penetrates more deeply into the dermis and is even less efficiently absorbed by melanin than the shorter wavelengths discussed previously. This allows for even safer treatment of patients with skin types IV, V, and even VI, and have made them the treatment of choice for patients with darker skin. They are significantly safer in the presence of a tan for patients with type II and III skin, and if the fluence is adjusted down for type IV. But even with the 1,064 laser, burns can occur when a tan is acquired after the initial testing and fluence is not adjusted down. High fluences are required to induce follicle injury, in the range of 30–60 J/cm². The Nd:YAG laser is less effective at treating light hair compared to the shorter-wavelength lasers mentioned previously, although at short pulse widths of 2–3 ms, type III patients can be treated effectively. In fact, for stubborn hairs not responding to a lower-wavelength laser, the deeper penetrating 1,064 wavelength can be very helpful. Pseudofolliculitis barbae, a disease commonly seen in darker skin types, is most effectively managed with the 1,064-nm Nd:YAG laser with longer pulse durations in the 20–30 ms range and lower fluences. All of the competitive current Nd:YAG laser devices are equipped with active cooling mechanisms.

QS-Nd:YAG

Q-switched 1,064-nm lasers are available for hair removal. They can treat darker skin types but generally do not produce long-term hair removal as the pulse durations are too short to sufficiently heat the entire follicular unit.

IPL

Nonlaser light sources that emit noncoherent, multiwavelength light in the 500–1,200 nm range are also used for hair removal. Many devices have filters in place to block out the shorter wavelengths in more darkly pigmented patients to prevent epidermal absorption and melanocyte damage. Wavelengths effective for hair removal range from 590 to

1,200 nm. Pulse durations are in the millisecond domain. The very large, rectangular spot sizes of most devices allow for rapid treatment of large areas but also make it difficult to treat concave or convex areas. Many devices have software that helps the practitioner decide which settings will be best for a given patient's skin type, coarseness of hair, and hair color. Devices have a wide variety of pulse durations, delay intervals, and wavelengths.

The Aurora (Syneron) device combines IPL and a bipolar radiofrequency current to damage the hair follicle. The company named the technology ELOS (Electro-Optical Synergy). The noncoherent pulsed light heats the follicle, which lowers the local impedance to the subsequent radiofrequency current and may create greater selectivity of the follicle.

Methods of Cooling

Epidermal cooling allows for higher tolerated fluences for all skin types, making laser hair removal more effective. The four major types of cooling are passive cooling with aqueous gel, forced air cooling, active contact cooling with a cooled glass or sapphire window, and dynamic active cooling with a cryogen spray.

Chilled aqueous gel cooling is the least effective form of epidermal protection as the cooling effect is limited and temporary, but it has a more closely matched index of refraction and acts as a heat and light wick.

Forced air cooling involves a continuous stream of air chilled to –5 degrees Celsius or cooler. It cools and protects epidermis, reduces pain of treatment, and may help reduce the noxious odor of singed hair.

Active contact cooling with water housed in glass or sapphire plates is more effective than gel and air cooling. The cooled surface may be in contact with the skin before, during, and after the laser pulse. The window must not be held for more than 0.5 s prior to the laser pulse or the hair shaft and bulb may be cooled excessively. In addition, water surface condensation may result in beam attenuation.

Dynamic active cooling with pulsed cryogen spray (usually, tetrafluoroethane with a boiling point of 26.2 degrees Celsius) utilizes evaporative cooling. Cryogen spray is non-toxic, nonflammable, and environmentally safe. The advantage of dynamic cooling is that it always gives the exact same cooling, no matter what the treatment speed of the operator. Disadvantages include some reduction of the light reaching the target due to scatter and reflection from the cryogen spray and the risk of pigment alteration from the cryogen spray itself.

Performing the Treatment

All topical anesthetic and makeup should be removed prior to treatment to reduce scatter of the light. The patient should be resting comfortably on a surgical table in a position that allows easy accessibility to the treatment areas. The patient and all staff should wear appropriate protective eyewear.

The use of a smoke evacuator is recommended as the plume of smoke is often bothersome to the patient and may irritate the mucous membranes of the surgeon, staff, and patient and may carry hazardous particles in it. If the laser is not equipped with an active cooling mechanism, cooling gel is applied liberally before the treatment. With contact cooling, the chilled plate attached to the handpiece must be firmly applied to the skin before and during pulse delivery. It should also be wiped clean every ten to twenty pulses to remove debris.

Using traction on the skin, with slight pressure applied with the handpiece, helps to provide uniform light delivery; decrease blood flow, which may compete for absorption of the light; and decrease the relative depth of the follicle. Pulses should be slightly overlapped as the beam profiles are generally Gaussian and give more energy in the center of the pulse than in the periphery.

The skin should be monitored five minutes after treatment is started. Perifollicular erythema and edema are desired and expected in most treatments. Whitening, vesiculation, or forced epidermal separation (Nikolsky's sign) signal epidermal damage. If these changes are observed, the operator should stop treatment and significantly lower the fluence, increase the pulse duration, and/or increase the cooling before continuing treatment. Close monitoring of patients during treatment is essential. Lower fluences should be used in parts of the body that have more of a tan than others.

Treatment Intervals and Total Number of Treatments Required

Treatment intervals are site-dependent: they can be spaced out every four to eight weeks for the face, axillae, and bikini areas and every ten to fourteen weeks for the chest, back, arms, and legs, where the resting, telogen phase is longer. Significant hair regrowth is often the best indicator for determination of retreatment intervals, especially for the latter sessions. The total number of treatments required varies depending on the site and the patient. In general, at least four to six treatments are required, and some patients may never achieve significant, long-term hair reduction (Figures 67.1 and 67.2).

Postoperative Care

Perifollicular edema usually lasts up to twenty-four hours, and erythema may occasionally persist up to one week. Application of ice immediately after treatment may reduce these reactions and provide patient comfort. If redness persists beyond ten days, low- to midpotency topical steroids may be used. Usually, analgesics are not required, unless an

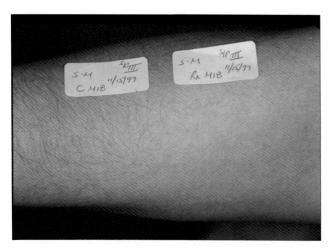

FIGURE 67.1: Patient's forearm: left side, untreated as control; right side, eighteen months after third treatment with 3-ms alexandrite laser.

extensive area has been treated. Rarely, perifollicular crusting can occur, which lasts seven to ten days. Patients should be counseled to use topical antibiotic ointment or petrolatum and to avoid picking or scratching until the crusting resolves. Rarely, purpura lasting two weeks can occur.

Hair may continue to grow for one to two weeks after treatment, until the hair is extruded from the follicle. In addition, hairs that were not in anagen at the time of treatment will grow over the next two to six weeks. Sun avoidance before, immediately after, and during the entire course of treatment is critically important. It takes two to three months for a tan to fade in many darker-skinned patients.

AVOIDING PITFALLS

Proper selection of patients during the consultation is the most important way of avoiding adverse events, especially pigmentary changes. Although they are safer with the long

wavelengths and long pulse durations, patients with an active tan should not be treated with any laser or light source. Patients with skin type II or greater should not be treated with the long-pulsed ruby laser, and type V and VI patients should be limited to the 1,064-nm laser or equivalently filtered IPLs.

The risk of postinflammatory hyperpigmentation can be reduced by avoiding inflammation during and immediately after the procedure. Utilizing longer wavelengths, longer pulse durations, bigger spot sizes, and adequate cooling all help reduce risks. The skin response should be observed closely during the entire treatment. If any signs of tissue damage are observed or the patient experiences significant pain, it is a sign that the energy is too high, the pulse duration is too short, or not enough cooling is being used. For dense hair-bearing areas, such as the back and chest, using lower fluences can reduce nonselective damage through excessive heat diffusion. However, using suboptimal fluences may actually lead, in a small percentage of patients, to a rebound effect, with denser, coarse hair growth.

Patients developing postinflammatory hyperpigmentation or hypopigmentation should be counseled that the vast majority of cases resolve, usually slowly over months to years. Strict sun avoidance is critical, and a bleaching cream can be applied twice daily to hasten the resolution.

For all laser wavelengths, the best results are obtained when the highest tolerated fluence and largest spot size are used. If there is significant concern about side effects in a particular patient, a test spot may be performed within or adjacent to the proposed treatment site. The skin should be observed immediately and one week after the test spot. If no side effects are noted at the one-week follow up, treatment can be initiated. Treatment of a few test spots at least one to three days before starting treatment is an excellent idea for all but the most fair skinned patients.

It is critical to always follow appropriate laser safety precautions, including the wearing of proper eyewear.

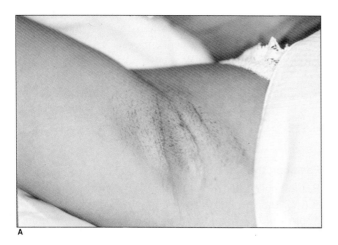
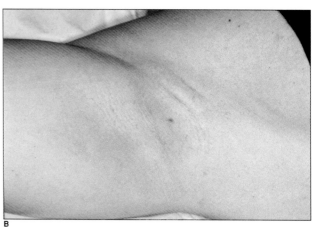

*FIGURE 67.2: **A**, Axilla pretreatment. **B**, Same axilla nine months after second treatment with 3-ms alexandrite laser.*

SUGGESTED READING

Dierickx CC. Hair removal by lasers and intense pulsed light sources. *Dermatol. Clin.* 2002;20:135–46.

Dierickx CC, Grossman MC. Laser hair removal. In: Goldberg D, ed., *Lasers and Lights*. Vol. 2. Elsevier Saunders, NY, NY; 2005:61–76.

Hair Removal Comparison Chart. Available at: http://www.miinews.com/pdf/Hair_Chart.pdf. 11-20-2007.

Liew SH. Laser air removal: guidelines for management. *Am. J. Clin. Dermatol.* 2002;3:107–15.

Rao J, Goldman M. Prospective, comparative evaluation of three laser systems used individually and in combination for axillary hair removal. *Dermatol. Surg.* 2005;31:1671–77.

Touma DJ, Rohrer TE. Persistent hair loss 60 months after a single treatment with a 3 millisecond alexandrite (755 nm) laser. *J. Am. Acad. Dermatol.* 2004;50:324–5.

Tsao SS, Hruza GJ. Laser hair removal. In: Robinson J, ed., *Surgery of the Skin*. Elsevier, NY, NY; 2004:575–88.

CHAPTER 68

Acne and Acne Scars: Laser and Light Treatments

E. Victor Ross

David Kiken

ACNE

Almost everyone experiences acne. If over-the-counter topical agents are ineffective, physicians prescribe antiacne creams, lotions, and/or gels. In a step-wise approach, stubborn cases are normally treated with oral antibiotics and, finally, by isotretinoin. Despite criticisms leveled against traditional antiacne remedies (i.e., drug resistance with antibiotics), creative dermatologists can usually manage acne using the full range of our present-day drug armamentarium. In fact, most dermatologists do not use light in the treatment of acne. However, all dermatologists encounter patients who either have severe acne that is unresponsive to traditional medications or, more commonly, chronic or intermittent acne that resists most therapies. In these circumstances, light therapy represents a viable treatment option, either as a monotherapy or as a complement to drugs. The following groups are especially good candidates for light: (1) the patient who fails oral antibiotic therapy and is unwilling or unable to tolerate isotretinoin; isotretinoin has been associated with suicide, and although no clear causality has been established, a teenager with volatile depression might undergo a trial of light before considering systemic retinoids; (2) the patient failing topical therapy who is unwilling or unable to take oral antibiotics; light may act as a medication-sparing agent in these cases; (3) a pregnant or nursing patient, or a woman actively trying to conceive; (4) patients sensitive to almost all topical remedies, especially topical retinoids; (5) the patient who resists or is noncompliant on at-home daily drug regimens; and (6) adult females with mild to moderate acne for whom a combination of hormonal therapy (i.e., BCP and possibly spironolactone), oral antibiotics, and topical retinoids has proved only partially effective.

Adult females comprise a great fraction of disgruntled acne patients. They (and some teenagers) often discontinue conventional medical therapy and resort to so-called alternative medicine approaches. Many acne sufferers are intrigued by products on the Internet or on TV infomercials. They are convinced of the ill effects of topical and systemic antiacne medications. Based on their real-life experience with technological marvels (cell phones, car-based GPS systems, etc.), they insist that there must be a better approach than pills, creams, and lotions.

Light treatment of acne is based on addressing the mechanisms that contribute to a typical acne lesion. Rather than considering individual acne lesions in treatment design, a rational approach aims to prevent new lesions by treating the entire affected area. Even with a severe acne outbreak, less than 1% of the surface area is involved. Treating specific acne lesions may accelerate the resolution of individual papules, comedones, and pustules, but (other than preprom or another big event) there is no practical role for this approach. The exception might be the patient who only experiences a few acneiform papules a month. In these cases, home-based lesion heating devices (i.e., Zeno, Tyrell Inc.) might prove useful.

One can photochemically, photothermally, and/or photoimmunologically modulate acne. Potential targets are the infundibulum, sebaceous gland, *P. acnes*, hair follicle, and epidermis. Figure 68.1 shows a typical sebaceous follicle in an acne-prone patient. No singular light chromophore exists for acne, although the abundance of sebum, bacteria, and hypervascularity of inflamed areas makes for potential selective acne lesion and/or sebaceous follicle damage. The sebaceous follicle is the site of lesion development. The most superficial portion of the sebaceous follicle (Figure 68.1), the acroinfundibulum, shows similar anatomy and keratinization to the adjacent epidermis. There is deposition of epidermal melanin, as seen in open comedones (black heads). Melanin is also found in the acroinfundibulum, but not in the lower parts of the follicle (with the exception of the hair shaft).

The infrainfundibulum is located deeper in the infundibulum, approximately 200 μm below the skin surface. This site of initial comedogenesis shows keratinocyte proliferation and accumulation of sloughed keratin and

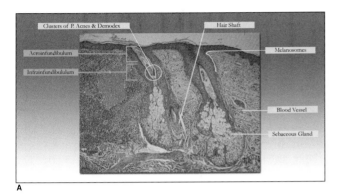
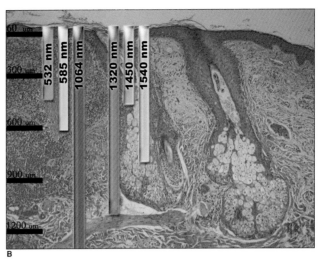

FIGURE 68.1: *Figures of enlarged sebaceous follicles associated with acne.* **A,** *The potential targets.* **B,** *Relative depths of penetration of various wavelengths. The visible light wavelengths selectively heat blood vessels and/or pigment, whereas the MIR wavelengths heat tissue water only.*

excessive sebum. The infrainfundibulum divides into numerous sebaceous ducts that connect to the lobules of the sebaceous glands. In an acne patient, sebaceous glands are much larger than in his or her nonacne counterparts. Sebaceous gland shrinkage invariably results in a decrease in acne severity, and perhaps the most attractive approach for long-term acne control is to decrease sebum output. Pore size is a constant concern among patients and is typically proportional to sebaceous follicle size.

In the pathogenesis of acne, the initial event is the formation of the microcomedo, and the genesis of most acne lesions is in the infrainfundibulum. One treatment approach is to normalize keratinization in the infrainfundibulum. This process is targetable pharmacologically, but among light devices, only the 1,450-nm laser has been shown to affect this region microscopically. Another approach, increasing epidermal turnover and desquamation (which, in turn, decreases keratin retention), can be accomplished by using visible light, whereby melanocytes in the dermal epidermal junction are damaged.

P. acnes only multiplies within the follicular canal and does not affect or invade normal skin. Its role in acne has been well documented, and destroying *P. acnes* is an intuitively attractive approach for acne treatment. However, no in vivo study has shown decreased *P. acnes* counts (via culture) after light- or other physical modality–based interventions for acne. On the other hand, decreased surface fluorescence has been observed after some light interventions. The major wavelength capable of photochemical killing of *P. acnes* is 410 nm (Soret band). Less absorptive Q bands (504 nm, 538 nm, 576 nm, and 630 nm) also kill *P. acnes* through endogenous porphyrin activation. There is little photochemistry activity beyond 670 nm.

There is a lymphohistiocytic infiltrate around even uninvolved enlarged sebaceous follicles in the acne-prone

patient. Anti-inflammatory mediators mitigate the severity of acne. Certain lasers have been shown to have an anti-inflammatory effect on acne. Thus, while some blue and red light therapies without aminolevulinic acid (ALA) might play a role in reducing acne bacteria counts, modulation of the immune response by these devices probably plays a more pivotal role in decreasing acne severity.

In taking a history, one should document the chronicity of disease and what remedies have been tried – often patients will have tried over-the-counter products. The physician must act like a good CSI agent, thorough in extracting all of the medications the patient has ever used. If the history is incomplete, invariably, the provider will write a prescription for a medication that has already failed in that patient. The physician must listen carefully to the patient, particularly with respect to what events are temporally related to relapses and remissions. Also, during the initial evaluation, one should inquire as to whether the patient is having a good or bad acne day, recalling the intrinsic volatility of acne. Is the acne in a teenager or an adult woman? The latter will typically have premenstrual flares.

In the physical exam, the types and distribution of lesions must be considered. Their location is very important: lesions on the back and chest might be more resistant to treatment than facial lesions. One should accurately determine the patient's expectations for therapy. Has the patient exhausted a long list of drug remedies and is approaching you as a last resort, or is the patient an acne newcomer who considers light the miracle cure he or she read about in a magazine or on the Internet? Ensure that the patient is aware of the financial commitment required for multiple light sessions. If the patient has insurance, make certain that he or she is aware of potentially covered therapeutics. If the office is a cash-only business, this consideration will not be as important. Still, most often, light works best as part of a broader treatment regimen.

There are several obstacles to integrating light into the traditional dermatology practice. Possibly the most important is the lack of insurance coverage. Most insurers do not underwrite experimental remedies. On the other hand, some carriers allow acne coverage on a case-by-case basis. This financial conundrum fundamentally changes the nature of the office visit and can compromise exploring the full buffet of light treatments. Treatment costs can transform light therapy into a boutique service only for the affluent. On the other hand, the financial investment often enhances patient compliance and may solidify the goals of treatment between patient and physician. Paying may enhance compliance with other parts of the therapeutic strategy, for example, if the patient is paying out of pocket for light therapy, he or she might be more willing to apply topical retinoids and possibly take oral antibiotics on a more regular basis. Another patient, however, given the expense, might set expectations unrealistically high; also, there is a risk that, particularly in a cosmetic practice, poor results in the acne arena might undermine patient credibility regarding other procedures in the practice.

Another drawback is the device cost to the provider. Although many devices used for acne can be applied for other conditions, those with a stable of lasers often are not treating large numbers of acne patients, but are rather concentrating on cosmetic applications. The medical dermatologist might be unwilling to invest in expensive technology.

Treatment Types

For each broad treatment type, a discussion of patient selection, predicted outcomes, techniques, advantages, drawbacks, and, finally, pearls is included. These are summarized in Table 68.1.

Low-Fluence Continuous Wave Sources

Devices include BLU U (DUSA), Omnilux (Photo Therapeutics Inc.), GentleWaves-588 nm (Light Bioscience), Aktilite (Photo-cure), with a wavelength of 630 nm and a total dose of 37 J/cm^2.

Patient selection: Patients should have mild to moderate acne without evidence of early scarring.

Predicted outcome: Predicted outcome is variable. Some patients experience remarkable decreases in acne number and severity within two to three treatments. However, other patients show little improvement.

Advantages: Procedures are painless, with virtually no side effects. There also may be a very mild photorejuvenation effect. Concurrent topical medications are allowed.

Specific techniques: At our center, we typically prescribe eight treatments with alternating red and blue light treatments (two treatments a week). The patient sits under the light (Omnilux) for approximately twenty minutes each session. The procedure is painless, and the patient continues any preexisting prescribed acne therapy. Microdermabrasion (i.e., Vibraderm) can be added to the regimen to complement the red/blue light therapy.

Drawbacks: One concern is possible photosensitization from oral drugs. These drugs have photoactivity with blue light and therefore should be used with caution. For most photosensitizers, the absorption and the action spectra are nearly equal, lying either in the visible or ultraviolet (UV) range, usually UV-A and UV-B.

Short-Pulsed Visible Light (1–50 ms)

This option has medium to high fluence (10–50 J/cm^2), with a power density of 1,000–5,000 W/cm^2. Short-pulsed visible (VIS) light technologies include pulsed dye laser (PDL), intense pulsed light (IPL), and the KTP laser. Multiple potential mechanisms of action are operative. One is temperature elevation in the hyperemic acne lesion as well as the DE junction (dermal epidermal junction). These technologies might also heat small hair follicles with subsequent diffusion to the sebaceous gland. Because of potential pumping of endogenous porphyrins in the Q bands, a second mechanism is photoactivation and singlet O$_2$ creation. Also, Demodex can be selectively coagulated with higher settings. The KTP laser, based on pulse length, pulse structure, and overall blood and pigment heating, mimics the typical green-yellow (GY) IPL output. The PDL with fluences sufficient for vascular or pigment dyschromia reduction has also been applied to facial acne.

Patient selection: Patients should be chronic acne patients with papules and pustules, plus coexisting vascular and pigment dyschromias.

Predicted outcomes: Outcomes are good for red and brow dyschromias. For acne lesions, reduction in number and severity of papule and pustules is highly variable.

Advantages: There is a reduction in dyschromias and overall skin rejuvenation.

Drawbacks: There are variable pain levels, risks of crusts with overtreatment, edema, and redness.

Low-Fluence PDL

The representative device for this approach is the N-lite (Euphotonics). Used with settings of about 2–3 J/cm^2 and a 0.35-ms pulse width, a series of four to eight weekly treatments has been shown to reduce acne papules and pustules for at least two months.

Patient selection: Patients should have mild to moderate acne and typically already be on a topical therapy program.

TABLE 68.1: Light Treatment Devices Used for Acne Treatment

Device	Wavelength Range (nm)	Possible Targets	Mechanism of Action	Pros	Cons
IPL	500–1200	blood, melanin *P. acnes*	1. HgB heating 2. *P. acnes* killing	may improve pigment and vascular dyschromias	possible pain and crusting
CW blue light (no ALA)	400–420	*P. acnes*	*P. acnes* killing	painless	only acne affected; minimal rejuvenation; short remission
CW red LED (no ALA)	600–650	*P. acnes*	*P. acnes* killing	painless	short remission; minimal rejuvenation
1,320 nm, 1,450 nm, and 1,540 nm		dermis, sebaceous gland	heating of sebaceous follicle and tissue water	possible cosmetic improvement in scars and wrinkles	pain
PDL (low fluence)	585	*P. acnes*, HgB	upregulation of TGFβ *P. acnes* killing	painless; may improve scars and wrinkles	only acne affected; no vascular or pigment clearance
PDL (high fluence)	585–595	*P. acnes*, HgB	*P. acnes* killing vascular reduction	will reduce redness; may improve scars and wrinkles	possible purpura; somewhat painful
KTP (high fluence)	532	*P. acnes*, HgB	*P. acnes* killing vascular reduction	may improve pigment and vascular dyschromias	possible pain and crusting
Visible light home therapy	broad-spectrum red and blue	*P. acnes*	*P. acnes* killing	painless; convenience of home site	efficacy may vary by specific device
Short contact ALA/PDT	CW	*P. acnes*	*P. acnes* killing, desquamation, immunomodulation	only slight pain; more effective than light alone	potential phototoxicity; cost
Short contact ALA/PDT	pulsed light source	HgB, melanin, *P. acnes*, PpIX in epidermis	*P. acnes* killing, erythema reduction, desquamation, immunomodulation	may potentiate destruction of telangiectases: More effective than light alone	pain, cost, Phototoxicity
Long contact ALA/PDT	CW light source	*P. acnes*, PpIX in epidermis, vasculature, and sebaceous gland	Desquamation, Sebaceous gland	Very effective	Acne flares, pain, cost, crusting, PIH, Phototoxicity

Predicted outcome: Outcome is very variable. We observed approximately 30 to 40% improvement after four treatments one month apart with settings of 2–3 J/cm². However, without concurrent topical therapy, there was a very high rate of relapse, with acne relapses occurring as early as three to four weeks after cessation of therapy.

Pros: This method is side effect–free and makes acne easy to treat. Treatment time is four to ten minutes. The mechanism of action is supported by a study (increase in TGF-β reduces inflammation).

Cons: There is a high rate of nonresponders and relapses.

Photopneumatic Therapy

This IPL device is coupled with suction, and the combination is thought to reduce *P. acnes* proliferation through photochemical inactivation as well as decrease follicular obstruction through removing sebaceous filaments.

Patient selection: Patient should have papules, pustules, and comedones.

Pros: This method is almost painless. Pores are emptied in real time; this immediate cleansing of the follicle might act as a good jump-start for other acne treatments. The forced sebum expression engages the patient and enhances compliance with slower-acting drugs.

Cons: Long-term remissions are unlikely when used as monotherapy. It is unclear how much the light component contributes to disease reduction.

Photo Dynamic Therapy (PDT)

By introducing ALA, the complexity of light protocols increases. The provider must choreograph the ALA application technique, ALA incubation time, and light source settings in a way to optimize outcomes, while minimizing pain and postirradiation photosensitivity. The patient must wait in the exam room (taking up coveted office space). Like all light strategies, another pitfall is an ill-advised subtherapeutic light treatment that delays initiation of isotretinoin in those patients with early scarring. Despite many articles extolling the virtues of ALA PDT in acne treatment, microscopic evidence is wanting. Data from only one study show microscopic sebaceous gland damage after ALA PDT. In this study, long application times and CW red light reduced acne severity, but with a high side effect profile. Unfortunately, these data have been creatively extrapolated to support more patient-friendly, short-contact pulsed light and CW techniques. However, there is no microscopic evidence that sebaceous gland damage plays a role in acne clearing with shorter-contact (less than a three-hour application time) approaches. Short-contact ALA PDT mechanisms of action remain unclear and most likely involve modulation of endogenous inflammatory mediators as well as desquamation of the epidermis.

We spend considerable time with patient education and propose two alternatives for treatment (based on acne severity and tolerance for downtime). In the first, one-hour incubations are followed by purpura-free PDL and then by CW red and blue light. Pain is typically minimal but can be managed with cold air. In the second, more aggressive (but more efficacious) scenario, ALA remains on the skin for three to four hours, followed by twenty minutes of CW red light therapy. The patient is counseled that significant redness, edema, and pain might occur with this second approach.

With PDT, regardless of the specific protocol, proposed mechanisms of action include destruction of bacteria, decreased sebaceous gland size, and increased keratinocyte shedding, and possibly a reduction in follicular obstruction. Although ALA is used almost exclusively in the United States, methyl aminolevulinate (MAL; Metvix, Galderma) is also available. A study comparing ALA and MAL creams found that after three-hour incubation times, the two compounds were equally effective, both showing about a 60% reduction in lesion counts after twelve weeks. MAL shows enhanced lipophilicity versus ALA and therefore is more likely to penetrate faster into skin. With ALA or MAL, the patient must be counseled regarding the risk of posttreatment phototoxicity. We prefer that the patient has a driver because of exposure to light on the way home from the clinic. Alternatively, we schedule treatments later in the day in the wintertime.

In the short-contact approach, the ALA solution is applied roughly one hour prior to irradiation. The sporadic nature of clearing, even with multiple treatments, is most likely linked to inadequate time for protoporphyrin IX (PpIX) formation in the sebaceous glands. When administered systemically, there is preferential accumulation of ALA in the sebaceous gland versus surrounding skin. However, with topical application and short incubation times, the sebaceous gland's location makes epidermal PpIX formation more likely. In support of the absence of PpIX fluorescence after short incubation times (less than three hours), we have observed that ALA PDT in this scenario is ineffective for sebaceous gland hyperplasia. However, longer incubation times and CW red light reduce lesion volume considerably.

In the long-incubation-time approach with CW red light, patients experience redness, swelling, and sometimes crusts lasting for two weeks. Postinflammatory hyperpigmentation and acne flares are also observed. Pain is best managed with devices that blow refrigerated air. In some cases, cold air is insufficient, and injectable anesthetics must be used. We have also used topical anesthetic cream over the ALA, but this step can accelerate ALA absorption. If the patient is willing to tolerate the downtime, the long-incubation-time/CW red light treatment regimen is by far the most predictably effective of all light acne treatments and the only one that achieves sustained isotretinoin-like results.

Patient selection: Optimal candidates present with pustules and papules, have failed other therapies, and will be compliant regarding sun avoidance.

Predicted outcomes: With long incubation times and CW red light, excellent results are expected. With shorter incubation times and red-blue with low-intensity approaches, intermediate results are normal, but outliers, either nonresponders or complete remissions, are sometimes observed (Figure 68.2). With short-contact and pulsed light CW devices, results are less reproducible, but side effect profiles are better.

Pearls: From a practical perspective, acne reduction should be enhanced by an increase in the ratio of sebaceous gland fluorescence to fluorescence in the epidermis. However,

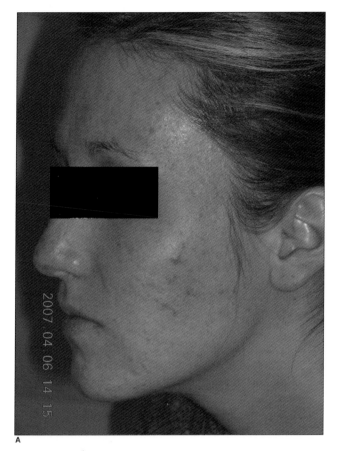 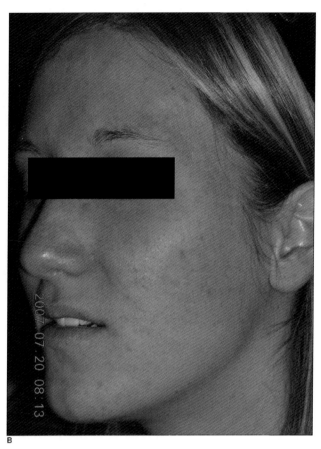

FIGURE 68.2: *Patient treated with 20% ALA and CW blue light (Omnilux blue, 48 J/cm²), three treatments spaced three weeks apart with sixty minutes' incubation time. **A**, Pretreatment. **B**, One month after the last treatment. Photos courtesy of Dr. Alex Itkin.*

to date, no one has found a practical way to favor PpIX formation in the gland. Marked sebaceous gland PpIX fluorescence is achieved only with prolonged incubation times, in which case, the epidermis typically shows high enough levels of fluorescence to cause significant desquamation and peeling, which can last for weeks and, in darker-skinned patients, is associated with postinflammatory hyperpigmentation. By using microdermabrasion followed by a ten-minute ALA application, one can increase the epidermal effect to that of a one-hour application. Although desirable in actinic keratoses treatment, this accelerated PpIX fluorescence does not aid in sebaceous gland damage and is therefore controversial in acne treatment.

Pearls: Inform the patient regarding the likelihood of an acneiform flare after treatment. Cold air can be used to minimize discomfort.

To maximize the efficacy–to–side effect ratio with ALA PDT, especially with deeply penetrating CW red light, an optimized approach includes lower light doses, fractionated treatments, and selective accumulation of ALA in the sebaceous glands versus the epidermis. For example, models and experiments suggest that it might be best to deliver treatment at one to two hours after ALA application, taking advantage of a possible micropore effect in the sebaceous follicles. Depilation prior to application might speed transport into the follicle and decrease epidermal damage. On the other hand, mild epidermal damage might speed epidermal turnover and at least provide a temporary benefit to acne due to a desquamative effect near the follicle orifice.

1,064-nm Laser

The 1,064-nm laser has a unique place in the absorption spectrum of major skin chromophores. There is some melanin and hemoglobin (HgB) absorption. With pulse stacking and higher fluences, water will also be heated such that damage can extend several millimeters into the dermis. With typical safe fluences (i.e., 10–50 J/cm² for millisecond–pulse width domains), single pulses of the Nd:YAG laser heat the sebaceous gland only 5 to 10 degrees Celsius. The lobules are heated only because they are embedded in the larger volume of heated tissue water. Severe damage to the gland in this setting (without selective fat heating) would cause considerable pain or possibly full-thickness dermal necrosis and scarring. A range of devices

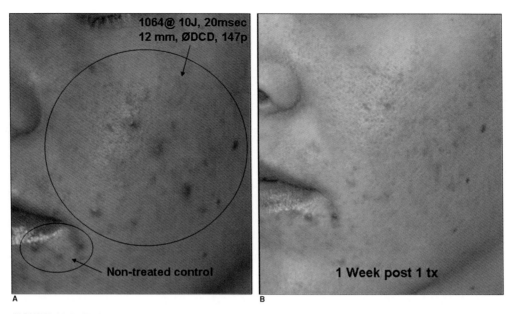

FIGURE 68.3: *Patient before and one week after treatment with long-pulsed Nd:YAG laser (GYAG, Candela), 20 J/cm², no cooling, three passes. Note that treated area has improved after one week. Photo courtesy of Nathan Uebelhoer, DO.*

has been used with pulse durations from 5 ns to 20 ms and fluences ranging from 3 to 50 J/cm² (Figure 68.3). The success of these systems supports the generally recognized tenet that any controlled heating of acne lesions can hasten their resolution. Unfortunately, there is no guarantee of long-term reduction after this accelerated clearing.

Midinfrared Lasers

Midinfrared (MIR) lasers heat different subsurface regions of skin, depending on cooling type, wavelength, pulse duration, and fluence. Water is the chromophore. The 1,450-nm laser equipped with cryogen spray cooling (dynamic cooling device; DCD) heats from about 200 to 500 μm below the surface. Recently, investigators have used confocal microscopy to show reduced sebaceous gland volume after treatment. The 1,450-nm laser was examined with multiple passes with lower fluences versus single passes with higher fluences. There were no significant differences in acneiform lesion reduction between the two groups. We noted in our studies that to see obvious microscopic thermal damage of the infundibulum or superficial portion of the sebaceous gland, fluences typically exceeded 14 J/cm², and the mean depth of damage was roughly 300 μm. Since most sebaceous glands reside subjacent to this level, the role of sebocyte damage with this approach is unclear. One report found a maximum of 18% reduction in sebum output after three 1,450-nm treatments – much less than for systemic isotretinoin, which may reduce sebum production by 60 to 90%. Most studies of MIR technologies have shown that pustules and papules respond better than comedones;

however, a recent study showed that comedones were the only lesion type to respond with a 1,320-nm laser. There was no change in sebum production with the 1,320-nm laser in acne. The nonfractional 1,540-nm laser has also been used in acne.

Patient selection: In general, the physician should reserve these wavelengths for more severe acne or for patients who have failed low-fluence continuous-wave therapy (without ALA).

Pros: Treatment is pigment-insensitive, and there is no requirement for strict sun avoidance before or after treatment.

Cons: The level of reported pain varies greatly, depending on the specific device and settings. With the 1,450-nm system, pigment disturbances have been reported with overcooling and overheating of skin. This risk is diminished by using lower cooling settings and lowered heating settings. With MIR lasers, there is a small chance of scarring and acne flares.

Pearls: With the 1,450-nm device, lower fluences and lower cooling settings are associated with less morbidity and similar efficacy as with higher settings. Recommended settings range from 8 J/cm² and 25 ms DCD to 14 J/cm² and 40–45 ms DCD.

Excimer Laser

The excimer laser has also been used for acne. On a practical level, the laser should be used with great caution because of the risk of carcinogenesis. Home UVB and UVA devices have also been applied for acne, but because of increased skin cancer risk, their use cannot be supported.

Home-Based Portable Heating Device

A home-based portable heating device (Zeno) is available for purchase for treatment of individual acne papules. The basis for lesion resolution is slow temperature elevation, which presumably kills *P. acnes* and increases release of follicular contents.

A special note regarding rosacea: rosacea can be quite frustrating to treat, and even after isotretinoin courses, the disease is susceptible to relapse. We use only high-fluence pulsed VIS light for rosacea. Although there may be an anti-inflammatory effect with light, the main goal is reduction of microvessel caliber. Before light treatment, we insist that the inflammatory component be as well controlled as possible. Rosacea is truly a disease in which laser and drugs work synergistically. Even with maximal drug control, flares sometimes occur after laser treatment. A short course of prednisone can reduce the risk of the flare – we usually give 40 mg one hour pretreatment and then 20 mg twice daily for two days.

Finally, a light source designed for selective sebaceous gland heating should emit around 1.2 or 1.7 μm. However, the ratio between water and sebum absorption coefficients is small at these wavelengths. But because the sebaceous gland should cool more slowly than the surrounding skin, selective destruction of the gland is theoretically possible with these wavelengths. These wavelengths are presently being explored as possible sebu-selective heating tools.

In general, most light acne treatments are performed monthly for three to four months (although large-scale studies have not been performed to optimize wavelength ranges, pulse durations, light doses, or treatment intervals). Also, in general, topical retinoids will accelerate the response to lasers and light. The exception is the patient with very sensitive skin. For these patients, mild salicylic acid preparations or sulfur preparations assist in acne clearing.

Complete acne remission with any painless light approach is uncommon. As a rule, we do not cure acne; rather, we treat it or wait for spontaneous involution. With most light therapies, improvement is incomplete and relapses are common. A recent well-performed split-face study (Orringer et al. 2007) is instructive in summarizing patient and provider experiences/biases with light and acne. In this study, a 1,320-nm device was found to reduce comedones but had no effect on papules or pustules. However, many patients were happy with the treatment and requested further therapy. The authors remarked that "in general, lesion counts were noted to wax and wane bilaterally, seemingly independent of the therapeutic intervention." In fact, despite no improvement in papules and pustules, many

subjects indicated a preference for this therapy as compared with so-called traditional drug treatments. The authors felt that it is possible that patients were able to pick up on improvements in their skin resulting from the laser treatments that could not be detected with the various objective means employed in our study. Alternatively, many other factors, such as the desire to please the investigators by giving positive responses, might have played a role in determining the patients' survey answers. In any case, the relatively positive view of the laser therapy among patients, despite minimal apparent clinical efficacy, underscores the potential importance and popularity of laser therapy for acne in the future if more optimal light sources and treatment protocols are developed.

Algorithm for Integration of Light in Acne Therapy

When and how does the dermatologist integrate light into his or her armamentarium? For the typical first-time acne patient, a logical approach is to start with topical remedies, adding oral antibiotics as necessary. In women, often an antiandrogen, such as spironolactone, and/or estrogens, such as Ortho Tri-Cyclen or Yasmin, are helpful. In resistant cases, the physician can add some light to the therapeutic mix, on a practical as well as pathophysiological basis.

Painless, easy treatments can be applied initially – early interventions might include low-fluence pulsed GY light sources or CW blue light sources (without ALA). If these treatments prove ineffective, one of the MIR lasers can be used, or short-contact ALA can be added to the pulsed or CW VIS light as a final approach, and the only one with isotretinoin-like effects, long-incubation-time ALA with CW light, is applied. Patients should be instructed that multiple sessions will be necessary for improvement with any of these devices. In any approach, recall that most patients outlive their acne so that buying time during the severe inflammatory phase might be an acceptable goal.

Cost

The cost of laser procedures varies widely, with most practitioners charging between \$200 and \$500 per treatment, depending on the type of treatment.

Conclusions

What approaches are most likely to yield long-term success in light-based acne therapy? We know that sebum output returns to normal after isotretinoin, and *P. acnes* returns. However, the infrainfundibulum keratinization process is still normalized, pointing to this as a possibly more important feature in any long-term acne solution. Acne does not occur when sebum output is low (but does not always occur when it is high). We may see, in the near future, more sebu-selective light sources and/or improved ways to achieve selective accumulation of photo-sensitiser in the gland. The ideal single device or drug-device combination would selectively destroy (or severely damage) the sebaceous gland without pain or other side effects.

ACNE SCARRING

Many acne patients show signs of acne scarring. Unfortunately, scarred patients often present to the dermatologist with active disease. This troubling situation, similar to trying to stop flooding when the dam is still in disrepair, requires that the physician address the active disease. Although past authors have suggested that dermabrasion, in particular, can assist in treating active disease as well as scars, this author considers any disease activity as a suboptimal background for initiating scar therapy.

Jacob et al. (2001) proposed a three-type scar system: ice pick, rolling, and boxcar. Ice pick scars are narrow, deep, sharply demarcated holes that extend into the deep dermis or subcutaneous layer. Rolling scars are usually wider than 4 to 5 mm and stem from tethering of otherwise normal looking skin. Boxcar scars are depressions with sharply demarcated vertical edges. Another classification scheme includes other scar designations, including macular scars (erythematous, white, or brown), elastolytic scars (like mini-striae), papular scars, and hypertrophic scars. Determining the types of scarring is critical in choosing a treatment course. Not all scars fit neatly into one of these categories; some scars are hybrid lesions, showing features of many scar types.

Once a treatment course has been established, preoperative photographs are taken. Photographs should be taken from several angles, including frontal, left, and right 45 degree and 90 degree angles, in addition to close-ups of particularly scarred areas. We normally take at least one flash-disabled photograph with sidelighting to accentuate surface irregularities. Preoperative photographs help gauge the final outcome and provide documentation for insurance companies for potential reimbursement.

A rational approach considers the microscopic anatomy of the scar. Rolling scars occur deep in the follicle and are the end product of inflammation that causes destruction of the subcuticular fat. These wider depressions are addressed by volume restoration, most commonly by a filler. For rolling scars, typically, a good first approach combines fillers such as hyaluronic acid, calcium hydroxylapatite (Radiesse, Bioform), or collagen (Cosmoderm or Cosmoplast, Inamed Aesthetics). Silicone has also been used as a volumizer, but only the microdroplet technique should be used.

Prior to filler placement, subcision can be performed. A Nokor 18-gauge needle is inserted from the periphery of the lesion. Then multiple swiping motions are made in the dermis like a windshield wiper, until the scar surface rises. An alternative technique uses a liposuction-like forward and backward motion. Bruising is commonly observed. Laser resurfacing will lead to short-term skin tightening, but often, this correction is quickly lost. A number of dedicated skin-tightening procedures can be applied (i.e., Thermage or Titan, Cutera; fractional IR, Palomar). Although sometimes helpful, predictable improvement is lacking, and the intervention should only be reserved for rolling scars or other scars with volume loss (atrophy).

For boxcar scars, fractional technologies should be considered first, depending on the patient's expectations and tolerance for downtime. Although not as effective as well–performed resurfacing procedures, fractional approaches have proved helpful for many boxcar scars and superficial ice pick scars. The best results are achieved with high densities (20 to 30% surface area per treatment) and deeper holes (>700 μm deep and 100–400 μm wide)(Figure 68.4). The number of available fractional technologies expands each month. Both nonablative and ablative approaches will reduce scarring. The conventional wisdom is that more sessions are required with nonablative technologies (3–5 sessions spaced apart 3–6 weeks) versus 1–2 sessions with ablative approaches (spaced 2–6 months apart). We have found that a speedier recovery makes nonablative fractional approaches a more popular choice among our patients. Needling has also been used, either with a manufactured roller (Roll CIT, Environ) or simply by repetitively impaling the skin into the deeper dermis with a 30-gauge, $\frac{1}{2}$-inch needle.

Long-pulse and millisecond domain Nd:YAG devices have been applied to acne scars. The Q-switched Nd:YAG laser beam is typically delivered at 2–4 J/cm^2 with a 4- to 6-mm spot and three passes per region (Figure 68.5). The end point is erythema – occasionally one will see fine punctuate petechiae. The treatments are only mildly uncomfortable, with the exception of male patients, in whom pulses over hair-bearing areas can be more painful. In applying the longer-pulse systems, multiple passes (usually three) are delivered at 20–50 J/cm^2. End points are mild erythema and edema. Care should be taken to avoid black-haired areas in male patients to avoid potential permanent hair reduction.

Ablative resurfacing represents a superb tool for scar improvement. The technique is often employed as the final procedure in a list of escalating interventions. We prefer the Er:YAG laser.

TECHNIQUES

For focal areas (i.e., cheeks or forehead), a topical anesthetic, such as EMLA or LMX, can be used for one to one and a half hours. If the patient is anxious, we add 1 mg of Ativan or 5 mg of oral Valium thirty minutes

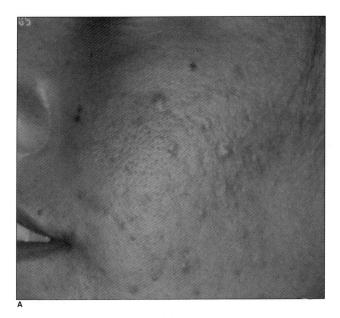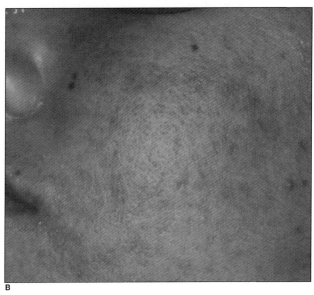

FIGURE 68.4: *Acne scars before and after three sessions of 1,540-nm fractional remodeling (10-mm spot, 10 ms, 50 mJ/mb, 600 mb/cm² [total]; Palomar Medical Technologies).*

prior to irradiation. Demerol (50–100 mg IM) and Vistaril (50 mg IM) are added if additional pain relief is required. The topical anesthetic remains on the skin until a focal area is treated, as the anesthetic effect wanes quickly after removal. We use a 1- or 2-mm spot size handpiece, focusing and defocusing the beam to achieve 20 to 60% effacement of individual scars. The operator moves the handpiece briskly in a pirouetting motion along the scar

perimeter. Spaces between scars are treated less aggressively, but almost always at least to the point of the dermis. A typical end point is about 50 to 80% effacement of the scar or exposure of the superficial sebaceous glands (Figure 68.6). If bleeding obscures the surface, thrombin spray is applied to the skin. Treatment must be carried out briskly – no more than five to ten minutes per 3 × 3 cm² region – or the topical anesthetic will not be adequate for pain

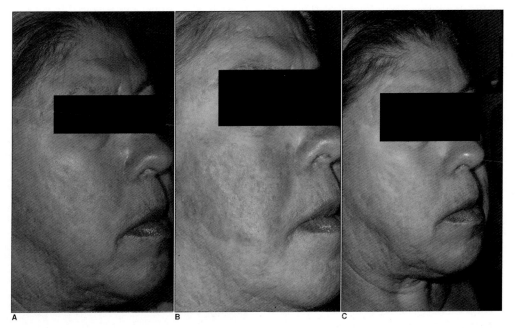

FIGURE 68.5: *Patient, A, before, B, just after, and, C, three months after Q-switched Nd:YAG laser, 4 J/cm², 6-mm spot, three passes per treatment, three treatments six weeks apart (MedLite C6, Con Bio).*

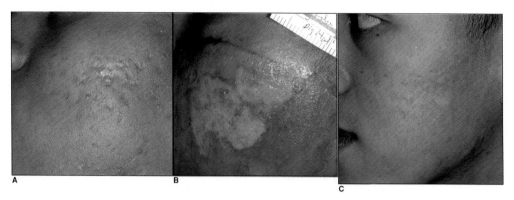

FIGURE 68.6: A, *Preacne scar.* B, *End point after Er:YAG laser; note the sebaceous lobules.* C, *Three months after treatment.*

control. Alternative anesthetic approaches are blocks combined with local anesthetics, tumescent approaches, or a general anesthetic. Combining fractional and ablative approaches is logical for maximizing efficacy. The fractional wounds create new collagen and may help to release the tethering of the skin. The ablative approach tapers the sharp edges of the scars. We have also used the plasma system (Portrait, Rhytec) and found that after one to two sessions two months apart with higher energies (3–4 J), modest reduction in acne scars was observed. The treatment was well tolerated. Anesthesia typically consists of topical lidocaine and the aforementioned cocktail of Ativan, Demerol, and hydroxyzine (Vistaril). We did encounter post inflammatory hyperpigmentation (PIH)in darker patients. One drawback of the treatment is that the beam size is fixed at 5 mm so that effacement of specific scar edges is difficult.

Punch grafts, punch elevations, and excisions can be used on small boxcar scars and ice pick scars. Punch excisions are immediately gratifying for small scars, for example, using a 2-mm punch for a 1.5-mm scar. However, with time, the scars often spread, and we do not routinely perform such surgery. Regarding punch grafts, the graft should be 0.5 mm larger than the recipient site. They are helpful only for smaller scars (3 mm or less). The grafts are harvested from the pre- or postauricular area and held in place with a Steri-Strip. Risks include graft necrosis (particularly in the glabella area or in smokers), loss of the graft, and edge irregularities at the skin surface as well as color and texture mismatch. Grafts should not be performed unless the physician plans to resurface the skin, preferably six to twelve weeks after graft placement. Resurfacing aids in homogenizing the region of the graft. The optimal interval between the surgical procedures and remodeling or resurfacing is typically four to eight weeks. Although the surgical and ablative interventions can be performed simultaneously, we prefer to wait to allow surgical wounds to heal.

For ice pick scars, typically the chemical reconstruction of skin scars (CROSS; also known as focal trichloroacetic acid) technique is used (Figure 68.7), potentially followed by ablative resurfacing two to three months later. Punch excisions can also be performed, but one must be careful to choose a punch just larger than the scar. A full range of punches from 1 to 4 mm with 0.5-mm increments should be available.

For macular red atrophic scars, the PDL with purpuric settings works best. The long-pulsed KTP laser and IPL improve redness and texture but require more treatment sessions than the PDL with purpuric settings. White macular scars are difficult to treat. The most common presentation is a confetti-like appearance, where the white scars are surrounded on the lower cheek by tanned skin. The most rewarding approach is depigmentation of the surrounding melasma-like skin. Topical steroids can be used along with topical hydroquinone preparations. These approaches typically are insufficient, in which case, chemical peels, laser peels, and fractional approaches can be helpful. Also, ablative and nonablative fractional devices can increase pigment homogeneiety. VIS light is effective at high fluences for some acne scars, but the improvement stems from reduction of dyschromias associated with telangiectasia and/or lentigines. One particular group of responders is atrophic

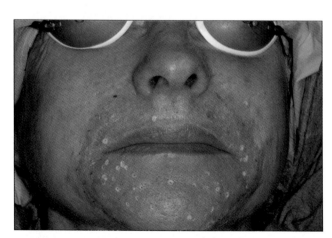

FIGURE 68.7: *Patient just after application of 100% TCA (CROSS technique).*

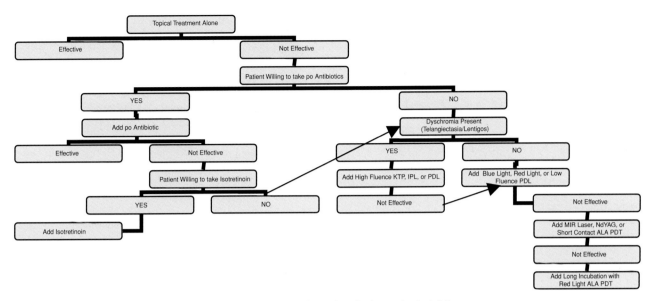

* For all interventions, addition of superficial peels (ie microdermabrasion) may be helpful.

FIGURE 68.8: Algorithm for treatment of Acne

pink scars. These scars respond uniquely well to purpuric settings with the PDL. For all scar types, a series of treatments with MIR or Nd:YAG lasers can be performed. These subsurface heating schemes typically achieve only mild scar reduction.

Test spots are prudent in any acne scar correction, particularly with surgical interventions. These smaller areas are somewhat predictive of overall outcomes and, more important, guide the patient through the healing process and give him or her firsthand knowledge regarding the nuances of healing and side effects. An algorithm for acne treatment is presented in Figure 68.8, and an algorithmic approach to acne scarring is presented in Figure 68.9.

We now have a large number of light treatments available for acne and acne scars. Used judiciously, within the context of available treatments, their roles will inevitably expand; however, more studies are needed to characterize mechanisms of action so that optimal light doses, treatment intervals, and numbers of treatments can be determined.

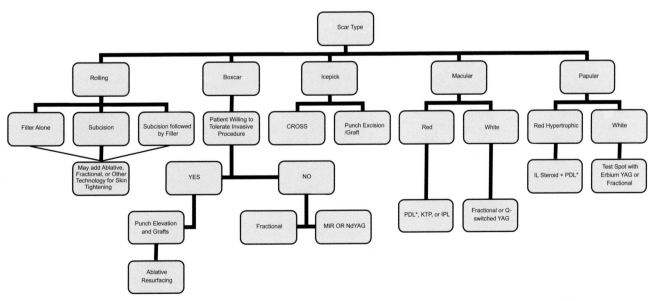

FIGURE 68.9: Algorithmic approach to acne scarring

SUGGESTED READING

Bogle MA, Dover JS, Arndt KA, et al. Evaluation of the 1,540-nm Erbium:Glass laser in the treatment of inflammatory facial acne. *Dermatol. Surg.* 2007;33:810–17.

Jacob CI, Dover JS, Kaminer MS. Acne scarring: a classification system and review of treatment options. *J. Am. Acad. Dermatol.* 2001;45:109–17.

Lee SY, You CE, Park MY. Blue and red light combination LED phototherapy for acne vulgaris in patients with skin phototype IV. *Lasers Surg. Med.* 2007;39:180–8.

Narurkar VA. Skin rejuvenation with microthermal fractional photothermolysis. *Dermatol. Ther.* 2007;20(Suppl 1):S10–S13.

Nestor MS. The use of photodynamic therapy for treatment of acne vulgaris. *Dermatol. Clin.* 2007;25:47–57.

Orringer JS, Kang S, Maier L, et al. A randomized, controlled, split-face clinical trial of 1320-nm Nd:YAG laser therapy in the treatment of acne vulgaris. *J. Am. Acad. Dermatol.* 2007;56:432–8.

Perez-Maldonado A, Runger TM, Krejci-Papa N. The 1,450-nm diode laser reduces sebum production in facial skin: a possible mode of action of its effectiveness for the treatment of acne vulgaris. *Lasers Surg. Med.* 2007;39:189–92.

Ross EV. Acne, lasers, and light. *Adv. Dermatol.* 2005;21:1–32.

Ross EV. Optical treatments for acne. *Dermatol. Ther.* 2005; 18:253–66.

Smolinski KN, Yan AC. Acne update: 2004. *Curr. Opin. Pediatr.* 2004;16:385–91.

Strauss JS, Krowchuk DP, Leyden JJ, et al. Guidelines of care for acne vulgaris management. *J. Am. Acad. Dermatol.* 2007; 56:651–63.

Uebelhoer NS, Bogle MA, Dover JS, et al. Comparison of stacked pulses versus double-pass treatments of facial acne with a 1,450-nm laser. *Dermatol. Surg.* 2007;33:552–9.

FAT AND CELLULITE REDUCTION

CHAPTER 69

Fat and Cellulite Reduction: General Principles

Molly Wanner
Mat Avram

Laser and light treatment of fat and cellulite is a new and burgeoning area of cosmetic practice. While liposuction remains the dominant procedure for effective large-volume fat removal, it is largely ineffective for the treatment of cellulite. Thus a variety of new light-based devices and technologies are emerging. Part of the reason for the proliferation of new technologies can be explained by the dearth of effective treatment options for cellulite currently. Nevertheless, this field is still in its infancy, and the efficacy of these devices is currently limited.

ETIOLOGY OF CELLULITE

Cellulite represents the orange peel– or cottage cheese–type dimpling of the buttocks, thighs, arms, breasts, and abdomen of women. It is present in up to 98% of postpubertal females and should be considered a normal secondary sex characteristic, rather than a pathologic condition. Although the etiology of cellulite is not completely understood, the best evidence supports cellulite being attributable to female subcutaneous fat architecture and hormones. The etiology of cellulite is a crucial component for developing effective technologies for improving its appearance. Many of the current treatments do not address its true physiology and thus are ineffective in improving its appearance.

Cellulite is far more common in females than males. Female superficial fat is characterized by large fat lobules with thin tissue septae. These features facilitate the herniation of female fat into the dermis, producing an undulating dermal-hypodermal interface clinically manifested as cellulite. By contrast, men typically have a thicker dermis, smaller fat lobules, and crisscrossing fat septae that frustrate fat protrusion into the dermis. These findings have been confirmed by cadaver studies, histology, and noninvasive imaging. There are other theories regarding the etiology of cellulite. Some attribute it to lymphatic and vascular alterations, while others attribute it to inflammatory factors. These alternative explanations for cellulite have little scientific evidence.

LASER- AND LIGHT-BASED THERAPY FOR FAT REMOVAL AND CELLULITE

Few scientific data show significant improvements in the appearance of cellulite or fat removal with any laser- or light-based technology. This reflects the reality that these treatments are, at best, only mildly effective. Because so many treatments have been proven ineffective to date, clinicians should regard claims of efficacy with skepticism. On the other hand, multiple new technologies are being developed within this field, and one or more of these devices may prove efficacious.

Infrared Light and Bipolar Radiofrequency

The VelaSmooth (Syneron Medical Ltd.) is a device approved by the Food and Drug Administration (FDA) that employs near- and midinfrared light, bipolar continuous wave radiofrequency, and suction and mechanical massage for improvement in the appearance of cellulite. Several studies have been performed that show a mild, temporary improvement after multiple treatments. The largest study examined thirty-five females who underwent biweekly treatments for four to eight weeks. At the completion of the eight weeks, there was a 0.8-inch decrease in thigh circumference by measurement. However, there were significant weaknesses with this study. No changes were demonstrated on histology. No noninvasive imaging techniques were performed to assess for a more objective improvement in the appearance of cellulite. Other studies showed similar mild, temporary improvement. Of the studies performed to date, the majority did not test for statistical significance.

Radiofrequency

The Alma Accent radiofrequency system (Alma Lasers) and the ThermaCool (Thermage Inc.) are FDA-approved devices for treatment of rhytids that utilize radiofrequency to treat cellulite. The ThermaCool is a unipolar radiofrequency device that is now being investigated for the treatment of cellulite. To date, no studies have been published demonstrating any efficacy. The Alma Accent is a unipolar and bipolar radiofrequency device. The unipolar mode of the Accent was evaluated in a study of twenty-six females that showed that it may influence the distance between the dermis and the muscle or fascia, suggesting an effect on the fibrous tissue in the fat; however, the study was small, and statistical significance was variable. Further studies will be necessary to assess what, if any, improvement it can achieve.

Laser and Massage

Triactive and SmoothShapes utilize a combination of massage and light. Triactive (Cynosure) is an FDA-approved, low-fluence, 810-nm diode laser and suction massage. SmoothShapes 100 (SmoothShapes) is a non-FDA-approved dual-wavelength laser that is combined with suction and massage. The FDA-approved Synergie Aesthetic Massage System (Dynatronics) employs massage with or without a 660- to 880-nm probe or 880-nm light pad. With respect to the massage and light devices, there are a few studies published about Triactive, suggesting minimal efficacy that is comparable with VelaSmooth. There are no data published in peer-reviewed journals assessing the Synergie Aesthetic Massage System and SmoothShapes devices.

Other Devices and Procedures

Several other devices and procedures attempt to ameliorate cellulite. None have demonstrated efficacy. Purporting to influence lymphatic and vascular drainage, Endermologie (LPG) is an FDA-approved device that employs massage, kneading the skin using a handheld device. To date, studies show marginal results. Similarly, intense pulsed light has been employed in the treatment of cellulite, with disappointing results, as well. Ultrasonic liposculpturing has not been definitively shown to improve cellulite, and skin necrosis from devascularization after extensive undermining has been reported. It remains to be seen whether such new devices as the UltraShape (see the following section), a noninvasive ultrasound device, or the recently described laser wavelengths that selectively target lipids will effectively treat cellulite.

REMOVAL OF ADIPOSE TISSUE

There have been a number of recent innovations for adipose tissue destruction, primarily using ultrasound or laser sources. Some of the methods are incorporated into liposuction, while others offer noninvasive alternatives. The noninvasive devices are unlikely to be used for removal of large areas of fat, and instead will be recommended for body contouring.

UltraShape is a non-FDA-approved, noninvasive, focused ultrasound system reported to decrease fat by 2.3 cm after three treatments in a study of thirty patients. This finding was statistically significant, with patients maintaining constant weight during the treatment period. Blisters were reported in one patient. Triglyceride levels were elevated, although they remained in the normal range. Liver ultrasound was done after the first, but not third, treatment and was found to be normal. Interestingly, fat is not directly removed by this device; rather, treatments effect a release of triglycerides, which are likely recycled to the liver. Further study will be needed as to potential short- and long-term side effects of the UltraShape. The consequences of the release of large amounts of triglycerides into the system are not well understood. If the triglycerides were to, for example, redistribute viscerally, there may be health effects as visceral fat distribution is associated with increased risk of coronary artery disease and stroke.

LipoSonix (LipoSonix Inc.) is another non-FDA-approved device that utilizes high-intensity, focused ultrasound to destroy fat. To date, there are no data published in peer-reviewed journals to demonstrate its efficacy.

Ultrasound has also been used in combination with liposuction (UAL), with results comparable to traditional liposuction, but with less physician exertion and fatigue. But many feel that the risks of complications with UAL are somewhat greater than with traditional tumescent liposuction. It has been suggested that ultrasonic liposculpturing with manual extraction of the cellular residues and intercellular substance may allow for more selective destruction of lipids.

Laser-Assisted Liposuction

The 1,064-nm Nd:YAG laser has been used for removal of adipose tissue. SmartLipo (Cynosure) is a 300-μm, 1,064-nm Nd:YAG laser fiber encased in a 1-mm microcannula that is inserted into the skin after tumescent anesthesia. The cannula is moved back and forth beneath the skin. The adipose tissue is not removed after the procedure. One study, using magnetic resonance imaging, found a statistically significant decrease in fat of 17%. Histologically, SmartLipo seems to degenerate adipocyte cell membranes, causing spilling of the internal contents. No change in triglyceride or lipid profiles has been reported after use of the Nd:YAG laser without liposuction. A variety of other companies have also developed fiber-delivered laser energy liposuction units similar to SmartLipo. The 1,320-nm wavelength delivered in very short pulse widths has also been shown to be very effective for lipolysis, and laser-assisted liposuction devices are now available from other well-established companies such as CoolTouch and Sciton.

A 635-nm, low-energy laser has been proposed for use in conjunction with liposuction, but it is unclear whether this combination improves standard liposuction. The CO_2 laser has been reported to vaporize fat; additionally, 1,210-nm and 1,720-nm laser wavelengths are able to selectively heat adipose tissue, but no devices associated with these wavelengths are commercially available.

CONCLUSION

With recent advances, adipose tissue may be able to be treated for the first time noninvasively and effectively. Noninvasive treatments raise a set of systemic health concerns, and further study of the safety of such devices in terms of crucial metabolic parameters, such as lipid and triglyceride levels, will be important. With the mild and often equivocal efficacy of currently available devices for cellulite, new advances in this field hold the promise of truly effective noninvasive treatment of fat and cellulite. To date, however, such devices are not available.

SUGGESTED READING

Adamo C, Mazzocchi M, Rossi A, Scuderi N. Ultrasonic liposculpturing: extrapolations from the analysis of in vivo sonicated adipose tissue. *Plast. Reconstr. Surg.* 1997;100:220–6.

Adcock D, Paulsen S, Jabour K, Davis S, Nanney LB, Shack RB. Analysis of the effects of deep mechanical massage in the porcine model. *Plast. Reconstr. Surg.* 2001;108:233–40.

Alster TS, Tanzi EL. Cellulite treatment using a novel combination radiofrequency, infrared light, and mechanical tissue manipulation device. *J. Cosmet. Laser Ther.* 2005;7:81–5.

Alster TS, Tehrani M. Treatment of cellulite with optical devices: an overview with practical considerations. *Lasers Surg. Med.* 2006;38:727–30.

Anderson RR, Farinelli W, Laubach H, et al. Selective photothermolysis of lipid-rich tissues: a free electron study. *Lasers Surg. Med.* 2006;38:913–19.

Avram MM. Cellulite: a review of its physiology and treatment. *J Cosmet. Laser Ther.* 2004;7:181–5.

Boyce S, Pabby A, Chuchaltkaren B, Brazzini B, Goldman MP. Clinical evaluation of a device for the treatment of cellulite: Triactive. *Am. J. Cosmet. Surg.* 2005;22:233–7.

Brown SA, Rohrich RJ, Kenkel J, Young L, Hoopman J, Coimbra M. Effect of low-level laser therapy on abdominal adipocytes before lipoplasty procedures. *Plast. Reconstr. Surg.* 2004;113:1796–9.

Collis N, Elliot LA, Sharpe C, Sharpe D. Cellulite treatment: a myth or reality: a prospective randomized, controlled trial of two therapies, endermologies, and aminophylline crea. *Plast. Reconstr. Surg.* 1999;104:1110–14.

Draelos ZD. Purported cellulite treatments. *Dermatol. Surg.* 1997;23:1177–81.

Draelos ZD. The disease of cellulite. *J. Cosmet. Dermatol.* 2005;4:221–2.

Fink JS, Mermelstein H, Thomas A, Tro R. Use of intense pulsed light and a retinyl-based cream as a potential treatment for cellulite: a pilot study. *J. Cosmet. Dermatol.* 2006;5:254–62.

Gasparotti M. Superficial liposuction: a new application of the Technique for aged and flaccid skin. *Aesthetic Plast. Surg.* 1992;16:141–53.

Goldman A, Schavelzon DE, Blugerman GS. Laserlipolusis: liposuction using Nd:YAG laser. *Rev. Soc. Bras. Cir. Plast.* 2002;17:17–26.

Grotting JC, Beckenstein MS. The solid-probe technique in ultrasound-assisted lipoplasty. *Clin. Plast. Surg.* 1999;2:245–54.

Igra H, Satur N. Tumescent liposuction versus internal ultrasonic-assisted tumescent liposuction. *Dermatol. Surg.* 1997;23:1213–18.

Kim KH, Geronemus RG. Laser lipolysis using a novel 1,064 nm Nd:YAG laser. *Dermatol. Surg.* 2006;32:241–8.

Kligman AM. Cellulite: facts and fiction. *J. Geriatr. Dermatol.* 1997;5:136–9.

Kulick M. Evaluation of the combination of radio frequency, infrared energy and mechanical rollers with suction to improve skin surface irregularities (cellulite) in a limited treatment area. *J. Cosmet. Laser Ther.* 2006;8:185–90.

Moreno-Moraga J, Valero-Altes T, Martinez Riquelme A, Isarria-Marcosy MI, Royo de la Torre J. Body contouring by noninvasive transdermal focused ultrasound. *Lasers Surg. Med.* 2007;39:315–23.

Neira R, Arroyave J, Ramirez H, et al. Fat liquefaction: effect of lower-level laser energy on adipose tissue. *Plast. Reconstr. Surg.* 2002;110:912–22.

Nootheti PK, Magpantay A, Yosowitz G, Calderon S, Goldman MP. A single center, randomized, comparative, prospective clinical study to determine efficacy of the VelaSmooth system versus the Triactive system for the treatment of cellulite. *Lasers Surg. Med.* 2006;38:908–12.

Nurnberger F, Muller G. So called cellulite: an invented disease. *J. Dermatol. Surg. Oncol.* 1978;4:221–9.

Pino ME, Rosado RH, Azuela A, et al. Effect of controlled volumetric tissue heating with radiofrequency on cellulite and the subcutaneous tissue of the buttocks and thighs. *J. Drugs Dermatol.* 2006;5:714–22.

Rossi ABR, Vergnanini AL. Cellulite: a review. *J. European Acad. Dermat. Venerol.* 2000;14:251–62.

Sadick N, Magro C. A study evaluating the safety and efficacy of the Velasmooth system in the treatment of cellulite. *J. Cosmet. Laser Ther.* 2007;9:15–20.

Sadick NS, Mulholland RS. A prospective clinical study to evaluate the efficacy and safety of cellulite treatment using the combination of optical and RF energies for subcutaneous tissue heating. *J. Cosmet. Laser Ther.* 2004;6:187–90.

Section 10

ULTRASONIC FAT REDUCTION DEVICES

CHAPTER 70

UltraShape Focused Ultrasound Fat Reduction Device

Karyn Grossman

ULTRASHAPE CONTOUR I TECHNOLOGY

Body contouring is one of the most popular cosmetic procedures today. While tumescent liposuction is certainly highly effective and very safe, there is still a search for less invasive means of effective body contouring. Some patients are still afraid of traditional surgical procedures, while others may not be able to afford the cost and/or opportunity cost of a more invasive procedure.

The UltraShape CONTOUR I system (UltraShape Ltd.), based on proprietary focused ultrasound technology, is the first clinically proven noninvasive fat cell lysis and body-contouring solution.

The UltraShape CONTOUR I uses a patented ultrasonic technology to deliver focused ultrasound energy at a precise depth within the subcutaneous fat layer. It selectively targets and lyses only adipose tissue, leaving critical surrounding structures, such as skin, blood vessels, nerves, and connective tissue, intact. The pulsed acoustic waves of ultrasonic energy converge in a confined focal volume, causing a selective mechanical destruction of fat cells. Mechanical, not thermal, effects are produced due to the precise acoustic parameters and pulsed energy delivery. It is this mechanical acoustic effect that allows for tissue selectivity to lyse adipocytes, while surrounding tissues remain unharmed. Precision and safety are reinforced by an integrated acoustic contact sensor (Figure 70.1), which provides real-time feedback on acoustic contact, thus ensuring proper transducer-to-skin contact and efficient energy delivery to the treatment area.

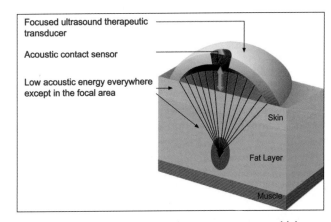

FIGURE 70.1: Integrated acoustic contact sensor, which provides real-time feedback on acoustic contact, thus ensuring proper transducer-to-skin contact and efficient energy delivery to the treatment area.

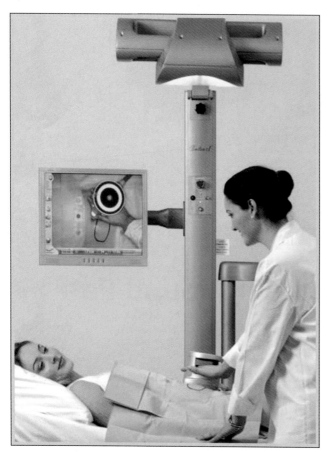

FIGURE 70.2: The UltraShape treatment being performed. The UltraShape system components shown include an illumination system with integrated computer-controlled video camera, a treatment monitor that guides the operator through the treatment, and a handheld transducer that delivers therapeutic ultrasound. A yellow dot indicates the location of the computer-generated target node per a preprogrammed treatment algorithm. Once the handpiece is correctly positioned over the target node, the green dot on the top of the transducer turns blue, indicating that the transducer is correctly positioned over the target node for treatment and that energy delivery can begin.

REAL-TIME TRACKING AND GUIDANCE SYSTEM

The UltraShape procedure (Figure 70.2) is guided by proprietary real-time tracking and guidance software designed to deliver uniform body-contouring results. The software maps the treatment area in three dimensions and guarantees adherence to a predetermined computer-controlled treatment algorithm. Key parameters of the computer-controlled treatment algorithm include the following:

1. Treatment is performed only within the marked treatment area.
2. Each point (node) is treated only once.
3. Each pulse of energy is delivered immediately adjacent to the prior pulse, ensuring complete uniform coverage over the entire treatment area.

This algorithm ensures complete and uniform energy delivery over the entire treatment area, minimizing the risk of double or overlapping pulses, which could then result in contour irregularities, isolated areas of increased lipoatrophy, or, in theory, a tissue injury. The tracking system also addresses the dynamic nature of the treatment area as it monitors and synchronizes patient position in real time, enabling the patient to move freely, without impacting the treatment.

The UltraShape CONTOUR I, version 2, was launched in June 2007. This second-generation technology offers improvements to both the operator and patient. First, it offers optimized acoustic output with adjustable power control to three levels. The default is to the highest level, but if the patient feels discomfort, the energy may be reduced to a nonpainful level. Second, it has new treatment tracking and guidance software, which includes optimized three-dimensional treatment mapping of the body curvature and superior tracking system stability and performance, resulting in reduced treatment time. Third, it has a new illumination system with LED technology and an integrated computer-controlled video camera, providing an easier UltraShape treatment experience for both the operator and patient. Last, it offers a new patient database to track and analyze all patient treatments.

NATURAL FAT CLEARANCE FOLLOWING TREATMENT

There has been concern that, after adipocytes are lysed in large quantity, the released triglycerides could adversely affect the body. The triglycerides should be released and processed by the body's natural physiological and metabolic pathways that handle fat during weight loss. UltraShape's published multicenter, controlled clinical study has shown that released triglycerides do not accumulate to any clinically significant extent in the blood or liver. One hundred sixty-four patients were treated with a single session of UltraShape and were followed for eighty-four days post-treatment. Blood and urinalysis were performed at days 0, 1, 3, 7, 14, 21, 28, 56, and 84. No clinically significant elevation of serum lipid profiles and no clinically significant changes in blood and urine tests were seen. Liver ultrasound was performed before and after treatment, and there were no treatment-induced changes to the liver seen. See Figure 70.3.

HISTOLOGIC STUDIES ON TISSUE EFFECTS OF ULTRASHAPE

UltraShape research using an ex vivo porcine model demonstrates immediate fat cell disruption after a single UltraShape treatment (Figure 70.4).

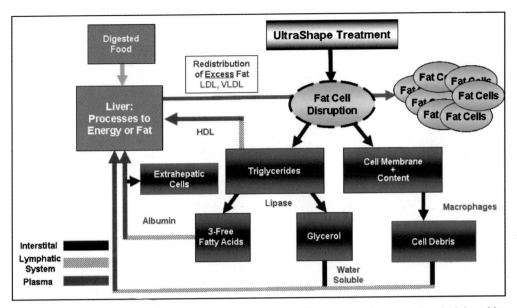

FIGURE 70.3: *The probable natural physiologic and metabolic process of clearing freed triglycerides released after UltraShape treatment.*

PATIENT SELECTION

As with any noninvasive procedure, it is important to select the right candidate and manage patient expectations carefully. The ideal candidate to undergo the UltraShape procedure is a motivated patient with realistic expectations. The patient should have the desire to reduce localized fat deposits and body circumference and improve his or her body shape without surgery or downtime. UltraShape patients should have a normal to overweight body mass index (BMI; less than 30) with localized fat deposits that measure at least 1.5 cm of fat thickness. Patients with greater BMI, overall diffuse fat distribution, or very large adipose deposits are less good candidates. However, greater circumference changes can be obtained with multiple treatments for patients with slightly larger localized areas of adiposity. Indicated treatment areas include the abdomen, flanks, and outer thigh/hip regions. Also, just as with liposuction, patients should be willing and able to maintain a healthy diet and exercise regimen to maximize their results. UltraShape is not a treatment for weight reduction, obesity, skin laxity, or patients with unrealistic expectations. Also, UltraShape is not currently a treatment for very thin deposits of fat less than 1.5 cm in thickness.

CURRENT PATIENT PREPARATION AND TREATMENT PROTOCOL

The UltraShape procedure is performed in an office-based environment; it requires no topical anesthesia or sedation, and the vast majority of patients report no pain or discomfort. There is no bruising, swelling, or downtime after the treatment, and patients may immediately resume

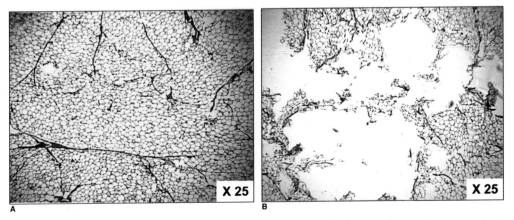

FIGURE 70.4: A, *Histology at 25 times magnification of untreated soft tissue.* **B,** *Histology at 25 times magnification of treated tissue, demonstrating acute fat cell lysis after a single treatment.*

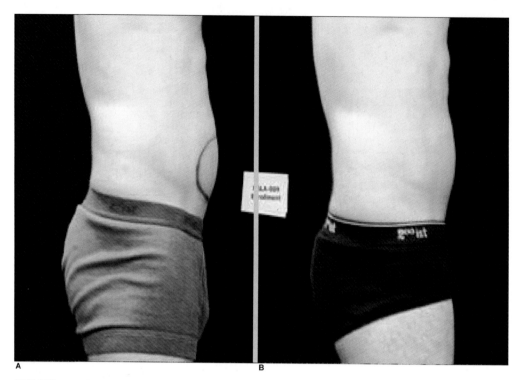

FIGURE 70.5: *Reduction of 3.5 cm of abdominal region. Photo courtesy of the Santa Monica Institute of Laser and Esthetic Surgery, Santa Monica, California.*

their daily routines. For those with stable body weights, there should be no need for maintenance treatments.

It is important to take consistent before and after photographs, make circumference measurements, and record weight change at each follow-up visit to document results and ensure that the patient is not gaining weight due to poor diet or lack of exercise. Also, one may want to document a constant weight so as to show that the results are due to treatment and not a generalized weight loss.

The patient's target treatment areas are assessed and marked in a similar way as for patients undergoing liposuction. When assessing and marking the targeted treatment area, the patient should stand straight up and look forward. Soft tissue deformities (unwanted fat deposits) should be evaluated from multiple views for best assessment. Palpate the perimeter of the area to identify exactly where the deformity begins and mark the precise area for treatment with a single line. Only soft tissue deformities with at least 1.5 cm of fat thickness should be treated, and not the adjacent flat or concave areas.

Proper patient positioning is a critical factor for successful treatment. It is important to position the patient so that the treatment area is as flat as possible, enabling complete transducer-to-skin contact and preventing adjacent anatomy from interfering with the transducer movement throughout the treatment. Once the patient is positioned on the treatment bed with a flat area marked for treatment, it is important to lift and reposition the soft tissue around the treatment area with soft positioning blocks and medical tape to maintain maximum fat thickness in the zone of treatment. These positioning and taping techniques have been shown to increase efficacy and reproducibility of results and should help reduce the risk of skin effects.

After proper positioning, the treatment drapes and markers are applied. The computer graphic program will walk the operator through the final setup, recognizing handpiece positioning. Once the treatment area and markers have been acquired, the real-time tracking and guidance system will guide the operator through the treatment per a preprogrammed treatment algorithm. The handpiece will be moved to the target on the screen, which then allows the operator to deliver energy. The target will then be moved to the adjacent area, and when the handpiece is placed on that exact location, the marker light will turn blue and the operator may deliver energy to the targeted node. The procedure should be able to be performed by appropriately trained and licensed medical personnel in the physician's office. To optimize results, patients should undergo a series of three UltraShape treatments spaced twenty-eight days apart. Maximum fat thickness and circumference reduction should be seen by thirty to sixty days after the final treatment.

CLINICAL RESULTS, EFFICACY, AND SIDE EFFECTS

Clinical results of UltraShape treatments (Figure 70.5) have been consistent in most published and presented literature.

In U.S. multicenter clinical trials, Teitelbaum et al. (2007) reported on 164 patients after a single treatment of the abdomen, flanks, or thighs. An average body circumference reduction of 2 cm was seen by day 14–21 and was sustained throughout the twelve-week follow-up. The reduction in fat thickness was 3 mm and was also sustained. No statistically significant weight loss was seen during this period; thus the circumference change was attributed to the treatment. No adverse effects were noted.

Clinical experience in the United Kingdom and Europe has led to a different algorithm, and treatments are performed to achieve greater results. The consensus seems to be to perform three treatments spaced thirty days apart. Greater fat reduction can be seen under these treatment parameters.

The effects of multiple treatments were reported by Moreno-Moraga et al. (2007), in whose study thirty patients received three treatments of the abdomen, flanks, and thighs at thirty-day intervals, with no adverse effects. A mean reduction in fat thickness of 2.28 cm was found, and a mean reduction in circumference of 3.95 cm was found in the treated areas at one month after final treatment. No statistically significant weight loss was noted.

Inglefield (2006) reported on a serious study of 148 patients treated with this three-treatment protocol and also found superior results. Mean circumference reduction after the three treatments was 8.5 cm for the abdomen, 5.2 cm for the lateral thighs, and 4.5 cm for the hips. The mean circumference reduction for all three areas was 6.3 cm. No statistically significant weight change was seen at the end of the follow-up period, and no significant adverse events were reported. Patient satisfaction was graded using a 0–5 scale, on which a score of 0 was poor and a score of 5 was excellent. A total of 93% of the patients rated good to excellent satisfaction after three treatments, while 5% reported poor satisfaction.

Ascher (2007) reviewed 130 patients who received one to three treatments to the abdomen, flanks, and/or thighs with a three-month follow-up period posttreatment. Results demonstrated that 92% of patients experienced a measurable circumference reduction and 73% of those patients had a 2- to 7-cm reduction in circumference. Patient satisfaction was evaluated based on patient self-ratings of not satisfied, moderately satisfied, or medium to very satisfied. A total of 88% of patients rated themselves as moderately to very satisfied, while 12% of patients reported that they were not satisfied after receiving one to three treatments. One patient experienced a blister, which resolved without sequelae. There was mild erythema or a stinging sensation observed in a small percentage of patients, which resolved within twenty-four hours.

The side effects and complications of UltraShape treatments have been limited in trials and clinical use. The most common side effects include mild erythema and occasional discomfort with treatment. The new settings allow for a reduction of intratreatment energies to decrease pain. Rare occurrences of blisters have been reported. These are most likely due either to treatment of areas with less than 1.5 cm of adipose tissue or to reflection of energy back from bone.

The UltraShape CONTOUR I received the CE mark in June 2005 and a Health Canada Medical License in May 2007, and it is currently distributed throughout forty-eight countries outside the United States. As of September 2007, the UltraShape CONTOUR I System is not cleared by the Food and Drug Administration for marketing in the United States.

SUGGESTED READING

Ascher B. Non-invasive lipolysis using focused ultrasound. Paper presented at: American Society for Aesthetic Plastic Surgery Meeting; 2007.

Grossman K, et al. Painless and noninvasive body contouring with the UltraShape. Paper presented at: American Society of Dermatologic Surgery Meeting; 2006.

Inglefield, C. Non-invasive body (fat) contouring using the Ultrashape Contour I System. Paper presented at: American Society of Plastic Surgeons Meeting; San Francisco, CA, Oct 30, 2006.

Moreno-Moraga J, Valero-Altés T, Riquelme AM, et al. Body contouring by non-invasive transdermal focused ultrasound. *Lasers Surg. Med.* 2007;39:315–23.

Teitelbaum S, Burns JL, Kubota J, et al. Non-invasive body contouring by focused ultrasound: safety and efficacy of the Contour I device in a multi-center controlled clinical study. *Plast. Reconstr. Surg.* 2007; 120:779–89.

CHAPTER 71

LipoSonix Ultrasound Device for Body Sculpting

Ernesto Gadsden

Maria Teresa Aguilar

BACKGROUND

High-intensity focused ultrasound (HIFU) was first used in research applications in 1942. Fry treated human subjects in 1958. It has since moved from being a research tool to an accepted part of the clinician's armamentarium. HIFU has been used clinically for many years to treat a variety of lesions in the liver, bladder, kidneys, prostate, breast, testes, uterus, and vasculature. Currently, several commercially available HIFU devices are available for these purposes. This chapter will address the next generation of HIFU devices for body sculpting, developed by LipoSonix Inc.

MECHANISMS OF ACTION OF HIFU

HIFU acts on tissue through two main mechanisms: thermal and thermomechanical effects. HIFU can reliably and predictably raise the temperature of the tissue in the focal zone to greater than 56 degrees Celsius to cause thermal toxicity. Shear forces, generated by the pressure wave and cavitation, can cause cellular disruption, but typically only in the focal area. It should be noted that because of the physics of HIFU technology, the mechanical effects will always be associated with temperature increases in tissue.

A unique property of HIFU, unlike other therapeutic energy modalities, is that the HIFU energy can be accurately controlled, including the depth of treatment. Numerous authors have shown that precise lesions can be reliably produced only in targeted locations, while the surrounding tissue outside of the HIFU focal zone is not affected. This is consistent with our research with the LipoSonix prototype.

METHODS

To date, we have successfully treated sixty-three adult volunteers with the LipoSonix device. Twenty of these subjects received abdominoplasties after various periods of residency; the remaining subjects were followed without surgical intervention for up to three months. Subjects were instructed not to change their diets, undertake weight loss programs, or alter their levels of regular exercise. As part of the clinical trial, subjects had blood drawn for extensive analysis. Also, aesthetic photographs were taken using standards developed by the ASAPS at baseline and at monthly intervals post-HIFU treatment. Waist circumference and weight data were also obtained on all subjects.

Treatment of the anterior abdomen routinely took well less than an hour (it should be noted that since our experience was in a clinical trial, we took extra time to query subjects as to their status and well-being). All subjects tolerated the HIFU treatments and subsequent post-HIFU healing process. There were no severe adverse events or device-related adverse events.

RESULTS

Blood samples were taken at baseline and at regular intervals post-HIFU. Extensive blood panels were analyzed on all human subjects treated as part of the LipoSonix trials in Mexico City. The blood panels included CBC, free fatty acids, total cholesterol, very low density lipoprotein, high-density lipoprotein, low-density lipoprotein, triglyceride, CPK, total bilirubin, AST, ALT, GGT, alk phos, CRP, uric acid, BUN, creatine, PT, PTT, INR, amylase, lipase, CPK-BB, CPK-MB, CPK-MM, leptin, and a chemistry panel (chem 12). There were no clinically significant changes in the blood profiles as compared to baseline, and all results were within normal limits of the central lab that processed the blood samples.

Gross pathology and histology of the abdominoplasty flaps demonstrated that the lesions created by HIFU treatment are consistently only within the targeted subcutaneous adipose tissue. There was no involvement of the skin or fascia. Even when changing the depth of the treatment layer or varying power output, the LipoSonix device always maintained an adequate safety margin from both the skin and abdominal muscles. Histology demonstrated a

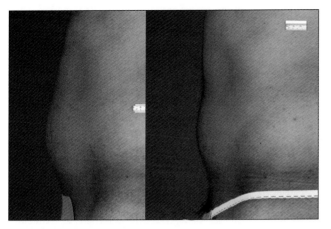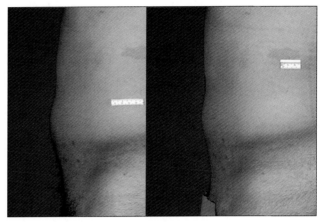

FIGURE 71.1: *Examples of two subjects treated with the LipoSonix prototype device, showing baseline (left) and one month post-HIFU (right).*

consistent, well-demarcated boundary between the treated and nontreated tissue at the predicted depths.

Of those subjects treated in the nonabdominoplasty arm of the research, we were able to document aesthetic improvement in a majority of the subjects (Figures 71.1 and 71.2). 92% of subjects treated with the latest optimized treatment regimen showed a reduction in waist circumference after only a single HIFU treatment. The amount of reduction was somewhat dependent on the distribution of adipose tissue in the body habitus of the subjects. 70% of subjects achieved at least a 2-cm reduction in waist circumference. Breaking down the clinical outcomes to specific treatment regimens (varying power and depth of treatment and number of layers treated), we found that up to 88% of subjects achieved an average waist reduction of over 3.7 cm from a single treatment session. The average change in body weight was insignificant.

A satisfaction survey was also given to the subjects to assess their perception of the procedure. Of those surveyed, 100% felt that the contour of their abdomen improved as compared to baseline; 92% reported that they would be very likely to return for a second treatment with the LipoSonix device. These are important findings as they speak to the device's ability to deliver a procedure that will meet the expectations of patients, and the high percentage of those willing to return for additional treatments is also important as it indicates that the procedure is well tolerated and will allow for multiple treatments on the same patient.

LIMITATIONS

We have only discussed treating the anterior abdomen. There are certainly other body parts where subcutaneous adipose could be treated with HIFU, including the hips, thighs, buttocks, back, and so on, and we have only targeted subcutaneous adipose tissue. There may be future cosmetic applications of HIFU such as treatment of cellulite or lipomas or skin tightening.

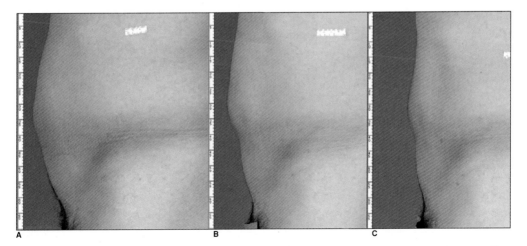

FIGURE 71.2: *Series of images taken of the same subject with the same camera settings at, A, baseline, B, one month post-HIFU treatment, and, C, three months post-HIFU treatment (right). The changes in the abdominal contour from baseline to both post-HIFU photos are evident.*

Another limitation of our experience was the lack of optimization of the treatment to the patient's adipose distribution; this was not done since this was a controlled clinical trial that sought a standardized treatment for all subjects. In clinical practice, it is reasonable to expect that clinicians will tailor the area, depth of treatment, and energy delivery to sculpt the adipose tissue based on the particular contours of the patient to improve clinical outcomes. In addition, little was done in this trial to optimize patient selection (other than meeting inclusion criteria); it may be possible to further improve the outcomes of treatment with the LipoSonix device by assigning patients to the appropriate treatment methods.

SUMMARY

The LipoSonix prototype has demonstrated an excellent safety record and easily appreciated clinical efficacy. The procedure and postprocedure courses are well tolerated by those we treated during this trial. The final clinical results were clearly demonstrable by objective measurements, in aesthetic photos, and by the subjects' own assessments of effectiveness. These data points, and the high marks obtained by the subject satisfaction survey, demonstrate that the LipoSonix prototype device can produce results acceptable to patients. The device may well become a valuable tool for office-based cosmetic procedures.

SUGGESTED READING

Adams WM, Higgins PD, Siegfired L, Paliwal BR. Chronic response of normal porcine fat and muscle to focused ultrasound hyperthermia. *Radiat. Res.* 1985;104:140–52.

Garcia-Murray E, Rivas OE, Stecco KA, Desilets CS, Kuns L, et al. The use and mechanism of action of high intensity focused ultrasound for adipose tissue removal and non-invasive body sculpting. *Plast. Reconstr. Surg.* 2005;116:222–3.

Garcia-Murray E, Rivas OE, Stecco KA, Desilets CS, Kunz L, et al. Evaluation of the acute and chronic systemic and metabolic effects from the use of high intensity focused ultrasound for adipose tissue removal and non-invasive body sculpting. *Plast. Reconstr. Surg.* 2005;116:151–2.

Linke CA, Carstensen EL, Frizzell LA, Elbadawi A, Fridd CW. Localized tissue destruction by high-intensity focused ultrasound. *Arch. Surg.* 1973;107:887–91.

Lynn J, Zwemer R, Chick A, et al. A new method for generation and use of focused ultrasound in experimental biology. *J. Ge Physiolo.* 1942;26:179–93.

ter Haar G, Sinnett D, Rivens I. High intensity focused ultrasound – a surgical technique for the treatment of discrete liver tumours. *Phys. Med. Biol.* 1989;34:1743–50.

PART FIVE

OTHER PROCEDURES

Section 1

SUTURE SUSPENSION LIFTS

CHAPTER 72

Suture Suspension Lifts: An Overview

Sorin Eremia

Suture suspension methods using ordinary sutures weaved in and out of tissues and/or looped around tissue have been around for some time, but have never been proven very practical or effective. Problems with tissue puckering and the sutures eventually cutting through the tissue that was pulled up and suspended seem to doom this type of approach. One version of such lifts, the curl lift, is still being used by some cosmetic practitioners, and one of its strongest proponents, Dr. Pierre Fournier, still promotes it, but in the past couple of years, only its latest version, which can incorporate barbed sutures.

The introduction of cogged sutures, originally with small barbs, to distribute tension and induce tissue fibrosis seemed like a revolutionary concept that might lead to better results. The initial attempts to perform face lifts using sutures with multiple barbs, cogs, or anchors that distribute tension over a greater surface started in Russia with the use of bidirectional polypropylene barbed sutures. The concept was introduced in Russia a decade ago, by Dr. Marlen Sulamanidze, as APTOS threads. It was introduced in the United States in 2000. A U.S. patent for similarly barbed sutures by Duke University plastic surgeon Dr. Gregory Ruff apparently preceded the APTOS thread concept and was the basis for the development of ContourThreads. The original Sulamanidze 2.0 polypropylene self-anchoring APTOS threads had bidirectional small barbs and floated freely in the subdermis. Subsequently, Wu (2004) described a method of looping a longer APTOS-type thread, suspending it, and tying it to temporal fascia. Though initially widely used, the APTOS threads have never received Food and Drug Administration (FDA) clearance in the United States. The APTOS sutures have been vastly modified over time (Figure 72.1) and are in use in many parts of the

world. Interested readers are encouraged to contact their inventors, Drs. Marlen and George Sulamanidze, for further information and training courses. The FDA-approved version, based on the Ruff U.S. patent, was a unidirectional, helical, barbed, polypropylene suture with a long, straight inserting needle attached at one end and a curved needle at the other. The suture had an increased number of short barbs over twenty-five helical twists (Figure 72.2). It was placed subdermally and secured to fascia through small incisions. The distal ends of two sutures are looped around temporal fascia and are tied together. Four to eight such sutures are used on each side of the face. Although the incisions are small and heal fast, there is swelling and puckering of the skin, and it takes a few days before the patient looks really close to normal. The one- to one-and-a-half-hour procedure could be done with local anesthesia, though some patients required sedation. It became commercially available in August 2004 as ContourThreads and was very aggressively marketed, with many proponents making predictions of long-term results and that such thread lifts would replace open minilifts altogether. Results with the initial version were not only disappointing, but there were problems with the knots and extrusions. Because of problems with extrusion of knots, a new double-armed suture was introduced, which reduced problems with extrusion, but other reports of annoying complications related to the sharp barbs and inserting needles, and breakage and migration of the permanent 2.0 polypropylene sutures, continued to surface. The addition of blind undermining to induce fibrosis appeared to improve duration of the results but also increased recovery time and risks. The better surgically trained users of ContourThreads eventually started to use them with open face lifts, where they seemed to

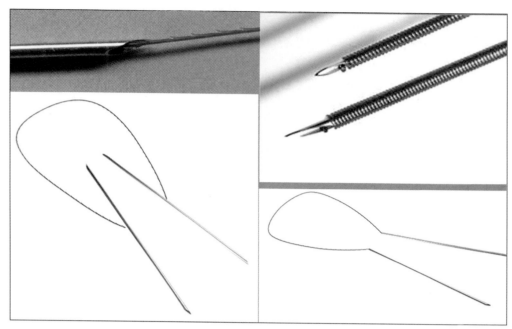

FIGURE 72.1: APTOS sutures.

have their best application. However, faced with mounting reports of problems, ContourThreads were suddenly pulled off the U.S. market in May 2007. The manufacturer reintroduced an absorbable version of the barbed suture in October 2007, but it is only marketed for wound closures.

Instead of relying on tiny directional barbs, in January 2004, the author designed a multianchor suspension suture by placing 7- to 9-mm bits of suture through each of five to nine simple square knots spaced 1 cm apart on an existing FDA-approved 2–0 absorbable monofilament suture. The bits of suture, stiff due to their short length,

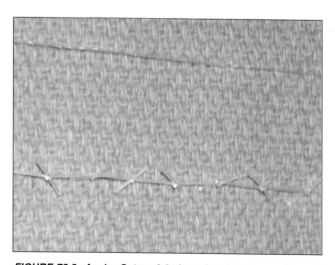

FIGURE 72.2: AnchorSuture 2.0 clear absorbable monofilament suture next to ContourThread barbed 2.0 clear polypropylene suture. Note the large size difference between anchors and barbs.

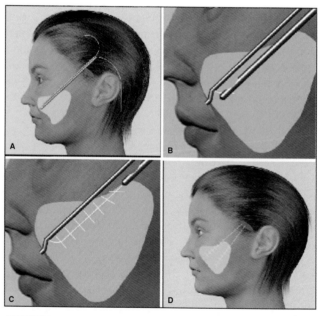

FIGURE 72.3: Anchor suture. There are six steps to placing the suture: A, insert the loaded suture passer in a deep subcutaneous plane, just over the SMAS; B, disengage the two components of the suture passer; C, pull back the larger component while holding the narrow component in place; this releases the section of suture with the anchors; the larger tube is pulled all the way out over the proximal needle end of the suture (the needle is a short, straight needle); D, a tug on the needle end of the suture engages the anchors, which bite into the tissue and can hold quite a bit of pull and tug. Next (not depicted), the narrow component is pulled out, leaving the distal end free floating. The needle end is used to pull up the tissues and is sutured to temporal fascia with the desired amount of pull.

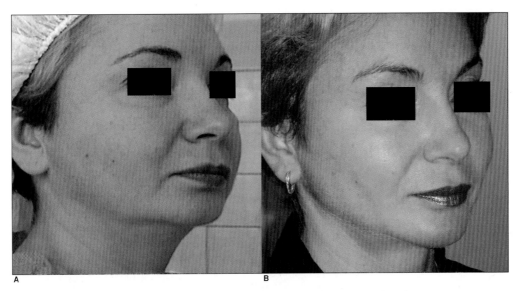

FIGURE 72.4: **A,** *APTOS.* **B,** *Suture lift. Photos courtesy of Drs. Marlen and George Sulamanidze.*

act like multiple anchors that open up at right angles to the main body of the suture, like multiple molly bolts that withstand significant tension. The author also devised a novel reusable instrument that allows simple, fast, atraumatic placement of his multianchor suture through a single entry point (Figure 72.3) and presented preliminary results at an American Society for Dermatologic Surgery course in September 2004. These sutures became known as multiknotted anchor sutures, or AnchorSutures for short. Short-term results were excellent. Due to deeper subcutaneous placement, just above the SMAS, there was far

less surface skin puckering than with the very superficially placed barbed threads. Recovery time was only one to two days, and with the use of a blunt inserter and slowly absorbable monofilament sutures, complications were largely avoided. Unfortunately, by twelve months, most of the initial correction was lost. Better results were obtained when combined with ablative and, to a lesser extent, nonablative skin treatments. The recent availability of fractional CO_2 resurfacing may now provide a good in-between alternative. The best application, however, was with open face lifts, allowing for better results with

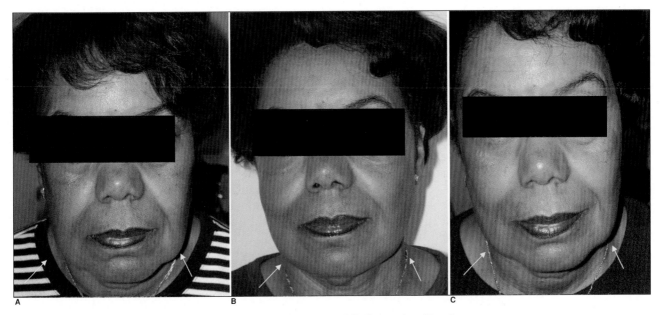

FIGURE 72.5: *Results of no-skin-excision, minimal-incision AnchorLift (knotted multianchor suspension lift) in an African American patient.* **A,** *Preoperative.* **B,** *Six months postoperative.* **C,** *Fifteen months postoperative. Note the remarkable initial improvement followed by eventual loss of correction.*

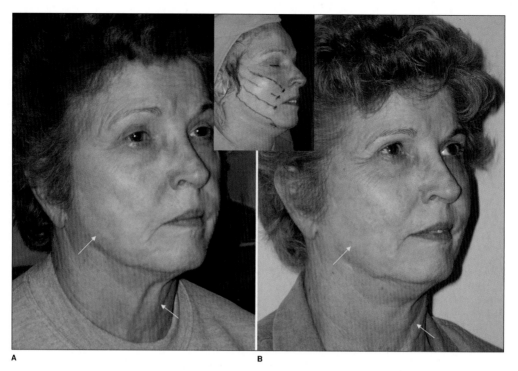

FIGURE 72.6: *Results of the same type of AnchorLift procedure as in Figures 72.1–72.5, with the addition of Thermage radiofrequency treatment immediately prior to the AnchorLift procedure. A, Preoperative. B, Twelve months postoperative. Note improvement in the neck area as well as improved volume, contour, and skin elasticity of the middle and lower face.*

conservative, or mini-, face lifts. These sutures are still in use today, but the suture company that was assembling them (Grams Suture) is no longer in business, and the sutures have to be assembled by hand from readily available PDS or Maxon by the physician's staff, which can be a bit time consuming, on one hand, but on the other, far less expensive than currently available commercially packaged alternatives. The inserting instrument is still available from Byron-Mentor or Beacon Medical.

In Europe and the rest of the world, while the modern versions of the APTOS sutures are best known, a variety of less expensive knockoff products are available and also used.

In the United States, the initial distributor of the APTOS threads, KMI, patented a cogged suture, called Silhouette Sutures, with multiple small (2 mm), slowly absorbable cones, fixed by knots on a permanent 3.0 polypropylene suture, which received FDA approval in early 2007. It is an intermediate concept between the Sulamanidze- or Ruff-style small barbed suture and the Eremia-style, larger, multianchor suture. Its chief proponent, the highly respected plastic surgeon Dr. Nicanor Isse, discusses Silhouette Sutures in Chapter 73. Currently, the Silhouette Sutures are the only FDA-approved suture being actively manufactured and distributed in the United States. Although relatively expensive, they are easy to use, and the author, who is also the inventor of the anchor suture, is

currently using Silhouette Sutures and finds them to be quite satisfactory. While Silhouette Sutures are primarily used for minimal-incision, pure suspension lifts, which, for most properly selected patients, appear to last one to two years, they can be used for supporting SMAS placation or for short SMAS flaps with conservative open lifts. Due to space limitations, only Silhouette Sutures are fully covered in this book.

In addition to use in the face and neck, various cogged sutures are being used for lifting other parts of the body such as breasts and buttocks. Initial results can be impressive, but the longevity of results from such procedures remains to be demonstrated. Non-U.S. readers, who may have multiple alternative cogged sutures available, should investigate the various options and applications in their respective countries. Figure 72.4 demonstrates representative lift results with APTOS, and Figures 72.5 and 72.6, with AnchorSutures.

SUGGESTED READING

Eremia S, Willoughby MA. Rhytidectomy. *Dermatol. Clin.* 2005; 23:415–30.

Eremia S, Willoughby MA. Novel face-lift suspension suture and inserting instrument: the use of large anchors knotted into a suture with an attached needle; an inserting device allowing for single entry point placement of the suspension suture. Preliminary report of 20 cases with 6–12 month follow up. *Dermatol. Surg.* 2006;32:335–45.

Eremia S, Willoughby MA. Management of SMAS: Plication, Imbrication, Deep-plane Face Lift. page 43–72. In: Moy R, ed., *Advanced Face Lifts*. New York: Elsevier; 2006.

Eremia S, Willoughby MA. Full FaceLift. page 117–142. In: Moy R, ed., *Advanced Face Lifts*. New York: Elsevier; 2006.

Lee S, Isse N. Barbed polypropylene sutures for midface elevation: early results. *Arch. Facial Plast. Surg.* 2005;7:55–61.

Lycka B, Bazan C, Poletti E, Treen B. The emerging technique of the antiptosis subdermal suspension thread. *Dermatol. Surg.* 2004;30:41–4.

Silva-Siwady JG, Diaz-Garza C, Ocampo-Candiani J. A case of Aptos thread migration and partial expulsion. *Dermatol. Surg.* 2005;31:356–8.

Sulamanidze MA. Removal of facial soft tissue ptosis with special threads. *Dermatol. Surg.* 2000;28:367–71.

Wu WTL. Barbed sutures in facial rejuvenation. *Aesthetic Surg. J.* 2004;24:582–7.

CHAPTER 73

Silhouette Sutures

Nicanor Isse

During facial aging, a series of physical and biochemical changes leading to tissue hypotrophy, sagginess, and wrinkles takes place not only at the level of the skin, but also at the level of fatty tissue, muscle, and so on. One of these changes is a decrease in the volume and elasticity of the tissue due to an alteration in collagen fiber formation.

The intermittent use of Silhouette Sutures is meant to prevent and treat tissue sagginess and reinforce the soft tissue of the face. The physical and chemical configuration of Silhouette Sutures will allow facial tissue repositioning by exerting traction on the soft tissue of the face, while, at the same time, new collagen fibers form around its structure.

The initial traction is produced by the presence of the slowly absorbing cones, which will be reinforced by the buildup of new collagen formation. After one year, the traction will be maintained by the collagen around and inside of a series of knots intercalated between the cones.

These sutures can be readjusted in the future (one and a half to two years after treatment) by pulling them from the temporal area, where all of them meet. Further sutures could be added at that time to reinforce the existing ones or to treat different areas.

SUTURE DESCRIPTION

1. Straight needle, six inches in length, allowing insertion of the suture into the soft tissue
2. Main suture
   a. The suture is a monofilament, nonabsorbable 3.0 polypropylene suture, 25 cm in length.
   b. The distal 10 cm of the sutures contains 11 knots, at approximately 10-mm intervals; each knot is intercalated with absorbable cones.
   c. The knotted polypropylene will exert a lasting soft tissue anchoring.
3. Cones
   a. The cones are a series of engaging elements, ten in total.

b. They are hollow structures about 1.12 mm diameter at the base and 2.50 mm in length.
c. They are made of copolymers of glycolic and lactic acid and are absorbable, taking approximately twelve months for complete absorption.
d. The polypropylene suture is inserted through the hollow cones like a Hawaiian necklace.
e. The cones are located in the distal 10 cm of the suture, between the first and last knots; the rest of the cones are intercalated with the knots.
f. They exert traction for about twelve to eighteen months.
4. Curved needle
   a. The curved needle is located in the proximal end of the suture and will secure the proximal end of the suture to the deep temporal fascia.

A patch or mesh is applied to the deep temporal fascia to prevent tearing or a cheese wire effect on the soft tissue of the temporal area. See Figure 73.1.

ANESTHESIA

The procedure is generally done under local anesthesia with intramuscular sedation. Local anesthesia could be applied in two ways:

- infiltration anesthesia immediately underneath each trajectory of the sutures
- nerve block anesthesia to each branch of the trigeminal nerve

SURGICAL TECHNIQUE

Access Incision

Incision location: The access incision is located in the temporal area, approximately 1 cm inferior to the superior temporal crest and 1–3 cm behind the hairline.

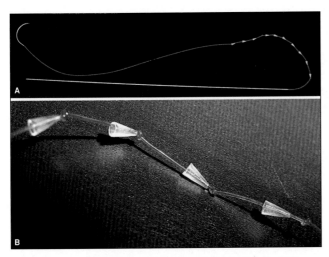

FIGURE 73.1: *Silhouette Sutures assembly:* **A,** *the straight needle, the 3.0 knotted polypropylene, the absorbable cones made of bipolymers of glycolic and lactic acids, and the curved needle;* **B,** *a close-up.*

Incision orientation: The superior end of the incision is approximately 1 cm behind the temporal hairline, and the lower portion of the incision is about 3 cm behind the temporal hairline.

Depth of the incision: The incision is deep down through the subcutaneous tissue and the superficial temporal fascia, down to the deep temporal fascia.

Dissection: A dissection is carried down between the superficial and deep temporal fascia, up to the level of the hairline. At this level, in the hair-bearing area, the sutures are located between the superficial and deep temporal fascia to prevent pressure alopecia in the hair-bearing area of the temple.

Reinforcement of the Deep Temporal Fascia

A patch, graft, or mesh (absorbable or not) is used to prevent shredding or tearing of the deep temporal fascia.

Exit Lines

These are the lines out of which all the sutures will come. Usually, there are two lines:

1. *Nasolabial line*: This line is located 5 mm lateral to the nasolabial groove.
2. *Jowl line*: After pulling the saggy jowls upward, until the skin appears smoothly elevated and even, a line is marked that joins the buccal commissure and the gonion of the mandible; the location of this line may vary to a lower location if there is heavy jowl formation.

Exit Points

There are a number of exit points located on or close to the exit lines. These will depend on the number of sutures employed during the procedure. Generally, the number of sutures used is six per side of the face (malar, submalar, cheek, and jowls).

1. Locations of the exit points
   a. Exit point 1 is located halfway between the ala of the nose and the oral commissure, and 5 mm lateral to the nasolabial groove.
   b. Exit point 2 is located 1 cm lower than the first and on the same nasolabial exit line.
   c. Exit point 3 is located at the junction of the nasolabial and jowl lines. Sometimes, if the jowls are heavy or large, this exit point will be located 1–1.5 cm lower.
   d. Exit point 4 is located 1 cm lateral to the third, on the jowl line.
   e. Exit point 5 is located 1 cm lateral to the fourth, on the jowl line.
   f. Exit point 6 is located 1 cm lateral to the fifth, on the jowl line.

2. Suture trajectory (skin marks)
   a. The two nasolabial sutures go from the lowermost portion of the temporal incision to exit points 1 and 2.
   b. Suture 3 (oral commissure or labiomental) goes to the uppermost end of the temporal incision.
   c. Sutures 4, 5, and 6, the jowl sutures, go inferiorly to suture 3, in the same order.
   d. Sutures 3, 4, 5, and 6 cross sutures 1 and 2 at the level of the zygoma.

Suture Deployment

The sutures are deployed at two different levels with regard to their location:

1. Temporal area deployment: The sutures are deployed between the superficial and deep temporal fascia (not in the subcutaneous tissue, hair-bearing area) to avoid pressure alopecia postoperatively. Once the straight needle reaches the anterior temporal hairline, the needle and suture become more superficial, into the subcutaneous tissue.

2. Facial deployment (malar, submalar, jowls): In these areas, the suture will be deployed in the subcutaneous tissue. Care is taken not to get too close to the dermis, to prevent dimpling of the skin, nor into the deep and fixed tissue, preventing the motion of the sutures. Due to the normal curvature between the malar and submalar areas, the needle at this level has a tendency to exit the

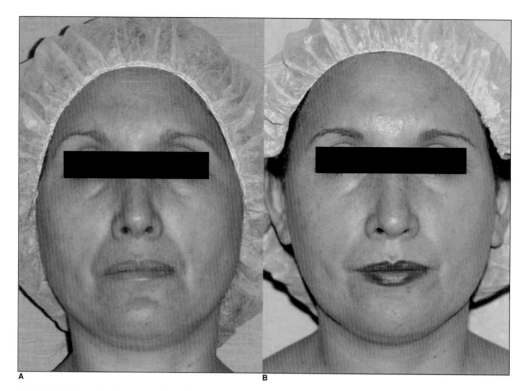

FIGURE 73.2: A, Pretreatment. B, 1.3 years after closed melopexy using six Silhouette Sutures per side, on the malar area, from midway between the nasolabial fold to the posterior portion of the jowls. The neck was not done.

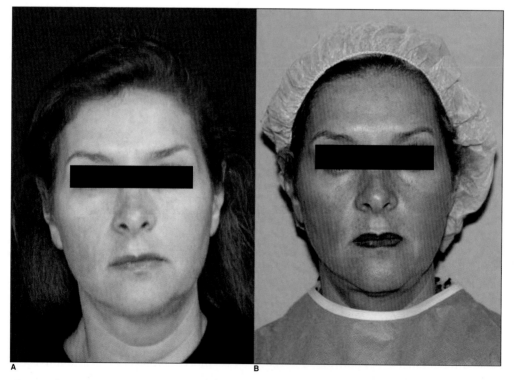

FIGURE 73.3: A, Pretreatment, 43-year-old patient. B, One year after closed melopexy using four Silhouette Sutures per side, on the malar area, from midway between the nasolabial fold to the posterior portion of the jowls. The neck was not done.

skin prematurely; lifting the submalar tissue to the level of the malar area will prevent an uneven insertion of the suture (Figures 73.2 and 73.3).

SUTURE TRACTION AND FIXATION

Although each suture's tension and traction are evaluated at the time of insertion, the final tension, traction, and adjustment are done at the very end of the procedure, when the sutures are tied in pairs into the deep temporal fascia, which was reinforced with mesh, either absorbable or non-absorbable. The temporal incision is closed in layers, the superficial fascia first to cover the mesh or patch and the skin.

DRESSING AND POSTOPERATIVE CARE

Immediately after surgery, a 1 × 5 inch Steri-Strip is applied to the malar-submalar and temporal areas in their entirety to support the soft tissue during the healing process, preventing or decreasing the chance of early soft tissue sagginess due to the cheese wire effect of the suture over the inflamed and fragile soft tissue of the face. The stitches on the temporal area are removed after five to seven days.

The patient is advised not to open the mouth wide and is instructed about no hard chewing and no puckering of the lips (smoking or drinking with straws) for about two weeks after surgery to prevent a cut-through effect of the suture on the tissue and to prevent inflammation, pain, and tenderness.

SUGGESTED READING

Isse NG. Elevating the midface with barbed polypropylene sutures. *Aesthetic Surg. J.* 2005;25:301–3.

Lee S, Isse N. Barbed polypropylene sutures for midface elevation. *Arch. Facial Plast. Surg.* 2005;7:55–61.

Moscoe ND, Isse N. The suture of the future? *Plast. Surg. Products.* 2007;4:44–6.

Sulamanidize MA, Fournier PF, Paikidze TG, et al. Removal of facial soft tissue ptosis with special threads. *Dermatol. Surg.* 2002;28:367–71.

PEELS AND MICRODERMABRASION

CHAPTER 74

Chemical Peels and Microdermabrasion

Suzan Obagi

Chemical peels are the oldest modality for skin resurfacing, having been in use for over centuries. Yet, technology continues to evolve with the introduction of newer resurfacing modalities such as dermabrasion, laser resurfacing, and, more recently, the trend toward noninvasive or so-called pixilated lasers. Interestingly, chemical peels have withstood the test of time and continue to play an important role in cosmetic dermatology. If used correctly, they can be tailored to treat almost any skin defect. Furthermore, they can be used in combination with laser resurfacing, dermabrasion, and surgical procedures to optimize the final outcome. Many physicians lack exposure and training in chemical peels in residency; however, it is an art that can be learned and can be very gratifying to both the physician and the patient.

INDICATIONS FOR CHEMICAL PEELS

The most important part of skin resurfacing is selecting the correct modality to address the patient's concerns. The physician must properly assess the patient to determine what needs to be addressed and the depth of peeling that will be needed to correct this. This is achieved by understanding skin anatomy, the depth of the cutaneous pathology being addressed, and the mechanisms of action of the various peeling agents.

As the largest organ, the skin has an important role as a barrier to environmental insults such as ultraviolet radiation, tobacco, temperature extremes, and pollution. Furthermore, there are internal influences on the skin such as hormones, inflammatory skin diseases, and systemic diseases. These factors give rise to actinic keratoses, solar lentigines, ephelides, dyschromias, rhytids, shallow or saucer-shaped scars, and photodamage, which are among the most common indications for resurfacing. Other indications include static rhytids, skin laxity, solar lentigines, so-called stretchable scars, photodamage, dyschromias, and enlarged pores.

PATIENT EVALUATION

As with any cosmetic surgery procedure, it is of paramount importance to evaluate and select the patient correctly. Patients seek cosmetic surgery for many reasons, ranging from the obvious to the subtle. Some patients are good at explaining their concerns and expectations, while others may not be able to verbalize their concerns. Regardless of what procedure the patient requires, it is important that the patient's expectations are in line with what the procedure will deliver. Thus it is very important that the physician present both what the procedure will achieve for the patient and what it will not. Sometimes the best way to convey this information is by showing the patient before and after photographs of the procedure in which they are interested.

The most challenging patients, and the ones who require the greatest degree of caution, are those who present with barely noticeable skin defects. These will tend to be the patients who are most likely to closely scrutinize results and to be disappointed in what they may perceive as not significant enough improvement. Most definitely, all patients should have standardized before and after photographs taken of them.

Every patient requires a thorough medical, social, and family history to identify potential problems. For example, certain medications may impact wound healing, such as prednisone or immunosuppressants, while others may indicate an underlying psychiatric disorder. The history of radiation treatment to the face or nicotine use may herald problems with wound healing as resurfaced skin requires intact and functioning pilosebaceous units and a good blood supply to reepithelialize correctly.

Additionally, it is important to inquire about the tendency to develop postinflammatory hyperpigmentation, hypertrophic or keloid scars, or poor wound healing.

The physical examination should take place in a well-lit room with no makeup on the patient's skin. Having an overhead, movable light fixture allows the physician to shine indirect lighting on the skin to highlight certain scars. During the examination, one should also exclude the presence of certain skin disorders that have the propensity to spread to traumatized skin (vitiligo, psoriasis, lichen planus, verrucae vulgaris, and plana). A more controversial issue is whether to screen patients who will be undergoing concomitant dermabrasion and laser resurfacing for viral diseases that may put the physician and surgical team at risk such as hepatitis B and C and HIV.

CONTRAINDICATIONS TO SKIN RESURFACING

The beauty of chemical skin resurfacing is that with the proper preoperative and postoperative skin conditioning as well as the proper procedure depth, patients of most skin types can be treated. However, special care is advisable when treating patients with darker complexions. Patients who are Fitzpatrick type III or darker are at risk for permanent hypopigmentation with procedures that reach the depth of the reticular dermis. These are the same patients who are at risk for a somewhat lengthy battle with postinflammatory hyperpigmentation with any procedure. To minimize this risk, the length of preoperative skin conditioning should be extended to three months and resumed immediately on reepithelialization of the skin.

When inquiring about medications, it is important to ask about isotretinoin (Accutane, Roche Laboratories Inc.) use and when it was last taken. The medical literature contains a small number of isolated case reports of hypertrophic scarring related to isotretinoin use in the perioperative period with dermabrasion and certain lasers. Therefore the general recommendation is to avoid laser resurfacing or dermabrasion for six to twelve months from the completion of a course of isotretinoin and to delay the start of isotretinoin for three months after any skin resurfacing. When it comes to skin peels, however, the author has published a large case series of patients undergoing medium-depth chemical peeling while using Accutane in the perioperative, which

showed no increased risk as compared to control patients. The use of isotretinoin in deeper peels was not studied; therefore caution is still recommended. Occasionally, skin resurfacing triggers a flare of acne or rosacea. To address this, systemic anti-inflammatory antibiotics, such as tetracycline, minocycline, or doxycycline, may be a safer alternative to isotretinoin.

The preceding issues are relative contraindications to skin resurfacing. However, absolute contraindications do exist. These include a significant propensity to keloid formation, active infection in the treatment area, pregnancy, and the inability to adhere to postoperative instructions.

EVALUATING SKIN TYPE

When resurfacing skin, the patient needs to be evaluated correctly to help in choosing the correct procedure and depth of treatment, and to help reduce postoperative complications. This evaluation needs to be performed in a standardized fashion. Skin color alone is insufficient in guiding the procedure depth. If one looks more closely, there are some important variations that exist even among patients of the same color.

Fitzpatrick phototype is simply a way to type the skin based on the ability to tan in response to ultraviolet (UV) exposure. In this classification, patients are categorized from I to VI as their skin color darkens and their ability to tan, rather than burn, increases. This classification is limited in that it does not address the degree of photodamage present or assist in selecting the correct procedure depth.

Glogau's classification attempts to objectively quantify the amount of photodamage present but fails to aid in selecting the procedure and the depth of treatment needed.

The Obagi skin classification system incorporates five variables that are important to address prior to any resurfacing procedures: skin color, oiliness, thickness, laxity, and fragility (Table 74.1). This system helps to identify which patients require a longer pre- and postoperative skin conditioning program, which patients are more likely to hyper- or hypopigment, which patients are prone to delayed healing, and which patients require a skin-tightening procedure (peels, lasers) over a planing procedure (dermabrasion). The evaluation of all five factors helps to maximize skin resurfacing results, while minimizing complications.

Patients with extensive photodamage need to be approached with caution. These patients are prone to postoperative pseudo-hypopigmentation following skin resurfacing. Once the treated area heals, the absence of photodamage may stand out in stark contrast to nearby photodamaged skin. This gives the appearance of hypopigmentation of the treated skin. However, when one compares the treated skin to other sun-protected areas, the color of the newly treated skin is not lighter than the patient's baseline. This occurs as the newly healed skin returns to a color closer to that of skin in sun-protected

TABLE 74.1: Obagi Skin Classification for Resurfacing

Skin Variable	Pre- and Postoperative Conditioning	Suitable Procedures and Potential Complications

Color	patients at *risk* for postoperative hypo- and hyperpigmentation:
	    darker-complexion Caucasian
	    lighter-complexion black, Indian, or Asian
	      require the following:
	aggressive conditioning before and after a procedure to minimize PIH[a]
	
	patients with more stable melanocytes:
	    lighter Caucasian
	    darker black, Indian, Asian patients
		resurfacing depth in at-risk patients can result in the following:
		
		hypopigmentation:
		• common superficial procedure: rare
		• medium-depth procedures: possible
		• deep procedures: more likely
		
		hyperpigmentation:
		• common
		
		best to keep procedures to papillary dermis or above

Oiliness	interferes with effectiveness of skin conditioning and should be controlled prior to surgery	topical treatments or low-dose systemic retinoids are needed to control and reduce surface oiliness prior to surgery unless oiliness is controlled, patients are more difficult to peel due to impaired penetration of peeling agents through oily skin do better with lasers or dermabrasion
Thickness	thin skin needs more stimulation of collagen synthesis with a good preconditioning regimen thick skin needs correction of skin function and stimulation of collagen synthesis	thin skin: lighter procedures such as Blue Peel or Er:YAG resurfacing medium-thickness skin: good for peels, dermabrasion, CO_2 laser, Er:YAG resurfacing thick skin: best for chemical peels, lasers, and dermabrasion
Laxity	long-term preconditioning stimulation of collagen and elastin production to prevent further laxity	skin laxity: medium-depth peel or several Blue Peels are ideal muscle laxity: face lift alone or in combination with a Blue Peel to correct any associated skin laxity
Fragility	aggressive stimulation to strengthen the skin	correlates with postsurgical scarring; in fragile skin, procedure depth should be limited to the papillary dermis

[a] Postinflammatory hyperpigmentation.

areas. This is not a complication, but it requires forewarning of the patient and blending in of the skin adjacent to the treated area to avoid lines of demarcation.

SKIN CONDITIONING

An appropriate skin care regimen can start improving the patient's appearance while he or she awaits the procedure. More important, the goal of skin conditioning, both before and after procedures, is to minimize wound-healing problems. Additionally, instituting an aggressive preconditioning program can help identify patients who may not be compliant with postoperative instructions if they quit their regimens once they develop the initial erythema and desquamation of a retinoid dermatitis.

There are many complex changes that occur as the skin ages. Aged skin shows a decline in collagen and elastin production in the dermis, which is much more prominent if there is significant photodamage, as well. Furthermore, photoaged skin will also have roughness, dyspigmentation, and keratinocyte atypia in direct correlation to the amount of damage. Therefore the goal of skin preconditioning is to restore the skin, as much as possible, to a normal state prior to wounding it. This is achieved by increasing dermal collagen production, regulating the melanocytes, normalizing keratinocyte atypia, and decreasing surface roughness (to allow more even acid penetration).

Skin conditioning should begin at least six weeks (longer in darker skin types) prior to any resurfacing procedure and should be resumed immediately after reepithelialization takes place. Six weeks is the epidermal turnover time – the time it takes for a keratinocyte to mature from the basal layer through the stratum corneum. Proper patient education about the initial erythema and scaling with the use of the topical regimen will help ensure patient compliance. These reactions are not harmful and, after initially peaking in two to three weeks, will slowly subside.

All resurfacing patients need to start a topical retinoid to enhance the rate of reepithelialization and to shorten wound-healing time. This can be achieved with tretinoin 0.05 to 0.1% (Retin-A, Ortho Biotech Inc.). Retinoids influence cell growth and differentiation, increase collagen and elastin production, and repair photodamaged skin.

Hydroquinone inhibits tyrosinase, a key enzyme in melanogenesis within the melanocytes. Hydroquinone 4% cream is used to suppress overactive melanocytes (melasma, lentigines) and to help blend in areas adjacent to that which will be treated. Twice daily application of hydroquinone is required since it has a half-life of twelve hours. Hydroquinone serves another important function: by decreasing the epidermal hyperpigmentation, it will unmask any dermal pigmentation that may be present. If dermal pigmentation is present, then one must choose a resurfacing modality that will reach the pigment. However, as will be discussed later, resurfacing procedures that penetrate into the reticular dermis are at increased risk for complications.

Acne-prone patients, very oily skinned patients, or those with severe dyschromias will require the use of a daily alpha-hydroxy acid, 6 to 8%. It helps acne by exfoliating the stratum corneum. The thinning of the stratum corneum also enhances the penetration of tretinoin and hydroquinone. Alpha-hydroxy acids can deactivate retinoids; therefore their application should be limited to the morning, rather than the evening. Examples of commonly used topical alpha-hydroxy acids include lactic acid and glycolic acid.

Patients must be instructed in the importance of daily sunblock to prevent further dyschromia and sun damage. Zinc oxide and titanium dioxide are physical sunblocks and are usually well tolerated by patients. The sunblock takes the place of a daily moisturizer and is applied to the skin after application of other creams but prior to applying any makeup. Tanning within six to eight weeks before surgery is highly discouraged since it stimulates melanin production.

Once reepithelialization of the wound is complete and the patient is able to tolerate the application of topical medications, it is important to resume the skin-conditioning program. Since reepithelialization time varies with wound depth, it may be as early as three days (with exfoliative procedures) to as late as fourteen days. Postinflammatory hyperpigmentation will not show up until three to four weeks after the procedure. Since there may be a delay until it shows up, it is easier to treat the skin prophylactically than to deal with this frustrating issue once it has occurred.

HERPES PROPHYLAXIS

Prior infection with herpes simplex virus (HSV) can result in a situation where the virus lies dormant for many years or decades, until some form of trauma triggers a reactivation. Reactivation of HSV can lead to devastating consequences as a result of disseminated cutaneous infection. Since all skin-resurfacing techniques have the potential to trigger HSV activation and replication, treatment is aimed at prevention of outbreaks. All patients receive valacyclovir (Valtrex, GlaxoSmithKline) 500 mg by mouth twice a day for seven to fourteen days (until the skin has fully healed), starting one day prior to the procedure for all patients. Patients with a history of frequent HSV outbreaks receive a dose of valacyclovir 1 g twice a day. The use of antibiotics or anti-*Candida* agents is best used only if an infection develops, rather than empirically on every patient.

CHEMICAL PEEL SKIN RESURFACING

Terminology

This chapter will describe peels based on their depth of penetration into the skin. Wounds confined to the epidermis (basal layer and above) will be called *exfoliation*. *Light peels* will refer to depths reaching the papillary dermis but not yet entering the reticular dermis. *Medium-depth peels* will refer to peels that have entered the superficial aspect of the reticular dermis. *Deep peels* extend into the midreticular dermis. The depth of peels is monitored by intraoperative signs, as will be discussed.

Mechanisms of Action

It is misleading to classify chemical peeling solutions as light or deep solutions based on their concentrations since there are many factors that affect peel depth. Acid concentration, the number of coats applied, skin thickness, percentage body surface area, skin preconditioning, and, in some cases, the duration of contact of the acid on the skin are the main variables. Rather, the trained physician knows to look at the peeling agents based on their mechanisms of action – either keratolytic agents or protein denaturants – rather than based on the concentration being used. The keratolytics are mainly used for superficial, exfoliative procedures, whereas the protein denaturants can be used for superficial or deeper peels.

Keratolytics

Keratolytics are acids that disrupt the adhesion between the keratinocytes, thus causing shedding of these layers. The two main acids used for exfoliative procedures are glycolic and salicylic acid. The role of these agents is to address superficial conditions such as roughness, acne, and mild dyspigmentation. These are oftentimes referred to as lunchtime peels as these exfoliative acids have the benefit of little to no downtime for the patient; in addition, there is no anesthesia requirement, and they are easy to perform. However, clinical results are seen only after numerous treatments, spaced several weeks apart. The results of these peels can be enhanced greatly by the addition of a good skin care regimen that the patient follows at home.

Microdermabrasion

While not a chemical peel, microdermabrasion falls under the category of a lunchtime procedure that utilizes a mechanical means to achieve keratolysis. The name *microdermabrasion* alludes to the mechanical sanding of the skin that is achieved with traditional dermabrasion, but at such a superficial level that it creates only minor skin wounding.

Most systems are based on a superficial abrading of the skin with a machine that forces crystal salts onto the skin while under vacuum suction, and draws them back up and into the machine. The contact of the skin with the crystals can be adjusted by increasing the power by which the crystals hit the skin and the power of the vacuum that pulls the skin up and into contact with the crystals. Alternatively, some systems rely on diamond-tipped tomes that manually abrade the skin to remove the surface layers.

The end point of most microdermabrasion procedures is to achieve a superficial exfoliation of the stratum corneum and maybe the uppermost layers of the epidermis. Some physicians advocate taking the treatment to the end point of pinpoint bleeding when treating over deeper wrinkles or acne scars. Caution is advised, however, as the visualization of pinpoint bleeding means that the papillary dermis has been reached. This increases the risk of adverse effects such as scarring or hyperpigmentation. This deeper type of treatment is best reserved for the physician and should not be delegated to an aesthetician or nurse.

Protein Denaturants

Trichloroacetic Acid Peels

Trichloroacetic acid (TCA) is the workhorse of chemical peels and has been used for over a century with relative safety. TCA works by causing protein coagulation and denaturation as it penetrates the skin. These are the proteins in the cells of the epidermis and dermis as well as the blood vessels. It is self-neutralized once it has coagulated a certain amount of protein. Therefore a subsequent application will then drive the peel deeper, until it is used up by coagulating proteins deeper down in the skin. When used correctly, it can be used to achieve a variety of peel depths, ranging from exfoliation to deep peels. Of outmost importance when using TCA is to make sure that the acid is purchased from a reliable source that uses the weight-to-volume (W:V) method to calculate concentration. There are four methods to calculate concentration, but the W:V method is by far the safest.

It is incorrect to refer to TCA peels as light or deep according to TCA concentration. As mentioned before, acid concentration is just one of the variables affecting peel depth. For example, 1 mL of 40% TCA applied to the face will result in penetration to the basal layer, while 6 mL of 40% TCA applied over the same body surface area will result in penetration to the middermis or deeper. Higher volumes will drive the peel even deeper.

With proper training, the physician can tailor peels to penetrate to certain depths, just as someone would dial up laser settings. One sees this as variations in peels that have risen up to give the physician more control over the peel. These are the modified TCA peels (Monheit's Jessner-TCA peel, Coleman's glycolic acid–TCA peel, Obagi's TCA–Blue Peel). These peels are designed to peel to a depth of the papillary dermis and into the most superficial aspect of the reticular dermis. Their main indications are for epidermal and upper dermal pathology: photodamage; actinic keratoses; lentigines; ephelides; fine rhytids; and very superficial, nonfibrotic scars. These peels will not address deeper scars or rhytids.

Monheit described a Jessner's-TCA peel employing the use of a keratolytic acid preparation – Jessner's solution – prior to the application of TCA. Jessner's solution consists of 14% each of resorcinol, salicylic acid, and lactic acid mixed in ethanol. The keratolytic effect of Jessner's solution allows for deeper and faster penetration of the subsequently applied 35% TCA. Rather than Jessner's solution, Coleman's glycolic acid–TCA peel uses 70% glycolic acid prior to the application of 35% TCA. These two peels will speed up the penetration of the TCA by disrupting the stratum corneum and the most superficial layers of the epidermis. The Obagi TCA–Blue Peel does the opposite. Obagi's TCA–Blue Peel combines a nonionic blue dye, glycerin, and a saponin with a specified volume of 30% TCA to yield either a 15 or 20%, or higher TCA–Blue Peel solution. The blue dye helps facilitate even application of the solution by staining the stratum corneum. The saponin is an emulsifying agent that creates a homogenous TCA-oil-water emulsion that penetrates the skin in a slower and more even fashion.

Phenol Peels

Phenol peels are used for deeper peels. In a fashion similar to TCA, phenol exerts its action by protein denaturation and coagulation; however, it quickly penetrates the skin to the level of the reticular dermis, thus requiring careful application. Serum phenol levels can quickly become elevated, resulting in systemic toxicity and cardiac arrhythmias. Phenol is partially detoxified in the liver followed by excretion by the kidneys. Therefore all patients must be cleared from a cardiac, renal, and hepatic standpoint preoperatively.

The percutaneous absorption of phenol is related to the body surface area treated, rather than the concentration used. To minimize toxicity, phenol peels are usually performed in small anatomic sections of the face with a fifteen-minute break before the application of the acid to the next anatomic unit. The face is usually treated in sections such as the forehead, right cheek, left cheek, nose and perioral, and the periorbital region. Intraoperative fluid hydration and cardiac monitoring are imperative.

Although any resurfacing modality that reaches the reticular dermis is at risk of causing permanent hypopigmentation, the traditional Baker-Gordon phenol peel resulted in an unacceptably high rate of permanent hypopigmentation, thus limiting its use to older, fair-skinned patients.

Weaker solutions of phenol (25 to 50%) can be used to achieve a lighter peel. However, the results are not better than TCA peels, and there still is a risk of systemic toxicity. Having said this, however, there are newer modifications of phenol peels in which the amount of croton oil has been reduced. This has dramatically reduced the amount of post-operative erythema, hypopigmentation, and scarring. Both Hetter and Stone independently described a modification of phenol peels that allows better control over depth of penetration. This has allowed patients with a variety of skin types to be treated with favorable results. While laser resurfacing with CO_2 and Er:YAG had largely replaced peels for the treatment of scars, the newer phenol peels are making a significant comeback.

Techniques

Glycolic Acid Exfoliation

It is important first to degrease the skin by cleansing it with alcohol or acetone, without vigorous rubbing. The glycolic acid, in concentrations of 50 to 70%, is used to coat the entire face quickly within fifteen to twenty seconds, using either gauze or a large cotton applicator. The application is timed so that the acid is left on for one to two minutes, then diluted with water or neutralized with sodium bicarbonate. The time of acid contact on the skin can be increased as tolerated in subsequent treatments. Caution is indicated when treating a patient using tretinoin or a topical alpha-hydroxy acid as the peel will penetrate much more quickly. These patients are better off starting with a thirty-second contact time and increasing it slowly at subsequent sessions.

While glycolic acid peels are considered light peels, unintended deeper peeling can occur if the acid is left on the skin for too long. A study has shown that 50 to 70% glycolic acid left in contact with the skin for fifteen minutes created a dermal wound identical to that seen with 35 to 50% trichloroacetic acid.

Salicylic Acid Exfoliation

Salicylic acid peels differ from glycolic acid peels in that there is no need to neutralize the peel. This increases the safety margin of this peel. Salicylic acid is also more lipophilic than glycolic acid. Thus it penetrates into acne lesions better than glycolic acid. Last, salicylic acid has anti-inflammatory properties, which make it better suited to treat inflammatory acne.

The peel is started first by degreasing the skin with acetone or alcohol. Salicylic acid in concentrations of 30 to 35% is applied evenly and washed off with water after six minutes. Since salicylic acid precipitates into a powder on the surface of the skin after solvent evaporation, it does not require neutralization. It is not unusual for the skin to tingle again once the skin is washed with water as some of the salicylic acid goes back into solution.

It is not recommended to apply salicylic acid peels to a large body surface area or under occlusion due to the real risk of developing salicylism. It is especially recommended that salicylic acid be avoided in pregnant females.

TCA Peels

TCA is usually used to peel to a depth greater than that of glycolic or salicylic acid. On application, TCA causes burning and stinging, which peaks in several minutes, then resolves. To reach the desired depth, however, several coats of TCA are usually required. This usually requires some type of anesthesia during the procedure.

Some physicians use electric fans or dynamic cooling units, which blow cold air onto the treated area. By far, patients receiving intramuscular or intravenous sedation tolerate the procedure better and allow the peel to proceed at a faster speed. Topical anesthesia does not offer enough pain relief once the peel exceeds the depth of the epidermis.

Monitoring of the intraoperative depth signs helps to gauge peel progression. All TCA peels will show these signs, but with stronger TCA peels or with well-conditioned skin, the signs will appear more quickly. Also, the use of Jessner's solution or glycolic acid peel prior to the application of the TCA will also speed up the penetration of the TCA; therefore physicians with minimal peeling experience are encouraged to start with relatively slower peeling techniques prior to proceeding to faster peels. This will help minimize the risk of penetrating deeper than expected. Anatomic variations in skin thickness must be a consideration with chemical peel resurfacing, just as with laser and dermabrasion.

Frosting is one of the first signs to appear as coagulation of epidermal and dermal proteins occurs. The frost starts off as light and nonorganized while the peel is epidermal in depth. As the peel progresses into the papillary dermis, the frost becomes a thin but even layer with a pink background (pink sign). The pink background is a sign that the superficial vascular plexus of the papillary dermis is still patent. The end point for the standard, papillary dermis–level peel is the level at which the pink sign is achieved, along with a thin, transparent, organized frost.

Continued application of the acid will result in vasospasm in the capillary loops of the papillary dermis. This will cause the blood flow in this area to cease and the pink background to disappear. The frost will appear as a solid white sheet (absence of the pink sign). A peel reaching this level implies that the whole papillary dermis is involved and the upper reticular dermis has been reached but not penetrated. This is the end point for a superficial reticular dermis peel. Since in darker-skinned individuals, the pink sign may be difficult to visualize, another sign, epidermal sliding, must be used to gauge depth.

Epidermal sliding indicates the point at which the peel has passed through the epidermis and entered the papillary dermis. Epidermal sliding refers to the exaggerated wrinkling of the skin when it is pushed or pinched, occurring when papillary dermal edema forms and disrupts the anchoring fibrils, thereby allowing the epidermis to move freely. This is only a transient sign and can be easily missed if attention is not paid to looking for it. This transient sign will disappear once the papillary dermis protein becomes coagulated and adherent to the epidermal coagulated proteins, indicating that the peel depth has reached the superficial reticular dermis. The pink background also disappears as the epidermal sliding sign disappears. In thick skin, epidermal sliding may not be very obvious, and the pink sign alone has to be used to indicate peel depth.

Further application of TCA will penetrate the reticular dermis. We recommend caution with performing peels to this level. At this point, the solid frost begins to take on a gray color. This is the maximum recommended depth for TCA peels. As with all resurfacing modalities that reach this depth, there is an increased incidence of scarring and hypopigmentation.

Intraoperative edema and protein coagulation give a gradual firmer texture to the skin, appreciated on pinching the skin. This textural change becomes more pronounced as the peel extends deeper or in patients with thick skin. Since firmness is a sign of peel depth, it is not present in superficial peels. Detecting the change in firmness intraoperatively is an acquired skill. All physicians are urged to develop this skill by assessing skin firmness in each peel performed.

Monheit's Jessner-TCA Peel

Monheit's Jessner-TCA peel is a medium-depth peel that employs a keratolytic agent prior to the application of the TCA. This peel emphasizes adequate degreasing of the skin, application of Jessner's solution, and the even application of a small volume of 35% TCA to create a light frost.

The facial skin is adequately degreased with gauze soaked with Septisol (Calgon Vestal Laboratories) then rinsed with water to allow for a more even peel. The face is further degreased by acetone. A 2 × 2 inch gauze or cotton-tipped applicator is used to apply Jessner's solution evenly, just enough to cause a very light frost. The 35% TCA is then applied to the skin in even strokes with either gauze or cotton-tipped applicators. It is important to allow the acid to neutralize prior to further application by waiting two to three minutes between applications. Any area that shows inadequate frosting can be retreated after a few minutes. To avoid lines of demarcation, the TCA should be feathered down along the jawline and should extend to the hairline.

Coleman's Glycolic Acid–TCA Peel

Coleman's glycolic acid–TCA peel, like Monheit's peel, is a medium-depth combination peel. The face is first cleansed with soap and water to degrease the skin. This is followed by the quick and even application of 70% unbuffered aqueous glycolic acid, which is left on for two minutes. It is then washed off with water to halt further penetration.

A small amount of 35% TCA is then applied to the skin in even strokes with gauze or cotton swabs. One should wait two to three minutes prior to retreating an area so that the TCA has fully penetrated.

Obagi's TCA–Blue Peel

The Obagi TCA–Blue Peel differs from the two previously mentioned peels as it does not start with a keratolytic step to alter the epidermal integrity prior to TCA application. The skin surface is gently cleansed with alcohol only; no further degreasing is necessary. The TCA–Blue Peel mixture is prepared immediately prior to use. The TCA–Blue Peel base (2 mL) is mixed with 2 mL of 30% TCA, to create a mixture of 15%; 4 mL of 30% TCA, to create a 20% solution; 6 mL of 30% TCA, to create a 22.5% solution; or 8 mL of 30% TCA, to create a 24% solution. The higher concentrations can be used, but only when the physician is more comfortable with skin peels. Both the 15% and 20% TCA–Blue Peel solutions are designed to be one coat that covers 5% of the body surface area (face or neck). In skin of normal thickness, it takes four coats of 15% TCA–Blue Peel to reach the papillary dermis, while it takes only two coats of the 20% mixture to reach the same depth. The number of coats must be tailored to skin thickness, with thinner skin requiring fewer coats and thicker skin requiring additional coats. The solution is applied evenly to the face, including the hairline, and is feathered down along the jawline. Any hair that is stained blue with the colored solution will return to its normal color after shampooing.

To allow the peel depth to be assessed, each coat is followed by a two- to three-minute waiting period before more TCA is applied. The end point of a papillary dermis peel is an even blue color, even frost, and pink background. If more TCA is applied, there will be a loss of the pink background, indicating penetration beyond the papillary dermis and into the superficial reticular dermis. This is the maximum recommended depth of a facial TCA–Blue Peel.

This peel can be used on the neck and chest, but caution is necessary as these areas are relatively poor in adnexal structures (needed for reepithelialization). Usually, one coat of 20% TCA–Blue Peel or two coats of 15% TCA–Blue Peel are evenly applied. The peel depth should be a continuum, with the deeper area up near the jawline and the lightest area down along the clavicles. This helps create a blending effect between the skin on the face and that on the chest.

HEALING AFTER CHEMICAL RESURFACING

Patients undergoing exfoliation with microdermabrasion, glycolic acid, or salicylic acid do not require any special home care regimen. Patients should expect a few days of flaking after each treatment. Rarely, patients may develop some crusting, which may be a sign of bacterial infection. This is easily treated with a nonneomycin containing topical antibiotic ointment three times a day until the crusting resolves. Patients should be encouraged to continue with their daily skin-conditioning regimens, or, if they do not tolerate this, a bland emollient for several days should suffice, along with a physical sunblock.

Regardless of which TCA peel is performed, home care regimens are identical. During the healing phase, patients can expect to look unsightly. The amount of swelling will vary among patients and is usually greatest in the periorbital area. Occasionally, this may be severe enough to warrant a short course of oral prednisone.

Patients will notice a progressive darkening and tightening of their skin into a masklike appearance with no associated pain. In fact, pain is usually a hallmark of infection or an area that has been traumatized. This must be addressed promptly. After four to five days, the skin will proceed to come off in sheets. Papillary dermis peels should heal in seven days, while peels reaching the superficial reticular dermis will take ten days to heal. Any healing time that is faster or more prolonged is a sign that the peel was either too superficial or too deep, respectively.

Starting the day after surgery, patients should cleanse their face twice a day with a mild cleanser, followed by the application of a cream such as Eucerin Cream (Beirsdorf Inc.), Cetaphil Cream (Galderma Laboratories Inc.), or Biafine (Ortho-Neutrogena). The goal of moisturization is to keep the skin slightly moist and comfortable. If patients feel excessive tightening of the skin, they should apply an ointment (Aquaphor Healing Ointment, Beirsdorf Inc.). The skin should be kept neither too dry nor too moist. All male patients should be encouraged to gently shave daily to minimize the risk of infection from beard hair.

Every four hours while awake, patients should perform compresses with an astringent solution (Domeboro Astringent Solution, Bayer Corp.), followed by reapplication of the emollient or ointment. Patients need to be instructed not to peel their skin prematurely as it may drive the wound deeper, uncover unhealed skin, and increase the risk for infection and scarring. If the skin is left to come off on its own, it will act as a bandage, which minimizes pain and the risk of infection. Patients can be given hydrocortisone 1% ointment to apply to pruritic areas if they arise. Patients should be encouraged to resume their skin-conditioning programs on reepithelialization of the skin. Absolute avoidance of sun exposure is recommended for the first four to six weeks postoperatively.

COMPLICATIONS OF SKIN RESURFACING

Skin-resurfacing risks and complications are identical whether they are from peels, lasers, or dermabrasion. Most of these complications, such as hypertrophic scarring, prolonged erythema (over three months), and pigmentary changes (Figure 74.1A), are related to wound depth and not specifically to the modality used. Other complications, such as infections and contact dermatitis, occur due to the impaired skin barrier function.

A good home hygiene regimen will help greatly reduce the risk of infection. This should minimize the need to use prophylactic antibiotics, which can alter the flora and favor the development of infection with less commonly seen bacteria such as *Pseudomonas aeruginosa* and other gram-negative organisms. Usually, infections are most commonly bacterial (*Staphylococcus aureus*), followed by yeast (*Candida*) or virus (HSV). Cultures and potassium hydroxide preps should be performed as indicated to identify the organism.

It is critical to recognize and treat an infection early to reduce the likelihood of scarring or delayed wound healing. Appropriate therapy should be directed at the most likely etiology while results are pending. Although the use of herpes prophylaxis has greatly decreased the incidence of viral infection, some patients can experience an outbreak even while on suppressive treatment. If a viral infection is suspected, patients should be treated with antiviral therapy dosed as if treating a herpes zoster infection (i.e., Valtrex 1 g three times a day for seven days).

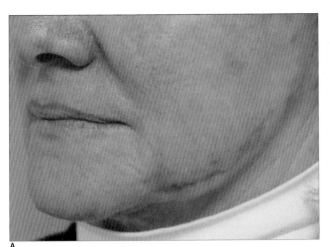
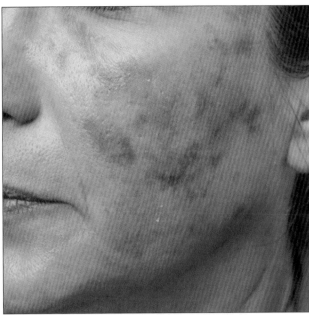

FIGURE 74.1: *Complications of chemical peeling.* **A**, *Hypertrophic scarring following chemical peel.* **B**, *Allergic contact dermatitis to propylene glycol.*

Allergic contact dermatitis to the postoperative skin care agents is oftentimes a challenging diagnosis (Figure 74.1B). Patients will usually complain of itching or burning of their skin, along with increased redness. These patients usually show normal wound healing until the allergic reaction occurs but then begin to show a setback in wound healing. The most likely culprits are propylene glycol or lanolins. One must rule out an early disseminated viral infection or *Candida*. If an allergic contact dermatitis is still the most likely diagnosis, the patient should stop all offending agents, cleanse the skin with water, and apply only white petrolatum to the skin. A topical midpotency steroid ointment can be used as long as it does not contain propylene glycol. These patients need to be followed every couple of days to monitor the wound-healing process.

Any procedure that reaches the reticular dermis, particularly true of aggressive phenol peels, can result in permanent hypopigmentation. While the color discrepancy may not be as apparent in lighter-skinned individuals, darker-skinned patients are more likely to notice any color discrepancy. Therefore patients of Fitzpatrick skin type III or greater should be warned of this possibility. This must be differentiated from the pseudo-hypopigmentation that is seen in photodamaged skin.

Postinflammatory hyperpigmentation, although transient, can overshadow the results of resurfacing. Thus it is better to anticipate this and treat it before it manifests by having patients resume their skin-reconditioning regimens once the wound has healed. However, if postinflammatory hyperpigmentation is difficult to clear with topical agents

alone, salicylic acid peels or microdermabrasion biweekly can help speed up resolution.

It is not unusual to see a flare of acne or rosacea postoperatively. Systemic anti-inflammatory antibiotics can help resolve the flare before scarring occurs. Systemic antibiotics (tetracycline, minocycline, doxycycline) should be used in combination with appropriate topical therapies.

Erythema lasting more than three weeks postoperatively is less common with peels than with laser resurfacing. It is seen commonly for several months following laser resurfacing, dermabrasion, and modified phenol peels. An area of persistent erythema is an ominous sign of an impending scar. This is more likely to occur in areas treated to the level of the reticular dermis or in areas that were traumatized during the wound-healing process. The treatment of this erythema consists of applying an ultrapotent topical steroid (betamethasone valerate, clobetasol, halobetasol, diflorasone) to the area two days out of each week for several weeks. Too much steroid use can have adverse effects; therefore close patient monitoring is needed. Flashlamp pulsed dye laser can be used for erythema that fails to respond to topical steroids. The goal with the pulsed dye laser is to treat at subpurpuric doses, but to treat frequently (every two to four weeks) until the erythema subsides.

One of the most dreaded complications of skin resurfacing is scarring. Scars can take a variety of morphologies such as atrophic, hypertrophic, or keloidlike. Oftentimes they are heralded by an area of pruritus, persistent erythema, delayed healing, or skin thickening. Early

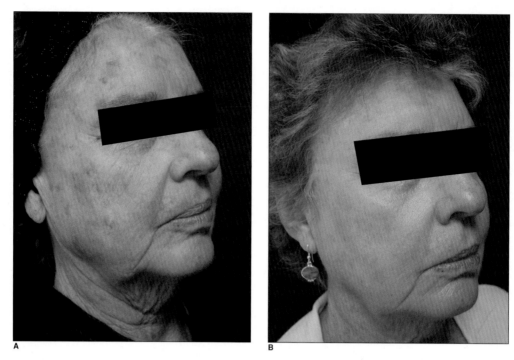

FIGURE 74.2: *Seventy-five-year-old female.* **A,** *Pretreatment.* **B,** *Three months post-QS-laser for lentigines and a Blue Peel to the level of the papillary dermis for skin tightening.*

detection and intervention is crucial. The area of impending scar formation should be treated with an ultrapotent topical steroid twice a day for three to four weeks. Care should be taken not to apply the steroid to normal skin as it may result in atrophy and telangiectasias. Intralesional steroid injections and manual massage should begin if the topical steroids fail to improve the scar. The thicker areas of the scar are injected at two- to four-week intervals with triamcinolone acetonide 1–10 mg/mL. The concentration used is based on scar thickness. Alternatively, a combination

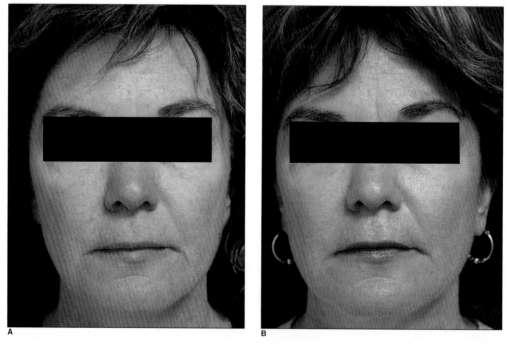

FIGURE 74.3: *Female patient.* **A,** *Pretreatment.* **B,** *Six weeks post–Blue Peel and upper blepharoplasty.*

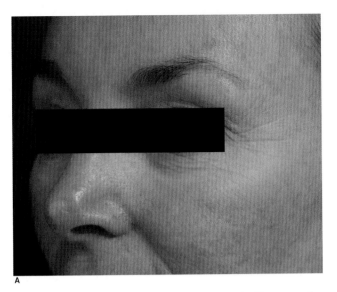
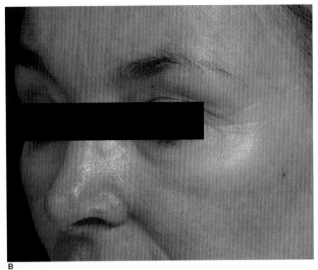

FIGURE 74.4: *Female patient.* **A**, *Pretreatment.* **B**, *Three months post–Blue Peel.*

of triamcinolone acetonide and 5-fluorouracil can be used. Some scars respond to flashlamp pulsed dye laser treatment performed biweekly at a low to moderate setting.

COMBINATION PROCEDURES

The art of chemical peeling is to be able to use it as a sole modality and, when needed, in combination with other resurfacing methods. Occasionally, patients will present with areas of focal scarring or deep rhytids. These patients benefit from a full-face, medium-depth peel in combination with a deeper resurfacing of the deeper defects. In these instances, the TCA peel is a great adjunct. In these cases, preoperative markings should be made to help demarcate the areas that will be treated more deeply from those to be treated more lightly. The peel should always be performed first, before any lasering or dermabrasion, to avoid having TCA penetrate the freshly resurfaced areas.

Light- to medium-depth peels can be performed during face lifts to safely improve skin appearance without compromising the flap. The peel should be performed after the face lift, with strict avoidance of the incisions. The peel should be of variable depth, with the deeper area in the central face (nonundermined skin), while becoming more superficial toward the lateral face. The maximum recommended depth of peels on undermined skin is the upper papillary dermis.

Approaching neck rejuvenation should be done with care as the neck has fewer adnexal structures, which are crucial to wound healing. Rather than a single deep peel, repeated papillary dermis–level peels at three-month intervals results in substantial improvement. More pronounced neck rhytids may benefit from a modified phenol peel using the Hetter VL formulation or from a series of minimally ablative fractional laser treatments.

CONCLUSION

Chemical peels are still an indispensable tool in skin rejuvenation (Figures 74.2–74.4). As laser technology has come and gone, peels have withstood the test of time. In fact, most physicians who regularly perform chemical peels would give up their skin resurfacing laser if they had to choose between peels or lasers. As with any procedure, optimizing results depends on proper procedure (or procedures) selection, proper patient evaluation, and the institution of appropriate skin care regimens.

SUGGESTED READING

Brody HJ, ed. *Chemical Peeling and Resurfacing*. 2nd ed. St. Louis: Mosby; 1997.

Coleman WP III, Futrell JM. The glycolic acid trichloroacetic acid peel. *J. Dermatol. Surg. Oncol.* 1994;20:76–80.

Hetter G. Examination of the phenol-croton oil peel: part IV. Face peel results with different concentrations of phenol and croton oil. *Plast. Reconstr. Surg.* 2001;105:1061–83.

Landau M. Cardiac complications in deep chemical peels. *Dermatol. Surg.* 2007;33:190–3; discussion 193.

Monheit, GD. The Jessner's-trichloroacetic acid peel: an enhanced medium-depth chemical peel. *Dermatol. Clin.* 1995; 13:277–83.

Obagi S. Pre- and postlaser skin care. *Oral Maxillofac. Surg. Clin. North Am.* 2004;16:181–7.

Obagi S, Obagi Z, Bridenstine JB. Isotretinoin use during chemical skin resurfacing: a review of complications. *Am. J. Cosmet. Surg.* 2002;19: 9–13.

Obagi ZE, ed. *Obagi Skin Health Restoration and Rejuvenation*. New York: Springer; 2000.

Obagi Z, Obagi S. Pearls for successful chemical peeling. *Cosmet. Dermatol.* 2004;17:363–71.

Obagi Z, Obagi S, Alaiti S, Stevens M. TCA-based Blue Peel: a standardized procedure with depth control. *Dermatol. Surg.* 1999;25:773–80.

Resnik SS, Resnik BI. Complications of chemical peeling. *Dermatol. Clin.* 1995;13:309–12.

Rullan PP, Lemon J, Rullan J. The 2-day light phenol chemabrasion for deep wrinkles and acne scars: a presentation of face and neck peels. *Am. J. Cosmet. Surg.* 2004;21:15–26.

Spencer L, Obagi S. Cosmetic dermatologic skincare: the essence of our training. *Cosmet. Dermatol.* 2007; 20: 663–9.

CHAPTER 75

Peeling Techniques from Europe

Michel Delune

Peels are one of the most popular cosmetic procedures you have to perform if your clinic is aesthetics oriented. Your patients will enjoy the procedure because it is cheap and the downtime can be adjusted to match the patient's social life. Nevertheless, you have to follow some basic but essential rules to ensure your patient's safety and avoid peeling complications such as postinflammatory hyperpigmentation (PIH) and hypertrophic scars.

First of all, why should one choose the peel from so many cosmetic procedures? The selection of a cosmetic procedure depends on multiple factors such as the goal of the procedure, the downtime your patient is willing to endure, the body area to be treated, the patient's skin type, the safety of the procedure, your own skill with the technique, and many other factors.

A chemical peel can be very superficial, with only a light exfoliation of the epidermis. It can also be deeper and penetrate to the mid- and deep dermis for severe acne scars or skin rejuvenation. Microdermabrasion is usually performed for epidermal damage only when dermabrasion will treat deep scars and severe signs of skin aging.

The skin improvement obtained with lasers or intense pulsed light (IPL) is often very outstanding, but it requires a very important investment for the practitioner. Moreover, technology is moving so fast that your laser or IPL unit will become obsolete before you finish paying for it, and this kind of device has no or a very poor secondhand market. Considering all these aspects, chemical peels remain a very valuable choice for the benefit of the patient.

The main goals and indications for a chemical peel are as follows:

- to exfoliate the superficial layers of the stratum corneum, improving skin brightness

- to treat superficial and moderate signs of intrinsic skin aging

- to take care of sun-damaged skin in treating fine lines and wrinkles

- to resolve pigmentary disorders associated with photo-damage and some skin types such as Asian and Hispanic skin

- to remove acne scars and even the skin surface

- to tighten loose skin and close enlarged pores

Pre- and postpeel skin conditioning is essential to prevent complications such as PIH and scarring. Moreover, it will speed up the healing process and give faster and better results. Skin conditioning has to be started six weeks before the peel and should be resumed for another four weeks at the end of the healing process. Skin conditioning is the workout of the skin. The goal of prepeel skin conditioning is to bring the skin to its best condition so that it can perfectly fulfill its job by the time of the procedure. Skin conditioning concerns both the epidermis and dermis. Epidermal targets are keratinocytes and melanocytes, while dermal targets are fibroblasts and dermal vascularization. The patient will have to follow several steps back to back, morning and night:

- *Step 1 – Preparation of the skin*: The goal of this step is to make the skin ready to receive active ingredients. It is a very easy step, using a cleanser, followed by a toner. A topical antibiotic might be added if the patient shows signs of active acne.

- *Step 2 – Melanocyte management*: At this stage, we want to prevent any PIH and to treat superficial pigmentary disorders. It is now the right time to use a bleaching agent such as hydroquinone (4 to 6%) or a hydroquinone substitute, such as arbutine, licorice, or azelaic acid.

- *Step 3 – Exfoliation of the skin*: We want to exfoliate the skin to regulate the keratinocyte cycle and to remove the dead cells of the stratum corneum. The most common exfoliating agents are fruity acids, mainly glycolic acid, to be used in a 4 to 6% solution. Should the patient complain about the dryness and sometimes severe exfoliation generated by glycolic acid, you can either mix it half-half with an aloe vera–based moisturizer or replace glycolic acid with phytic acid, which is less of an irritant.

- *Step 4 – Fibroblast activity stimulation and dermal vascularization improvement*: This step is essential to stimulating elastin and collagen fiber production and to having more glycoaminoglycans in the dermis to match the patient's skin needs. The best agent to use for this step is retinoic acid in a concentration to adapt to the skin's damage (0.05 to 0.1%). Finally, a combination of retinoic acid and hydroquinone can give a very nice blending effect, if needed.

WHAT PEELING SOLUTION TO CHOOSE?

There are so many peeling solutions on the market today that it could be quite difficult for a beginner to make the right choice. The choice has to be based on two basic rules: how deep do you want to go, and what kind of downtime will be acceptable for the patient? If you want to treat deep acne scars or severe photodamage, you will have to penetrate the dermis. If you want to improve skin brightness and very superficial lines, you can stay epidermal. Should your patient be ready for a ten- to fourteen-day downtime, you can go deep; if he or she wants a short downtime, you cannot.

The question is, do we really need so many different peeling solutions in our cosmetic practices? My answer is definitely no. Let me share with you the way I make my decision, which is based on the depth I want to reach:

- *Superficial epidermal exfoliation*: glycolic acid peel in a light concentration (20 to 35%)
  - *Main indication*: skin refreshment and skin brightness improvement
  - *Downtime*: twenty-four to forty-eight hours
- *Mid- and deep epidermis*: glycolic acid (50 to 70%) or modified trichloroacetic acid (TCA) 15%
  - *Main indication*: fine lines, epidermal melasma, open pores
  - *Downtime*: three to five days
- *Upper dermis*: modified TCA 15 to 20%
  - *Main indication*: photodamage, pigmentary disorders, fine lines and wrinkles, superficial and moderate acne scars, enlarged skin pores
  - Downtime: five to eight days
- *Deep dermis*: plain TCA 30% or modified phenol
  - *Main indication*: severe photoaging, deep acne scars, loose skin, uneven skin surface
  - *Downtime*: ten to fourteen days

In case of acne, I will use a salicylic acid peel (20 to 30%) with a downtime of two to four days. This choice is dictated by the fact that salicylic acid has a very strong keratolytic and sebostatic effect, which is essential for acne management.

PEELING TECHNIQUE

Regardless of the peeling solution you intend to use, it is essential to consider the two following points.

Do I Need to Neutralize the Peel, or Is It a Self-Neutralizing Peel?

In the previous peeling agent list, the only one that needs to be neutralized is the glycolic acid peel. Most glycolic acid brands have their own postpeel neutralizers, which I suggest you use. Otherwise, you can use plain water. All other mentioned peels are self-neutralizing.

What Are My End Points?

Each peeling solution has its own end points, which you have to know before you start. I strongly recommend reading the manufacturer's instructions to be sure you understand when to stop your peeling application. If you are relatively inexperienced with peels, seek a hands-on demonstration, especially with deeper peels.

FREQUENTLY ASKED QUESTIONS ABOUT PEELING TECHNIQUE

- How many coats should be applied?
  - What is important is not the number of coats, but the observation of your end points. As soon as you begin to reach them, stop applying the solution and neutralize it right away (only if you use glycolic acid).
- How is the peeling solution applied?
  - You have to follow your road map. I always start on the forehead, followed by the left cheek, the chin, the right cheek, the nose's wings, the upper lip, and the eyelids.
  - Follow the manufacturer's instructions to learn if you have to use Q-tips or a brush or gauze.
- When can I perform the next peel?
  - The deeper you go, the longer the healing process will be. You can perform a superficial peel every other week, whereas you have to wait at least three months between two deep peels.
- What is the difference between a conventional and a modified TCA peel?
  - A conventional TCA peel will penetrate faster and deeper into the skin, making your peeling management more difficult and risky, with a higher risk of potential complications.
  - A modified TCA peel is made of conventional TCA plus a base made of different ingredients, slowing down

the speed of penetration of the TCA and allowing you to observe your end points.

- What are the most common end points?
  - Depending on your peeling solution, it can be frost, erythema, microcrystals, or epidermal sliding. Please refer to the manufacturer's instructions, or better yet, observe someone experienced with that particular peel perform it.

POSTPEEL CARE

You are not done with your patient when the peeling procedure is over. Postpeel management is essential to prevent complications.

Basic postpeel care is to apply a moisturizer three times a day after having cleaned the skin very gently with a soft cleanser. You have to inform your patient that he or she will be ugly for a couple days, with some swelling and darker spots on the skin. He or she will start to peel around the mouth, and you have to teach the patient not to pick. Should the patient have a history of cold sores, do not forget to give him or her acyclovir or comparable antivirals, as a prevention, to be started three days before the peel and continued five days after the peel. Always follow the basic principle in dermatology: if the skin is becoming wet, you have to dry it; if the skin is becoming dry, you have to moisturize it.

In case of oozing, ask your patient to apply compresses loaded with a solution of aluminium acetate. If your patient comes back with very thick scabs, apply additional moisturizer and be very cautious in removing the scabs, and avoid pulling them off. Teach your patient how essential sun protection is, as well.

RESULTS

In my experience, the best results I have obtained with peels were for pigmentary disorder management, fine lines and wrinkles, acne scars, photoaging, and loose skin.

I have to make special mention about combined procedures such as a face lift plus peeling. A peel will never replace a face lift but can be a very nice complement to the surgery. We know very well that surgical face rejuvenation will work on the muscles and excess skin, while peels will work on skin structure. Another nice example of combined procedures is to touch up the results of a peel with fillers to treat deep wrinkles and BOTOX for expression lines.

CONCLUSION

Chemical peeling is a wonderful tool to use in any cosmetic practice. It is very cheap for the patient who cannot afford other techniques such as laser and IPL or cosmetic surgery. It is safe, as long as you follow the basic rules, as explained in this chapter.

Never rush while performing a peel. Also, do not give false hope to your patient; let your patient know if he or she has unrealistic expectations. Finally, be safe.

Section 3

MESOTHERAPY: INJECTION LIPOLYSIS

CHAPTER 76

Mesotherapy: Injection Lipolysis

Adam M. Rotunda

The term *injection lipolysis*, which is most popularly ascribed, suggests injectable methods which "activate" adipocytes to mobilize their fatty acid stores without affecting the integrity of their cell membranes. The focus of this chapter and indeed the preponderance of literature on the subject of injectable treatments for fat relate to agents that *completely ablate* or *destroy fat by breaking down or solubilizing the fat cell membrane*. Adipolytic therapy is therefore a technique that describes the subcutaneous injection of pharmacologically active detergents to chemically ablate localized adipose tissue. In addition to *injection lipolysis*, numerous names have been ascribed to the technique, including *mesotherapy*, *Lipodissolve®*, and *mesolipolysis*. It has therefore been proposed that the terms *injection adipolysis* or *adipolytic therapy* most accurately describe injectable methods that employ detergents to reduce fat. The most well studied component of these treatments is sodium deoxycholate (DC), a biologic detergent. Unless noted elsewhere, this compound is present in all formulations that include phosphatidylcholine (PC)

To date, no European or United States regulatory body has approved a pharmaceutical grade, subcutaneously injected preparation indicated to treat fat. As such, there are neither standardized practices, nor formal teaching of the technique in post-graduate residency training programs. Therefore, physicians worldwide have been teaching one another through continuing education conferences or peer-reviewed publications. In the US, the most commonly used agents, phosphatidylcholine (PC) and deoxycholate

(DC), are typically obtained from compounding pharmacies. In Europe, Lipostabil®, Sanofi-Aventis, is commonly used. It is imperative that treating physicians inquire about the status of this procedure with their malpractice carrier, and become informed (and likewise appropriately consent patients) of the literature, risks, benefits, and alternatives of this (as of yet) unapproved practice.

RECENT BEGINNINGS

PC for localized fat ablation emerged on the international scene after Patricia Rittes, a dermatologist in São Paolo, Brazil, published her findings using Lipostabil transcutaneously into infraorbital fat pads. The results were significant – "cosmetic improvement occurred in all patients" – as were the accompanying photographs. Similar outcomes have been replicated in two additional studies by independent authors.

PC

PC is a soy-derived phospholipid composing about 40% of the mammalian cell membrane, forming lipid bilayers that protect the cell from its environment. PC is water-insoluble, and thus aqueous (injectable) PC solutions require a solvent (commonly, DC) to dissolve PC in water. Lipostabil was manufactured by Natterman International GMBH in Europe and consisted of PC (5%), DC (2.5%), and minute quantities of dl-alpha-tocopherol (vitamin E),

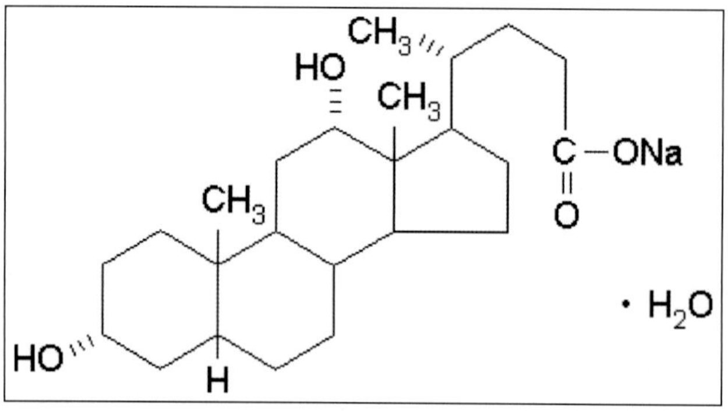

FIGURE 76.1: *Chemical structure of sodium deoxycholate.*

sodium hydroxide, ethanol, and benzyl alcohol, in sterile water. This medication is approved in European countries as Lipostabil N (Sanofi-Aventis), indicated for intravenous delivery as a treatment for dyslipidemia, for fat emboli, and as an anticirrhotic because of PC's serum lipid–reducing and hepatic antifibrotic effects.

Rittes and a growing consortium of physicians who share their experiences at international conferences and in the literature have used the PC formulation (as Lipostabil or compounded formulations) to treat localized fat deposits, including lipomas; so-called buffalo humps; jowls; and submental, truncal, and extremity fat. While instructive and, to a large degree, responsible for the popularity of the treatment, these innovators' experiences and data require confirmation by controlled, randomized, double-blind studies to enact wider acceptance in the medical community.

PC has long been speculated to be the active ingredient in adipolytic therapy. It was assumed that PC's effects of lowering lipids in serum could account for its effect subcutaneously. As of this writing, this theory has not been verified. There is no evidence (experimentally or clinically) to support the lipolytic effects of PC alone (without DC) in subcutaneous tissue. In fact, the most recent peer-reviewed evidence suggests that DC is the major, if not the only, agent responsible for the fat-ablative effects in adipolytic therapy.

DC

DC (Figure 76.1) has been used by investigators as a laboratory detergent for decades and by pharmaceutical companies as a physiologically compatible solvent for intravenous formulations, including Amphocin (Pfizer) and Lipostabil. DC is a secondary bile acid produced by intestinal bacteria after the release of primary bile acids (i.e., cholic acid) in the liver. Bile acids are stored in the gall bladder and secreted into the duodenum, where various free and conjugated bile acids function as detergents to solubilize ingested lipids. A majority (90 to 95%) of DC is subsequently reabsorbed, but the amount that is excreted can be replaced by ab initio synthesis from cholesterol in the liver. As bile acids

are end products of cholesterol, they are not subsequently degraded into other catabolites. Approximately 1 g of DC is present at any time in an adult human, confined mostly to the enterohepatic circulation. However, DC is present in the peripheral blood (estimated at 0.56 μmol/L) and can be elevated in patients with certain liver conditions or after surgery.

Clinical experience with a pharmacy-compounded DC without PC was recently published. Six subjects with one or more lipomas (1–4 cm) had between one and four intralesional injections of DC at various concentrations (1%, 2.5%, or 5%), at various treatment intervals (between two weeks and six months). Although the study was open-label and dosing was not standardized, all treated lipomas decreased in area in a range from 37% to 100%. Activity was seen with as little as one injection and at the lowest concentration of DC (1%). Results of a randomized, double-blind, clinical trial comparing the safety and efficacy of a PC-DC formulation versus a DC-only formulation for submental fat revealed no significant differences between the two treatments. These data suggest that PC may not be necessary for fat ablation and, furthermore, does not confer any clinical benefit (i.e., reduction of adverse events).

Histology of animal and human tissue exposed to DC as well as PC-DC combinations demonstrates cell lysis, acute inflammation, and necrosis. Despite these untoward effects microscopically, there are no published reports describing surface irregularities, contracture, dimpling, or necrosis. No laboratory abnormalities have been described in patients receiving DC or PC-DC formulations. There are reports of gastrointestinal discomfort (including nausea, vomiting, and diarrhea) in patients receiving high volumes of PC-DC, which is consistent with the adverse events described in the *Physician's Desk Reference* for oral PC. It may be that bolus administration of PC subcutaneously (at doses lower than those orally) stimulates these cholinergic reactions, but additional safety testing is required to verify this theory. Although most of the subsequent discussion is applicable to any adipolytic therapy technique (i.e., using PC-DC combinations or DC alone), specific guidelines on medication preparation will assume that PC is not used.

INDICATIONS AND PATIENT SELECTION

Indications

Indications are relatively small, localized fat deposits on the trunk and/or extremities; especially responsive are the upper posterior arms, lateral waist, outer hips, upper back (bra strap fat), and submental (anterior neck) fat (Figures 76.2 and 76.3). Anecdotally, fat on the inner or anterior thighs and lower legs is best not treated. Patients considered candidates for liposuction are not candidates for adipolytic therapy. Both the patient and physician should be realistic that these treatments are not a replacement for liposuction.

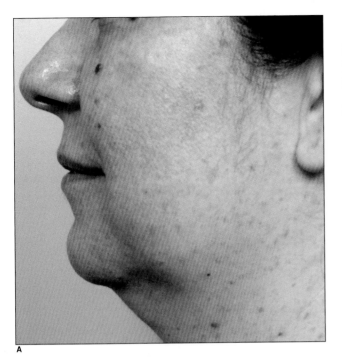
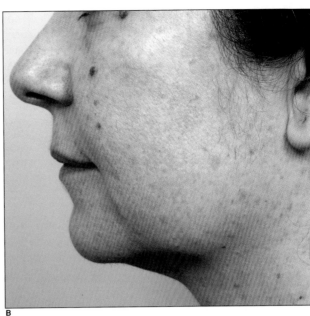

Figure 76.2: **A,** *Profile of subject at baseline.* **B,** *Same subject two months after five monthly, 1-mL subcutaneous injections of 1% deoxycholate into the submental fat.*

Dimpling and irregularity after liposuction are good indications for the procedure, where repeat liposuction would otherwise not be considered desirable.

Patients often inquire whether the effects are permanent. Just as liposuction-aspirated fat will not regrow, chemically ablated fat cells will not return. Yet, neither technique eliminates completely all the fat in the target areas; fat may recur in the treated site should the patient gain weight.

Selection Demographics

Males or females between the ages of eighteen and seventy-five years can be treated. Body mass index should be less

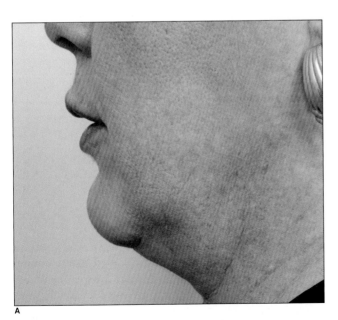
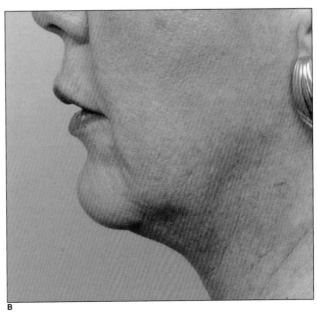

FIGURE 76.3: **A,** *Profile of subject at baseline.* **B,** *Same subject two months after five monthly, 1-mL subcutaneous injections of 1% deoxycholate into the submental fat.*

than 28. Patient should have maintained a stable body weight for the last six months (i.e., plus or minus 5% of initial consultation weight). Serum studies are usually not necessary, unless, during the initial screening, the patient reports a comorbid medical condition. Patients should have normal blood counts, serum lipids, and liver and renal function.

Ethical Considerations

The patient or his or her legally authorized representative should read, comprehend, and sign an informed consent before any study-specific screening or treatment is conducted.

Contraindications

Female patients who are pregnant, breast-feeding, or of childbearing potential who are not observing adequate contraceptive precautions during the treatment are contraindicated. Patients with significant overlying skin laxity, photodamage, inflammatory dermatoses (any sites), or platysmal banding (submental) are also contraindicated. Prior cholecystectomy or current liver disease, including acute or chronic hepatitis, cirrhosis, and so on, eliminates candidacy for the treatment, as does a known bleeding or coagulation disorder and known seropositivity to HIV. History of or current respiratory, cardiovascular, or neurological disease; uncontrolled hypertension; or other medical conditions; and psychiatric, addictive, or other disorders that would compromise the ability of the patient to give informed consent and/or comply with multiple treatments serve as contraindications. Patients currently taking (or within two weeks) oral anticoagulants (e.g., Coumadin, aspirin intake greater than 81 mg/day) should be warned about increased ecchymosis risk or possible hematomas at injection sites. Patients currently taking bile acid sequestrants (e.g., cholestyramine and colestipol) or with a known sensitivity to any components of the medication (i.e., lidocaine) are contraindicated. Darkly pigmented skin types (i.e., Fitzpatrick types IV–VI) are at increased risk for postinflammatory hyperpigmentation; keloid or hypertrophic scar–prone patients should be forewarned. Inability to appreciate that multiple visits (typically two to three monthly treatments) are necessary before patients see and/or feel a local change in the volume of the treated area also contraindicates a patient.

TREATMENT PROTOCOL

Materials required include the following:

1. 30-gauge, 0.5-inch needles for injection and 18-gauge, 1-inch needles for withdrawing medication

2. depending on the total volume, several 1-, 3-, or 5-mL syringe(s); even if larger volumes are used, multiple 5-mL syringes are preferred since high thumb pressures are required for a 10-mL syringe; for this reason, pneumatic or electronic handheld mesoguns are available, but they are relatively costly

3. surgical marking or eyeliner pen for mapping of injection sites

4. isopropyl alcohol with cotton/gauze

5. sodium deoxycholate (1%, 10 mg/mL) in sterile water (i.e., water for injection with 0.9% benzyl alcohol)

6. lidocaine (1%) without epinephrine

The DC and lidocaine are mixed prior to injecting. A 3:1 ratio of DC and lidocaine is drawn into the same syringe (i.e., 0.75 mL or 3.75 mL of DC is mixed with 0.75 mL or 1.25 mL of lidocaine for a total volume of 1.0 mL or 5.0 mL, respectively). A white precipitate may become evident transiently but should resolubilize spontaneously or with a gentle mix of the syringe. It is unadvisable to order premixed compounded medication; the stability and activity of these solutions are not currently known.

Patients are made comfortable either sitting upright or lying down, and the treatment site is exposed. Topical anesthetic is usually not used, but this can be offered to the patient. Once the skin is cleaned thoroughly with alcohol and marked according to the subsequent spacing guidelines, the site is injected.

Volume and spacing of injections depend on the anatomic site treated. Specifically,

1. Truncal fat and extremity fat (i.e., abdomen, waist, posterior upper arms, bra strap fat [posterior upper back]): 0.4-mL solution spaced 1.5 cm apart

2. Submental or facial (jowls) fat: 0.25- to 0.33-mL solution spaced 1 cm apart (Figure 76.4)

3. Lipomas: with the first injection starting at one end of the lipoma, 0.4 mL of solution is injected every 1.5 cm

4. Liposuction contour irregularities: 0.4 mL of solution is injected every 1.5 cm into the protuberant fat

The injection depth is midsubcutaneous to circumvent migration of the solution into the dermis above and the fascia below. For lipomas, the needle is directed into the middle of lipomas. The skin may be pinched for more accurate needle placement.

Patients are treated typically every four weeks, although some authors recommend as short as two and as long as eight weeks between sessions. A standard treatment regimen is four to six consecutive sessions (or less, depending on the patient's response), and final evaluation is performed two months after the last session (to allow for

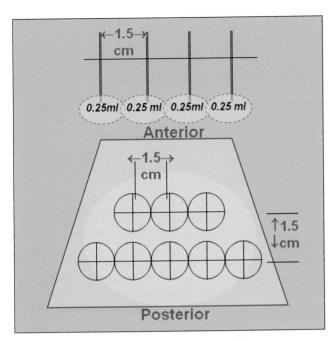

FIGURE 76.4: *Injection pattern for submental fat.*

residual swelling to subside). Generally, several treatments are required before results are seen or felt by the patient.

Total volume injected per session is patient-dependent, as it varies per site and surface area. In general, patients should have a maximum of two sites (i.e., both arms and both thighs) treated per session to minimize patient discomfort and overall dose. Using the mixing protocol described previously, a patient may receive upward of 40 mL if multiple sites are injected per treatment (i.e., 10 mL into each hip, 10 mL into each arm), but as little as several milliliters should the submentum or a lipoma be treated.

Evaluation

Pre- and posttreatment photography, circumferential measurements (where applicable), and patient feedback are used to assess results. However, photography cannot convey the desired "firmer, tighter" sensation most patients experience after treatment. Comparing the photographs of pre- and posttreatment profiles with patients is a useful and gratifying exercise.

AFTERCARE

Immediate

The injected site should be monitored for several minutes so that pressure can be applied to minor injection site bleeding. Cleanse the injected area with isopropyl

alcohol or hydrogen peroxide to remove residual bleeding and/or pen marks. Use of a cold pack may comfort some patients.

At Home

The patient is instructed to continue cold pack care on the hour for ten minutes over the next several hours and, if necessary, to take extra strength acetaminophen (no NSAIDs) if there is persistent discomfort. Patients should use sunblock or completely avoid sun exposure in the injected site for up to three days after treatment. Some clinicians recommend that pressure garments similar to those worn after liposuction be worn for three to five days, especially for truncal treatments.

ANTICIPATED ADVERSE EVENTS

Local Effects

Immediately after Injection to Day 1

Some patients experience mild tenderness, burning, or itching. Most patients do not feel discomfort aside from mild to moderate focal tenderness once the effect of the anesthesia subsides (approximately one hour). Erythema and moderate edema will persist.

Days 2–3

Edema will be moderate to significant, as will focal tenderness, although erythema will dissipate after this time period. The swelling is often described by patients as "jellylike." Cutaneous anesthesia may begin and persist until most of the swelling subsides. Patients should be reassured that a majority of swelling subsides after three days. Patients may experience some ecchymoses at this time, which may fade slowly over the week. First treatments are best performed immediately prior to a weekend of social inactivity. After the first treatment, patients will know what to expect and are usually comforted to know that the reactions after subsequent treatment are often less apparent (should similar volumes be injected).

Day 3 to One Week

Tenderness and edema gradually resolve, but may persist to a milder degree, along with superficial anesthesia, beyond this period.

Weeks 2–4 and Beyond

Most anticipated adverse events have passed at this point, although a firm, minimally tender, subcutaneous nodule ("raisin") may be felt at the injection site. Patients are reassured that the nodule is ablated fat that will disappear slowly as the site recovers. Rarely, localized nodularity persists beyond four to six weeks.

Systemic Effects

Despite significant volumes per session (60 mL and more total) using the DC-lidocaine described previously, the author has never had a patient experience gastrointestinal or other effects described by some authors in patients injected with PC-DC combinations of less volume. Nevertheless, as rigorous safety data have not been published, it is prudent to remain conservative in total dose. Published and ongoing studies with DC alone (as well as PC-DC) reveal no systemic alterations in serum chemistries, lipids, or blood counts at these doses.

PREVENTING AND TREATING COMPLICATIONS

The adverse events described are expected and should be explained as such to the patient before the procedure and as a reminder throughout the treatment course. These effects are consistent between hundreds of patients, whether the clinician uses DC-lidocaine or PC-DC formulations. The reactions are likely a by-product of the detergent (necrotic) effects of DC on the adipose tissue, release of cellular debris, influx of inflammatory mediators, and subsequent host repair.

Despite a (yet undefined) degree of detergent migration, and evidence for muscle and collagen necrosis in vitro microscopically, there are no reports of adverse events related to muscle weakness or other deep soft tissue damage. Perhaps this is due to dilution of the medication in vivo, or the relative selectivity of the detergent toward fat. However, the author is aware of several anecdotal incidents of dermal necrosis leading to superficial ulceration, likely a result of inadvertent superficial injection. Properly placed and dosed medication will significantly reduce the risk of necrosis.

Hyperpigmentation has been reported and is likely due to too superficial an injection and/or too large a volume injected per site. The brisk inflammatory reaction will lead to postinflammatory pigmentation in darker skin types or those who do not take proper precautions (such as sun avoidance) after the treatment.

Ecchymoses are more likely to occur in patients on blood thinners of any type (pharmaceutical or over the counter) but are potential risks for any patient.

Persistent nodularity (longer than two months) is more likely to occur in patients receiving multiple high-volume injections in the same location. The author has not witnessed any patient with permanent nodularity; it is unknown at this point whether intralesional steroids or hyaluronidase, treatments offered by some clinicians, are effective. Patience, reassurance, and regular follow-up

visits until disappearance of the nodules have been the rule.

CONCLUSION

The concept of injectable fat loss has inspired numerous reports (in peer-reviewed literature as well as the lay press), although the procedure is still considered fringe and is viewed with skepticism by many. The outcome of standardized, placebo-controlled studies will ultimately determine whether it becomes an accepted therapeutic option for localized fat. Furthermore, only through the standard rigor required for regulatory submission and approval will this procedure ever truly be considered safe and effective for the desired indication.

Should this chapter have been a practical introduction that motivates you to consider this technique, it cannot be emphasized enough that managing patient expectations is critical to the satisfied patient (and, by extension, physician). It is the author's experience that ill-conceived expectations (based on the assumption that the photographs depicting dramatic before and after results in now infamous mesotherapy marketing campaigns are true) will limit patient satisfaction. Selection of only those very healthy, physically fit, and patient patients is the most prudent way to explore this novel technique.

SUGGESTED READING

Ablon G, Rotunda AM. Treatment of lower eyelid fat pads using phosphatidylcholine: clinical trial and review. *Dermatol. Surg.* 2004;30:422–8.

Atiyeh BS, Ibrahim AE, Dibo SA. Cosmetic mesotherapy: between scientific evidence, science fiction, and lucrative business. *Aesth. Plast. Surg.* 2008;32:842–9.

Bahar RJ. Bile acid transport. *Gastroenterol. Clin. North Am.* 1999;28:27–58.

Bechara FG, Sand M, Altmeyer P, Hoffmann K. Intralesional lipolysis with phosphatidylcholine for the treatment of lipomas: pilot study. *Arch. Dermatol.* 2006;142:1069–70.

Duncan D, Hasengschwandtner F. Lipodissolve for subcutaneous fat reduction and skin retraction. *Aesthetic Surg. J.* 2005;25:530–43.

Duncan D, Rubin JP, Golitz L, et al. Refinement of technique in injection lipolysis based on scientific studies and clinical evaluation. *Clin. Plast. Surg.* 2009;36:195–209.

Hasengschwandtner F. The non-surgical liposculpture. *J. Cosmet. Dermatol.* 2005;4:310–15.

Hasengschwandtner F. Injection lipolysis for effective reduction of localized fat in place of minor surgical lipoplasty. *Aesthetic Surg. J.* 2006;26:125–30.

Hexsel D, Serra M, Mazzuco R, Dal'Forno T, Zechmeister D. Phosphatidylcholine in the treatment of localized fat. *J. Drugs Dermatol.* 2003;2:511–18.

Jones MN. Surfactants in membrane solubilisation. *Int. J. Pharm.* 1999;177:137–59.

Klimov AM, Konstantinov VO, Lipovetsky BM, et al. Essential phospholipids versus nicotinic acid in the treatment of patients with type IIb hyperlipoproteinemia and ischemic heart disease. *Cardiovasc. Drugs Ther.* 1995;9:779–84.

Kopera D, Binder B, Toplak H, Kerl H, Cerroni L. Histopathologic changes after intralesional application of phosphatidylcholine for lipoma reduction: report of a case. *Am. J. Dermatopathol.* 2006;28:331–3.

Lieber CS, Weiss DG, Groszmann R, et al. Veteran Affairs Cooperative Study of the polyenylphosphatidylcholine in alcoholic liver disease. *Alcohol Clin. Exp. Res.* 2003;27:1765–72.

Motolese P. Phospholipids do not have lipolytic activity. A critical review. *J Cosmet. Laser. Ther.* 2008;10:114–8.

Myers P. The cosmetic use of phosphatidylcholine in the treatment of localized fat. *J. Cosmet. Dermatol.* 2006;19:416–20.

Odo MEY, Cuce LC, Odo LM, Natrielli A. Action of sodium deoxycholate on subcutaneous human tissue: local and systemic effects. *Dermatol. Surg.* 2007;33:178–89.

Palmer M, Curran J, Bowler P. Clinical experience and safety using phosphatidylcholine injections for the localized reduction of subcutaneous fat: a multicentre, retrospective UK study. *J. Cosmet. Dermatol.* 2006;5:218–26.

Rittes PG. The use of phosphatidylcholine for correction of lower lid bulging due to prominent fat pads. *Dermatol. Surg.* 2001;27:391–2.

Rittes PG. The use of phosphatidylcholine for correction of localized fat deposits. *Aesthetic Plast. Surg.* 2003;27:315–18.

Rose PT, Morgan M. Histological changes associated with mesotherapy for fat dissolution. *J. Cosmet. Laser Ther.* 2005;7:17–19.

Rotunda AM, Ablon G, Kolodney MS. Lipomas treated with subcutaneous deoxycholate injections. *J. Am. Acad. Dermatol.* 2005;53:973–8.

Rotunda AM, Avram MM. The importance of caution in the use of unregulated anticellulite treatments. *Arch Dermatol.* 2009;145:337.

Rotunda AM, Kolodney MS. Mesotherapy and phosphatidylcholine injections: historical clarification and review. *Dermatol. Surg.* 2006;32:465–80.

Rotunda AM, Suzuki H, Moy RL, Kolodney MS. Detergent effects of sodium deoxycholate are a major feature of an injectable phosphatidylcholine formulation used for localized fat dissolution. *Dermatol. Surg.* 2004;30:1001–8.

Rotunda AM, Weiss SR, Rivkin LS. Randomized double-blind clinical trial of subcutaneously injected deoxycholate versus a phosphatidylcholine-deoxycholate combination for the reduction of submental fat. *Dermatol. Surg.* 2009;35:792–803.

Salles AG, Valler CS, Ferreira MC. Histologic response to injected phosphatidylcholine in fat tissue: experimental study in a new rabbit model. *Aesthetic Plast. Surg.* 2006;30:479–84.

Salti G, Ghersetich I, Tantussi F, et al. Phosphatidylcholine and sodium deoxycholate in the treatment of localized fat: a double-blind, randomized study. *Dermatol. Surg.* 2008;34:60–6.

Schroder D, Buttenschon K, Herrmann F, Brede S. Is there a drug treatment approach for prevention and therapy of fat embolism syndrome? *Klin. Wochenscr.* 1991;69:229–33.

Schuller-Petrovic S, Wölkart G, Höfler G, et al. Tissue-toxic effects of phosphatidylcholine/deoxycholate after subcutaneous injection for fat dissolution in rats and a human volunteer. *Dermatol. Surg.* 2008;34:529–4.

Treacy P, Goldberg D. Use of phosphatidylcholine for the correction of lower lid bulging due to prominent fat pads. *J. Cosmet. Laser Ther.* 2006;8:129–32.

Victor S. Phosphatidylcholine works. *Skin Allergy News* 2003;34:12.

Wiedmann TS, Kamel L. Examination of the solubilization of drugs by bile salt micelles. *J. Pharm. Sci.* 2002;91:1743–64.

Yagina Odo YME, Cuce LC, Odo LM, et al. Action of sodium deoxycholate on subcutaneous human tissue: local and systemic effects. *Dermatol. Surg.* 2007;33:178–89.

Young VL. Lipostabil: the effect of phosphatidylcholine on subcutaneous fat. *Aesthetic Surg. J.* 2003;23:413–17.

Index